SIXTH EDITION

T0210342

DERMATOLOGY SECRETS

SIXTH EDITION

DERMATOLOGY SECRETS

EDITORS

WHITNEY A. HIGH, MD, JD, MEng
Professor
University of Colorado School of Medicine
Aurora, Colorado

LORI D. PROK, MD
Associate Professor
University of Colorado School of Medicine
Aurora, Colorado

ELSEVIER

Elsevier
1600, John F. Kennedy Blvd.
Ste 1800
Philadelphia,PA 19103- 2899

DERMATOLOGY SECRETS, SIXTH EDITION

ISBN: 978-0-323-67323-5

Notices

Practitioners and researchers must always rely on their own experience and knowledge in evaluating and using any information, methods, compounds or experiments described herein. Because of rapid advances in the medical sciences, in particular, independent verification of diagnoses and drug dosages should be made. To the fullest extent of the law, no responsibility is assumed by Elsevier, authors, editors or contributors for any injury and/or damage to persons or property as a matter of products liability, negligence or otherwise, or from any use or operation of any methods, products, instructions, or ideas contained in the material herein.

International Standard Book Number 978-0-323-67323-5

Content Strategist: Marybeth Thiel
Content Development Manager: Meghan Andress
Content Development Specialist: Angie Breckon
Publishing Services Manager: Shereen Jameel
Project Manager: Nadhiya Sekar
Design Direction: Bridget Hoette

Printed in the United States of America

Last digit is the print number: 9 8 7 6 5 4 3

Working together
to grow libraries in
developing countries

www.elsevier.com • www.bookaid.org

CONTRIBUTORS

Brian J. Abittan, MD,
Icahn School of Medicine at Mount Sinai
New York, New York

Israel David Andrews, MD, FAAD
Associate Program Director
Pediatric Dermatology
Phoenix Children's Hospital
Phoenix, Arizona;
Assistant Professor
Pediatrics
Mayo College of Medicine
Scottsdale, Arizona;
Clinical Assistant Professor
Department of Child Health
University of Arizona College of Medicine
Phoenix, Arizona

Eileen L. Axibal, MD
Department of Dermatology
University of Colorado
Aurora, Colorado

Scott D. Bennion, MS, MD, FAAD
Associate Clinical Professor
Dermatology
University of Colorado
Health Science Center
Denver, Colorado;
Associate Clinical Professor
Department of Medicine
University of Washington Medical School
Spokane, Washington

Kristen G. Berrebi, MD
Pediatric Dermatology Fellow
Department of Dermatology
University of Colorado Denver
Denver, Colorado

Sylvia L. Brice, MD
Associate Professor
Department of Dermatology
University of Colorado School of Medicine
Aurora, Colorado

Mariah R. Brown, MD
Associate Professor
Department of Dermatology
University of Colorado
Aurora, Colorado

Anna L. Bruckner, MD, MSCS
Associate Professor
Dermatology and Pediatrics
University of Colorado School of Medicine
Aurora, Colorado

Joanna M. Burch, MD
Pediatric Dermatologist
Department of Dermatology
Kaiser Permanente
Centennial, Colorado

Michael R. Campoli, MD, PhD, FAAD, FACMS
Mohs Surgery and Cutaneous Oncology
Fairview Medical Group
Minneapolis, Minnesota

Ali Damavandy, MD
Department of Dermatology
Georgetown University
Washington Hospital Center
Washington, DC

Brittney DeClerck, MD
Assistant Professor
Pathology and Dermatology
University of Southern California
Los Angeles, California

Nazanin Ehsani-Chimeh, MD
Dermatology Resident
University of Colorado
Denver, Colorado

Steven E. Eilers, MD
Mohs Micrographic Surgery and Cutaneous Oncology Fellow
Dermatology
Skin Laser and Surgery Specialists of NY and NJ
Hackensack, New Jersey

Colby C. Evans, MD
Strategic Adviser
Dermatology
US Dermatology Partners
Austin, Texas

James E. Fitzpatrick, MD
Professor (retired)
Department of Dermatology
University of Colorado Denver
Aurora, Colorado

Andrew Fischer, MD
Resident Physician
Department of Dermatology
University of Colorado
Denver, Colorado

Emilie Fowler, BS
Professor (retired)
Department of Dermatology and Cutaneous Surgery
Miami Itch Center
University of Miami School of Medicine
Miami, Florida

Sheila Friedlander, MD,
Professor
University of California San Diego
Department of Dermatology
San Diego, California

David J. Goldberg, MD
Director
Dermatology
Skin Laser and Surgery Specialists of NY and NJ;
Clinical Professor
Dermatology
Icahn School of Medicine at Mount Sinai
New York, New York

Gary Goldenberg, MD
Professor
Goldenberg Dermatology
Assistant Clinical Professor
Dermatology
Icahn School of Medicine at Mount Sinai
New York, New York

Robert O. Greer, Jr. DDS, ScD
Professor and Chair
Diagnostic and Biological Sciences
University of Colorado School of Dental Medicine;
Professor
Pathology, Medicine, and Dermatology
University of Colorado School of Medicine
Aurora, Colorado

Deborah B. Henderson, MD, MPH
Staff Dermatologist
Dermatology Clinic
Evans Army Community Hospital
Fort Carson, Colorado

Whitney A. High, MD, JD, MEng
Professor
University of Colorado School of Medicine
Aurora, Colorado

William D. James, MD
Paul Gross Professor of Dermatology
University of Pennsylvania
Philadelphia, Pennsylvania

Meena Julapalli, MD, FAAP, FAAD
Assistant Professor
Dermatology
University of Colorado School of Medicine
Denver, Colorado

Rohit K. Katial, MD
Professor of Medicine
National Jewish Health
University of Colorado
Denver, Colorado

Richard A. Keller, MD
Chief of Dermatology/Mohs Surgery
Dermatology Service
Audie L. Murphy Memorial Veterans Hospital;
Adjunct Professor
Dermatology
University of Texas Health Science Center
San Antonio, Texas

John Y.M. Koo, MD
Professor Emeritus
Department of Dermatology
University of California, San Francisco
San Francisco, California

Shannan E. McCann, MD, FAAP, FAAD
Pediatric Dermatologist
San Antonio Uniformed Services Health Education
    Consortium
San Antonio, Texas

Thomas J. McIntee, MD
Pediatric Dermatologist
Department of Dermatology
Marshfield Clinic
Marshfield, Wisconsin

Misha D. Miller, MD, FAAD, FACOG
Assistant Professor
Dermatology
Obstetrics and Gynecology
University of Colorado
Aurora, Colorado

Nicola Natsis, BA
University of California San Diego
School of Medicine
Rady Children's Hospital Division of Pediatric and
    Adolescent Dermatology
San Diego, California

Scott A. Norton, MD, MPH, MSc
Chief of Dermatology
Children's National Medical Center
Washington, DC;
Professor of Dermatology and Pediatrics
George Washington University
Washington, DC

Theresa R. Pacheco, MD
Associate Professor
Dermatology
University of Colorado
Aurora, Colorado

Andrew T. Patterson, MD
Resident Physician
Dermatology
San Antonio
Uniformed Services Health Education Consortium
    (SAUSHEC)
San Antonio, Texas

Grant Plost, MD
Pediatric Dermatology Fellow
University of Colorado School of Medicine
Children's Hospital Colorado
Aurora, Colorado

Lori D. Prok, MD
Associate Professor
University of Colorado School of Medicine
Aurora, Colorado

Theodore Rosen, MD,
Professor of Dermatology
Department of Dermatology
Baylor College of Medicine
Chief, Dermatology Service
Michael E. DeBakey VA Medical Center
Houston, Texas

Karl M. Saardi, MD
Physician
Dermatology
Georgetown University Hospital
Washington, DC

Curt P. Samlaska, MD, FACP, FAAD
Assistant Professor
Department of Medicine
University of Nevada School of Medicine
Las Vegas, Nevada

Marc Serota, MD
Resident Physician
Department of Dermatology
University of Colorado School of Medicine
Aurora, Colorado

Stephen Thomas Spates, MD
Director
Mohs Surgery Center
The Dermatology Group
Tricenna
West Orange, New Jersey

Ryan A. Stevens, MD
Dermatologist
Ephiphany Dermatology
Phoenix, Arizona

Leslie A. Stewart, MD
Dermatologist
Greenwood Village, Colorado;
Adult and Pediatric Dermatology
Greenwood Village, Colorado

Elizabeth Swanson, MD
Dermatologist
Pediatric Dermatologist
Advanced Dermatology Skin Cancer and Laser
   Surgery Center
Centennial
Colorado

Quinn Thibodeaux, MD
Dermatologist
San Francisco, CA

Carla X. Torres-Zegarra, FAAP, MD
Assistant Professor
Dermatology and Pediatrics
The University of Colorado
Denver, Colorado

Jeffrey B. Travers, MD, PhD
Professor and Chairman
Pharmacology and Toxicology
Wright State University
Dayton, Ohio

George W. Turiansky, MD, COL (ret.), MC, USA
Professor of Dermatology
Dermatology Department
Uniformed Services University of the Health Sciences
Bethesda, Maryland

William L. Weston, MD
Professor Emeritus of Dermatology
University of Colorado School of Medicine
Aurora, Colorado

Wendi E. Wohltmann, MD
Program Director
Dermatology
San Antonio Uniformed Services Health Education
   Consortium
San Antonio, Texas

Gil Yosipovitch, MD
Department of Dermatology and Cutaneous Surgery
Miami Itch Center
University of Miami School of Medicine
Miami, Florida

Matt Zirwas, MD
North American Contact Dermatitis Group
Columbus, Ohio;
Dermatologists of Central States
Bexley Office
Bexley, Ohio

PREFACE

"I cannot teach anybody anything, I can only make them think."

Socrates, 470–399 BC

Drs. Fitzpatrick and Morelli prefaced prior editions of this text with this quote from Socrates. We continue this tradition with the sixth edition of *Dermatology Secrets Plus*. We were blessed to learn from these two "greats" in the field of dermatology. We are forever indebted for their expertise, tireless dedication to patient advocacy, commitment to teaching, and love of the specialty. These educators taught us to think critically about dermatology and to explore teaching of the subject to others; the concept, organization, and content of this book are a tribute to them.

The Socratic method examines a concept via sequential interrogatories. In academic practice and medicine, the technique is used to augment classroom teaching and the reading of medical literature. Rather than rote memorization, questions posed in this book invite the reader to carefully consider an answer, with the goal being to understand, diagnose, and treat dermatologic disease. Moreover, because dermatology is a visual specialty, we chose photographs of disease states in their most illustrative form.

Socrates also said, "Education is the kindling of a flame, not the filling of a vessel," and more recently, Winston Churchill said, "Perfection is the enemy of progress." Ergo, this edition of *Secrets* focuses upon questions that students of dermatology will be asked by teachers. It is not comprehensive. Answers are kept purposefully short and may not include every asserted theory on a subject. Instead, this is an exploratory framework upon which to build knowledge. Readers are encouraged, even challenged, to refer to one of many fully comprehensive textbooks of dermatology to build upon their education, particularly as interest in the field foments.

Whitney High, MD, JD, MEng
Lori D. Prok, MD

CONTENTS

X EMERGENCIES AND MISCELLANEOUS PROBLEMS

TOP 100 SECRETS

1. Ichthyosis vulgaris, with an incidence of 1:250, is the most common ichthyosis.
2. Multiple Lisch nodules (melanocytic hamartomas of the iris) are pathognomonic of neurofibromatosis-1.
3. Hypomelanotic macules are a useful diagnostic skin sign for tuberous sclerosis in infants with seizures.
4. Squamous cell carcinoma is the most common cause of death in adults with recessive dystrophic epidermolysis bullosa.
5. Seborrheic dermatitis can be found not only on the scalp but also on the face around the eyebrows, nares, external auditory canal, central chest, and axillae.
6. Pityriasis rosea has oval papules and plaques that tend to orient along skin tension lines ("Christmas tree" pattern).
7. Skin barrier dysfunction is a basic component of atopic dermatitis pathophysiology.
8. Dilute bleach baths are an effective therapy to decrease *Staphylococcus aureus* colonization in atopic dermatitis.
9. Eighty percent of contact dermatitis reactions are due to irritation, and 20% are due to allergic causes.
10. Patch testing is a reliable way to distinguish between allergic and irritant contact dermatitis.
11. Immunobullous diseases are acquired and are due to autoantibodies directed at protein components of the epidermis or dermoepidermal junction.
12. Direct immunofluorescent studies on biopsies from perilesional skin are required to diagnose and differentiate between the immunobullous diseases.
13. Systemic corticosteroid withdrawal is a common implicating factor in precipitating the onset of generalized pustular psoriasis in patients with classic plaque-type psoriasis.
14. Erythema toxicum neonatorum, a benign pustular eruption on a background of erythema, develops in about 20% of neonates shortly after birth.
15. The primary lesion of lichen planus is a flat-topped, pruritic, purple, polygonal papule.
16. Lichen planus frequently demonstrates the isomorphic response (Koebner phenomenon), which refers to the development of new lesions in sites of minor trauma.
17. Cutaneous sarcoidosis occurs in 20% to 35% of patients with sarcoidosis.
18. Heerfordt's syndrome, or uveoparotid fever, is a variant of sarcoidosis presenting as uveitis, facial nerve palsy, fever, and parotid gland swelling.
19. Consider a fixed drug eruption in a patient who presents with bullous or hyperpigmented lesions that are recurrent at the same site.
20. The clinical signs of a potentially life-threatening drug eruption include high fever, dyspnea or hypotension, angioedema and tongue swelling, palpable purpura, skin necrosis, blistering, mucous membrane erosions, confluent erythema, and lymphadenopathy.
21. Cytoplasmic antineutrophil cytoplasmic antibody (c-ANCA) is found in up to 90% of patients with granulomatosis with polyangiitis (Wegener's granulomatosis); high titers often correlate with increased disease activity.
22. Pretibial myxedema is associated with Graves' disease.
23. Life-threatening calciphylaxis usually occurs in the setting of renal disease.
24. Phototoxic reactions clinically and symptomatically resemble sunburn, while photoallergic reactions resemble dermatitis.
25. Photosensitive drug reactions may occur in either the ultraviolet A (UVA) or ultraviolet B (UVB) spectrum. Because UVA passes through window glass, patients may develop photosensitive drug reactions even while they are in their homes or cars.
26. Sunlight stimulates human epidermal melanocytes to increase melanin synthesis and stimulates increased melanocyte transfer of melanosomes to keratinocytes. This melanocyte response to sunlight is called *tanning*.
27. The action spectrum of sunlight that causes tanning is the ultraviolet spectrum (wavelengths 290 to 400 nm).
28. Lesions of erythema nodosum occur most commonly on the anterior lower legs (shins), while lesions of erythema induratum occur most commonly on the posterior lower legs (calves).
29. In widespread subcutaneous fat necrosis of the newborn, it is prudent to monitor calcium levels for the first 3 to 4 months of life.
30. An inflamed or scaly bald spot in a school-aged child should be considered tinea capitis unless proven otherwise.
31. Bacterial resistance to benzoyl peroxide does not occur. Benzoyl peroxide used concomitantly with antimicrobial therapy for acne (as a leave-on or as a wash) is effective in limiting antibiotic resistance.
32. Drug-induced acne is caused most often by anabolic corticosteroids. It is differentiated from acne vulgaris by its sudden onset, distribution mainly on the upper trunk, and its monomorphous pustular appearance without comedones.

33. Gottron's papules (erythematous to violaceous papules over the knuckles) are a cutaneous finding that strongly supports a diagnosis of dermatomyositis.
34. Between 10% and 50% of adult patients that present with dermatomyositis have an underlying malignancy.
35. Chronic urticaria is most often idiopathic and not due to an allergic etiology, but it has an autoimmune basis in up to 50% of cases.
36. In angioedema without urticaria, one should screen for both hereditary and acquired angioedema by obtaining a C4 level.
37. Erythema infectiosum, caused by parvovirus B19, is characterized by bright erythema of the cheeks ("slapped cheeks") and a lacy erythematous eruption that most commonly affects the extremities.
38. Gianotti-Crosti syndrome and papular acrodermatitis of childhood are synonyms for a viral eruption characterized by the acute onset of a symmetrical, erythematous papular eruption that is accentuated on the face, extremities, and buttocks.
39. Asymptomatic shedding occurs in both orolabial and genital herpes simplex virus infections.
40. Postherpetic neuralgia is a common complication of herpes zoster, especially in older individuals.
41. Most human papillomavirus (HPV) infections are not carcinogenic, but persistent infections with some genotypes, especially HPV-16 and HPV-18, are associated with a high risk of epithelial neoplasia.
42. Syphilis is a sexually transmitted disease produced by the spirochete *Treponema pallidum* ssp. *pallidum* that can also be transmitted from the mother to the fetus.
43. Atypical mycobacteria infections are acquired from ubiquitous acid-fast bacilli that are found in soil, water, and domestic and wild animals. The presentation of these infections is variable, leading to frequently missed diagnoses.
44. Patients with tuberculoid leprosy have a high degree of immunity against *Mycobacterium leprae* and have few skin lesions and few organisms in their skin, while patients with lepromatous leprosy have low immunity against *M. leprae* and have many skin lesions and millions of organisms in their skin.
45. Azole antifungal agents block the cytochrome P-450 enzyme lanosterol 14-α demethylase, which depletes ergosterol from cell membranes, whereas allylamine antifungals block ergosterol production through inhibition of squalene epoxidase.
46. The differential diagnosis of lymphocutaneous (sporotrichoid) spread includes *SLANTS:* **S**porotrichosis, **L**eishmaniasis, **A**typical mycobacteria, **N**ocardia, **T**ularemia, and cat-**S**cratch disease.
47. While most cases of leishmaniasis seen in the United States are acquired elsewhere, a form of cutaneous disease caused by *Leishmania mexicana* may be acquired in central Texas and Oklahoma, nicknamed "Highway 90 disease" by those familiar with its distribution.
48. The brown recluse spider (*Loxosceles reclusa*) is the most common cause of dermonecrotic arachnidism.
49. *Cheyletiella* is a nonburrowing mite that presents as "walking dandruff" on pets and manifests as nonspecific pruritic papules and plaques on affected patients.
50. Acanthosis nigricans is a common condition, and most cases are associated with insulin resistance. Paraneoplastic acanthosis nigricans is rare, may be of explosive onset, and associated with tripe palms and the sign of Leser-Trélat (multiple eruptive seborrheic keratoses).
51. The presence of eruptive xanthomas indicates the presence of high levels of serum triglycerides.
52. Bilirubin has a strong affinity for tissues rich in elastic tissue, which is why it accumulates earliest in the sclera of the eye, followed by the skin (especially the face), hard palate, and abdominal wall.
53. Clinically apparent jaundice is not noticeable until the serum bilirubin exceeds 2.0 to 2.5 mg/dL in an adult.
54. Small vascular lesions called angiokeratoma corporis diffusum are most commonly found in a bathing suit distribution area. These angiokeratomas are characteristic of Fabry's disease, a genetic disorder that affects the kidney.
55. Nephrogenic systemic fibrosis is a recently described disease characterized by papules, plaques, and thickened skin of the trunk and extremities. It is associated with impaired renal function and deposition of gadolinium in tissues from gadolinium-based contrast media.
56. Atypical molluscum contagiosum manifestations in the HIV-infected population include giant molluscum, disseminated lesions, confluent lesions, lesions distributed in atypical sites such as the perianal area, and lesions mimicking warts, skin cancers, and keratoacanthomas.
57. The classic tetrad of pellagra all start with the letter D: **d**iarrhea, **d**ermatitis, **d**ementia, **d**eath.
58. Casal's necklace is the distinctive photosensitive eruption seen in pellagra that presents as a "necklace" around the neck.
59. There is an increased risk of melanoma in patients with giant congenital melanocytic nevi (greater than 40 cm in diameter adult predicted size). These melanomas often arise in the dermis and in childhood (before age 10 years).
60. Patients with a large number (>100) of atypical melanocytic nevi should be followed closely for the possible development of melanoma.
61. Kasabach-Merritt syndrome (platelet trapping and consumption coagulopathy associated with a vascular tumor) is seen with kaposiform hemangioendothelioma and tufted angioma.
62. Dermatofibromas often demonstrate dimpling with lateral pressure. This has been called a "dimple" or "Fitzpatrick" sign.
63. The presence of pigmentation extending onto the nail fold from a band of linear melanonychia (Hutchinson's sign) is a strong indication for biopsy and histopathologic evaluation of the nail matrix to evaluate for acral melanoma.

64. Mycosis fungoides is an indolent epidermotropic cutaneous lymphoma.
65. Sézary syndrome is the term applied to the leukemic subtype of cutaneous T-cell lymphoma.
66. Merkel cell carcinoma is an aggressive neuroendocrine malignancy of the skin with frequent recurrences and metastasis.
67. Epithelioid sarcoma is an aggressive soft tissue malignancy that most commonly presents on the volar distal extremities of young adults as a slow-growing dermal or subcutaneous nodule.
68. Approximately 9% of all patients who die from internal malignancy will demonstrate metastatic tumors in the skin.
69. Reducing ultraviolet radiation exposure is the single best strategy for reducing skin cancer.
70. Approximately 2% total body surface area (TBSA) requires 1 fingertip unit (FTU) or 0.5 gram of topical steroid medication. One percent of the patient's TBSA can be estimated as one palmar surface, including the fingers.
71. The safe total maximum dose of 1% lidocaine for adults is 7 mg/kg if combined with epinephrine and 4.5 mg/kg if given without epinephrine.
72. Damage to the temporal branch of the facial nerve when cutaneous surgery is performed will result in an ipsilateral brow ptosis and ipsilateral lack of forehead animation.
73. Mohs micrographic surgery is indicated for cutaneous carcinomas arising on the face and other sites where the maximal preservation of normal skin and cosmesis are important goals.
74. The wavelengths of common lasers are as follows: potassium-titanyl-phosphate (KTP), 532 nm; pulsed dye, 585 nm; ruby, 684 nm; alexandrite, 755 nm; diode, 810 to 1450 nm; neodymium (Nd):yttrium-aluminum-garnet (YAG), 1064 nm; erbium:YAG, 2490 nm; and carbon dioxide, 10,600 nm.
75. The pulsed dye laser is the gold standard for treatment of vascular lesions, although KTP, Nd:YAG, and alexandrite lasers are also useful.
76. Narrowband UVB is now the phototherapy treatment of choice for psoriasis, other inflammatory skin disease, vitiligo, and possibly mycosis fungoides (patch stage), given its superior efficacy to broadband UVB and decreased side effects compared with psoralen UVA therapy.
77. Phototherapy exerts its effects primarily through immunomodulation (T-cell apoptosis within the epidermis and dermis, and suppression/depletion of Langerhans cells within the epidermis).
78. Systemic retinoids, which are used for the treatment of many cutaneous diseases, including acne vulgaris, psoriasis, and disorders of keratinization, are very potent teratogenic drugs.
79. The *TORCHES* infections are **T**oxoplasmosis, **O**ther (varicella-zoster virus, parvovirus B19), **R**ubella, **C**ytomegalovirus, **H**erpes simplex virus and **H**IV, **E**nteroviruses and **E**pstein-Barr virus, and **S**yphilis.
80. The classic triad of congenital rubella syndrome consists of congenital cataracts, deafness, and congenital heart malformations.
81. Pyogenic granulomas are neither pyogenic nor granulomatous; they are neovascularizations, likely in response to minor trauma and/or growth factors.
82. Aging of the skin may be divided into that due to intrinsic aging (normal maturity and senescence) and that secondary to extrinsic aging (external factors such as ultraviolet light).
83. Xerosis (dry skin, asteatosis, dermatitis hiemalis) is the most common geriatric dermatosis and the most frequent cause of pruritus in the elderly.
84. The umbilical area is preferentially affected in pemphigoid gestationis and can be a clue to the diagnosis.
85. Circinate balanitis is a cutaneous manifestation of reactive arthritis (formerly known as "Reiter's disease").
86. Oral smokeless tobacco keratoses have little malignant potential, and the vast majority of such lesions are reversible if the tobacco habit is discontinued.
87. HPV is considered causal in nearly 20% of oral squamous cell carcinomas.
88. Erythema may be more difficult to appreciate on darkly pigmented skin, and this must be considered during clinical examination.
89. Pigmentation of the oral mucosa, benign-appearing palmoplantar macules, or multiple longitudinal pigmented streaks of the nails may represent normal variants in persons with darker skin types.
90. Many cutaneous diseases may present with follicular accentuation or other unusual clinical aspects in persons with darker skin types.
91. Skin signs of toxic epidermal necrolysis, a life-threatening mucocutaneous disease, include diffuse and severe skin tenderness and "cayenne pepper" nonblanching erythema that evolves into widespread blistering and superficial ulcers.
92. Contact dermatitis is the most common form of occupational skin disease, with irritant contact dermatitis being more common than allergic contact dermatitis.
93. Patients with delusions of parasitosis have monosymptomatic hypochondriacal psychosis; their other mental functions are typically normal.
94. Munchausen syndrome is a chronic factitious disorder in which patients totally fabricate their symptoms, self-inflict lesions, or exaggerate or exacerbate a preexisting physical condition.
95. Trauma is the most common cause of splinter hemorrhages of the nail.
96. Squamous cell carcinoma is the most common malignant tumor of the nail unit.
97. Cantharidin ($C_{10}H_{12}O_4$), a vesicant therapy for molluscum contagiosum and warts, is a semipurified extract from blister beetles from the family Meloidae.

98. The nine-banded armadillo (*Dasypus novemcinctus*) is an animal reservoir in the United States for *Mycoacterium leprae*, the cause of leprosy.
99. Tungiasis refers to parasitization by the gravid female flea (*Tunga penetrans*), which burrows into the skin where the eggs mature, and she passes them through an opening in the skin to the environment.
100. It has been calculated that we shed about 35,000 skin cells per minute, which calculates to more than 50 million per day!

STRUCTURE AND FUNCTION OF THE SKIN

Scott D. Bennion

CHAPTER 1

KEY POINTS: ANATOMY AND FUNCTION OF SKIN

1. The skin is composed of an epidermis, dermis, and subcutis (composed mainly of subcutaneous fat).
2. The four primary functions of skin are:
   - Barrier function and prevention of desiccation
   - Immune surveillance
   - Temperature control
   - Cutaneous sensation
3. The main cell types in the epidermis are melanocytes, keratinocytes, Langerhans cells, and Merkel cells.
4. Genetic mutations in critical adhesion molecules cause inherited blistering diseases that are usually evident at birth (e.g., epidermolysis bullosa simplex [EBS]).
5. Autoimmune diseases characterized by autoantibodies to critical adhesion molecules produce acquired blistering diseases (e.g., pemphigus vulgaris).

1. Name the three layers of the skin. What composes them?

The epidermis, dermis, and subcutis (subcutaneous fat). The **epidermis** is the outermost layer and is composed primarily of keratinocytes, or epidermal cells. Beneath the epidermis lies the **dermis**, which is composed primarily of collagen but also contains adnexal structures, including the hair follicles, sebaceous glands, apocrine glands, and eccrine glands. Numerous blood vessels, lymphatics, and nerves also traverse the dermis. Below the dermis lies the **subcutis,** or subcutaneous layer, which consists of adipose tissue, larger blood vessels, and nerves. The subcutis may also contain the base of hair follicles and sweat glands (Fig. 1.1).

2. How many layers are there in the epidermis? How are they organized?

The epidermis has four layers: the basal cell layer, spiny cell layer, granular cell layer, and cornified layer (Fig. 1.2). The basal cell layer **(stratum basalis)** is composed of columnar or cuboidal cells that are in direct contact with the basement membrane, the structure that separates the dermis from the epidermis. The basal cell layer contains the germinative cells, and, for this reason, occasional mitoses may be present.

The three layers above the basal cell layer are histologically distinct and demonstrate differentiation of the keratinocytes as they move toward the skin surface and become "cornified." Just above the basal cell layer is the spiny cell layer **(stratum spinosum),** so called because of a high concentration of desmosomes and keratin filaments that give the cells a characteristic "spiny" appearance (Fig. 1.3A). Above the spiny layer is the granular cell layer **(stratum granulosum).** In this layer, keratohyalin granules are formed and bind to the keratin filaments (tonofilaments) to form large electron-dense masses within the cytoplasm that give this layer its "granular" appearance.

The outermost layer is the cornified layer **(stratum corneum),** where the keratinocytes abruptly lose all of their organelles and nuclei. The keratin filaments and keratohyalin granules form an amorphous mass within the keratinocytes, which become elongated and flattened, forming a lamellar array of "corneocytes." The corneocytes are held together by the remnants of the desmosomes (dense bodies) and a "cementing substance" released into the intracellular space from organelles called Odland bodies.

3. Do other types of cells normally occur in the epidermis?

In addition to keratinocytes, three other cells are normally found in the epidermis. The **melanocyte,** the most common, is a dendritic cell situated in the basal cell layer. There are approximately 36 keratinocytes for each melanocyte. This cell's function is to synthesize and secrete melanin-containing organelles called melanosomes.

The next most common cell is the **Langerhans cell,** which is a bone marrow–derived, antigen-presenting cell that has very important immune surveillance functions. On light microscopy, these dendritic cells are primarily distributed in the stratum spinosum. Langerhans cells were first described by Paul Langerhans in 1868 while he was still a medical student.

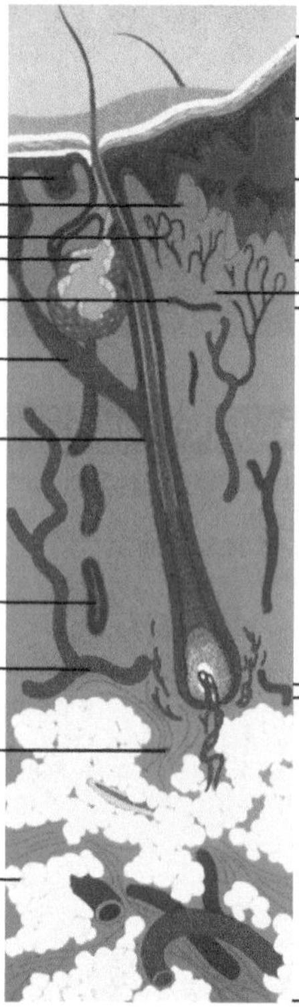

Epidermis (raised to show papillary dermis)

Rete ridge

Papilla

Papillary capillary loops

Sebaceous gland (cutaway view)

Superficial or subpapillary plexus of blood vessels

Arrector pili muscle

Hair follicle

Papillary dermis

Periadnexal dermis

Reticular dermis

Dermal duct of eccrine sweat gland

Deep plexus of blood vessels

Loose connective tissue of subcutaneous fat layer (connective tissue septum)

Lobules of adipose tissue

Subcutaneous fat layer

Fig. 1.1 Structure of the skin.

Also located in the epidermis in small numbers are **Merkel cells.** They are in contact with nerve fibers and are involved in tactile discrimination. Ultrastructurally, Merkel cells contain electron-dense bodies that are also found in the amino acid precursor uptake and decarboxylation cells of endocrine glands. Merkel cells have recently been shown to be derived from epidermal stem cells.

Perdigoto CN, Bardot ES, Valdes VJ, et al. Embryonic maturation of epidermal Merkel cells is controlled by a redundant transcription factor network. *Development.* 2014;141:4690–4696.

4. What is apocopation?
   Apocopation is the process by which melanocytes transfer melanosomes to keratinocytes. In this process, the tips of the melanocytic dendritic processes are phagocytized by the keratinocytes.

5. Are stem cells found in the epidermis?
   Yes. Epithelial stem cell populations have been found in the adult hair follicle, sebaceous gland, and epidermis. This has been an area of intense research in recent years because of the potential to treat a number of genetic diseases.

Forni MF, Trombetta-Lima M, Sogayar MC. Stem cells in embryonic skin development. *Biol Res.* 2012;45:215–222.

6. Describe the structure of the basement membrane zone (BMZ).
   The BMZ is not normally visible by light microscopy in sections stained with hematoxylin-eosin, but can be visualized as a homogeneous band measuring 0.5 to 1.0 mm thick on periodic acid–Schiff staining. Ultrastructural studies and immunologic mapping demonstrate that the BMZ is an extremely complex structure consisting of many components that function to attach the basal cell layer to the dermis (Fig. 1.3B). Uppermost in the BMZ are the cytoplasmic tonofilaments of the basal cells, which attach to the basal plasma membrane of the cells at the hemidesmosome. The hemidesmosome is attached to the lamina lucida (LL) and lamina densa of the BMZ via anchoring filaments. The BMZ,

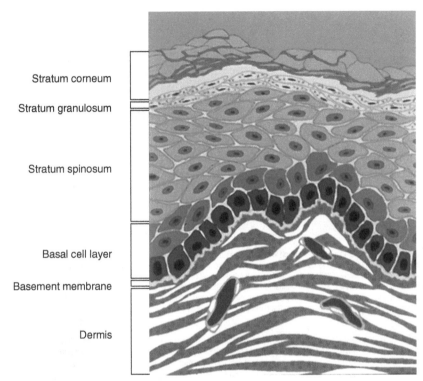

Stratum corneum

Stratum granulosum

Stratum spinosum

Basal cell layer

Basement membrane

Dermis

Fig. 1.2 Epidermal layers and papillary dermis.

in turn, is anchored to the dermis by anchoring fibrils that intercalate among the collagen fibers of the dermis and secure the BMZ to the dermis. The importance of these structures in maintaining skin integrity is demonstrated by diseases such as epidermolysis bullosa (EB), in which they are congenitally missing or damaged.

Natsuga K, Watanabe M, Nishie W, Shimizu H. Life before and beyond blistering: the role of collagen Xvii in epidermal physiology. *Exp Dermatol.* 2019;28(10):1135–1141.

7. How is the structure of the epidermis related to its functions?

The three most important functions of the epidermis are protection from environmental insult (barrier function), prevention of desiccation, and immune surveillance. The stratum corneum is an especially important cutaneous barrier that protects the body from toxins and desiccation. Although many toxins are nonpolar compounds that can move relatively easily through the lipid-rich intracellular spaces of the cornified layer, the tortuous route among cells in this layer and the layers below effectively forms a barrier to environmental toxins. The process of shedding the stratum corneum also plays an important role in the removal of microbes. Ultraviolet light, another environmental source of damage to living cells, is effectively blocked in the stratum corneum and the melanosomes. The melanosomes are concentrated above the nucleus of the keratinocytes in an umbrella-like fashion, providing photoprotection for both epidermal nuclear DNA and the dermis.

The prevention of **desiccation** is another extremely important function, as extensive loss of epidermis is often fatal (e.g., toxic epidermal necrolysis). In the normal epidermis, the water content decreases as one moves from the basal layer to the surface, comprising 70% to 75% of weight at the base and decreasing to 10% to 15% at the bottom of the stratum corneum.

Immune surveillance against foreign antigens is a function of the Langerhans cells that are dispersed among the keratinocytes. Langerhans cells internalize external antigens and process these antigens for presentation to T lymphocytes in the lymph nodes. Inflammatory cells (i.e., neutrophils, eosinophils, lymphocytes) are also capable of intercepting and destroying microorganisms in the epidermis.

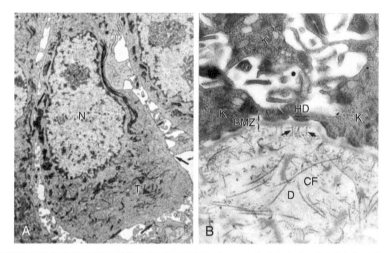

Fig. 1.3 A, Keratinocyte. An electron micrograph illustrates the ultrastructural components of a typical keratinocyte in the stratum spinosum, including the nucleus (*N*), tonofilaments (*T*), and desmosomal intercellular connections (*arrow*) that give this layer its "spiny" appearance. **B,** Basement membrane zone (*BMZ*). At the interface of the basal keratinocytes (*K*) of the epidermis and dermis (*D*) is the BMZ. The keratinocytes are attached to the BMZ by hemidesmosomes (*HD*). The BMZ is composed of the lamina lucida, which is the upper clear area, and the lamina densa, which is the dark area just below the lamina lucida. Anchoring fibrils (*arrows*) bind the BMZ to the dermis by intercalating among the collagen fibers (*CF*) of the dermis.

8. **What structural components of the epidermis are involved in blistering diseases?**
   In the epidermis, the keratinocytes are bound to each other by a desmosomal complex. These complexes consist of the desmosome and the tonofilaments of the cytoplasm that are made of cytokeratins. In the upper stratum spinosum, the tonofilaments are composed mainly of keratins 1 and 10. Congenital abnormalities in these keratins produce structural weakness between keratinocytes, producing a disease called **epidermolytic ichthyosis** (epidermolytic hyperkeratosis). Abnormalities in keratin types 5 (KRT5) and 14 (KRT14) in the basal cell layers lead to a mild blistering disease named **epidermolysis bullosa simplex** (EBS) (Fig. 1.4). **Pemphigus** is an acquired group of blistering diseases of the epidermis in which autoantibodies directed against antidesmosomal proteins produce damage to the desmosomes (see Chapter 10).
   The skin diseases associated with antibodies and damage to the desmosomes and their characteristics are listed in Table 1.1.

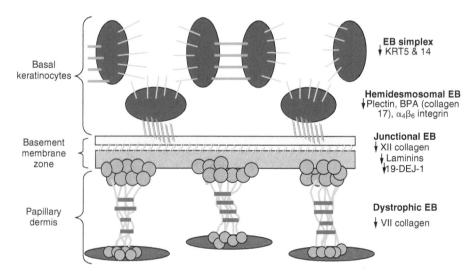

Fig. 1.4 This diagram of the dermal-epidermal junction illustrates the affected levels in the various types of epidermolysis bullosa (*EB*). *BPA*, bullous pemphigoid antigen.

Table 1.1 Diseases associated with antibodies and damage to desmosomes

DISEASE INVOLVED	CLINICAL APPEARANCE AND LOCATION	MAIN DERMOSOMAL MOLECULES
Pemphigus vulgaris	Oral and diffuse superficial flaccid blisters with ulcers	Desmogleins 1 and 3 (Dsg1 and 3) and plakoglobin
Pemphigus foliaceus	Diffuse superficial blisters and crusting	Desmoglein 1 (Dsg1)
Pemphigus vegetans	Vegetating, weeping lesions in the intertriginous areas	Desmoglein 3 (Dsg3)
Pemphigus Desmoglein 3 (Dsg3)	Erythematosus	Butterfly eruption with Blistering in malar areas
Paraneoplastic pemphigus	Diffuse erythema multiforme–like painful eruption	Desmoplakins 1 and 2 (Dsg1 and 2), bullous pemphigoid antigen 1 (BP230), plectin, desmogleins 1 and 3 (Dsg1 and 3), envoplakin, periplakin
Immunoglobulin A pemphigus	Pustular or vesiculopustular eruption	Desmogleins 1 and 3 (Dsg1 and 3), desmocollin 1

9. **Are there hereditary diseases of the BMZ and dermis that cause blistering and damage to the skin?**
   Yes. There is a complex group of inherited diseases in which the skin is friable and bullous lesions occur, often with subsequent scarring (see Chapter 6). The two subgroups within this group are junctional EBs (JEBs) and dystrophic EBs (DEBs). Like the EBS diseases, which affect the epidermal layers, these diseases occur because the vital structural elements of the BMZ and dermis are missing, causing the skin to separate easily and blister. In JEBs, the separation occurs within the LL of the BMZ. Decreased amounts or abnormalities in the LL components, such as laminins I and V, 19-DEJ-1 protein, XII collagen, plectin, XVII collagen (bullous pemphigoid [BP] antigen), and $\alpha_4\beta_6$ integrin, have been identified in this group.
   In the DEB group, separation occurs below the BMZ in the dermal layer, and a decreased amount or absence of type VII collagen has been noted. As a rule, the deeper in the skin the separation occurs, the more severe the clinical picture with increased scarring and loss of function. DEB patients typically have severe deforming scars and decreased life span (see Fig. 1.4).

10. **Are there acquired blistering diseases of the BMZ and dermis?**
   Yes. There are several diseases in which blistering occurs secondary to disruption of the structures of the BMZ and dermis. As with the epidermal blistering diseases, antibodies to the hemidesmosomes and other structures within the BMZ and dermis cause separation of the skin and blistering. In the uppermost portion of the BMZ, the LL, hemidesmosomes bind the

Table 1.2 Skin diseases associated with antibodies and damage to basement membrane structures and dermis

DISEASE	CLINICAL APPEARANCE AND LOCATION	BASEMENT MEMBRANE MOLECULE INVOLVED
Bullous pemphigoid	Tense blisters diffusely	Bullous pemphigoid antigens 1 (BP230) and 2 (BP180)
Pemphigoid (herpes) gestationis	Urticarial blisters with pruritus in late pregnancy	BP antigen 2 (BP180 or collagen XVII antigen)
Epidermolysis bullosa acquisita	Friable skin and blistering knees, elbows, and sites of increased pressure	Type VII dermal collagen (anchoring fibril antigen)
Bullous lupus erythematosus	Blistering face and trunk with flairs of systemic lupus erythematosus	Type VII dermal collagen and lamins 5 and 6
Linear IgA bullous disease	Tense vesicles in annular and target-like patterns on the trunk	BP antigen 2 (BP180 or collagen XVII antigen) and 97 kDa

basal keratinocytes to the basement membrane. BP is a classic example of an acquired blistering disease in which antihemidesmosomal antibodies are produced and appear to induce inflammation and subsequent damage of the hemidesmosomes, causing a blister to develop between the cells and the basement membrane.

A partial list of the skin diseases associated with antibodies and damage to the basement membrane structures and dermis is provided in Table 1.2.

11. What abnormalities in structural components of the basement membrane are involved in bullous skin diseases?
Structures within the basement membrane can be congenitally absent or decreased in number, or, as with the epidermal desmosomes, they can be affected by antibodies directed against them. In the uppermost portion of the BMZ, in the LL, hemidesmosomes bind the basal keratinocytes to the basement membrane. **BP** is an acquired blistering disease in which antihemidesmosomal antibodies are produced. These antibodies appear to induce inflammation and subsequent damage to the hemidesmosomes, causing a blister to develop between the cells and the basement membrane.

12. What is the function of the sebaceous gland?
The sebaceous gland is a holocrine gland that is a part of the pilosebaceous unit. The lipid-producing cells within the sebaceous gland are called sebocytes. Its function is to produce **sebum** that accounts for 90% of the skin surface lipids. Sebum is a combination of wax esters, squalene, cholesterol esters, and triglycerides and it is secreted through the sebaceous duct into the hair follicle, where it covers the skin surface, possibly as a protectant. Sebum may also have antifungal properties. Sebaceous glands are located everywhere on the skin except the palms and soles.

Hinde E, Haslam IS, Schneider MR, et al. A practical guide for the study of human and murine sebaceous gland in situ. *Exp Dermatol.* 2013;22:631–637.

13. How do the eccrine sweat glands and apocrine sweat glands differ?
Embryologically, eccrine glands derive from the epidermis and are not part of the pilosebaceous unit. The eccrine sweat glands function in temperature regulation via secretion of sweat, a combination of mostly water and electrolytes, which evaporates and cools the skin. Their ducts pass through the dermis and epidermis to empty directly onto the skin surface. Eccrine glands are located everywhere on the skin surface except on modified skin areas, such as the lips, nail beds, external auditory canal, and glans penis. Eccrine sweat glands are found only in higher primates and horses.

Apocrine glands originate from the same hair germ that gives rise to the hair follicle and sebaceous gland. The apocrine duct empties into the follicle above the sebaceous gland. Their anachronistic function is to produce scent. They are located primarily in the axillae and perineum, and their activity is sex hormone dependent. The breast and cerumen glands are both modified apocrine sweat glands.

14. What causes axillary body odor?
Axillary body odor is due to the production of short- and medium-chain volatile fatty acids, 16-androstene steroids, and thioalcohols from apocrine secretions that are actually odorless. Bacteria from the genus *Cornybacterium* are thought to be responsible for the production of these malodorous molecules.

James AG, Austin CJ, Cox DS, et al. Microbiological and biochemical origins of human axillary odour. *FEMS Microbiol Ecol.* 2013;83:527–540.

15. How is the dermis organized?
The dermis is organized into two distinct areas: the papillary dermis and the reticular dermis. The superficial **papillary dermis** is a relatively thin zone beneath the epidermis. On light microscopy, it is composed of thin, delicate collagen fibers and is highly vascularized. The hair follicles are enveloped by a **perifollicular dermis** that is contiguous with, and morphologically resembles, the papillary dermis. Collectively, the papillary dermis and perifollicular dermis are called the **adventitial dermis,** although this term is rarely used in dermatology texts.

The deeper zone is the **reticular dermis,** which comprises the bulk of the dermis. It is less vascular than the papillary dermis and demonstrates thick, well-organized collagen bundles.

16. What are the components of the dermis?
The main cell type in the dermis is the fibroblast. The fibroblast produces the main components of the dermis, including collagen (70% to 80%) for resiliency, elastin (1% to 3%) for elasticity, and proteoglycans to maintain water within the dermis. The bulk of the collagen within the dermis consists of types I and III and is organized into collagen bundles that mostly run horizontally throughout the dermis.

The elastic fibers are interspersed among the collagen fibers with three identified subtypes. Mature thicker elastic fibers are primarily found in the reticular dermis and demonstrate a predominantly horizontal orientation. At the junction of the papillary and reticular dermis, horizontally oriented elastic fibers called elaunin fibers are found in abundance. Oxytalan fibers, which are thought to be important in anchoring the epidermis, are small elastic fibers found primarily in the papillary dermis and are usually oriented perpendicularly to the skin surface (Fig. 1.5).

The proteoglycans (primarily hyaluronic acid) comprise the amorphous ground substance around the elastic and collagen fibers.

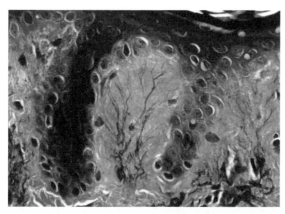

Fig. 1.5 Thin, vertically oriented oxytalan fibers in the papillary dermis as demonstrated by a Verhoeff–Van Gieson stain. (Courtesy James E. Fitzpatrick, MD.)

17. What are the functions of the dermis?
    - Temperature regulation through control of cutaneous blood flow and sweating, achieved by the dermal vessels and eccrine sweat glands
    - Mechanical protection of underlying structures, achieved primarily by the collagen and hyaluronic acid
    - Innervation of the skin that mostly occurs in the dermis and is responsible for cutaneous sensation

18. Which structural component of the dermis is involved in congenital and autoimmune skin diseases?
    Collagen. Antibodies against **type VII collagen,** which makes up the anchoring filaments within the dermis, are found in the autoimmune diseases **bullous systemic lupus erythematosus** (SLE) and **acquired EB.** Antibodies to laminins 5 and 6, which are also located in the anchoring filaments, are found in bullous SLE patients. The anchoring filaments function to bind the basement membrane to the dermis, and damage to this collagen results in blister formation below the basement membrane. Clinically, blistering damage beneath the basement membrane causes significant scarring in contrast to blisters in the epidermis or above the basement membrane that do not cause scarring. **Congenital dystrophic EB**, in which there is a congenital paucity or absence of type VII collagen and anchoring fibers, can result in severe scarring. The most severe form of this disease, recessive dystrophic EB, is associated with "mitten" deformities of the hands and feet, severe scarring of the upper respiratory and gastrointestinal tracts, and early death (Fig. 1.6A).

    Congenital abnormalities in the various collagens in the dermis, especially types I and III, are found in several of the Ehlers-Danlos syndromes. The cutaneous manifestations of these syndromes are hyperextensibility of the skin, easy bruising, and poor healing with resultant wide scar formation (Fig. 1.6B).

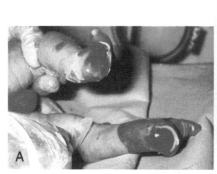

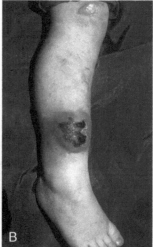

Fig. 1.6 A, Epidermolysis bullosa of a newborn. **B,** Ehlers-Danlos syndrome. A large hematoma with poor healing secondary to minor trauma of the lower extremity.

19. **How does the vasculature of the dermis function in temperature control?**

    Body temperature is regulated, in part, through control of dermal blood flow. Lowering body temperature is accomplished through increased blood flow in the vascular plexus in the high papillary dermis, allowing heat to be removed through radiation from the skin. The dermal vasculature is composed of a superficial and deep plexus of arterioles and venules that are interconnected by communicating vessels (Fig. 1.7). The incoming blood flow to the superficial capillary plexus in the upper dermis can be decreased by increased smooth muscle tone in the ascending arterioles, or it can be shunted directly from the arterioles to the venous channels in the deeper plexus systems via glomus bodies, which are modified arterioles surrounded by multiple layers of muscle cells. During cold temperatures, decreased blood flow to the papillary dermis, in essence, shunts the blood away from the skin surface and decreases heat loss from the body. The hot flashes that typically occur in menopausal women are caused by instability of this system. Periodic dilation of the skin capillaries allows increased blood flow to the skin, which is perceived as heat.

20. **How is the skin innervated?**

    The innervation of the skin recapitulates the blood flow: large, myelinated, cutaneous branches of the musculocutaneous nerves branch in the subcutaneous tissue to form a deep nerve plexus in the reticular dermis. Nerve fibers from the deep plexus ascend to form a superficial subpapillary plexus. Nerves from these plexuses innervate the skin either as free nerve endings or as corpuscular receptors. The free nerve endings may terminate in the superficial dermis or on Merkel cells in the epidermis. Free nerve endings function as important sensory receptors. They transmit touch, pain, temperature, itch, and mechanical stimuli. These exist in the papillary dermis as individual fibers surrounded by **Schwann cells.** The other type of receptor in the skin is the **corpuscular receptor.**

21. **Name the two main corpuscular (encapsulated) nerve receptors found in the skin**
    - **Meissner corpuscle:** Found in highest concentration on the papillary ridge of glabrous skin. It is a touch receptor. "Mucocutaneous end organs" is the name applied to similar corpuscular nerve receptors found on the areola, labia, glans penis, clitoris, perianal canal, eyelids, and lips.
    - **Pacinian corpuscle:** Found in acral areas in the deep dermis and subcutaneous tissue. It has a very distinct capsule associated with multiple lamellated wrapping cells that surround a myelinated axon with an "onion-like" appearance on cross-section (Fig. 1.8). Pacinian corpuscles are mechanoreceptors that respond to vibration.

        Some textbooks list other corpuscular nerve receptors including the Ruffini corpuscle (rare, expanded, myelinated, afferent fibers that connect to collagen in digits), Golgi-Mazzoni corpuscles (laminated like Pacinian corpuscles, found on fingers with simpler organization), and Krause end bulbs (encapsulated myelinated endings found in the papillary dermis).

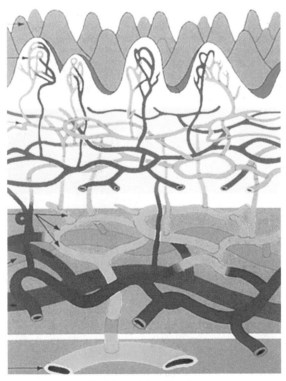

Fig. 1.7 Vasculature of the skin.

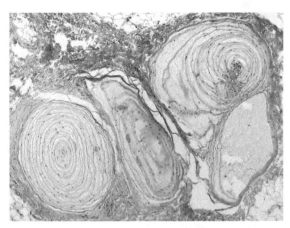

Fig. 1.8 Pacinian corpuscle demonstrating characteristic onion-like appearance on cross-section (H&E).

22. Is loss of cutaneous sensation very serious?

The importance of skin innervation is best illustrated by diseases that destroy cutaneous nerves. The archetypical disease is **Hansen's disease (leprosy).** This disease attacks and destroys cutaneous nerves, resulting in severe mutilation of the extremities after years of unperceived trauma.

23. How is the subcutis organized?

The subcutis, or subcutaneous fat, is arranged into distinct fat lobules, which are divided by fibrous septae composed primarily of collagen. Blood vessels, nerves, and lymphatics are also found in the fibrous septae. In addition to its role as a caloric reserve, the subcutaneous fat serves as a heat insulator and shock absorber.

24. Does the skin have a microbiome?

Yes, the skin microbiome is complex, and the bacterial population varies according to the area sampled. There appears to be a multifaceted interaction between the skins immune system and resident flora.

SanMiguel A, Grice EA. Interactions between host factors and the skin microbiome. *Cell Mol Life Sci.* 2016;72(B):1499–1515.

25. Are there any specific diseases directly linked to the bacterial microbiome?

Yes, overgrowth of Cutibacterium acnes in the pilosebaceous unit upregulates multiple proinflammatory cytokines, leading to inflamed lesions in acne vulgaris. In atopic dermatitis, overgrowth and colonization of *Staphylococcus aureus* stimulates the production of interleukin-4 an immunoglobulin E promoting cytokine.

Saba, AM, Yosipovitch G. Skin pH: from basic science to basic skin care. *Acta Derm Venereol.* 2013;93:261–267.

26. Does the pH of the skin play a part in skin barrier function?

Yes. The phrase "acid mantle" was first proposed by two German doctors in 1928 and appears to have a significant role to play in skin barrier function, and in multiple skin diseases such as atopic dermatitis and acne.

Surber C, Humbert P, Abels C, et al. The acid mantle: a myth or an essential part of skin health? *Curr Probl Dermatol.* 2018;54:1–10.

27. How do pH changes affect certain skin conditions?

The skin microbiome lives in an acidic pH of around 5, and this environment inhibits the growth of many pathogenic bacteria.

Schmid-Wendtner M-H, Korting HC. The pH of the skin surface and its impact on the barrier function. *Skin Pharmacol Physiol.* 2006;19:296–302.

28. How does the clinician utilize the basic interaction between pH and the microbiome?

Raising the pH of the skin appears to exacerbate several inflammatory skin conditions. Maintaining a relatively acidic pH (<7.0) through decreased washing with harsh high pH (alkaline) soaps, and instead using mild synthetic detergent soaps, helps lessen the severity of these conditions.

CHAPTER 2

MORPHOLOGY OF PRIMARY AND SECONDARY SKIN LESIONS

Elizabeth Swanson

1. Why do dermatologists use words that no one else understands?

   The language of dermatology is unique. It encompasses terms that rarely, if ever, are used in other medical specialties. The use of these correct dermatologic terms is important to accurately describe skin lesions to dermatologists during telephone calls and during rounds and teaching. A good description of a skin lesion enables the listener to formulate a series of differential diagnoses, whereas a poor one does not.

2. But why are the descriptions so long?

   Use of appropriate terminology and important clues, such as configuration and skin distribution, effectively paints an accurate picture for the listener. Use of vague terms—spot, bump, rash, and lesion—is not helpful. Such vocabulary is counterproductive to formulating an accurate differential diagnosis. "Grouped vesicles on an erythematous base" immediately suggests herpes simplex, and "brown, friable 'stuck-on' papules" accurately describes seborrheic keratoses. "Well-demarcated, erythematous plaques with micaceous, silvery scales located on extensor surfaces" is suggestive of psoriasis. "Violaceous, polygonal papules with Wickham's striae located on flexural surfaces" is consistent with lichen planus. On the other hand, "red, scaly rash on the foot" describes an enormous, nebulous group of disorders.

3. How can I possibly learn the language of dermatology?

   First, learn the definitions of the various primary, secondary, and special skin lesions. Each of these groups consists of a short list of terms that specifies basic types. Then, follow this simple template when describing skin lesions:
   - Size
   - Color or additional descriptive terms (e.g., pigmentation, shape)
   - Type of primary, secondary, or special skin lesion (e.g., papule, macule)
   - Arrangement (e.g., grouped lesions)
   - Distribution (e.g., truncal, generalized). This template provides a systematic way to add adjectives to the type of lesion. Repetition is key; practice using the template when describing skin lesions.

4. What is a primary skin lesion?

   It is the initial lesion that has not been altered by trauma, manipulation (scratching, scrubbing), or natural regression over time. Examples include:
   - Macules
   - Wheals
   - Papules
   - Vesicles
   - Plaques
   - Bullae
   - Patches
   - Pustules
   - Nodules
   - Cysts

5. How is each of the primary lesions defined?

   See Table 2.1.

6. How do you determine whether a lesion is flat or raised?

   Palpation is the most reliable method, but side-lighting also helps. It can be difficult to distinguish a macule from a papule or a patch from a plaque in a photograph, and it is one of the limiting factors in teledermatology.

7. How does a primary lesion differ from a secondary lesion?

   Secondary skin lesions are created by scratching, scrubbing, or infection. They may also develop normally with time. For example, the primary lesion in a sunburn is a macular erythema (although it could also be a blister), but with resolution, scale and increased pigmentation become prominent. Examples of secondary lesions include:
   - Crusts
   - Scale
   - Ulcers

(Text continues on p. 15)

Table 2.1 Primary skin lesions

PRIMARY LESION	DEFINITION	MORPHOLOGY	EXAMPLES
Macule	Flat, circumscribed skin discoloration that lacks surface elevation or depression		Café-au-lait Vitiligo Freckle Junctional nevi Ink tattoo
Papule	Elevated, solid lesion <0.5 cm in diameter		Acrochordon (skin tag) Basal cell carcinoma Molluscum contagiosum

Continued on following page

Table 2.1 Primary skin lesions (*Continued*)

PRIMARY LESION	DEFINITION	MORPHOLOGY	EXAMPLES
Plaque	Elevated, solid "confluence of papules" ($>$0.5 cm in diameter) that lacks a deep component		Bowen's disease Mycosis fungoides Psoriasis Eczema Tinea corporis
Patch	Flat, circumscribed skin discoloration; a very large macule		Port wine stain Vitiligo
Nodule	Elevated, solid lesion $>$0.5 cm in diameter; a larger, deeper papule		Rheumatoid nodule Tendon xanthoma Erythema nodosum Lipoma Metastatic carcinoma

Wheal

Firm, edematous plaque that is evanescent and pruritic; a hive

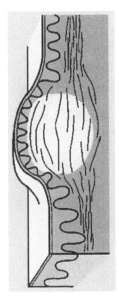

Urticaria
Dermographism
Urticaria pigmentosa

Vesicle

Papule that contains clear fluid; a blister

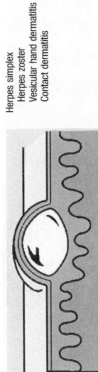

Herpes simplex
Herpes zoster
Vesicular hand dermatitis
Contact dermatitis

Bulla

Localized fluid collection >0.5 cm in diameter; a large vesicle

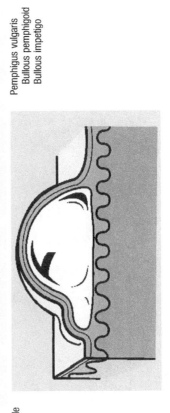

Pemphigus vulgaris
Bullous pemphigoid
Bullous impetigo

Continued on following page

Table 2.1 Primary skin lesions (*Continued*)

PRIMARY LESION	DEFINITION	MORPHOLOGY	EXAMPLES
Pustule	Papule that contains purulent material		Folliculitis Impetigo Acne Pustular psoriasis
Cyst	Nodule that contains fluid or semisolid material		Acne Epidermal inclusion Trichilemmal cyst

- Fissures
- Excoriations
- Scars
- Erosions
- Postinflammatory dyspigmentation

8. How are secondary skin lesions defined?
   See Table 2.2.

9. What is a maculopapular eruption?
   A dermatitic lesion that is composed of both macules and papules. Maculopapular eruptions are commonly seen with viral exanthems and drug-induced reactions. The cutaneous eruption of measles is an example of a maculopapular eruption.

Table 2.2 Secondary skin lesions

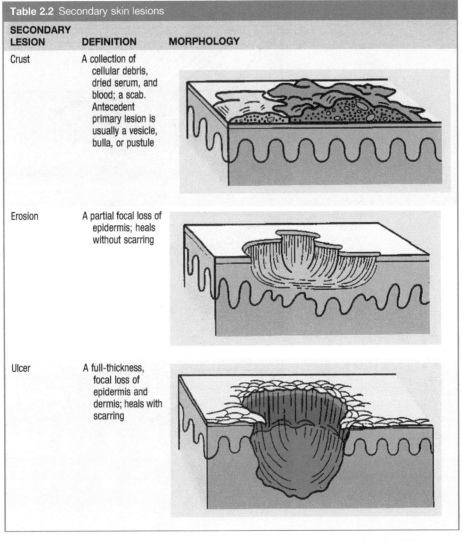

SECONDARY LESION	DEFINITION	MORPHOLOGY
Crust	A collection of cellular debris, dried serum, and blood; a scab. Antecedent primary lesion is usually a vesicle, bulla, or pustule	
Erosion	A partial focal loss of epidermis; heals without scarring	
Ulcer	A full-thickness, focal loss of epidermis and dermis; heals with scarring	

Continued on following page

Table 2.2 Secondary skin lesions (*Continued*)

SECONDARY LESION	DEFINITION	MORPHOLOGY
Fissure	Vertical loss of epidermis and dermis with sharply defined walls; crack in skin	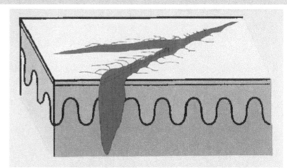
Excoriation	Linear erosion induced by scratching	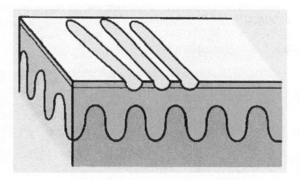
Scar	A collection of new connective tissue; may be hypertrophic or atrophic. Scar implies dermoepidermal damage	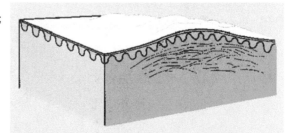
Scale	Thick stratum corneum that results from hyperproliferation or increased cohesion of keratinocytes	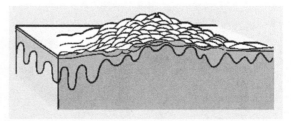

10. Give some examples of special skin lesions.
    • Telangiectasias
    • Purpura
    • Petechiae
    • Comedones
    • Burrows
    • Target lesions

11. What are telangiectasias?
    Telangiectasias (Fig. 2.1) are small, dilated, superficial blood vessels (capillaries, arterioles, or venules) that blanch (disappear) with pressure.

12. Are telangiectasias pathognomonic for a certain disease?
    No. Telangiectasias may occur in many cutaneous disorders, including connective tissue diseases such as dermatomyositis, systemic lupus erythematosus, and progressive systemic sclerosis. They are also commonly seen as a consequence of chronic ultraviolet radiation and topical steroid usage. Telangiectasias may also be seen in tumors such as a noduloulcerative basal cell carcinoma, which is classically described as a pearly colored papule with telangiectasias and central ulceration.

13. What is a burrow?
    A burrow (Fig. 2.2) is an elevated channel in the superficial epidermis produced by a parasite, such as the mite *Sarcoptes scabiei*. Scabies burrows characteristically are located on the wrists and in fingerwebs; the diagnosis is confirmed by demonstrating the mite microscopically in skin scrapings. The dog and cat hookworm, *Ancylostoma braziliense*, may also produce a serpiginous burrow; however, demonstrating the organism is more difficult. The human hookworm penetrates the skin with a papular lesion and does not typically produce a burrow.

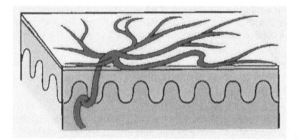

Fig. 2.1 Telangiectasia.

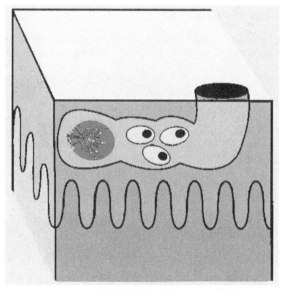

Fig. 2.2 Scabies burrow.

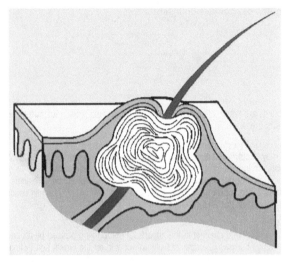

Fig. 2.3 Comedo.

14. What is a comedo?

A comedo (Fig. 2.3) is a folliculocentric collection of sebum and keratin. Comedonal acne characteristically consists of both open (blackheads) and closed (whiteheads) comedones. When the contents of a closed comedo are exposed to air, a chemical reaction occurs, imparting the black color to an open comedo.

15. What is the difference between petechiae and purpura?

The size of the lesion is the major difference. Both petechiae and purpura result from extravasation of red blood cells into the dermis; hence, they do not blanch with pressure. Petechiae, however, are much smaller than purpura; they are <5 mm in diameter.

16. What are targetoid (target) lesions?

Targetoid lesions typically consist of three zones. The first zone consists of a dark or blistered center (bull's-eye) that is surrounded by a second, pale zone. The third zone consists of a rim of erythema. Target lesions classically are found in patients with erythema multiforme (Fig. 2.4).

17. List some of the additional descriptive adjectives used in dermatology that refer to color or pigmentation.

- **Depigmented:** Absence of melanin, a lack of color. Depigmented macules and patches are commonly found in vitiligo.
- **Hypopigmented:** Lighter-than-normal skin color; normal number of melanocytes but decreased production of melanin by the melanocytes. The ash-leaf macule of tuberous sclerosis is an example of a hypopigmented macule.

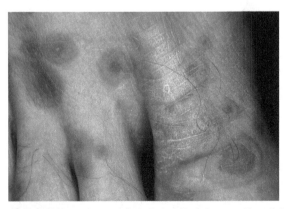

Fig. 2.4 Targetoid lesions. Patient with classic erythema multiforme demonstrating lesions resembling a "bull's-eye." Note that some lesions demonstrate a small, centrally placed blister. (Courtesy Fitzsimons Army Medical Center teaching files.)

- **Hyperpigmented:** Darker-than-normal skin color. Junctional nevi and café-au-lait macules (neurofibromatosis) are hyperpigmented macules.
- **Erythematous:** Showing redness of the skin.

18. How do atrophy and lichenification differ?

Atrophy (Fig. 2.5) is thinning of the epidermis, dermis, or subcutis (fat). Epidermal atrophy can manifest as a fine, cigarette-paper wrinkling of the skin, the appearance of telangiectasia, or even the development of stretch marks on the skin surface. Dermal and fat atrophy can cause a depression in the skin surface.

A **lichenified lesion** (Fig. 2.6) is a focal area of thickened skin produced by chronic scratching or rubbing. The skin lines are accentuated, resembling a washboard (Fig. 2.7).

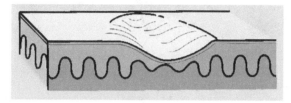

Fig. 2.5 Atrophy.

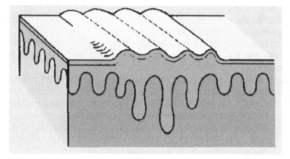

Fig. 2.6 Lichenification.

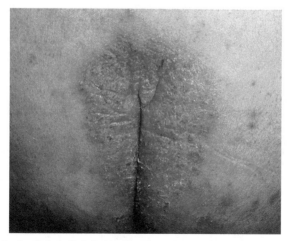

Fig. 2.7 Lichen simplex chronicus. Patient with atopic dermatitis and secondary lichenification manifesting as thickened skin with accentuation of skin markings. Secondary excoriations are also present. (Courtesy Fitzsimons Army Medical Center teaching files.)

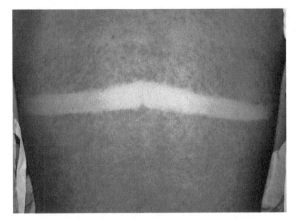

Fig. 2.8 Koebner (isomorphic) phenomenon. Patient with acute explosive psoriasis demonstrating restriction of lesions to the site of minor trauma in the form of a sunburn. (Courtesy William L. Weston, MD, collection.)

19. Do skin diseases have characteristic arrangements or configurations?

Some, but not all, cutaneous diseases demonstrate characteristic arrangements or configurations of lesions. Commonly used adjectives include:

- **Annular:** Used to describe lesions that are ring shaped. Annular plaques are typical findings in granuloma annulare, tinea corporis (ringworm), and erythema marginatum.
- **Gyrate:** From the Latin *gyratus*, which means "to turn around in a circle," gyrate skin lesions are rare presentations. Gyrate erythema that resembles wood grain or topographic maps is seen in erythema gyratum repens, which usually heralds the presence of an internal malignancy.
- **Dermatomal:** Used to describe lesions that follow neurocutaneous dermatomes. The classic example is herpes zoster (shingles), which demonstrates grouped vesicles on an erythematous base in a dermatomal distribution.
- **Linear:** More than 20 diseases may demonstrate linear configurations. One example is allergic contact dermatitis to poison ivy; it characteristically demonstrates linear erythematous papules or vesicles.
- **Grouped:** Papules, pustules, or blisters (vesicles or bullae) may demonstrate grouped configurations. A typical example is herpes simplex, which demonstrates grouped vesicles on an erythematous base.

20. What is the Koebner (isomorphic) phenomenon?

The Koebner (isomorphic) phenomenon describes the process by which traumatizing the epidermis of a patient with a certain preexisting skin disease will cause the same skin disease to form in the traumatized skin. Noticing this skin finding is helpful when creating a differential diagnosis. Only certain diseases are associated with a Koebner phenomenon; lichen planus, lichen nitidus, and psoriasis (Fig. 2.8) are examples.

21. Do skin diseases characteristically occur in certain locations?

Yes. This is the reason that a complete skin examination should be performed on all patients. Seborrheic dermatitis characteristically occurs on the scalp, nasolabial folds, retroauricular areas, eyelids, eyebrows, and presternal areas; it tends to spare the extremities. Psoriasis may resemble seborrheic dermatitis, but it characteristically demonstrates a different distribution, usually involving the extremities (elbows, knees), intergluteal fold, scalp, and nails.

KEY POINTS: PRIMARY AND SECONDARY LESIONS

1. The clinical diagnosis of skin disease is accomplished by a complex appreciation of the primary and secondary skin lesions, distribution, color, arrangement, and body site.
2. Palpation of skin lesions is an underappreciated physical skill that augments the visual clues.
3. Not all lesions can be diagnosed by the initial physical examination and the presence or absence of symptoms (e.g., pruritus, burning); history and clinical course are often required to establish a diagnosis.
4. Not all skin diseases can be diagnosed in a single or even multiple visits.

BIBLIOGRAPHY

Cox NH, Coulson IH. Diagnosis of skin disease. In: Burns S, Breathnach SM, Cox N, et al. *Rook's textbook of dermatology*. 7th ed. Malden, MA: Blackwell; 2004:5.1–5.10.

Rapini R. Clinical and pathologic differential diagnosis. In: Bolognia JL, Jorizzo JL, Rapini R, eds. *Dermatology*. London: Mosby; 2003:3–12.

CHAPTER 3

DIAGNOSTIC TECHNIQUES

Stephen Thomas Spates

1. **What is the most sensitive office laboratory test for diagnosing dermatophyte infections of the skin?**

   Microscopic examination of a potassium hydroxide (KOH) preparation of scrapings taken from the affected area is the most sensitive office laboratory test. A study of 220 specimens examined by both KOH and culture demonstrated positive KOH preparations and positive cultures in 45% of samples, a positive KOH preparation and negative culture in 52% of samples, and a negative KOH preparation and a positive culture in only 3% of samples. However, cultures can be useful because other studies have shown a 5% to 15% increase in positive specimens by culturing KOH-negative materials. Moreover, it is important to realize that the diagnostic accuracy of the KOH preparation depends on the skill of the individual performing the test. The cellophane adhesive tape method (see below) may increase accuracy of the test, even by inexperienced performers, by decreasing artifact and clumping of cells in the preparation.

Lefler E, Haim S, Merzbach D. Evaluation of direct microscopic examination versus culture in the diagnosis of superficial fungal infections. *Mykosen*. 1981;24:102–106.

Raghukumar S, Ravikumar BC. Potassium hydroxide mount with cellophane adhesive tape: a method for direct diagnosis of dermatophyte skin infections. *Clin Exp Dermatolo*. 2018;43(8):895–898.

2. **How is a KOH examination performed?**

   The highest rate of recovery of organisms occurs in specimens taken from the tops of vesicles, the leading edges of annular lesions, or deep scrapings from the nails suspected to be infected with fungi. The site should be swabbed with an alcohol pad or water and scraped with a no. 15 blade. In some instances, such as the scalp or nail, a curette may be more effective. The moist corneocytes are then easily transferred from the blade to a glass slide. One or two drops of KOH (10% to 20%) are added, and a coverslip is applied to the specimen. The KOH preparation is gently warmed, but not boiled, and then examined under the microscope. It is important to focus back and forth through the material so that the refractile hyphae can be visualized. Fungal hyphae can be recognized by their regular cylindrical shapes with branching and the presence of septae that may demonstrate a subtle greenish hue (Fig. 3.1). A pencil eraser or pen cap gently applied to the surface of the coverslip may enhance keratinocyte breakdown, especially for clumped specimens. If no organisms are observed initially, waiting 10 to 15 minutes may aid visualization.

3. **What laboratory tests are useful for diagnosing tinea capitis?**

   Testing for fluorescence in the affected area using a Wood's light is the quickest technique. If the hair fluoresces yellow-green, then a fungal infection is likely. However, lack of fluorescence does not exclude tinea capitis, because *Trichophyton tonsurans* accounts for 80% to 95% of scalp ringworm infections in the United States, and it does not fluoresce. Therefore, examination of KOH-treated infected hair is more sensitive and can also be rapidly performed. The best results are obtained when broken-off hairs are examined, because these are the ones infected by hyphae and arthrospores. Most dermatophytes, such as *T. tonsurans*, grow within the hair shaft (endothrix), and a few minutes are required to let KOH break down the hair shaft and visualize the infection. Finally, the diagnosis can also be proved by fungal cultures. The easily broken, infected hairs are embedded in the media. The specimen can be obtained using a no. 15 blade, curette, or hemostat.

4. **What is a Wood's light or lamp? How is it useful in skin diseases?**

   A Wood's light produces invisible long-wave ultraviolet radiation, or "black light," at a wavelength of 360 nm. When this light strikes the surface of the skin or urine, fluorescence is produced in some disorders. This fluorescence is best observed in a completely dark room. The Wood's lamp is useful in diagnosing cases of several skin conditions: tinea capitis (see preceding text), tinea versicolor (dull yellow fluorescence), erythrasma (coral red fluorescence; Fig. 3.2), and *Pseudomonas* infections of the skin (green fluorescence). It is also useful as a screening test in porphyria cutanea tarda, as the urine fluoresces a coral red color (Fig. 3.3). The Wood's light may also be used in certain disorders of pigmentation. In patients with hyperpigmentation, it is used to localize the site of the pigment because it accentuates superficial epidermal pigment, whereas deeper dermal pigment is unchanged. It is also used in patients with vitiligo because it demonstrates complete depigmentation. Finally, it can be used to delineate the borders of melanocytic lesions, such as lentigo maligna, prior to surgery.

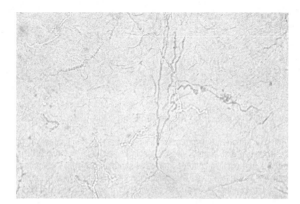

Fig. 3.1 Refractile and cylindrical hyphae traversing KOH preparation of skin scraping.

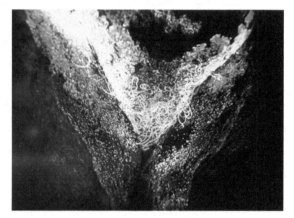

Fig. 3.2 Wood's light examination of the groin area demonstrating classic coral red fluorescence associated with erythrasma. (Courtesy John L. Aeling, MD.)

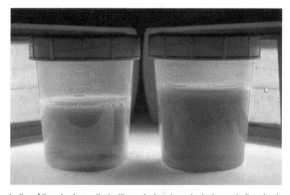

Fig. 3.3 Wood's light examination of the urine in a patient with porphyria cutanea tarda demonstrating classic coral red fluorescence with normal urine specimen exhibited for comparison. (Courtesy James E. Fitzpatrick, MD.)

5. **Name common culture media used for isolating dermatophytes.**
Dermatophyte test media (DTM) and Sabouraud's dextrose agar, with or without antibiotics (e.g., Mycosel agar, Mycobiotic agar), are the two most common types of culture media used. Many dermatologists prefer DTM because it has the advantage of a color indicator that changes the media from yellow to red when a dermatophyte is present. DTM is 95% to 97% accurate in differentiating dermatophytes from nondermatophytes. Sabouraud's dextrose agar is

a standard in mycology laboratories and also in many dermatologists' offices. It consists of dextrose (energy source), peptone (protein source), and agar (for a firm surface). Antibiotics can be added to suppress bacterial contaminants, and cycloheximide is added to suppress yeasts and nondermatophytes. Plain Sabouraud's agar is an especially good culture medium for *Candida albicans*.

6. Describe a simple test for tinea versicolor other than a KOH preparation.

Clear cellophane tape preparations are an excellent diagnostic testing material because the organism is found in the upper stratum corneum. First, the skin is scraped to ensure that there is adequate scale. The tape is applied over the scale and then mounted on a glass slide and examined under a microscope. Clusters of short hyphae and yeasts are seen producing a "spaghetti and meatballs" pattern. Methylene blue may also be added to the slide, selectively staining the organism and thus enhancing visualization (Fig. 3.4). It is important to note that *Malassezia globosa* and *M. furfur*, the most common etiologic agents of tinea versicolor, cannot be cultured on any of the routine fungal media kept in most laboratories.

Martin AG, Kobayashi GS. Yeast infections: candidiasis, pityriasis (tinea) versicolor. In Fitzpatrick TB, Eisen AZ, Wolff K, et al, editors. *Dermatology in general medicine*. 4th ed. New York, NY: McGraw-Hill; 1993, 2462–2467.

7. What is a Tzanck preparation or smear?

A Tzanck smear is a standard technique for the rapid diagnosis of herpes simplex virus (HSV) or varicella-zoster virus infections. It cannot distinguish between these two agents, nor can it distinguish between HSV subtypes (HSV type 1 or 2). It is performed by scraping the base of a fresh blister with a scalpel blade and then spreading the adhering cells and material onto a glass slide. The slide is then stained with a Giemsa, Wright, or Sedi stain. The typical multinucleated giant cells or atypical keratinocytes with large nuclei are then easily visualized (Fig. 3.5).

Micheletti RG, Dominquez AR, Wanat KA: Bedside diagnostics in dermatology: parasitic and noninfectious diseases, *J Am Acad Dermatol* 77(2):221–230, 2017.

8. What is the best method of diagnosing scabies?

The best method is to scrape a burrow and demonstrate the parasite inside it. A classic burrow appears as an irregular, linear, slightly elevated lesion, best found on the flexor wrists, fingerwebs, and genitalia. Eighty-five percent of adult male patients with scabies will have mites on the hands or wrists. Occasionally, the mite can be seen with the naked eye as a small dot at one end of the burrow. Following the application of mineral oil, on either the blade or skin, the burrow is scraped vigorously with a no. 15 scalpel blade, but not so vigorously as to draw blood. The mineral oil is collected from the skin and blade and transferred to a glass slide, which is then examined under the microscope. The diagnosis is established by identifying either the fecal pellets (scybala), eggs, or the mite itself (Fig. 3.6).

Leung AKC, Lam JM, Leong KF. Scabies: a neglected global disease. *Curr Pediatr Rev.* 2020;16(1):33–42.

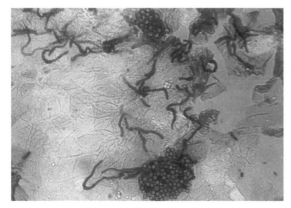

Fig. 3.4 A positive cellophane tape preparation of tinea versicolor that has been stained with methylene blue. The characteristic clusters of spores and short hyphae are demonstrated. (Courtesy James E. Fitzpatrick, MD.)

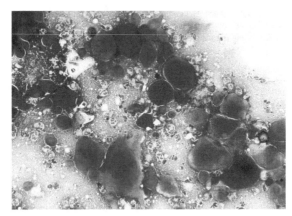

Fig. 3.5 A positive Tzanck preparation demonstrating large multinucleated keratinocytes. The nuclei of normal keratinocytes are the size of neutrophils, which are the other cells present in this preparation. (Courtesy James E. Fitzpatrick, MD.)

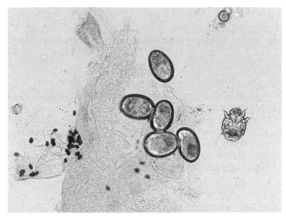

Fig. 3.6 A positive scraping for scabies showing an immature mite, eggs, and numerous fecal pellets. (Courtesy James E. Fitzpatrick, MD.)

9. How do you diagnose mite bites acquired from an animal?

   Clinically, patients present with pruritic red bumps, most commonly on the arms, breasts, and abdomen. The most common sources of these animal mites are cats infested with *Cheyletiella* species. This nonburrowing mite exhibits "bite and run" tactics, so it is not likely to be found on the patient's body. The key to making the diagnosis is to have the animal examined by a veterinarian who is familiar with these parasites. The diagnosis is established by a cellophane tape preparation taken from the cat, dog, or rabbit, demonstrating either the six-legged larval form or the eight-legged adult. Unlike the scabies mite, *Cheyletiella* has well-developed, clawlike mouth parts.

10. How do you diagnose lice infestation?

   Lice infestation is caused by *Pediculus humanus capitis* (head louse), *P. humanus corporis* (body louse), or *Phthirus pubis* (pubic louse). Lice can be identified by eye or by using a hand lens, but they can be very difficult to locate. If body lice infestation is suspected, examination of the seams of clothing is more likely to be diagnostic than is examining the skin. Lice will appear as brownish-gray specks. Head and pubic lice are more often seen in hairy areas and are often found with their mouth parts embedded in the skin with outstretched claws grasping hairs on either side. Usually more numerous are nits (eggs), which are white-gray oval structures smaller than 1 mm in size and firmly attached to the hair shaft. Eggs that are near the junction of the hair shaft and the skin are indicative of active or recent infection. Since hair casts are white and may resemble nits, it is sometimes necessary to examine possible nits under the microscope to prove their identity (Fig. 3.7).

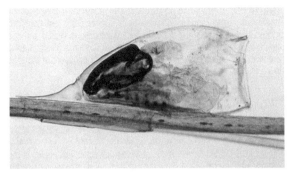

Fig. 3.7 Microscopic examination of a hair shaft demonstrates an empty hair louse egg that is glued to the hair shaft. (Courtesy James E. Fitzpatrick, MD.)

11. What is the diagnostic test of choice for a patient presenting with a suspected syphilitic chancre on his penis?

   Dark-field examination of the chancre is the most specific test for the diagnosis of syphilis. This test is typically positive unless the patient has applied or ingested antibiotics. In addition to primary syphilis, dark-field microscopy can also be used to diagnose all of the mucocutaneous lesions of secondary syphilis. However, it is less reliable for examining specimens from the mouth or rectum because of the high prevalence of commensal, nonpathogenic treponemes in these locations that may be mistaken for *Treponema pallidum*, the agent of syphilis. The best specimen for dark-field examination is serous fluid expressed from the base of the chancre following cleaning with sterile saline and clean gauze. The specimen then should be immediately evaluated for the organism's characteristic corkscrew morphology and flexing, hairpin motility. If a patient is suspected of having a syphilitic chancre and a dark-field evaluation is negative, it should be repeated at least once before the diagnosis is excluded. Fluorescent antibody microscopy, although not widely available, offers a sensitive alternative and has the advantage that it does not require live organisms and it can be done on fixed slides. This technique utilizes antibodies to *T. pallidum*.

12. How is secondary syphilis diagnosed?

   As with primary syphilis, the most specific test is dark-field microscopy. Special stains on skin biopsies are diagnostic as well. More often, screening tests for syphilis such as nontreponemal serologic tests are utilized; usually, a rapid plasma reagin or a Venereal Disease Research Laboratory (VDRL) test is ordered. Nontreponemal serologic tests for syphilis detect antibodies to reagin, a cholesterol-lecithin-cardiolipin antigen that cross reacts with antibodies present in the sera of patients with syphilis. These antibodies are not specific for syphilis and should always be confirmed by a specific test for syphilis, usually a fluorescent treponemal antibody–absorption (FTA-ABS) or the microhemagglutination–*T. pallidum* test. Nontreponemal serologic tests for syphilis are positive in almost all cases of secondary syphilis. Adequate treatment causes the titer to decline to low titers or nonreactivity.

Domantay-Apostol GP, Handog EB, Gabriel MT. Syphilis: the international challenge of the great imitator. *Dermatol Clin*. 2008;26:191–202.

13. How long do serologic tests for syphilis remain positive?

   Nontreponemal test antibody titers (e.g., VDRL) are reported quantitatively in the form of the highest positive titer. This titer correlates with disease activity, and treated patients may demonstrate negative results or very low titers. More than 50% of patients will be seronegative 1 year after treatment. A patient with a positive treponemal test (e.g., FTA-ABS) is less likely to revert to negative, and only 24% of patients will be seronegative 1 year after treatment; both treated and untreated patients may demonstrate positive serologic tests for the rest of their lives.

14. In patients with symptomatic gonococcal urethritis, how efficacious is a Gram stain of the exudate in comparison to a culture utilizing selective media for gonococcus?

   A Gram stain of a urethral discharge in symptomatic males is an excellent method of diagnosing gonorrhea. A positive Gram stain showing multiple neutrophils, some containing clusters of gram-negative diplococci with the sides flattened toward one another, is cited as having a sensitivity of 98%. With such a Gram stain, a culture is expensive and adds little diagnostic yield (about 2%). Cultures are usually done in males with a urethritis and a negative or nondiagnostic Gram stain of the urethral exudates. In women suspected of having gonorrhea, the site of choice for obtaining specimens is the endocervix. However, Gram-stained smears are relatively insensitive (30% to 60%), and their interpretation is difficult. A culture on selective media is essential to diagnose gonorrhea in women.

Holder NA. Gonococcal infections. *Pediatr Rev* 2008;29:228–234.

15. What is the best way to diagnose allergic contact dermatitis?

The diagnostic test of choice is a properly applied and correctly interpreted patch test. Contact dermatitis is divided into irritant or allergic subtypes. Allergic contact dermatitis is immunologically mediated and is an acquired sensitivity that affects only certain individuals. Irritant contact dermatitis is not immunologically mediated and is due to chemical damage of the skin. For example, excessive hand washing or exposure to battery acid will involve almost everyone exposed in such fashion.

Goossens A. Recognizing and testing allergens. *Dermatol Clin.* 2009;27:219–226.

KEY POINTS: DIAGNOSIS OF FUNGAL INFECTIONS

1. Microscopic examination of KOH-treated clinical material (epidermal scale, hair, nails) is more sensitive in experienced hands than are cultures for establishing the diagnosis of dermatophyte infections.
2. The Wood's light is very specific but not sensitive for establishing the diagnosis of tinea capitis because the majority of cases are produced by *Trichophyton tonsurans*, a species that does not fluoresce.
3. Dermatophyte test medium is excellent for establishing the diagnosis of a dermatophyte infection but will miss most infections by yeast such as *Candida* species.
4. When examining or culturing hairs in suspected cases of tinea capitis, pluck or remove the broken hairs, which are infected, and not the intact hairs.

KEY POINTS: BIOPSY TECHNIQUES

1. Shave biopsies are often poor choices for melanocytic lesions such as dysplastic nevi or melanoma, as they may fail to allow full and complete microscopic assessment of the lesion.
2. An incisional biopsy is used to remove the thickest or clinically most worrisome portion of a larger lesion not amenable to complete removal for diagnostic pathologic examination.
3. When splitting a punch biopsy, the specimen is cut through the dermal rather than the epidermal side to reduce crush artifact.

16. How are patch tests applied?

The suspected allergen is usually placed in an appropriate vehicle at an appropriate concentration. The patch test allergens are usually purchased in prepared forms, but less common allergens can be prepared individually. The allergens are placed in special wells that are taped against the skin of the back for 48 hours and then removed. It is important to instruct patients to keep the testing area completely dry. This skin area is then examined 24 to 72 hours after the patch is removed for a reading. A strong positive reaction has erythema, infiltration, papules, and vesicles. A bullous reaction is extremely positive. Interpretation of patch tests and correlation with the clinical disease are complex and usually performed by dermatologists.

17. In what diseases is a skin biopsy helpful?

A skin biopsy with routine hematoxylin-eosin staining is the best diagnostic technique for many cutaneous neoplasms that cannot be diagnosed visually. It is also helpful in many inflammatory skin disorders, especially those in which a specific diagnosis cannot be made from clinical examination, blood tests, or scrapings of the skin. The skin biopsy is a common office procedure, and specimens may also be submitted for more advanced studies such as immunofluorescence, electron microscopy, special stains, cultures, or polymerase chain reaction studies.

18. When are shave biopsies indicated?

The choice of the biopsy technique requires knowledge of basic dermatology, most specifically where in the skin the pathology is likely to be located. A shave biopsy is usually the most superficial of the skin biopsies and particularly useful when the lesion is in or close to the epidermis. A shave biopsy is best for pedunculated, papular, or otherwise exophytic lesions. It is particularly useful for diagnosis of basal cell and squamous cell carcinomas, seborrheic keratoses, warts, intradermal nevi, and pyogenic granulomas. Shave biopsies are often poor choices for biopsies of melanocytic lesions such as dysplastic nevi or melanoma. Unlike punch biopsies, shave biopsies only require a clean, nonsterile field and do not require sutures.

19. What are the indications for punch biopsies?

A punch biopsy utilizes a round knife that takes a cylinder of tissue including the epidermis, dermis, and often the subcutaneous fat. Although punch biopsies from 2 to 10 mm in diameter can be used, the most common diameter is 4 mm. A larger punch biopsy may be useful if the specimen is to be divided for culture or other procedures. When splitting the biopsy, the specimen is cut through the dermal rather than the epidermal side to reduce crush artifact. A larger punch biopsy of the skin is also helpful in the diagnosis of cutaneous T-cell lymphoma and for scalp biopsies, where a generous specimen is often necessary to establish the diagnosis. The surgical defect left by punch biopsies may be allowed to heal in secondarily, but most dermatologists close the defect with a single suture.

20. Describe the indications for an excisional or incisional biopsy.

Excisional or incisional biopsies are usually elliptical in shape and typically deeper than punch biopsies. An excisional biopsy is the complete removal of a lesion into the fat, followed by layered closure of the skin. It is particularly helpful in the complete removal of malignancies, such as malignant melanoma, basal cell carcinoma, and squamous cell carcinoma. Excisional biopsies can also be performed when the cosmetic result is felt to be superior to that of a punch biopsy. An incisional biopsy is the incomplete or partial removal of a lesion. If a suspected malignancy is felt to be too large to remove with simple surgery, an incisional biopsy is used to remove the thickest or clinically most worrisome portion for diagnostic pathologic examination. It is also useful for diagnosing panniculitis, sclerotic, or atrophic lesions in which it is important to compare normal adjacent skin to that of the lesion, and to lesions with active expanding borders, such as pyoderma gangrenosum.

21. Define and describe direct immunofluorescence of the skin.

Direct immunofluorescence (DIF) of the skin is a histologic stain for antibodies or other tissue proteins in skin biopsy specimens. A skin sample obtained from the patient is immediately frozen in liquid nitrogen or placed in special media to preserve the immunoreactants. Arrangements should be made to ensure proper and timely transport to the immunofluorescence laboratory. Once received, the tissue is sectioned and then incubated with antibodies to human immunoglobulins or complement components that have been tagged with a fluorescent molecule to allow their visualization. The samples are then examined with a fluorescence microscope, where fluorescence indicates that immunoreactants were deposited in the patient's tissue. The specific immunoreactants present, and the pattern and intensity of staining, are used to determine the diseases most likely to be associated with the DIF findings.

Diercks GF, Pas HH, Jonkman MF. Immunofluorescence of autoimmune bullous diseases. *Surg Pathol Clin*. 2017;10(2):505–512.

22. Name some skin diseases in which DIF is helpful in making a diagnosis.

Many of the immunobullous diseases are associated with specific DIF findings: bullous pemphigoid, herpes gestationis, cicatricial pemphigoid, epidermolysis bullosa acquisita, dermatitis herpetiformis, linear IgA bullous dermatosis, and the various types of pemphigus. In addition, DIF may be helpful in evaluating cutaneous and systemic lupus erythematosus, other collagen vascular diseases, vasculitis such as Henoch-Schönlein purpura (Fig. 3.8), and certain types of porphyria.

23. How does indirect immunofluorescence of the skin differ from DIF of the skin?

Indirect immunofluorescence studies test for the presence of circulating autoantibodies in the serum, in contrast to DIF studies, which test for the presence of autoantibodies deposited in the skin. The serum from the patient is incubated with an appropriate normal substrate such as monkey esophagus, rat bladder, or human skin. The substrate is incubated with fluorescein-labeled antibodies directed against the antibody in the tissue. The specimen is then examined under a fluorescence microscope. By running this test at various dilutions, the amount of circulating antibody can be determined and reported as a titer. Titers are useful in some diseases, such as pemphigus vulgaris, in determining disease activity and treatment.

24. Is ELISA ever used for the diagnosis of immunobullous disease?

Yes. In recent years, the enzyme-linked immunosorbent assay (ELISA) has been increasingly used for the diagnosis and differentiation of various forms of pemphigus, based on the presence of immunoglobulin (IgG) autoantibodies directed against desmoglein-1 (dsg-1) and desmoglein-3 (dsg-3), which are proteins found in the intercellular

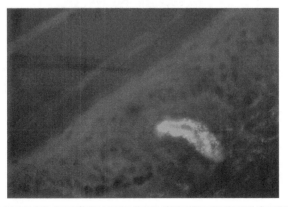

Fig. 3.8 Direct immunofluorescent study demonstrating granular deposits of IgA within a blood vessel of a patient with Henoch-Schönlein purpura. (Courtesy James E. Fitzpatrick, MD.)

junctions between keratinocytes. The ELISA is also, but less commonly, used to detect IgG autoantibodies against BP180 and BP230, which are the major antigens associated with bullous pemphigoid. The ELISA is both more specific and sensitive when compared to indirect immunofluorescence testing.

Witte M, Zillikens D, Schmidt E. Diagnosis of autoimmune blistering diseases. *Front Med (Lausanne)*. 2018;5:296.

25. How are bacterial skin cultures performed, and when are they useful?

Bacterial cultures are useful when active infection of the skin is suspected. Bacterial cultures demonstrate high yields in superficial infections such as impetigo, ecthyma, and infected ulcers, and lower yields in cellulitis. When culturing superficial infections, the involved area should first be cleaned with an alcohol pad and then thoroughly swabbed. A higher concentration of bacteria may be found at the point of maximal inflammation. The best results in cellulitis are obtained when the leading edge is injected with nonbacteriostatic saline using a 20-gauge needle mounted on a tuberculin syringe. The aspirate may be sent for culture while still in the syringe if it can be taken to the laboratory immediately, or the aspirated material may be submitted in a bacterial culturette.

26. What are some new technologies that may help improve dermatologists' ability for the accurate early detection of melanoma?

The optimal method to identify melanoma is a full skin examination by a trained clinician and the removal of any suspicious lesion(s). However, detecting melanoma early and limiting the unnecessary removal of benign lesions remain a challenge. There are technologies newly available that can act as a useful adjunct to biopsy: Whole body, high-resolution, digital photographic imaging can detect changes in lesions over time or the appearance of new-onset findings between visits. Dermoscopy allows the use of a handheld device to utilize magnification and a light source to appreciate features of a lesion that cannot be appreciated visually during a skin examination (Fig. 3.9). Multispectral imaging captures imaged data by examining a lesion with different wavelengths of light, which may reveal information about the visualized lesion that the eye itself fails to appreciate. Some of these devices are able to generate a probability score, which can support a decision to perform a biopsy based on how atypical a lesion is deemed. Confocal scanning laser microscopy creates in vivo images of skin lesions. The technology is based on the fact that early melanoma and benign lesions will have different reflective properties. The result is an image that is comparable to an actual pathology specimen.

Angelucci DD. Diagnosis: melanoma. *Dermatology World* (a publication of the American Academy of Dermatology Association). 2014; May, 20–24.

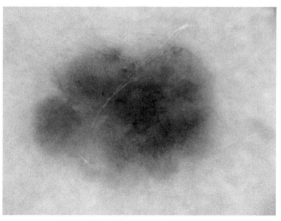

Fig. 3.9 Dermatoscope image of an atypical (dysplastic) nevus demonstrating asymmetry, irregular outline, and multiple shades of brown. (Courtesy Wendi Wohltmann, MD.)

DISORDERS OF KERATINIZATION

Lori D. Prok

CHAPTER 4

1. **What are the ichthyosiform dermatoses?**
   The ichthyosiform dermatoses are a heterogeneous group of disorders presenting with excessive scaling of the skin. The inherited forms of the ichthyoses are most common, although the condition can occur secondary to other diseases.

2. **What does "ichthyosis" mean?**
   The term *ichthyosis* is derived from the Greek root *ichthy,* meaning fish, indicative of the scales on the skin of affected individuals.

3. **How are the congenital (inherited) ichthyoses classified?**
   The classification is clinically based, and distinguishes between syndromic and nonsyndromic forms of inherited icthyoses. This classification system is likely to change in coming years as more data are collected regarding the genetic basis of these disorders.

Yoneda K. Inherited ichthyosis: syndromic forms. *J Dermatol.* 2016;43(3):252–263.
Takeichi T, Akiyama M. Inherited ichthyosis: non-syndromic forms. *J Dermatol.* 2016;43(3):242–251.
Hernández-Martín A, González-Sarmiento R. Recent advances in congenital ichythosis. *Curr Opin Pediatr.* 2015;27(4):473–479.

4. **How common are the major inherited nonsyndromic ichthyoses? How are they inherited?**
   - **Ichthyosis vulgaris:** Incidence of 1:250; autosomal dominant
   - **X-linked ichthyosis:** Incidence of 1:6000; X-linked recessive
   - **Epidermolytic ichthyosis:** Incidence of 1:300,000; autosomal dominant
   - **Congenital ichthyosiform erythroderma (CIE):** Incidence of 1:100,000; autosomal recessive
   - **Lamellar ichthyosis:** Incidence of 1:300,000; autosomal recessive
   - **Harlequin fetus:** Rare; autosomal recessive

Dreyfus I, Chouquet C, Ezzedine K, et al. Prevalence of inherited ichthyosis in France: a study using capture-recapture method. *Orphanet J Rare Dis.* 2014;9:1.
Hernandez-Martin A, Garcia-Doval I, Aranegui B, et al. Prevalence of autosomal recessive congenital ichthyosis: a population-based study using the capture-recapture method in Spain. *J Am Acad Dermatol.* 2012;67(2):240–244.
Kurosawa M, Takaga A, Tanakoshi A, et al. Epidemiology and clinical characteristics of bullous congenital ichthyosiform erythroderma (keratinolytic ichthyosis) in Japan: results from a nationwide survey. *J Am Acad Dermatol.* 2013;68(2):278–283.

5. **What features help differentiate the most common inherited ichthyoses?**
   Both clinical and histologic features are helpful in the diagnosis of ichthyoses (Table 4.1). Onset of symptoms, anatomic location of skin changes, birth history, and the condition of the infant's skin at birth are helpful clues. In some instances, a skin biopsy can be diagnostic.
   Ichthyosis vulgaris (Fig. 4.1A,B) usually develops around school age and is characterized by generalized xerosis and scale, with characteristic sparing of the flexural skin. Additional findings include follicular accentuation (keratosis pilaris), hyperlinearity of palms and soles, and a personal or family history of atopy. Rare patients may have an associated palmar-plantar keratoderma. Skin biopsy demonstrates a decreased granular cell layer associated with moderate hyperkeratosis.
   X-linked ichthyosis, in contrast, is usually present by 1 year of age, affects the posterior neck with "dirty"-appearing scales, and spares the palms and soles (Fig. 4.1C). The skin changes—gradually worsening with age—with the neck, face, and trunk ultimately developing thick, brown scales. The disease is caused by a defect in steroid sulfatase, an enzyme important in cholesterol synthesis and vital for normal development and function of the stratum corneum. Accumulation of cholesterol sulfate and a lack of tissue cholesterol ensue, leading to a disturbance in steroid hormone metabolism. Skin biopsy of X-linked ichthyosis is rarely diagnostic and demonstrates a normal granular layer with hyperkeratosis.

6. **What genetic defect is responsible for X-linked ichthyosis (XLI)?**
   Ninety percent of patients with XLI have deletions in the *STS* gene on chromosome Xp22.3, leading to steroid sulfatase deficiency and the classic phenotype of XLI. However, some patients have larger deletions at this site, encompassing neighboring genes. These patients present with more complicated forms of XLI representing contiguous gene deletion syndromes (OMIM [Online Mendelian Inheritance in Man] #308100).

Table 4.1 Clinical features of the major inherited nonsyndromic ichthyoses

DISORDER	ONSET	TYPE OF SCALE	SITES	HISTOLOGY	OTHER FINDINGS	DEFECT
Ichthyosis vulgaris	Childhood	Fine	Palms, soles, extensors	Diminished granular layer	Atopy, keratosis pilaris	Filaggrin
X-linked ichthyosis	Birth or infancy	Coarse, brown	Neck, face, trunk, flexors	Normal granular layer	Corneal opacities	Steroid sulfatase
Keratinopathic ichthyosis (epidermolytic hyperkeratosis)	Birth	Erosions/bullae, coarse, verrucous	Generalized, especially flexors	Epidermolytic hyperkeratosis	Foul odor, pyogenic infections	Keratin
Autosomal recessive congenital ichthyosis Congenital ichthyosiform erythroderma (CIE) Lamellar ichthyosis	Birth	Fine, white, with erythroderma Platelike, dark, erythroderma	Generalized with flexors, palms, soles	Increased granular layer, focal parakeratosis Increased granular layer, hyperkeratosis	Ectropion, nail dystrophy, poor growth, alopecia	Transglutaminase ALOXE3/ ALOX12B ABCA12 CYP4F22 NIPAL4
Harlequin fetus	Birth	Massive thick plates	Generalized	Massive compact hyperkeratosis	Ectropion, eclabium, ear and limb deformities	ACBA12

7. What additional phenotypes may patients with XLI contiguous gene syndromes exhibit?
   Hypogonadotropic hypogonadism and anosmia (Kallmann's syndrome), chondrodysplasia punctata, short stature, and/or ocular albinism may be present in these patients in addition to ichthyosis.

8. What important birth history may be obtained in patients with XLI?
   Labor may be protracted or fail to progress when the fetus is affected with XLI. This is directly related to the defect in steroid sulfatase, which leads to abnormal steroid hormone metabolism. Female carriers may also exhibit asymptomatic corneal opacities.

9. Name the hereditary syndromes presenting with ichthyosis as a component.
   See Table 4.2.

10. What is a collodion baby?
    A collodion baby is a newborn infant whose skin looks like a "baked apple," with a shiny, tough, membrane-like covering. This term describes a phenotype that occurs in several types of ichthyosis. Although CIE is the most common underlying condition (Fig. 4.1D), lamellar ichthyosis, Netherton's syndrome, Conradi's syndrome, and others may also present as a collodion baby. Collodion babies may also go on to have normal skin. These infants are at increased risk for infections and fluid and electrolyte imbalances due to cutaneous fissures and impaired barrier function of the skin. Treatment in a high-humidity environment with frequent application of petrolatum allows gradual sloughing of the collodion membrane. Manual debridement and keratolytics are not recommended.

Chan A, Godoy-Gijon E, Nuno-Gonzalez, et al. Cellular basis of secondary infections and impaired desquamation in certain inherited ichthyoses. *JAMA Dermatol.* 2015;151:285–292.

11. What is a harlequin fetus?
    The most severe manifestation of congenital ichthyosis, the harlequin fetus, is born with massive hyperkeratotic plates associated with limb deformities, rudimentary ears, ectropion, and eclabium (Fig. 4.2). These infants rarely survive beyond the first week of life. The use of acitretin in harlequin ichthyosis may be lifesaving, although side effects are numerous and may be severe.

Ahmed H, O'Toole EA. Recent advances in the genetics and management of harlequin ichthyosis. *Pediatr Dermatol.* 2014;31(5):539–546.

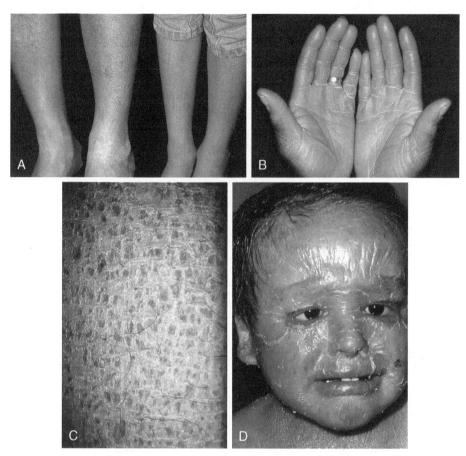

Fig. 4.1 A, Grandfather and granddaughter with ichthyosis vulgaris. **B,** Palmar hyperkeratosis, a finding often associated with ichthyosis vulgaris. **C,** X-linked ichthyosis, showing characteristic coarse, brown scales. **D,** Young child with congenital ichthyosiform erythroderma demonstrating diffuse erythema and scale. (A, B, and D, courtesy James E. Fitzpatrick, MD.)

12. Name several conditions associated with acquired ichthyosis.
    See Table 4.3.
    - **Malignancy:** The pathogenesis of the skin changes associated with malignancies is unknown, although reduced dermal lipid synthesis, malabsorption, and immunologic abnormalities have been identified.
    - **Nutritional and metabolic disorders:** Many of nutritional problems involve abnormal vitamin A metabolism. Chronic renal failure may result in hypervitaminosis A, which produces rough, scaly skin. Hypovitaminosis A produces follicular hyperkeratosis and dry skin.
    - **Drugs and other therapies:** Medications produce ichthyosis by various mechanisms. Niacin, triparanol, butyrophenones, dixyrazine, and nafoxidine alter cholesterol synthesis. Cimetidine and retinoids are antiandrogenic and reduce sebum secretion (Fig. 4.3).

Dalcin D, Beecker J. Acquired ichthyosis. *J Cutan Med Surg*. 2018;22(6):608.

13. Are laboratory tests helpful in the diagnosis of ichthyoses?
    In general, no. However, with recent advancements in genetic testing and microarray analysis, genetic testing is becoming easier and more readily available for this group of disorders. In ichthyosis vulgaris, cultured keratinocytes demonstrate absent or reduced filaggrin keratohyalin granules, and fail to react to antifilaggrin monoclonal antibodies. The defective enzyme in X-linked ichthyosis, steroid sulfatase, can be assayed in cultured keratinocytes, fibroblasts,

Table 4.2 Hereditary syndromes with ichthyosis

SYNDROME	CLINICAL FEATURES	SKIN FINDINGS	DEFECT
Conradi-Hünermann disease (chondrodysplasia punctata)	Chondrodysplasia punctata, limb defects, cataracts, cardiovascular and renal abnormalities, mental retardation	Congenital ichthyosiform erythroderma (CIE), whorled hyperpigmentation, palmoplantar keratoderma	Sterol isomerase emopamil–binding protein
CHILD (congenital hemidysplasia with ichthyosiform erythroderma and limb defects) syndrome	Hemidysplasia and limb defects with sharp midline demarcation	CIE	NAD(P)H steroid dehydrogenase–like protein
Sjögren-Larsson syndrome	Spasticity, mental retardation, retinal degeneration	Lamellar scales	Fatty aldehyde dehydrogenase
Chanarin-Dorfman syndrome (neutral lipid storage disease)	Fatty liver, myopathy, cataracts, deafness, CNS defects	CIE	Impaired long-chain fatty acid oxidation
Netherton's syndrome	Trichorrhexis invaginata (bamboo hairs), atopy, aminoaciduria	Ichthyosis linearis circumflexa	SPINK5 gene
Refsum's disease	Cerebellar ataxia, peripheral neuropathy, retinitis pigmentosa	Like ichthyosis vulgaris	Phytanoyl-CoA hydroxylase
Multiple sulfatase deficiency	Metachromatic leukodystrophy, hepatosplenomegaly	Like X-linked ichthyosis	Sulfatase modifying factor-1 gene
Trichothiodystrophy (PIBIDS)	Photosensitivity, ichthyosis, brittle hair, intellectual impairment, decreased fertility, short stature	CIE	Xeroderma pigmentosa D or B gene
KID (keratitis-ichthyosis-deafness) syndrome	Keratitis, neurosensory deafness, alopecia	Grainy, spiculated scaling	Connexin 26 gene

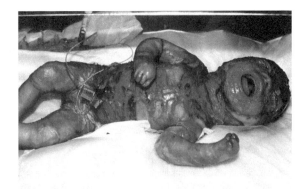

Fig. 4.2 Fatal case of harlequin fetus demonstrating large, fissured, keratotic plates. (Courtesy Fitzsimons Army Medical Center teaching files.)

Table 4.3 Conditions associated with acquired ichthyosis

MEDICATIONS	MALIGNANCIES	NUTRITIONAL DISORDERS	METABOLIC DISORDERS	MISCELLANEOUS DISORDERS
Butyrophenone	Non–Hodgkin's	Essential fatty acid	Chronic renal failure	Systemic lupus
Cimetidine	lymphoma	deficiencies	Hypothyroidism	erythematosus
Clofazimine	Hodgkin's	Hypervitaminosis A	Panhypopituitarism	Sarcoidosis
Dixyrazine	lymphoma	Hypovitaminosis A		Leprosy
Isoniazid	Carcinoma of solid	Kwashiorkor		Dermatomyositis
Nafoxidine	organs	Pellagra		HIV infection
Niacin	Mycosis fungoides			Polycythemia
Triparanol	Leukemia			Haber's syndrome
Allopurinol	Lymphosarcoma			
Retinoids	Rhabdomyosarcoma			
	Kaposi's sarcoma			
	Leiomyosarcoma			
	Multiple myeloma			

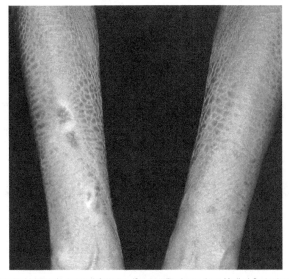

Fig. 4.3 Acquired ichthyosis due to clofazimine. (Courtesy Fitzsimons Army Medical Center teaching files.)

leukocytes, or skin scales. Low levels of cholesterol sulfate in blood can be detected by the increased mobility of low-density lipoproteins on serum protein electrophoresis. Female heterozygotes can be detected by Southern blot hybridization from peripheral blood leukocytes. The gene has been mapped to the short arm of the X chromosome (Xp22.3). Several of the rarer ichthyosiform syndromes are also associated with enzyme deficiencies detectable in cell cultures.

Scharschmidt TC, Man MQ, Hatano Y, et al. Filaggrin deficiency confers a paracellular barrier abnormality that reduces inflammatory thresholds to irritants and haptens. *J Allergy Clin Immunol.* 2009;124(3):496–506.

14. Is prenatal diagnosis of congenital ichthyosis possible?
    Prenatal diagnosis is available for many of the congenital ichthyoses, if one is suspected, based on family history. Fetal skin biopsy performed at 19 to 21 weeks will demonstrate early development of a thickened stratum corneum, normally not present until 24 weeks. This is useful in lamellar ichthyosis, epidermolytic ichthyosis, Sjögren-Larsson syndrome, and harlequin fetus. Lamellar ichthyosis may also be detected via a transglutaminase activity assay from a fetal skin sample. Epidermolytic ichthyosis, known to result from mutations in keratins 1 and 10, can be detected by direct gene sequencing done on chorionic villus sampling in the second trimester. Cultured chorionic villi cells or

amniocytes will demonstrate the enzyme deficiency in XLI, Sjögren-Larsson syndrome, and Refsum's disease. A high ratio of maternal urinary estrogen precursors in a male fetus also suggests the diagnosis of XLI. Trichothiodystrophy can be identified by unscheduled DNA synthesis in cultured amniocytes exposed to ultraviolet light. Recent advances in prenatal ultrasonography have also aided in prenatal diagnosis of some ichthyosiform disorders.

Brandão P, Seco S, Loureiro T, Ramalho C. Prenatal sonographic diagnosis of Harlequin ichthyosis. *J Clin Ultrasound.* 2019;47 (4):228–231.

Sheth JJ, Bhavsar R, Patel D, Joshi A, Sheth FJ. Harlequin ichthyosis due to novel splice site mutation in the ABCA12 gene: postnatal to prenatal diagnosis. *Int J Dermatol.* 2018;57(4):428–433.

Luu M, Cantatore-Francis JL, Glick SA. Prenatal diagnosis of genodermatoses: current scope and future capabilities. *Int J Dermatol.* 2010;49(4):353–361.

Tourette C, Tron E, Mallet S, et al. Three-dimensional ultrasound prenatal diagnosis of congenital ichthyosis: contribution of molecular biology. *Prenat Diagn.* 2012;32(5):498–500.

15. How is ichthyosis treated?

Acquired ichthyosis usually improves with treatment of the underlying condition. Congenital ichthyosis is difficult to treat, especially in its severe forms. Topical emollients containing glycolic acid, lactic acid, urea, or glycerin may partially improve dryness and scaling. Topical tretinoin (Retin-A) is effective but poorly tolerated due to irritation. Oral retinoids, including isotretinoin, etretinate, and acitretin, are very effective, but relapses after treatment cessation are common. The use of oral retinoids is limited by major side effects (including teratogenic effects), and chronic use, which is often required in congenital disorders, is associated with hyperostoses. Blistering may indicate bacterial infection and should be cultured and managed with oral antibiotics. The foul odor present in epidermolytic ichthyosis may be due to bacterial colonization and can be improved by the use of antibacterial soap.

Limmer AL, Nwannunu CE, Patel RR, Mui UN, Tyring SK. Management of ichthyosis: a brief review. *Skin Therapy Lett.* 2020;25(1):5–7.

16. What is Hailey-Hailey disease?

Hailey-Hailey disease, also known as benign familial pemphigus, is an autosomal dominant condition in which mutations in the *ATP2C1* gene result in abnormal intracellular calcium signaling. It is characterized histologically by acantholysis (loss of cohesion between keratinocytes) and clinically by patches of minute vesicles that break and form crusted erosions.

17. How does Hailey-Hailey disease present?

Skin changes consisting of localized patches of minute vesicles and erosions start in areas of friction, usually the neck, groin, and axilla (Figs. 4.4 and 4.5). Patches spread peripherally with serpiginous borders and show central healing with hyperpigmentation or granular vegetations. Onset of lesions is often delayed until the second or third decade. Associated symptoms include itching, pain, and foul odor.

18. Do any factors exacerbate the skin changes of Hailey-Hailey?

Physical trauma, heat, or sweating worsen skin lesions. Patients have reported the onset of new lesions within hours of wearing restrictive shirt collars, tight bra straps, and electrocardiogram electrodes. Most patients report a worsening of lesions in the summer.

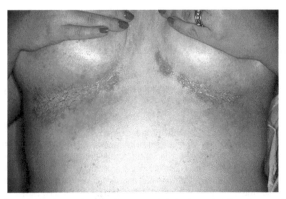

Fig. 4.4 Patient with Hailey-Hailey disease demonstrating characteristic involvement of flexural areas of inflammatory crease.

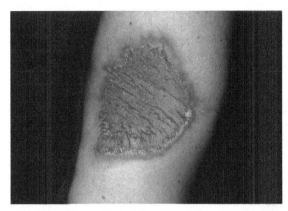

Fig. 4.5 Hailey-Hailey disease showing a patch of minute vesicles, erosions, and crusting in the antecubital fossa.

19. **Which diseases may be confused with Hailey-Hailey disease?**
Eczema, impetigo, fungal or viral infections, pemphigus vulgaris, pemphigus vegetans, or Darier's disease. The recurring, chronic nature of Hailey-Hailey disease, lack of oral and ocular involvement, and intertriginous predilection help to differentiate these conditions.

20. **How is Hailey-Hailey disease treated?**
Topical steroids are generally helpful in relieving burning and itching. Both *Staphylococcus aureus* and *Candida albicans* infections may exacerbate lesions, requiring treatment with appropriate antibacterial and antifungal agents. Recalcitrant cases have been treated with localized steroid injections, carbon dioxide laser, dermabrasion, topical cyclosporine, dapsone, vitamin E, ultraviolet radiation, methotrexate, thalidomide, vitamin D analogs, imiquimod, and numerous other topical and systemic medications, with variable results.

Mizuno K, Hamada T, Hashimoto T, Okamoto H. Successful treatment with narrow-band UVB therapy for a case of generalized Hailey-Hailey disease with a novel splice-site mutation in ATP2C1 gene. *Dermatol Ther.* 2014;27(4):233–235.
Sárdy M, Ruzicka T. Successful therapy of refractory Hailey-Hailey disease with oral alitretinoin. *Br J Dermatol.* 2014;170(1):209–211.
Varada S, Ramirez-Fort MK, Argobi Y, Simkin AD. Remission of refractory benign familial chronic pemphigus (Hailey-Hailey disease) with the addition of systemic cyclosporine. *J Cutan Med Surg.* 2014;18(5):1–4.

21. **What is Darier's disease?**
Darier's disease, also known as keratosis follicularis and Darier-White disease, is a dominantly inherited disorder of keratinization caused by mutations in the *ATP2A2* gene, resulting in dysfunction of intracellular calcium signaling. Typically, the disease presents in the first or second decade of life. Microscopically, it is characterized by distinctive changes of both premature keratinization and acantholysis.

22. **How is Darier's disease diagnosed?**
The diagnosis is based on clinical manifestations and histologic features. The primary lesions are flesh-colored papules that may coalesce into plaques and develop tan, scaly crusts (Fig. 4.6). These keratotic papules are located in "seborrheic areas," such as the chest, back, ears, nasolabial folds, scalp, and groin. Thick, foul-smelling, warty masses can develop. Flat, wartlike papules may be seen on the dorsa of distal extremities, and 1- to 2-mm punctate keratoses may be present on the palms and soles. Oral and rectal mucosal surfaces often demonstrate small, cobblestone-like papules. The diagnosis can be confirmed by skin biopsies that reveal acantholytic dyskeratosis.

23. **Are there any nail or hair changes in Darier's disease?**
Nails demonstrate longitudinal ridging, as well as red and white longitudinal streaks. Distal nail edges show V-shaped notching and subungual thickening. Rarely, alopecia results from extensive scalp involvement.

24. **Is Darier's disease difficult to treat?**
Complete clearing of Darier's disease is rare. Soothing moisturizers containing urea or lactic acid reduce scaling and irritation. Salicylic acid in a propylene glycol gel and topical retinoids are also effective in reducing crusts and scale, although retinoids may need to be initiated on an alternate-day schedule in combination with midpotency topical steroids to minimize irritation. Aggravating factors such as heat, humidity, sunlight, and lithium should be avoided. Infection should be prevented with antibacterial soaps and treated with antibiotics. Oral retinoids are effective, but toxicity limits their use; intermittent use may be preferable, such as starting the medication before a summer holiday to prevent sun-induced exacerbations. Recalcitrant verrucous lesions have been treated with dermabrasion, carbon dioxide laser vaporization, surgery, and numerous topical preparations.

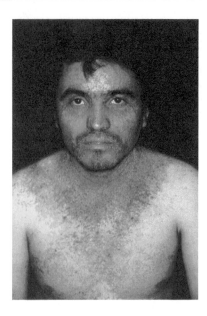

Fig. 4.6 Darier's disease. Confluent, crusted papules involving the face, scalp, and chest.

Cooper SM, Burge SM. Darier's disease: epidemiology, pathophysiology, and management. *Am J Clin Dermatol.* 2013;4(2):97–105.
Zamiri M, Munro CS. Successful treatment with oral alitretinoin in women of childbearing potential with Darier's disease. *Br J Dermatol.* 2013;169(3):709–710.

25. What is axillary granular parakeratosis?

Axillary granular parakeratosis is an uncommon distinctive acquired disorder of keratinization. As the name implies, it usually presents in the axillae, although other intertriginous sites such as in the inframammary and inguinal areas have also been reported. Clinically it presents as asymptomatic or pruritic red, tan, or brown patches (Fig. 4.7). The diagnosis is established by a biopsy that demonstrates a characteristic histologic pattern of marked hyperkeratosis with retained nuclei (parakeratosis) and keratohyalin granules in the stratum corneum. The pathogenesis is not understood, but it has been postulated that topical antiperspirants, deodorants, or pomades may interfere with the degradation of profilaggrin precursor to filaggrin.

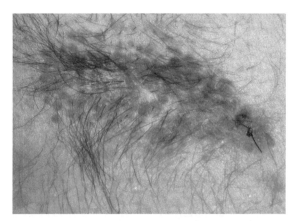

Fig. 4.7 Axillary granular parakeratosis demonstrating reddish-brown hyperkeratotic coalescent papules. (Courtesy Fitzsimons Army Medical Center teaching files.)

KEY POINTS: DISORDERS OF KERATINIZATION

1. Ichthyosis vulgaris, with an incidence of 1:250, is by far the most common ichthyosis.
2. CIE and lamellar ichthyosis (autosomal recessive congenital ichthyosis) are the two disorders of keratinization that are most likely to present as a collodion baby.
3. Topical emollients containing glycolic acid, lactic acid, urea, and glycerin are the mainstay of therapy in mild disorders of keratinization.
4. Oral retinoids are the most effective therapy for severe ichthyoses, but their use is limited by side effects of chronic use.

CHAPTER 5

NEUROCUTANEOUS DISORDERS

Israel David Andrews

NEUROFIBROMATOSIS

1. **What are the two main forms of neurofibromatosis?**
   Neurofibromatosis type 1 (NF-1 or von Recklinghausen's disease) and neurofibromatosis type 2 (NF-2). NF-1 accounts for 90% of all cases of neurofibromatosis and affects approximately 1 in 2600–3000 individuals. NF-2 is a genetically distinct entity with a prevalence of 1 in 25,000. Both conditions have autosomal dominant inheritance with 50% of cases representing sporadic (de novo) mutations.

KEY POINTS: DIAGNOSTIC CRITERIA OF NEUROFIBROMATOSIS TYPE 1

Two of the following criteria are required for a diagnosis of NF-1:
- Six or more café-au-lait macules >5 mm in diameter in prepubertal children and >15 mm in diameter in postpubertal individuals
- Two or more neurofibromas of any type or one plexiform neurofibroma
- Freckling in axillary or inguinal regions
- Two or more Lisch nodules (melanocytic hamartomas of the iris)
- Optic glioma (nerve tumor affecting the optic nerve)
- Distinctive osseous lesion, such as sphenoid wing dysplasia or thinning of long bone cortex, with or without pseudarthroses
- First-degree relative with NF-1.

National Institutes of Health Consensus Development Conference. Conference statement: neurofibromatosis. *Arch Neurol.* 1988;45:575–578.

2. **Where is the gene for NF-1 located? What protein does it encode? What is the function of this protein?**
   The NF-1 gene is a large gene mapping to chromosome 17q11.2. It encodes a protein called neurofibromin, which functions as a tumor suppressor by inhibiting the Ras signal. Ras promotes mitogen-activated protein kinase (MAPK) pathways, which contribute to cell survival and proliferation. Mutations in neurofibromin remove the inhibition of the Ras-MAPK pathway promoting tumor growth.

Abramowicz A, Gos M. Neurofibromin in neurofibromatosis type I—mutations in NF1 gene as a cause of disease. *Dev Period Med.* 2014;18:297–306.

3. **What is the earliest manifestation of NF-1?**
   Café-au-lait macules (CALMs) and axillary/inguinal freckling are the earliest **cutaneous** sign of NF-1. These sharply defined, light brown patches may be present at birth but more commonly appear by the first year of life (Fig. 5.1). They are noted initially by 4 years or less in all affected children and within the first year in 82% of cases. Osseous dysplasia, such as sphenoid wing dysplasia, and plexiform neurofibormas may be present at birth or arise earlier than CALMs but can go undetected until later in life.

Boyd KP, Korf BR, Theos A. Neurofibromatosis type 1. *J Am Acad Dermatol.* 2009;61:1–14.

4. **What is Crowe's sign? When does it develop?**
   Crowe's sign is freckling of the axillae or other body folds. It develops in 90% of NF-1 patients, usually by age 3 to 5 years. These lesions are not really freckles, but multiple small café-au-lait macules.

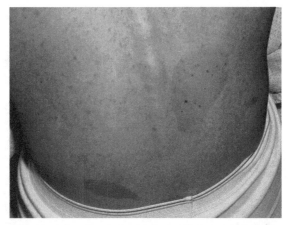

Fig. 5.1 Multiple café-au-lait macules >5 mm in diameter. *(Courtesy Fitzsimons Army Medical Center teaching files.)*

KEY POINTS: NEUROCUTANEOUS DISORDERS

1. Multiple Lisch nodules are pathognomonic of NF-1.
2. NF-1 should be considered in patients presenting at any age with six or more café-au-lait macules.
3. NF-2 most commonly presents with deafness or tinnitus related to underlying vestibular schwannomas.
4. The two genetic loci for tuberous sclerosis are on chromosomes 9 and 16 coding for TSC1 (hamartin) and TSC2 (tuberin), respectively.
5. In virtually all cases of Sturge-Weber syndrome, the facial capillary malformation involves the V1 and/or the V2 distribution of the trigeminal nerve.
6. Hypomelanotic macules are a useful diagnostic skin sign for tuberous sclerosis in infants with seizures.

5. When do neurofibromas appear in NF-1?

Neurofibromas usually start to develop just before or during puberty but increase in size and number in early adult life. They are soft, pink, or skin-colored papules, nodules, or tumors distributed mainly over the trunk and limbs (Fig. 5.2). They increase in size and number with age and can range from a few to thousands, with the highest density occurring over the trunk.

6. What is a plexiform neurofibroma?

Plexiform neurofibromas are neurofibromas that grow longitudinally along a nerve involving multiple fascicles. Lesions are usually congenital and can grow rapidly in childhood. They can be deep or superficial and present with overlying skin hypertrophy, hyperpigmentation, and hypertrichosis. They are a major cause of morbidity and are often disfiguring (Fig. 5.3).

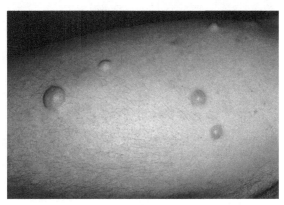

Fig. 5.2 Multiple peripheral neurofibromas.

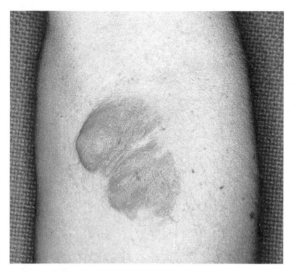

Fig. 5.3 Soft baglike lesion of a plexiform neurofibroma.

7. **Why is it necessary to follow patients with plexiform neurofibroma(s)?**
Studies examining the behavior of plexiform neurofibromas have found a rate of malignant degeneration between 3% and 15%. The sudden onset of rapid growth, acute pain, or neurologic deficit in an associated plexiform neurofibroma may be a sign of malignant transformation into a malignant peripheral nerve sheath tumor (MPNST).

8. **What are Lisch nodules?**
Melanocytic hamartomas of the iris. When multiple, these lesions are pathognomonic of NF-1, occurring in more than 90% of patients by the second decade. They are best seen on slit lamp examination (Fig. 5.4).

9. **What is the most common central nervous system (CNS) tumor occurring in NF-1?**
Optic pathway gliomas, which are typically low-grade astrocytomas, occur in 15% of patients before 6 years of age. They can occur anywhere on the optic pathway, and a majority are asymptomatic. A minority of children become symptomatic with visual disturbance, but advanced tumors involving the hypothalamus can present with precocious or delayed puberty which can alert the clinician to their presence.

Guillamo JS, Creange A, Kalifa C, et al. Progrnostic factors of CNS tumours in neurofibromatosis 1 (NF-1): a retrospective study of 104 patients. *Brain* 2003;126:152.
Lewis RA, Gerson LP, Axelson KA, et al. Von Recklinghausen neurofibromatosis. II. Incidence of optic gliomata. *Ophthalmology.* 1984;91:929.

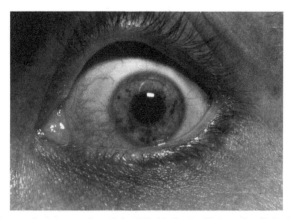

Fig. 5.4 Lisch nodules presenting as numerous brown lesions of the iris. (Courtesy Fitzsimons Army Medical Center teaching files.)

10. What are the most common skeletal abnormalities in NF-1?

Scoliosis and macrocephaly are the most common skeletal abnormalities in NF-1. Pseudoarthrosis, or false joint formation following nonunion of bone following fracture, is a highly suggestive finding of NF-1. NF-1 is the most common cause of pseudoarthrosis, accounting for up to 50%–80% of cases. Long bone and sphenoid wing dysplasia are less common and are usually present at birth.

Elefteriou F, Kolanczyk M, Schindeler A, et al. Skeletal abnormalities in neurofibromatosis type 1: approaches to therapeutic options. *Am J Med Gen A.* 2009;149A:2327–2338.

11. What is segmental NF?

Formerly known as NF-5, segmental NF is due to a post-zygotic mutation in the NF-1 gene leading to somatic mosaicism. It can present with CALMs and neurofibromas involving a block-like or blaschkolinear pattern with midline demarcation, and in 30% of patients, there may be extra-cutaneous systemic manifestations.

Garcia-Romero MT, Parkin P, Lara-Corrales I. Mosaic neurofibromatosis type 1: a systematic review. *Pediatr Dermatol.* 2016;33:9–17.

12. How frequently should patients with NF-1 be assessed? What should this assessment include?

An annual assessment is usually sufficient. The clinical examination should include a blood pressure measurement (hypertension occurs in 6% due to renovascular stenosis or pheochromocytoma) and a full neurologic examination. Children should receive an annual eye exam until the age of 10; surveillance for scoliosis, precocious puberty, and hypogonadism; and regular developmental assessments. Additional investigations should be guided by symptoms or physical signs. Lifelong follow-up is recommended for the surveillance of MPNSTs.

Drappier J-C, Khosrotehrani K, Zeller J, et al. Medical management of neurofibromatosis 1: a cross sectional study of 383 patients. *J Am Acad Dermatol.* 2003;49:440–444.

13. What are the diagnostic criteria for NF-2?

The diagnostic criteria are met by an individual who has:
- Bilateral vestibular schwannomas before age 70 **or** unilateral vestibular schwannomas **and** first-degree relative with NF-2
- First-degree relative with NF-2 **or** unilateral eighth nerve mass **and** any two of the following: neurofibroma, meningioma, glioma, schwannoma, or juvenile posterior subcapsular lenticular opacity.

14. Where is the gene for NF-2? What is the gene product?

The *NF-2* gene is located on chromosome 22q12.1. It encodes a cytoskeletal protein, merlin (also called schwannomin), which acts as a tumor suppressor.

15. What are the most common presenting symptoms of NF-2? What are the most common cutaneous symptoms of NF-2?

Hearing loss or tinnitus related to underlying vestibular schwannomas is the presenting symptom in the majority of patients, developing at a mean age of 20 years. Other presenting symptoms relate to underlying CNS tumors (20% to 30%), skin tumors (12.7%), and ocular abnormalities (12.7%). Cutaneous lesions arise in 70% of patients with NF-2; they are fewer in number when compared to NF-1 (<10) and include hyperpigmented plaques, nodular schwannomas, and neurofibromas.

Asthagiri AR, Parry DM, Butman JA, et al. Neurofibromatosis type 2. *Lancet.* 2009;373:1974–1986.

16. What is Legius syndrome?

Legius syndrome is an NF-1-like syndrome due to a mutation in the *SPRED1* gene. It shares many features with NF-1, including multiple CALMs, inguinal freckling, and macrocephaly, but lacks cutaneous neurofibromas and CNS tumors. SPRED1 is also a negative regulator of RAS/RAF and MAPK signaling pathway. This diagnosis should be considered in the differential for NF-1.

TUBEROUS SCLEROSIS

17. Wheat is the genetic etiology of tuberous sclerosis?

There are two separate genes linked to tuberous sclerosis: *TSC 1*, located on chromosome 9, encoding a protein called hamartin; and *TSC 2*, located on chromosome 16, encoding a protein called tuberin.

Curatolo P, Bombardieri R, Jozwiak S. Tuberous sclerosis. *Lancet.* 2008;372:657–668.

18. What is the function of hamartin and tuberin? Why is this important clinically?

Hamartin and tuberin are tumor suppressors that work synchronously to inactivate the mammalian target of rapamycin (mTOR). mTOR is a protein that promotes cellular growth and tumor formation. The targeting of mTOR with both systemic and topical mTOR inhibitors, such as rapamycin (sirolimus), has led to reduction in size of renal and pulmonary tumors, as well as cutaneous angiofibromas associated with tuberous sclerosis.

19. What is the inheritance of tuberous sclerosis?

Inheritance is autosomal dominant, with high penetrance but variable expression. A majority of affected individuals (80%) represent sporadic mutations; however, genetic testing should be offered to asymptomatic parents to elucidate carrier status and for the purposes of family planning.

20. What is the earliest skin sign of tuberous sclerosis?

Hypomelanotic macules (Fig. 5.5) are present at birth or in early infancy; these lesions aid in the diagnosis of infants with convulsions. Best seen with Wood's lamp exam, they are polygonal or ash-leaf in shape, ranging in size from 1 to 3 cm and numbering 1 to 100. Occasionally, 1- to 3-mm confetti-like white spots scattered over the trunk and limbs accompany them. Additional skin signs of tuberous sclerosis include facial angiofibromas, periungual fibromas (Koenen tumors), and the shagreen patch (connective tissue nevus).

21. What are the major noncutaneous findings of tuberous sclerosis?

Noncutaneous major features of tuberous sclerosis include multiple retinal nodular hamartomas, cortical tubers, subependymal nodules, subependymal giant cell astrocytoma, renal angiomyolipoma, cardiac rhabdomyoma, and lymphangioleiomyomatosis.

22. What is the correct term for the facial papules seen in tuberous sclerosis?

Angiofibromas consist of collagen arranged concentrically around hair follicles, blood vessels, and plump stellate-appearing fibroblasts (Fig. 5.6). Angiofibromas do not derive from a sebaceous origin, making adenoma sebaceum a misnomer. Facial angiofibromas appear at 4 to 9 years of age as macules, increase in size and number during puberty, and tend to involve the nasolabial folds, central face, chin, and forehead. Koenen tumors are a variant of angiofibromas that develop after puberty and project from the nail folds (periungual) or beneath the nail plate (subungual) (Fig. 5.7).

23. What is a shagreen patch?

A shagreen patch is a connective tissue nevus that appears as an irregularly thickened, slightly elevated, skin-colored plaque commonly located over the lumbosacral area. Fibromatous plaques are also frequently found on the forehead (Fig. 5.8).

24. What are tubers, and where do they occur?

Tubers are nodules of glial proliferation and are the characteristic CNS lesion of tuberous sclerosis. They may occur anywhere in the cerebral cortex, basal ganglia, and ventricular walls (subependymal nodules), and their number and size correlate with clinical features of seizures and intellectual impairment. Cortical tubers are often dense when compared to normal brain tissue and are best detected with magnetic resonance imaging (MRI). Subependymal nodules may calcify and are readily detectable with computed tomography scanning. Fifty percent of plain skull radiographs taken in later childhood also reveal bilateral areas of calcification in the brain.

25. What signs of tuberous sclerosis may be revealed on funduscopic examination?

Retinal hamartomas may occur in 50% of patients. They may be seen as white streaks along the retina or elevated multinodular lesions near the optic disc. Ocular lesions in tuberous sclerosis do not lead to visual loss.

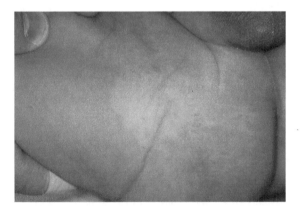

Fig. 5.5 Ash-leaf macule in an infant.

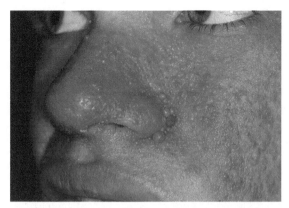

Fig. 5.6 Facial angiofibromas in tuberous sclerosis (adenoma sebaceum).

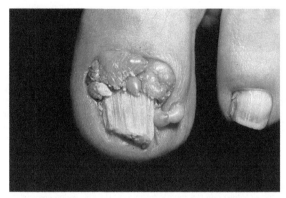

Fig. 5.7 Koenen tumors (periungual fibroma) of the great toenail with associated nail dystrophy. (Courtesy Fitzsimons Army Medical Center teaching files.)

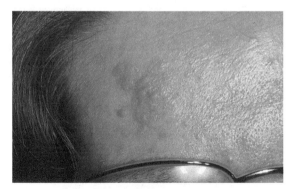

Fig. 5.8 Fibromatous plaque on the forehead of a patient with tuberous sclerosis.

26. Which systemic finding, characteristic of tuberous sclerosis, may be present at birth, but not later in life?

Cardiac rhabdomyomas, which can be present at birth in up to 80% of infants with tuberous sclerosis, typically involute in the first 3 years of life and disappear completely by adulthood.

27. Can renal involvement occur in tuberous sclerosis?

    Yes. Renal angiomyolipomas and cysts are common tumors in the kidney. They may be multiple and bilateral and are usually asymptomatic.

28. What is the prognosis for patients with tuberous sclerosis?

    The prognosis is variable and dependent on the severity of the clinical manifestations. In severe cases, death may occur from epilepsy, infection, cardiac failure, or, rarely, pulmonary fibrosis.

STURGE-WEBER SYNDROME

29. Name the essential components of the Sturge-Weber syndrome. How is it inherited?

    A facial capillary malformation (CM) (formerly port-wine stain) and cerebral capillary-venous malformations (C-VMs) (formerly leptomeningeal angiomatosis). Ocular involvement is common, and all three systems (skin, eye, and CNS) share neuroectodermal origin. Sturge-Weber syndrome (SWS) is not inherited and is due to somatic mosaic activating mutations in *GNAQ*.

Shirley MD, Tang H, Gallione CJ, et al. Sturge-Weber syndrome and port-wine stains caused by somatic mutation in GNAQ. *N Engl J Med.* 2013;368:1971–1979.

30. Does the location of the capillary malformation affect the likelihood of developing SWS?

    A patient with a CM in the V1 distribution of the trigeminal nerve has a 10% risk of developing SWS; bilateral involvement of V1, or involvement of V2 and V3 along with V1, increases the risk of developing SWS to 25% (Fig. 5.9). A patient with a CM in the V1 distribution should be closely followed for the development of extracutaneous manifestations associated with SWS.

31. What are the complications of leptomeningeal C-VMs? At what age does epilepsy manifest?

    Both the C-VM of the cerebral meninges as well as the underlying neocortex can become calcified, resulting in cerebral atrophy. These cortical changes represent the pathogenesis of epilepsy in 75% to 90% of cases, intellectual impairment (particularly in those with severe epilepsy), and, occasionally, contralateral hemiplegia. Epilepsy presents between the second and seventh months of life, although it may be delayed until later in childhood.

Thomas-Suhl KA, Vaslow DF, Maria BL. Sturge-Weber syndrome: a review. *Pediatr Neurol.* 2004;30:303–310.

32. What investigations confirm leptomeningeal C-VM?

    MRI with gadolinium contrast is the preferred imaging technique to identify leptomeningeal C-VM and its extent. While controversy exists as to which age this should be performed in high-risk patients, a normal MRI in the first few months of life does not rule out SWS.

33. Do ocular complications occur in the SWS?

    Ocular complications occur in 30% to 70% of cases and include capillary malformations of the conjunctiva, iris, and choroid (ipsilateral to the facial port wine stain), and glaucoma. These complications may be associated only with a facial CM involving the V1 distribution and do not necessarily imply SWS. Glaucoma most commonly begins in the first 2 years of life; hence, regular ophthalmologic review from birth is vital in patients with V1 or eyelid CMs.

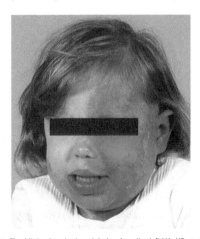

Fig. 5.9 Sturge-Weber syndrome. The bilateral port wine stain involves the left V1, V2, and V3 regions and right V3 region.

34. Are there additional complications in the SWS?

Yes. An increased prevalence of hypothyroidism and growth hormone deficiency has been reported in patients with SWS, necessitating close endocrinologic follow-up in patients demonstrating symptomatology.

Lo W, Marchuk DA, Ball KL, et al. Brain Vascular Malformation Consortium National Sturge-Weber Syndrome Workgroup: updates and future horizons on the understanding, diagnosis, and treatment of Sturge–Weber syndrome brain involvement. *Dev Med Child Neurol.* 2012;54:214–223. Erratum in: *Dev Med Child Neurol* 2012;54(10):957.

35. How can a facial capillary malformation be treated?

The pulsed dye laser (wavelength = 585/595 nm) is the most effective treatment modality. Regular laser treatments may result in significant fading and may also help prevent the soft tissue hypertrophy that gradually develops within many port wine stains.

ATAXIA-TELANGIECTASIA

36. What is the inheritance of ataxia-telangiectasia?

Inheritance is autosomal recessive with the defective gene located on chromosome 11. It encodes an ataxia-telangiectasia mutated gene *(ATM)* that gives rise to a protein member of the phosphatidylinositol 3-kinase family.

37. What is the earliest clinical sign of ataxia-telangiectasia?

Progressive cerebellar ataxia due to degeneration of Purkinje cells, beginning at age 12 to 18 months. Choreoathetoid movements, hypotonia, dysarthria, and abnormal eye movements gradually develop, and intelligence frequently declines.

Smith SL, Conerly SL. Ataxia-telangiectasia or Louis-Bar syndrome. *J Am Acad Dermatol.* 1985;12:681–696.

38. Name the typical skin sign of ataxia-telangiectasia.

Mucocutaneous telangiectases. These begin on the bulbar conjunctiva and ears between 2 and 6 years of age and may progress to involve the periorbital skin, trunk, extremities, body folds, and other mucosal surfaces.

39. What are the two most common causes of death in ataxia-telangiectasia?

B- and T-cell immunodeficiencies give rise to the two most common causes of death in ataxia-telangiectasia: sinopulmonary infections and hematologic malignancy. Breast cancer, premature aging, and sensitivity to ionizing radiation are also increased risk factors for morbidity and mortality in these patients.

NEUROCUTANEOUS MELANOCYTOSIS

40. What are the essential features of neurocutaneous melanocytosis (NCM)? Is it always symptomatic?

NCM is characterized by a cutaneous congenital melanocytic nevus (CMN) with melanotic rests in the brain or meninges. Up to one-quarter of patients may be asymptomatic (positive imaging but no symptoms) or present with hydrocephalus and seizures, spinal cord compression, or developmental delay.

41. What high-risk features of CMN would increase risk for neurocutaneous melanosis?

Size and number of satellite lesions are the most important risk factors for NCM. There is a fivefold increased risk of NCM in patients with large or giant (≥40 cm) CMN and in patients with ≥ 20 satellite nevi. The risk for NCM is also increased in patients with multiple medium-sized CMN.

42. How is NCM diagnosed?

MRI scanning done before 6 months of age is the most appropriate investigation in high-risk babies.

43. What else are patients with NCM at risk for?

Patients with NCM are also at risk for CNS melanoma. While a majority of melanotic rests in the brain or meninges are benign, malignant transformation has been reported in 2% to 3% of affected patients.

Acknowledgment

Some of the clinical photographs were kindly provided by Drs. William Weston and Joseph Morelli.

CHAPTER 6

MECHANOBULLOUS DISORDERS

Anna L. Bruckner

1. **What are mechanobullous disorders?**
   Mechanobullous disorders, either inherited or acquired, are skin conditions characterized by blister formation (vesicles, bullae, and resultant erosions) due to mechanical trauma to the skin and/or mucous membranes. Common friction blisters that develop on the feet due to tight-fitting shoes or boots are an example of acquired lesions. Inherited mechanobullous disorders are rare, and most are classified as a form of epidermolysis bullosa (EB). In EB, deficient or abnormal proteins that hold the skin together lead to a lower threshold for blister formation. Minimal or minor trauma is needed to produce vesicles, bullae, and erosions in individuals with EB. The remainder of this chapter will focus on EB and its complications.

2. **Where do the blisters that form in EB occur in the skin?**
   The blistering of EB generally occurs at the level of the dermal-epidermal junction, where the epidermis joins with the dermis (Fig. 6.1). This interface is also called the basement membrane zone (BMZ). Depending on the type of EB, the blister can arise in the basal keratinocytes just above the BMZ, through the BMZ, or in the superficial dermis below the BMZ.

3. **How is EB classified, and what are the major modes of inheritance?**
   EB is classified into four major types based on where the blister arises in relation to the BMZ. Subtypes are based on clinical characteristics, mode of inheritance, the targeted protein, and the specific genetic mutation. Table 6.1 reviews the classification and inheritance of the most common forms of EB.

Has C, Bauer JW, Bodemer C et al. Consensus reclassification of inherited epidermolysis bullosa and other disorders with skin fragility. *Br J Dermatol*. 2020 Feb 4. https://doi.org/10.1111/bjd.18921.

4. **Describe the typical skin findings in EB simplex.**
   In the **localized** form, blisters and erosions are most common on the hands and feet. This can present at any age, but a common scenario is the individual may go undiagnosed until he or she is in a situation that produces increased mechanical stress on the skin, such as marching in the military (Fig. 6.2). The **generalized** form usually presents at birth and can be extensive. In the generalized severe subtype (formerly called Dowling-Meara), blisters tend to occur in annular clusters (Fig. 6.3). The affected areas generally heal without scarring, but dyspigmentation of the skin is common. The blistering of EB simplex tends to improve as the individual ages.

5. **How do mutations in KRT5 and KRT14 cause the autosomal dominant forms of EB simplex?**
   KRT5 and *KRT14* encode the structural proteins keratin 5 and 14 that are expressed in the basal keratinocytes. These intermediate filaments link together, forming a structural network similar to the frame of a house. The most common mutations in either *KRT5* or *KRT14* produce disease through a **dominant negative effect.** The mutation leads to an abnormal protein that is incorporated into the structural network but is unable to withstand mechanical stress. This inherent weakness in the intermediate filaments leads to blistering in the basal keratinocytes in the autosomal dominant forms of EB simplex.

Coulombe PA, Lee CH. Defining keratin protein function in skin epithelia: epidermolysis bullosa simplex and its aftermath. *J Invest Dermatol*. 2012;132:763–775.

6. **What are the clinical findings in junctional EB (JEB) generalized?**
   At birth, the amount of blistering can vary. Over time, persistent erosions occur, with the central face and buttocks being commonly affected (Fig. 6.4). These erosions are often associated with excessive granulation tissue. Blisters and erosions also affect the mouth and airway, producing symptoms of hoarseness and stridor. A tracheostomy may be needed to maintain the patency of the upper airway. Hypoplasia of the dental enamel leading to dental anomalies is also seen. Infants with JEB generalized severe (previously known as the Herlitz subtype) also have severe failure to thrive, anemia, and a high risk for sepsis. JEB generalized severe is considered a lethal disease. The average life span is 6 months.

7. **How does JEB with pyloric atresia differ from other forms of JEB?**
   In most cases, JEB with pyloric atresia is caused by mutations in the genes that encode the adhesion protein $\alpha_6\beta_4$ integrin. In addition to affecting the skin and nails, stenosis or atresia of the pyloris can occur. The amount of skin

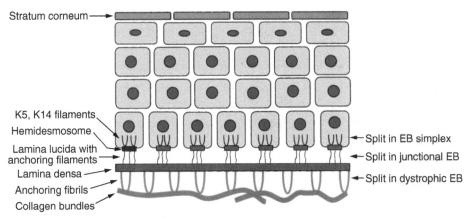

Stratum corneum

K5, K14 filaments
Hemidesmosome
Lamina lucida with anchoring filaments
Lamina densa
Anchoring fibrils
Collagen bundles

Split in EB simplex
Split in junctional EB
Split in dystrophic EB

Fig. 6.1 A schematic of the epidermis and basement membrane zone, showing the major sites of blister formation in epidermolysis bullosa *(EB)*. (Courtesy James E. Fitzpatrick, MD.)

Table 6.1 Classification and inheritance of the most common forms of EB.

MAJOR EB TYPE	MAJOR EB SUBTYPE	MINOR EB SUBTYPE	AFFECTED GENE(S) (PROTEIN)	TYPICAL INHERITANCE
Simplex	Basal	Localized	*KRT5* (keratin 5), *KRT14* (keratin 14)	AD
		Generalized intermediate	*KRT5* (keratin 5), *KRT14* (keratin 14)	AD
		Generalized severe (formerly called Dowling-Meara)	*KRT5* (keratin 5), *KRT14* (keratin 14)	AD
		With muscular dystrophy	*PLEC1* (plectin)	AR
Junctional	Generalized	Generalized severe (formerly Herlitz)	*LAMA3, LAMB3, LAMC2* (laminin-332)	AR
		Generalized intermediate (formerly non-Herlitz)	*LAMA3, LAMB3, LAMC2* (laminin-332), *COL17A1* (type 17 collagen)	AR
		With pyloric atresia	*ITGA6, ITGB4* ($\alpha_6\beta_4$ integrin), *PLEC1* (plectin)	AR
Dystrophic	Dominant	Generalized	*COL7A1* (type VII collagen)	AD
	Recessive	Generalized severe	*COL7A1* (type VII collagen)	AR
		Generalized intermediate	*COL7A1* (type VII collagen)	AR
Kindler syndrome			*FERMT1* (also called *KIND1*, kindlin-1)	AR

AD, Autosomal dominant; *AR,* autosomal recessive; *EB,* epidermolysis bullosa.

involvement varies, but extensive erosions on the extremities at birth are common when the phenotype is severe. Loss-of-function mutations are usually lethal, but less severe mutations produce milder skin findings. Many of these patients have involvement of the urinary tract, which may be more severe than their skin disease.

Schumann H, Kiritsi D, Pigors M, et al. Phenotypic spectrum of epidermolysis bullosa associated with $\alpha_6\beta_4$ integrin mutations. *Br J Dermatol.* 2013;169:115–124.

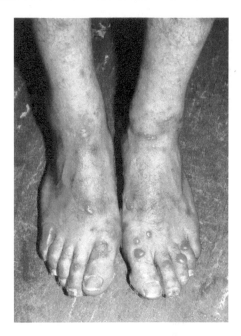

Fig. 6.2 Localized blistering on the feet occurring in an infantry soldier. This exacerbation was produced by a long forced march. (Courtesy Fitzsimons Army Medical Center teaching files.)

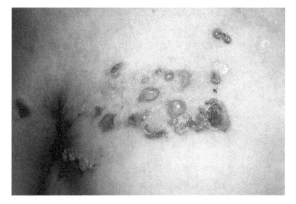

Fig. 6.3 Epidermolysis bullosa simplex generalized, demonstrating annular blistering on the chest.

8. What are the clinical findings in dystrophic EB?

Blisters and erosions typically present at birth. Because the blisters arise in the superficial dermis, they heal with scarring. The recessive form of the disease is more severe. Blisters occur in a generalized distribution, and over time the scarring leads to joint contractures and fusion of the fingers and toes, called pseudosyndactyly (Fig. 6.5). Oral and esophageal involvement causes feeding problems and esophageal strictures. Anemia, poor nutrition, and osteopenia are common complications of recessive dystrophic EB (RDEB). The dominant form of the disease is less severe and tends to be more localized. Atrophic scarring occurs over affected areas, usually the dorsal hands and feet, knees, and elbows.

Bruckner-Tuderman L. Dystrophic epidermolysis bullosa: pathogenesis and clinical features. *Dermatol Clin.* 2010;28:107–114.

9. What is the most serious late complication of RDEB?

Individuals with RDEB have an increased risk of developing squamous cell carcinomas (SCCs) as they age. These SCCs typically occur on the extremities (Fig. 6.6) and are quite aggressive. Involvement of the regional lymph nodes is not uncommon at the time of diagnosis. Metastatic SCC is the most common cause of death in adults with RDEB

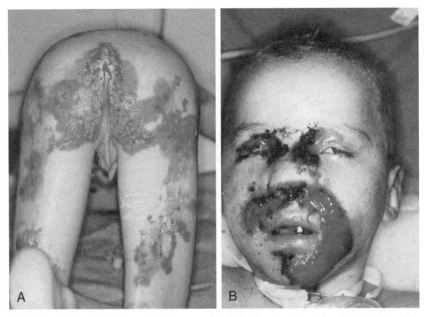

Fig. 6.4 A and **B,** Junctional epidermolysis bullosa generalized severe. Chronic central facial erosions are characteristic.

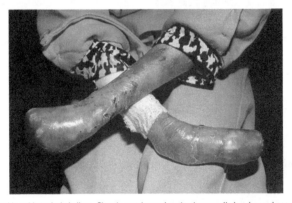

Fig. 6.5 Recessive dystrophic epidermolysis bullosa. Chronic scarring and contracture results in advanced pseudosyndactyly with loss of function.

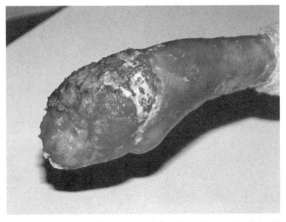

Fig. 6.6 Large ulcerative squamous cell carcinoma arising in the hand of a patient with recessive dystrophic epidermolysis bullosa. (Courtesy John L. Aeling Collection.)

generalized. The risk of developing SCC begins in adolescence and increases thereafter, from 7.5% by age 20 to 67.8%, 80.2%, and 90.1% by ages 35, 45, and 55, respectively. The risk of death due to SCC in these patients is estimated to be 38.7% by age 35, 70% by age 45, and 78.7% by age 55.

Fine JD, Johnson LB, Weiner M, et al. Epidermolysis bullosa and the risk of life-threatening cancers: the National EB Registry experience. *J Am Acad Dermatol.* 2009; 60:203–211.

10. What is Kindler syndrome?

Kindler syndrome is an ultra-rare form of EB that is characterized by blistering that improves with age, mucosal inflammation, photosensitivity, and poikiloderma. The cause of Kindler syndrome is autosomal recessive mutations in the *FERMT1* gene. These mutations cause an alteration in the actin cytoskeleton-extracellular matrix and result in variable planes of blister formation at or close to the BMZ. Because of the mucosal inflammation, patients with Kindler syndrome can have significant dental issues, as well as esophageal, anal, and genitourinary stenoses.

Lai-Cheong JE, McGrath JA. Kindler syndrome. *Dermatol Clin.* 2010;28:119–124.

11. How is EB diagnosed?

In newborns and infants, clinical findings are not reliable in diagnosing the EB type and subtype. In older children and adults, characteristic physical findings can establish a working diagnosis. While skin biopsies were relied on in the past, genetic testing is preferred nowadays.

If performed, skin biopsies are taken from an induced blister for immunofluorescence (IF) and electron microscopy (EM) studies. IF includes immunomapping, which uses a limited panel of antibodies to known BMZ proteins to map the level of the blister (Fig. 6.7). This can be followed by the use of a larger panel of antibodies specific to the proteins affected in EB, evaluating if their expression if present, reduced, or absent. EM is another way to determine the level of the blister in relation to the BMZ. It also provides information about the morphology of BMZ structures (Fig. 6.8). Genetic testing is increasingly common, especially with the advent of next-generation sequencing panels that allow for the parallel analysis of multiple known genes.

Bruckner AL, Murrell DF. Diagnosis of epidermolysis bullosa. In: Hand JL, Corona R, editors: *UpToDate*. Waltham, MA: UpToDate Inc. Available at: https://www.uptodate.com/contents/diagnosis-of-epidermolysis-bullosa. Accessed August 23, 2020.

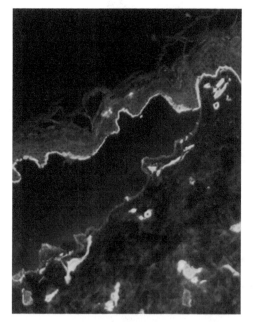

Fig. 6.7 Immunomapping using a fluorescent marker for laminin. Note that laminin *(bright line)*, which is normally found on the dermal side of the basement membrane zone, is on the roof of the blister. This is consistent with a diagnosis of dystrophic epidermolysis bullosa. (Courtesy James E. Fitzpatrick, MD.)

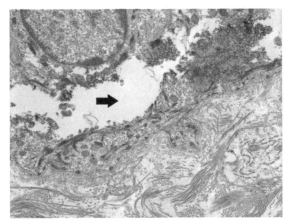

Fig. 6.8 Electron microscopy study of an induced blister in epidermolysis bullosa simplex demonstrating a split *(arrow)* in the cytoplasm of the basilar keratinocyte. (Courtesy James E. Fitzpatrick, MD.)

12. How is EB treated?

At this time, there is no cure for EB. However, a focus on wound care and recognizing and treating complications has greatly improved the prognosis and quality of life for many patients. The current standard of wound care is the use of nonadherent dressings to help blisters heal and decrease trauma to the skin. Bathing can be quite painful for these children, and adding 1 cup or more of pool salt to a full tub of water has been found to help alleviate the pain with bathing.

In variants with oral manifestations, such as JEB and RDEB, meticulous oral hygiene with close dental follow-up is essential. Capping, crowns, and restorations can be helpful. Blended foods or liquid nutritional supplements are necessary for patients with RDEB to help minimize trauma to the esophagus and meet the caloric needs generated by chronic wound healing. Hand deformities in dystrophic EB can be surgically corrected, but the recurrence rate is high. Supporting the psychosocial needs of affected patients and their families is important. The Dystrophic EB Research Association (DebRA) (www.DebRA.org) provides both clinical information and a plethora of resources to support patients and families. The representatives at DebRA can refer new patients to a multidisciplinary EB clinic where a variety of specialists work together to address the complex needs of patients with EB.

Several emerging therapies for EB, including genetic therapy and protein replacement therapy, are being studied at this time.

KEY POINTS: MECHANOBULLOUS DISORDERS

1. Epidermolysis bullosa (EB) is a group of inherited disorders characterized by fragility of the skin and mucous membranes.
2. The key clinical findings of EB are blisters and erosions that arise in areas of minor mechanical trauma.
3. There are four major types of EB (EB simplex, junctional EB, dystrophic EB, and Kindler syndrome) differentiated by the level of blister formation in relationship to the basement membrane zone.
4. Severe forms of EB are complicated by nonskin manifestations, including nutritional compromise, poor growth, anemia, and osteopenia.
5. Squamous cell carcinoma is the most common cause of death in adults with recessive dystrophic EB.
6. Immunofluorescent microscopy, electron microscopy, and genetic studies are used to diagnose the EB type and subtype.
7. The management of EB consists of wound care, monitoring for and treating complications, and psychosocial support for the patient and his/her family.

Acknowledgment

The author acknowledges the prior contributions of Drs. H. Alan Arbuckle and Ronald E. Grimwood to this chapter.

CHAPTER 7

PAPULOSQUAMOUS SKIN ERUPTIONS

Nazanin Ehsani-Chimeh, Meena Julapalli, and Jeffrey B. Travers

1. Name the papulosquamous skin eruptions.
   Papulosquamous skin disorders are inflammatory reactions characterized by red or purple papules and plaques with scale. These diseases include psoriasis, pityriasis rubra pilaris (PRP), seborrheic dermatitis, pityriasis rosea, and pityriasis lichenoides et varioliformis acuta (PLEVA). Lichen planus and lichen nitidus are also considered papulosquamous disorders (see Chapter 12).

2. What is psoriasis?
   Psoriasis is a common, genetically determined, inflammatory, and hyperproliferative skin disease. Although there are morphologic variations, the most characteristic lesions consist of chronic, well-demarcated, dull-red plaques (Fig. 7.1A) with silvery scale found commonly on extensor surfaces and the scalp (Fig. 7.1B).

3. What is the incidence of psoriasis?
   Psoriasis is estimated to occur in about 2% to 3% of the population worldwide. The most recent U.S. data suggest a prevalence of 3.2% among adults ages 20 and older with an estimated 7.4 million adults affected in 2013. It is less common, in descending order, in African Americans (1.9%), Hispanics (1.6%), and others (1.4%).

Rachakonda TD, Schupp CW, Armstrong AW. Psoriasis prevalence among adults in the United States. *J Am Acad Dermatol.* 2014; 70:512–516.

4. List the different types of psoriasis
   The different clinical presentations of psoriasis can be separated by morphology or location.

Morphologic Variants	*Locational Variants*
Chronic plaque psoriasis	Scalp psoriasis
Guttate psoriasis	Palmoplantar psoriasis
Pustular psoriasis	Inverse psoriasis
Erythrodermic psoriasis	Nail psoriasis
Psoriatic arthritis	

5. What is guttate psoriasis?
   Guttate psoriasis is a variant of psoriasis usually seen in adolescents and young adults. It is characterized by crops of small, droplike, psoriatic papules and plaques (Fig. 7.2A). The word "guttate" is derived from the Latin *gutta*, which means "drop." This type of psoriasis is often found in association with streptococcal pharyngitis. One-third of patients can progress to chronic plaque type psoriasis.

Ko HC, Jwa SW, Song M, Kim MB, Kwon KS. Clinical course of guttate psoriasis: long-term follow-up study. *J Dermatol.* 2010;37 (10):894–899.

6. What is inverse psoriasis?
   Inverse psoriasis refers to psoriasis that involves intertriginous areas (axillae, groin, umbilicus). This distribution is opposite to the usual extensor distribution of psoriasis vulgaris. Psoriatic lesions with both distributions sometimes can be found in the same patients. Clinically, psoriatic lesions found in these "inverse" distributions often do not have scale but consist of sharply demarcated red plaques that may become macerated and eroded (Fig. 7.2B). Treatment of inverse psoriasis usually involves low-potency (nonfluorinated) topical corticosteroids or topical calcineurin inhibitors.

7. Does pustular psoriasis refer to psoriasis that is secondarily infected?
   No. The pustular forms are uncommon, less stable variants of psoriasis. Instead of erythematous plaques with silvery scale as seen in typical psoriasis, pustular psoriasis is characterized by superficial pustules, often with fine desquamation (Fig. 7.3). Although triggers such as infection can precipitate a flare of pustular psoriasis, the pustules

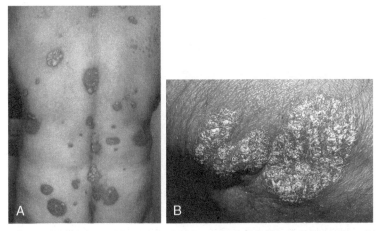

Fig. 7.1 Psoriasis vulgaris. **A,** Numerous well-demarcated scaly plaques on the trunk. **B,** Close-up of elbow involvement demonstrating typical, well-demarcated red plaques with silvery scale. (Panel A courtesy Fitzsimons Army Medical Center teaching files.)

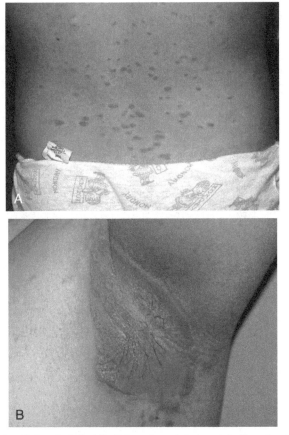

Fig. 7.2 A, Guttate psoriasis on the lower back of a child with the acute onset of numerous droplike erythematous papules. This type of psoriasis is associated with streptococcal infections, probably through the immune-stimulating effects of exotoxins secreted by the bacteria. *(Courtesy William L. Weston, MD, Collection.)* **B,** Inverse psoriasis involves intertriginous areas such as the axilla, as shown here. Note the lack of silvery scale seen in psoriasis vulgaris. (Courtesy James E. Fitzpatrick, MD.)

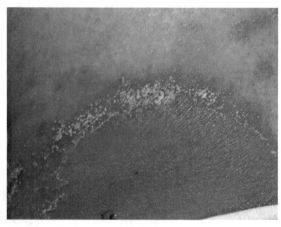

Fig. 7.3 Pustular psoriasis demonstrating superficial pustules on a well-defined erythematous plaque. (Courtesy John L. Aeling Collection.)

are sterile. A mutation in IL36RN has recently been described in patients with generalized pustular psoriasis. In addition to topical corticosteroids, patients often need systemic treatments, such as retinoids, immunosuppressives, or phototherapy, to keep their disease under control.

8. Is there a genetic basis for psoriasis?
Although a specific genetic abnormality has not been identified, psoriasis is generally considered to be a genetically determined disease. There are reports of striking family pedigrees that suggest an autosomal dominant inheritance, but with only partial penetrance. Keep in mind that psoriasis is probably not a single disease, but a family of diseases involving epidermal hyperproliferation. More than 40 independent genome-wide psoriasis susceptibility loci have been identified; however, further study is needed to determine the importance and significance of these findings.
  The external environment presumably plays a role in the clinical expression. The strongest evidence for the importance of external factors in the expression of psoriasis is seen in acute guttate psoriasis, which often occurs in association with streptococcal pharyngitis.

Mahil SK, Capon F, Barker JN. Genetics of psoriasis. *Dermatol Clin.* 2015;33:1–11.

9. If one of my relatives has psoriasis, what is the chance that I will get psoriasis?
A large questionnaire-based study out of Germany revealed that a child has a 41% chance of developing psoriasis if both parents are affected, in contrast to 14% if one parent is affected or 6% if a sibling is affected. Twin studies indicate that there is a two to three times increased risk of psoriasis in monozygotic twins compared to dizygotic twins.

Farber EM, Nall ML. The natural history of psoriasis in 5,600 patients. *Dermatologica.* 1974;148(1):1–18.

10. Name the types of psoriatic arthritis
Although the exact incidence of psoriatic arthritis is unknown, an estimated 5% to 30% of patients with psoriasis suffer from psoriatic arthritis. The arthritis may precede, accompany, or, more commonly, follow the development of the skin disease. The five types of psoriatic arthritis are:
- Asymmetric oligoarthritis, monoarthritis (60% to 70%)
- Symmetric polyarthritis (15%)
- Distal interphalangeal joint (DIP) disease (5%)
- Destructive arthritis (5%)
- Axial arthritis (5%)

Tintle SJ, Gottlieb AB. Psoriatic arthritis for the dermatologist. *Dermatol Clin.* 2015;33:127–148.

11. Describe the clinical features of the psoriatic arthritis.
Asymmetric arthritis, the most common form of psoriatic arthritis, usually involves one or several joints of the fingers or toes. The appearance of this type of arthritis can be similar to subacute gout and include "sausage-like" swelling of a digit due to involvement of the proximal and DIP joints and the flexor sheath (Fig. 7.4). Symmetric polyarthritis

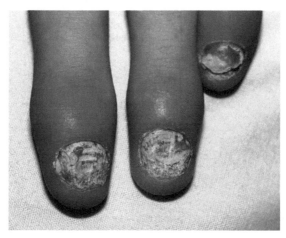

Fig. 7.4 Distal psoriatic arthritis in an 11-year-old patient. Note the extensive nail changes. (Courtesy William L. Weston, MD, Collection.)

resembles rheumatoid arthritis, but tests for rheumatoid factor are negative, and the condition is clinically less severe than rheumatoid arthritis. Although not common, DIP joint disease of hands and feet is the most classic presentation of arthritis with psoriasis. Destructive arthritis (arthritis mutilans) is a rare, severely deforming arthritis involving predominantly fingers and toes. Gross osteolysis of the small bones of the hands and feet can result in shortening, subluxations, and, in severe cases, telescoping of the digits, resulting in an "opera glass" deformity. Axial arthritis of the spine, which resembles idiopathic ankylosing spondylitis, manifests by itself or with peripheral joint disease. Management of psoriatic arthritis includes nonsteroidal antiinflammatory drugs, physical therapy, and, in more recalcitrant cases, systemic treatments such as methotrexate and biologic agents.

12. What are the abnormal nail findings seen in psoriasis? Which is most common?
    A careful examination of the nails should be part of the skin exam, especially when evaluating a rash that might be psoriasis. Characteristic nail changes are found in 25% to 50% of psoriatics. These changes include nail pitting, discoloration, onycholysis, subungual hyperkeratosis, and nail deformity. Nail pitting, the most common nail finding in psoriasis, consists of small, discrete, punched-out depressions on the nail surface (Fig. 7.5). Circular areas of nail bed discoloration that resemble oil drops are often seen under the nail plate (hyponychium). The nail can become thin and brittle at the distal edge with separation from the nail bed (onycholysis) or thickened with subungual debris. Ridges, grooves, or even frank deformity of the nail plate can also be seen.

13. Are there other nonskin manifestations of psoriasis?
    Recent studies have confirmed that psoriasis is associated with medical and psychiatric comorbidities. Patients with psoriasis have a higher incidence of obesity, diabetes mellitus, hypertension, hypercholesterolemia, and myocardial

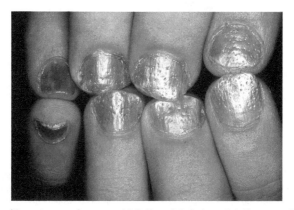

Fig. 7.5 Nail pitting is one of the most common changes associated with psoriasis. As demonstrated here, even nail polish cannot hide these discrete pits.

infarction. Rates of Crohn's disease and ulcerative colitis are also increased in patients with psoriasis. In addition, the emotional distress of having a severe skin disease may have a profoundly negative psychological impact. Depressed mood, anxiety, suicidal ideation, and clinical depression are found at a higher incidence in psoriatic patients.

14. You are working in a dermatology clinic, seeing a patient with a rash that is possibly psoriasis. Outside the room, the attending asks if you noticed any evidence of the "Koebner phenomenon" or an "Auspitz sign" when you examined the patient. What are these?

    The Koebner phenomenon (isomorphic response) is the development of a cutaneous eruption at the site of physical trauma (scratch, surgical wound, tattoo, or sunburn). Other skin conditions that exhibit the Koebner phenomenon include lichen planus, lichen nitidus, and vitiligo. Patients with psoriasis should be warned of this tendency before subjecting themselves to cosmetic procedures involving physical trauma (such as having a tattoo).

    The Auspitz sign is the presence of small bleeding points seen on a psoriatic lesion when the scales are removed. This bleeding is due to thinning of the epidermis (suprapapillary plates) between the elongated rete ridges. Note that it is not a good idea to attempt to elicit these two signs on your psoriatic patients.

15. Name three types of drugs that precipitate or exacerbate psoriasis

    Beta-blocking agents, antimalarials (i.e., hydroxychloroquine), and lithium. All three can precipitate or exacerbate psoriasis. These medications should be used with caution in psoriatics.

16. What other factors can provoke or exacerbate psoriasis?

    Infection (especially streptococcal pharyngitis as well as HIV), hypocalcemia, stress, alcohol consumption, smoking, and obesity have been shown to induce or aggravate psoriasis.

17. Do systemic corticosteroids help psoriasis?

    Although treatment with systemic corticosteroids rapidly clears psoriasis, the disease usually "breaks through," requiring higher doses of corticosteroids. If systemic corticosteroid treatment is withdrawn, the psoriasis usually relapses and may worsen. This "rebound" worsening of psoriasis may even result in a severe flare-up of erythrodermic (total body) or generalized pustular psoriasis.

18. What topical medications are used to treat psoriasis?

    Patients with limited disease (usually <5% of their body surface) can often be managed on topical agents alone. Although systemic corticosteroids generally should not be used, topical corticosteroids are a first-line treatment. For plaques, medium- to high-potency corticosteroids used daily can result in a rapid response, often controlling the inflammation and itching. Unfortunately, the relief is often temporary, and tolerance can occur. Side effects include atrophy and telangiectasias, especially if high-potency topical preparations are used on the face or intertriginous areas (see also Chapter 49).

    Calcipotriene and calcipotriol, vitamin D_3 analogs, have shown efficacy in mild to moderate psoriasis or for severe psoriasis when used in combination preparations with betamethasone. Due to the possibility of systemic absorption resulting in changes in calcium homeostasis, vitamin D_3 analogs should be limited to a maximum dosage of 100 g/wk. The keratolytic salicylic acid can be used to soften thick scale in cases of severe scalp psoriasis. Coal tar can also be effective due to its antiinflammatory and antipruritic properties, and tar shampoo preparations are available over the counter. However, tar preparations have taken on a more secondary role in topical therapy due to staining skin and clothes.

Menter A, Korman NJ, Elmets CA, et al. Guidelines of care for the management of psoriasis and psoriatic arthritis. Section 6: treatment of patients with limited disease. *J Am Acad Dermatol.* 2011;65:137–174.

19. How is ultraviolet radiation used to treat psoriasis?

    It has been known for centuries that sunlight exposure can improve psoriasis. Two forms of ultraviolet radiation are used clinically: ultraviolet B (UVB, 290 to 320 nm) and ultraviolet A (UVA, 320 to 400 nm) combined with an oral photosensitizer, psoralen plus UVA (PUVA). Compared to PUVA, use of UVB, particularly narrowband UVB (311 nm), results in less incidence of side effects and is often used first in the treatment of light-sensitive psoriasis (see also Chapter 54). Excimer laser (308 nm) has also been used for localized disease with some efficacy.

20. What systemic drugs are used to treat psoriasis?

    Methotrexate, cyclosporine, and retinoids (i.e., acitretin). Because of the potential side effects of these agents, their use should be carefully considered by the physician and patient. Methotrexate suppresses DNA synthesis by inhibiting the enzyme dihydrofolate reductase. In addition to its antimitotic effects, methotrexate inhibits neutrophil function. Side effects include bone marrow suppression, stomach upset, and hepatotoxicity. Concurrent administration of folic acid to reduce the risk of pancytopenia and gastrointestinal side effects is controversial due to conflicting studies about folic acid reducing the efficacy of methotrexate. Although the incidence of hepatic fibrosis and cirrhosis is low with cumulative doses less than 1.5 g, liver function tests are not a reliable indicator of methotrexate-induced hepatotoxicity. In patients with other risk factors for hepatotoxicity, a liver biopsy to monitor for hepatic fibrosis and cirrhosis may be considered. However, due to the infrequent nature of this consequence, routine liver biopsies for all patients on prolonged courses of methotrexate are no longer recommended. Methotrexate should be avoided in psoriatic patients who have underlying liver disease, renal disease, or are heavy drinkers. Patients who take methotrexate should be aware of its interactions with many other medications.

The antilymphocytic drug cyclosporine can be used for severe psoriasis. It has a relatively rapid onset of action, but side effects such as hypertension, nephrotoxicity, hepatotoxicity, oncogenicity, and hypertrichosis limit its use as a long-term agent. The doses used, 3 to 5 mg/kg/day, are usually lower than the dosages used to inhibit organ transplant rejection.

Systemic retinoids such as acitretin are first-line agents in pustular psoriasis and also may be used to treat chronic plaque psoriasis. Unlike methotrexate and cyclosporine, retinoids do not suppress the immune system. Rather, retinoids likely mitigate the epidermal hyperproliferation seen in psoriasis. Acitretin is a potent teratogen and must be avoided in women of childbearing age. Other systemic treatments include biologic agents, which will be covered in the next question (see also Chapter 56).

Aithal GP, Haugk B, Das S, et al. Monitoring methotrexate-induced hepatic fibrosis in patients with psoriasis: are serial liver biopsies justified? *Aliment Pharmacol Ther.* 2004;19:391–399.

Chladek J, Simkova M, Vaneckova J, et al. The effect of folic acid supplementation on the pharmacokinetics and pharmacodynamics of oral methotrexate during remission-induction period of treatment for moderate-to-severe plaque psoriasis. *Eur J Clin Pharmacol.* 2008;64:347–355.

21. What biologic agents may be used in the treatment of psoriasis?

Biologic agents are proteins derived from living cells that are used to modulate specific portions of the aberrant immune response that leads to psoriasis. They are administered by subcutaneous, intramuscular, or intravenous injection. Tumor necrosis factor-α (TNF-α) inhibitors (etanercept, adalimumab, and infliximab), interleukin (IL)-12/-23 inhibitors (ustekinumab), as well as IL-17 inhibitors (secukinumab, ixekizumab, and brodalumab) are used in the treatment of refractory or extensive psoriasis. The TNF-α inhibitors block the proinflammatory action of TNF-α, a potent cytokine that mediates the formation of psoriatic plaques. Risks of TNF-α inhibitors include increased susceptibility to infections, such as reactivation of tuberculosis or hepatitis B, and higher rates of malignancy such as lymphoma.

Another biologic agent is ustekinumab, a humanized antibody against the p40 subunit found in the cytokines IL-12 and IL-23. In particular, the inhibition of IL-23 blocks the T-cell pathway (Th17) implicated in the pathogenesis of psoriasis.

Although these systemic psoriasis therapies may be more effective, care must be exercised in their use, especially because the long-term side effects of biologic agents are not completely clear, particularly in children.

22. Describe the rash of PRP.

PRP is a rare disease in which the primary abnormality appears to be hyperproliferation of the epidermis. Five variants have been described, the most common being type I, the classic adult-onset form. In this type, the eruption commonly begins on the head and neck as orange-red, slightly scaly macules and thin plaques. The rash extends in a cephalocaudal fashion, and within several weeks, red, perifollicular papules with central plugs develop in the lesions. The scalp often develops extensive yellowish scale. The palms and soles become thickened and yellow, which is called keratoderma. This results in a well-demarcated, very characteristic "PRP sandal" (Fig. 7.6A). Although total body involvement (erythroderma) is not uncommon, the rash of PRP often has characteristic skip areas of normal skin ("islands of sparing") (Fig. 7.6B). Considering that the rash usually looks very impressive, it is surprising that patients often complain of only mild irritation and pruritus.

23. Although PRP can occur at any age, in what decades is it most often seen? What is the prognosis?

PRP has a bimodal age distribution, with the highest incidence in the fifth and sixth decades and a smaller peak in childhood. The prognosis is variable, but usually, 80% of patients clear spontaneously in several years.

24. How is PRP treated?

Treatment strategies for PRP depend on the extent of involvement and how much the patient is bothered. Lubrication with emollients and topical corticosteroids is rarely helpful. The treatment of choice is oral retinoids, with methotrexate being reserved for retinoid-resistant cases. There have also been reports of the successful utilization of biologics with PRP in select cases.

Ivanova K, Itin P, Haeusermann P. Pityriasis rubra pilaris: treatment with biologics—a new promising therapy? *Dermatology.* 2012;224:120–125.

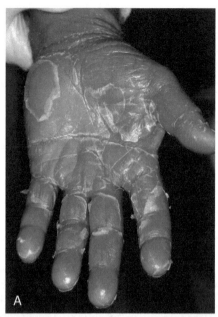

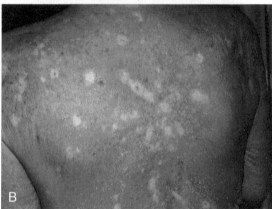

Fig. 7.6 Pityriasis rubra pilaris. **A,** Characteristic thickened scaly palms. (Courtesy Johanna Burch Collection.) **B,** Extensive involvement in adult showing characteristic salmon color and "islands of sparing."

KEY POINTS: PAPULOSQUAMOUS DISORDERS

1. Psoriasis classically has symmetrical, red plaques with silver-white scale on the elbows, knees, and scalp.
2. Nail changes in psoriasis can mimic those seen with a dermatophyte fungal infection.
3. Pityriasis rubra pilaris has large areas of red to orange-red plaques with islands of sparing, and hand/foot thickened skin.
4. Seborrheic dermatitis can be found not only on scalp but also on the face around the nares, central chest, axillae, and even on the penis.
5. Pityriasis rosea has oval papules and plaques that tend to develop along skin lines ("Christmas tree" pattern) with trailing scale (scale does not reach the end of the lesion).

25. Describe the distribution of the "seborrheic areas."
    Seborrheic areas have a rich supply of sebaceous glands and include the scalp, face, central chest, and intertriginous areas. Skin diseases that can have a "seborrheic distribution" include seborrheic dermatitis, psoriasis, Darier's disease, and pemphigus foliaceus.

26. What does seborrheic dermatitis look like?

Seborrheic dermatitis is a chronic dermatitis with a typical morphologic appearance of red plaques with greasy, yellow scales, distributed in the seborrheic areas. Scalp involvement is almost universal. Facial involvement is common and manifests itself as erythema and scaling on the medial sides of the eyebrows, glabella, and nasolabial folds. Ocular involvement (blepharitis and conjunctivitis) and ear involvement (external auditory canal and posterior auricular scalp) are also frequently seen. Visible scalp desquamation, commonly known as dandruff, is probably the precursor and/or a mild form of seborrheic dermatitis.

Naldi L, Rebora A. Clinical practice. Seborrheic dermatitis. *N Engl J Med.* 2009;360:387–396.

27. What causes seborrheic dermatitis?

Seborrheic dermatitis is probably a hypersensitivity response to common skin yeasts, of the genus *Malassezia* *(Pityrosporum)*. Seborrheic dermatitis may be more severe when associated with HIV infection, the use of dopamine antagonist antipsychotics, and Parkinson's disease.

28. How can you differentiate between seborrheic dermatitis and psoriasis of the scalp?

The differentiation between these two disorders can be difficult. However, in contrast to seborrheic dermatitis, scalp psoriasis is often patchy, consisting of thicker plaques with silvery scale. The rest of the skin should be examined, including the nails, to look for other evidence of psoriasis. The patient should also be questioned about a possible family history of psoriasis.

29. How is seborrheic dermatitis treated?

Although treatment of seborrheic dermatitis is suppressive, it is not curative. The scalp is best treated with medicated shampoos (ketoconazole, selenium sulfide, zinc pyrithione, and tar). Patients should be instructed to leave the shampoo on their scalp for at least 5 minutes before rinsing (or two or three songs for patients who are inclined to sing in the shower). Use of a medium- or high-potency topical steroid solution on the scalp is often helpful for patients who experience burning or pruritus or have resistant areas. Facial seborrheic dermatitis is very responsive to low-potency topical corticosteroids (hydrocortisone) or topical antifungal creams.

30. What is pityriasis rosea? Describe the characteristic rash

Pityriasis rosea is an acute, benign, self-limiting disorder that most commonly affects teenagers and young adults. The eruption has a characteristic pattern, and 70% of cases start with a single 2- to 4-cm, sharply defined, thin, oval plaque on the trunk or, less commonly, on the neck or proximal extremities. Within a few days to weeks, crops of similar-appearing, although usually smaller, papules follow the initial "herald patch" (Fig. 7.7). The eruption characteristically involves the trunk and proximal extremities, usually sparing the face, palms, soles, and scalp. Lesions on the trunk tend to run parallel to the lines of skin cleavage, resulting in a "Christmas tree" pattern. The lesions usually resolve within several weeks to a month but may persist longer. Except for a mild prodrome, affected

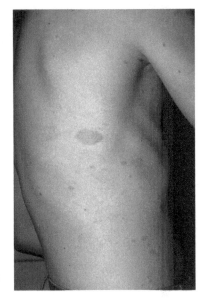

Fig. 7.7 Pityriasis rosea. A young adult demonstrates a characteristic large herald patch near the axilla associated with numerous oval secondary lesions that follow skin lines.

patients are usually asymptomatic. The lesions of pityriasis rosea often have "trailing scale" (e.g., collarette of scale that does not extend to the border of the lesion), and papular variants can be seen, especially in children.

Drago F, Broccolo F, Rebora A. Pityriasis rosea: an update with a critical appraisal of its possible herpesviral etiology. *J Am Acad Dermatol.* 2009;61:303–318.

31. What is the cause of pityriasis rosea?

Although the etiology of pityriasis rosea is unknown, the occasional prodromal symptoms, characteristic disease course, tendency for lifelong immunity, seasonal variance, and reports of epidemics all point to an infectious (viral) agent. Some studies suggest that human herpesvirus-6 and/or -7 are the causative agents. Treatment consists of reassurance, emollients, and antipruritic agents for symptomatic patients. Ultraviolet radiation treatment (sunshine or UVB) hastens the disappearance of the eruption.

32. In the dermatology clinic, you evaluate a 20-year-old man who has been referred from the primary care clinic with a diagnosis of pityriasis rosea. He has a rash that looks like pityriasis rosea, but he complains of fevers, myalgias, and swollen lymph glands. He remembers having an ulcer on his penis several months ago. What test do you recommend?

The eruption of secondary syphilis can mimic pityriasis rosea, although patients often have systemic manifestations such as fever, lymphadenopathy, headache, or bone pain. Unlike pityriasis rosea, secondary syphilis often involves the palms, soles, and mucous membranes. A sexual history should be elicited in such patients, and a rapid plasma reagin (RPR) or Venereal Disease Research Laboratory (VDRL) test should be obtained. Because syphilis is readily treated, and because untreated syphilis can result in life-threatening cardiovascular and neurologic sequelae, many dermatologists customarily obtain an RPR or VDRL test on every sexually active patient who presents with a pityriasis rosea–like eruption.

33. What is pityriasis lichenoides et varioliformis acuta?

PLEVA (or Mucha-Habermann disease) is a rare disease characterized by crops of polymorphous lesions on the trunk, thighs, and upper arms. The eruption consists of red-brown papules that can become purpuric, scaly, and even necrotic (Fig. 7.8). The patients usually are asymptomatic, although itching and low-grade fevers and malaise are not uncommon. Individual lesions resolve in several weeks leaving postinflammatory hyper- or hypopigmentation and occasionally scars. The clinical course of PLEVA often waxes and wanes and can last months to years.

Khachemoune A, Blyumin ML. Pityriasis lichenoides: pathophysiology, classification, and treatment. *Am J Clin Dermatol.* 2007;8:29–36.

34. How is PLEVA treated?

Oral antibiotics (erythromycin or tetracycline) have been suggested, but no controlled studies exist. Phototherapy and immunosuppressive agents, such as methotrexate, have been used for recalcitrant or severe cases.

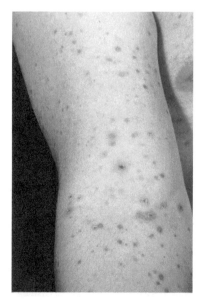

Fig. 7.8 Pityriasis lichenoides et varioliformis acuta. Characteristic polymorphic appearance with red scaly papules, hemorrhagic papules, and necrotic papules.

CHAPTER 8

ECZEMATOUS DERMATITIS

Thomas J. McIntee

1. **What is eczematous dermatitis?**
   Eczematous dermatitis is the clinical diagnosis used to designate a broad category of skin disorders that manifest with intensely pruritic, scaly, erythematous macules, papules, vesicles, or plaques, often with poorly defined margins. The base term *eczema* is taken from the Greek *ekzema* meaning "to boil over." Eczema tends to have overlapping clinical phases: acute (vesicular), subacute (scaling and crusting), and chronic (lichenified) phases. Oozing, crusting, scaling, fissuring, and lichenification frequently accompany the primary lesions. Nearly one-fourth of all presenting dermatology complaints involve a form of eczematous dermatitis.

2. **Are there different types of eczematous dermatitis?**
   Included in the category of eczematous dermatitis are the following:
   1. Atopic dermatitis (AD) (eczema)
   2. Nummular dermatitis
   3. Contact dermatitis—allergic and irritant
   4. Seborrheic dermatitis
   5. Diaper dermatitis
   6. Autosensitization dermatitis (Id Reaction)
   7. Photodermatitis
   8. Perioral dermatitis
   9. Juvenile plantar dermatosis

3. **Are eczema and AD the same disorder?**
   Eczema and *AD* are terms frequently used interchangeably to describe a chronic, often familial, relapsing, pruritic skin disorder with clinical manifestations of xerosis, inflammation, and lichenification. Many dermatologists prefer to use the term *atopic dermatitis* to avoid confusion with other eczematous dermatoses.

4. **What is atopy?**
   The term *atopy* is derived from the Greek word *atopos*, meaning "out-of-place," and refers to the predisposition to develop AD, asthma, and allergic rhinitis commonly known as the atopic triad.

5. **How common is AD?**
   The prevalence of AD in the United States has increased over the past 50 years to 6%–13% in the general population and 8.7%–18.1% in children. Higher prevalence rates are found in developed, more urban countries. The increased prevalence of AD over time and the difference between more and less developed nations has been supported by the "hygiene hypothesis." This theory postulates that a protective effect is incurred with antigenic exposure from day care settings, endotoxins, unpasteurized farm milk, dog and farm animals, and nonpathogenic microbes; early antigenic stimulation encourages immune tolerance, leading to a lower incidence of various allergic diseases including AD, asthma, and allergic rhinitis, and autoimmune diseases such as diabetes and inflammatory bowel disease.

6. **What are the diagnostic criteria for AD?**
   Several sets of criteria for the diagnosis of AD have been developed based on the initial criteria proposed by Hanifin and Rajka in 1980. The American Academy of Dermatology 2014 Atopic Dermatitis Work Group presented the following recommendation of diagnostic criteria (Table 8.1).

7. **What is the etiology of AD?**
   The pathogenesis of AD is not completely understood; expert consensus postulates that a complex interaction of skin barrier dysfunction, exaggerated immune response, inherited susceptibility, and environmental factors combine to produce the phenotype of AD. Important in skin barrier integrity is profilaggrin, which degrades to filaggrin (FLG), an essential protein for proper terminal differentiation of the epidermis, organization of keratin cytoskeleton elements, and skin barrier formation—essentially the "mortar" between corneocytes. Filaggrin degradation products constitute natural moisturizing factor that enhances epidermal hydration and barrier function. Impaired skin barrier function leads to increased transepidermal water loss (TEWL) and allows entry of various irritants, microbes, and allergens together promoting keratinocyte release of cytokine mediators. This initiation of the type 2 helper T cell (Th2) immune cascade and concomitant release of Th2, Th22, and Th17 cytokines (interleukin [IL]-4, IL-13, IL-22, IL-31) appear to modulate the epidermal barrier function and, along with elevated IgE, acutely lead to the clinical manifestations of AD. Type 1 helper T cell (Th1) cytokines become more prevalent in chronic-phase AD. While loss-of-function FLG mutations are not essential in AD, an estimated 50% of moderate and severe AD patients have FLG null alleles while conversely 40% of individuals with null FLG alleles do not have AD.

Table 8.1 Atopic dermatitis diagnostic criteria

Essential features—must be present
1. Pruritus
2. Eczema (acute, subacute, chronic)
   a. Typical morphology and age-specific patterns
      i. Infants and children—facial, neck, and extensor involvement
      ii. Any age group—current or previous flexural lesions
      iii. All groups—sparing of groin and axillary regions

Important supporting features (seen in most cases)
1. Early age of onset
2. Personal or family history of atopic disease
3. IgE reactivity
4. Generalized xerosis

Exclusionary conditions
1. Scabies
2. Seborrheic dermatitis
3. Allergic or irritant contact dermatitis
4. Ichthyoses
5. Cutaneous T-cell lymphoma (CTCL)
6. Psoriasis
7. Photodermatoses
8. Immunodeficiency with cutaneous findings
9. Erythroderma of other etiologies

8. Is itch a primary or a secondary manifestation of AD?
   AD is frequently called "the itch that rashes." Life-altering intense pruritus is a major component of AD, often affecting sleep and activities of daily living.

9. Why does AD itch?
   There is not yet full understanding of pruritus in AD, but essential is the recognition of the embryologic ectodermal-derived origin of both the nervous system and skin. While no single neuropeptide is responsible for pruritus, chemical mediators associated with pruritus and acting on nerve endings or keratinocytes directly are found in the skin; substance P, IL-2, and IL-31, acetylcholine, prostanoids, calcitonin, and gene-related peptide are produced by mast cells, keratinocytes, T lymphocytes, and nerve fibers. Keratinocytes and mast cells release a neuropeptide, nerve growth factor, increasing the sensitivity of cutaneous itch receptors. These sensitized nerve endings have an increased transmission of stimuli interpreted as pruritus (allokinesis). Multiple studies have failed to show histamine as a major contributor to AD pruritus.

10. What are factors that lead to pruritus in AD?
    See Table 8.2.

11. Are antihistamines the answer for the AD itch?
    Numerous studies have failed to show benefit with nonsedating antihistamines in controlling AD itch. Sedating antihistamines such as hydroxyzine may offer benefit with nighttime sedation. Topical treatment utilizing corticosteroids and calcineurin inhibitors have shown itch score reductions of up to 78% and 36%, respectively. Crisaborale is a new phosphodiesterase (PDE-4) inhibitor that has demonstrated benefit with AD itch. Cyclosporine has

Table 8.2 Pruritus

ENDOGENOUS FACTORS	EXOGENOUS FACTORS
Perspiration	Warm environments
Xerosis	Wool fibers
Physical exertion	Soaps, detergents
Emotional stress	Hot water
	Atopic dermatitis flare
	Contact with allergens

proven to be the most effective short-term systemic treatment in refractory AD pruritus, but long-term use has problematic side effects. Narrowband ultraviolet B (UVB) light (311 nm) can be an effective long-term itch management option. Dupilumab, a monoclonal antibiody to IL-4 and IL-13, is reported to have significant benefit for patients with atopic itch. Maintenance of skin moisturization and emollient therapy should be the cornerstone of pruritus treatment.

12. **Will AD lead to other types of atopic disease?**
AD is the first manifestation of the atopic triad (also known as the "atopic march") consisting of AD, allergic rhinitis, and asthma. Up to 70% of patients with moderate to severe AD will develop allergic rhinitis and 50% will develop some form of asthma. Those AD patients with filaggrin mutations are at higher risk of subsequent asthma development. It is believed that epicutaneous exposure to allergens (e.g., dust mites) in AD patients leads to airway disease. Diligent skin barrier protection and inflammation control appears to lower the risk of progression of the atopic march.

13. **How does AD present by age?**
While AD typically presents in childhood, it may present at any age; 60% to 88% of AD patients have their first AD outbreak by 1 year of age, 70% to 95% by school entry at age 5.
AD may be classified into three phenotypic phases:
1. Infantile (2 months to 2 years)
   - Symptoms: Intense pruritus.
   - Distribution: Often symmetric. Cheeks (Fig. 8.1A), forehead, ears (Fig. 8.1B), and scalp, extensor surfaces of extremities and trunk (often exacerbated due to friction from crawling).
   - Morphology: Erythema, papules, vesicles, oozing, and crusting. Dry scale as opposed to greasy scale in seborrheic dermatitis. Postinflammatory hypo/hyperpigmentation is common.
   - Course: Dermatitis clears in half of the patients by age 3.
2. Childhood (2 years to puberty)
   - Symptoms: Intense pruritus.
   - Distribution: Wrists, ankles, neck, posterior thighs, buttocks, antecubital and popliteal fossae (Fig. 8.1C,D).
   - Morphology: Poorly defined, erythematous, scaly patches, frequently studded with crust, exudate, and erosions. Lichenification may be present in antecubital and popliteal fossae. Nummular patches may also be evident. Postinflammatory hypo/hyperpigmentation common.
   - Course: Two-thirds of patients clear by age 6.
3. Adult pattern
   - Symptoms: Chronic pruritus.
   - Distribution: Face, neck, arms, back, and flexures.
   - Morphology: Thick, dry, lichenified plaques (Fig. 8.1E) without exuberant weeping, crusting, or oozing. Generalized xerosis. Acral surface fissures, scale, and vesicles are not uncommon. Facial central pallor may be evident.
   - Course: Adult pattern less likely to clear.

14. **What physical findings are associated with AD?**
   - Xerosis due to skin barrier dysfunction and increased TEWL.
   - Keratosis pilaris: Follicular-based erythematous hyperkeratotic papules, especially on dorsal arms, anterior thighs, buttocks, and upper back.
   - Pityriasis alba: Hypopigmented patches with fine scale, particularly on the medial/malar cheeks in children with darker skin types.
   - Hyperlinear palm and sole creases.
   - Dennie-Morgan pleats (extra skin folds on lower eyelids—often glazed and hyperpigmented) (Fig. 8.2A).
   - Dermatographism: Exuberant reaction to skin friction. May vary from slight vascular flare to frank edema/vesicle formation (Fig. 8.2B).
   - Vascular abnormalities: Skin pallor, low finger and toe temperatures, pronounced vasoconstriction on exposure to cold.
   - Eye findings: Keratoconjunctivitis may be found in up to 30% of children with AD, posterior > anterior subcapsular cataracts, keratoconus.

15. **What factors provoke or exacerbate AD?**
   - Wool clothing: Wool fibers stimulate intense itching via allokinesis. Larger fibers induce more pruritus.
   - Clothing made of blended or synthetic fabrics and shirt collar tags.
   - Prolonged bathing/hot water bathing: Promotes TEWL.
   - Soaps, especially soaps with a high (basic) pH.
   - Infection: *Staphylococcus aureus* skin colonization releases superantigens, triggering dermatitis flares.
   - Climate extremes: Heat, cold, low humidity, and high humidity.
   - Contact allergens: Pet hair, especially cat dander.

16. **Does breast feeding prevent AD?**
Breastfeeding provides numerous health benefits to infants and should be *strongly encouraged*. Breastfeeding appears to provide a modest risk reduction (33%) in the onset of AD in high-risk infants (familial predisposition) who are breast-fed during the first 4 months of life. Infants not at high risk of AD development do not appear to have a difference in AD

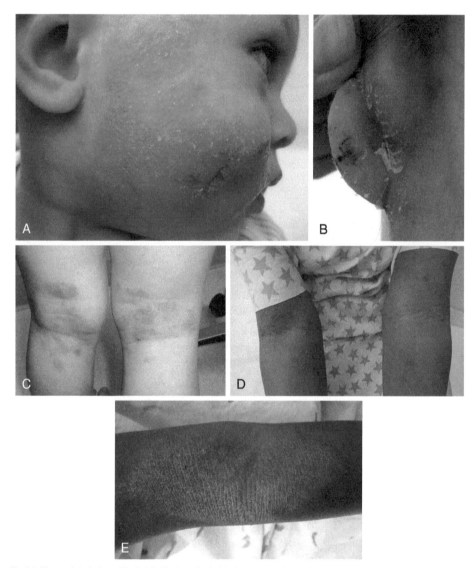

Fig. 8.1 Phases of atopic dermatitis. **A,** Infantile phase. Typical erythematous, oozing, and crusted plaque seen on the cheek of an infant with atopic dermatitis. **B,** Infantile/childhood phase. Scaly, crusted, fissured erythematous patches in postauricular sulcus and at earlobe insertion. **C** and **D,** Childhood phase. Pink, scaly, crusted patches in the popliteal and antecubital fossae. **E,** Adolescent/young adult phase. Lichenified, dry antecubital plaque in an adolescent.

occurrence if breast-fed versus formula fed. Antigen avoidance diets for nursing mothers are not currently recommended.

17. Does avoidance of certain foods prevent AD?

   Numerous studies have failed to demonstrate food allergy causality of AD. Similarly, dietary restriction has not been shown to prevent AD. Food allergy testing is generally not recommended in AD patients unless directed by a pertinent history of suspect food exposure and allergic symptoms. Food elimination diets attempting to effect AD control in children have been reported to lead to impaired growth and development; extreme diet restriction has resulted in kwashiorkor and marasmus. In contrast, early introduction of foods, including peanut, may increase tolerance and lower food allergy risk.

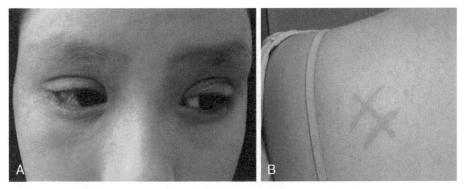

Fig. 8.2 Atopic dermatitis–associated skin findings. **A,** Dennie-Morgan pleats—lower eyelid edema and lichenification resulting in appearance of additional transverse skin folds. **B,** Dermatographism from stroking skin with cotton applicator stick.

18. Are skin infections a concern with AD?

Secondary infection is the most common complication of AD due to the disrupted epidermal barrier and dysfunctional immune response. Protective skin antimicrobial peptide levels are reduced in AD, in part due to production inhibition by inflammatory cytokines. AD children are colonized with *Staphylococcus aureus* three times as often as non-AD children. Colonization as well as superinfection with *S. aureus* are thought to be a driver of AD disease in part due to superantigen stimulation (Fig. 8.3A). Treatment of suspected infection with antistaphylococcal antibiotics should include culture confirmation with antibiotic sensitivity. Dilute sodium hypochlorite (bleach) baths taken on a regular basis are widely accepted as a safe, effective therapy to decrease *S. aureus* colonization. Herpes simplex infection in AD—eczema herpeticum—is a feared complication with potential significant ocular and systemic morbidity. Intravenous antiviral therapy is frequently required in children afflicted with herpes simplex virus (HSV)–infected AD (Fig. 8.3B,C). Molluscum contagiosum also occurs more frequently in AD patients.

19. What are effective treatments for AD?

- Avoid triggers!
- Moisturize by hydration of the skin and immediate application of moisturizers after bathing. Moisturizers containing ceramides, glycerin, and dimethicone have shown benefit in AD patients. Ointments and thick creams are more effective in barrier protection than lotions. White petrolatum is a very effective and low-cost moisturizer in children who typically tolerate the "greasy" feeling better than adults.
- Optimal bathing frequency and duration are unclear. Expert opinion generally recommends up to once-daily bathing to remove serous crust as long as moisturizers are applied immediately after bathing and bathing is of short duration. Excessively warm water temperatures should be avoided.
- Limit soap use to mild, unscented soaps on hairy or oily areas.
- Wear 100% cotton clothing when possible with attention to coverage of affected areas.
- Humidifier use to keep ambient humidity between 35% and 40% may help with pruritus.
- Topical corticosteroids are the treatment of choice for subacute or chronic lesions.
- Twice-daily use of corticosteroids is recommended but has been shown to be only minimally more effective than once-daily use. Application in the evening may have more benefit than morning application.
- Corticosteroids can safely be used on skin colonized by bacteria.
- Use the lowest strength topical steroid required to achieve inflammation and pruritus relief. High-potency topical steroids may be used to achieve rapid control if needed; lower strength topical therapies should be instituted when skin improvement is seen. Use occlusive vehicles (ointments, emollient creams) on dry and/or exposed lesions.
- For acutely inflamed and weeping skin, wet-wrap dressings are soothing, antipruritic, cleansing, hydrating, and cooling. Application of a topical corticosteroid as the base topical treatment enhances effectiveness.
- Topical calcineurin inhibitors (TCIs), for example, tacrolimus and pimecrolimus, are effective immunomodulator therapies. U.S. Food and Drug Administration guidelines recommend limiting use to 2 years of age and older, and the products are labeled with a black box warning regarding theoretical increased risk of lymphoproliferative disorders with use. TCIs should not be used in Netherton's syndrome due to high transcutaneous absorption. Crisaborale, a PDE-4 inhibitor, has shown promise in chronic eczema control; stinging and tingling with application can be problematic.
- If secondary impetiginization is evident, skin bacterial culture is indicated. Appropriate limited antibiotic therapy should be judiciously used if infection is suspected. Alternatively, dilute bleach baths may be sufficient antimicrobial therapy and can be used for decolonization maintenance.

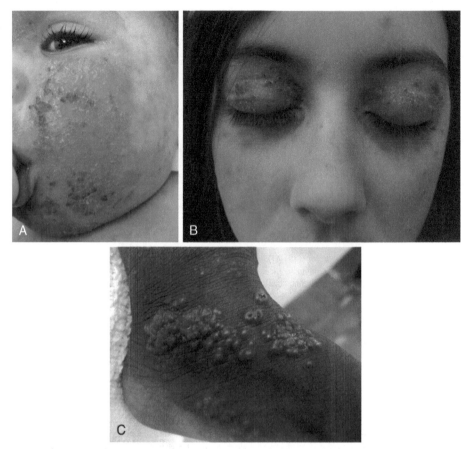

Fig. 8.3 A, Crusted, secondary impetiginized eczema. **B,** Periocular eczema herpeticum in an adolescent girl. **C,** Eczema herpeticum due to herpes simplex virus type 1 (HSV-1) on the foot of a toddler. Note umbilicated and eroded vesicles, typical for HSV cutaneous infection.

- Severe and recalcitrant AD may require systemic treatment with cyclosporine, azathioprine, methotrexate, mycophenolate mofetil, or dupilumab.
- Skin-directed phototherapy, specifically narrowband UVB 311 nm, is an effective treatment for more severe cases of AD and provides excellent pruritus relief.

20. **Describe wet-wrap therapy**
    An effective method for enhancing the penetration and effectiveness of topical anti-inflammatory medications to areas of widespread dermatitis is wet-wrap therapy, also known as "two-pajama treatment" (a type of wet-to-damp dressing especially suited for young children).
    - At bedtime, take two pairs of cotton pajamas and soak one pair in warm water.
    - Apply a mild- or moderate-strength topical corticosteroid to involved skin immediately after bathing.
    - Don the wet (wrung-out) pajamas.
    - Put the dry pair on top of the wet pair and wear while sleeping.
    - Upon waking, remove pajamas, bathe, apply moisturizers, and get dressed.
    - Modify this therapy as the "two-socks," "two-gloves," "two-caps," "two-shirts," or "two-pants" treatment as the distribution of lesions dictates.
    - A modification of the wet-wrap method used for adolescents and adults is to don a sauna suit or nylon exercise suit over the wet cotton layer directly in contact with the skin and topical steroid therapy. The trapped body heat enhances penetration of topical therapy and emollients. Caution should be exercised in those patients with heat intolerance or cardiovascular compromise. Sauna suit use duration should not exceed 8 hours per treatment.

21. Is "hand dermatitis" a specific diagnosis?

The term "hand dermatitis" is used generically to indicate an eczematous eruption on the palmar surface. Irritant and allergic contact dermatoses, id reactions, AD, psoriasis/eczema overlap, and infection can all appear similar with eczematous changes to the palms.

22. What is acute palmoplantar eczema?

Acute palmoplantar eczema accounts for up to 20% of hand dermatitis. It has also been called dyshidrotic eczema, pompholyx, and acute vesiculobullous hand eczema. Eighty percent of patients develop crops of clear, deep-seated, tapioca-like vesicles on the palms and sides of the fingers (Fig. 8.4). Another 10% also have sole involvement, whereas the remaining 10% have only sole involvement. Erythema may be absent, and heat and prickling sensations may precede attacks. Nails may become dystrophic. Pruritus may be intense. Contact dermatitis and id reaction should be explored if clinically indicated as potential etiologies.

23. How can acute palmoplantar eczema be managed?

Most attacks resolve spontaneously within 1 to 3 weeks. Protective gloves, bland emollients, and 15-minute soaks twice daily containing 0.25% acetic acid are beneficial. Bullae and large blisters can be lanced with a scalpel blade or medical needle to relieve pain and pruritus. Potent topical corticosteroids can be used with or without occlusion for moderate or severe acute disease. Soaking hands in warm water before applying superpotent steroids and then applying white cotton gloves overnight is especially helpful. Periodically, systemic corticosteroids are indicated for symptomatic relief. Steroid-sparing agents such as cyclosporine, dapsone, and methotrexate are potential therapies in recalcitrant disease. Keratolytics, tar, and bath PUVA can help chronic and/or hyperkeratotic disease.

24. Describe the typical presentation of nummular eczema (nummular dermatitis)

Nummular dermatitis presents as an abrupt onset of small edematous papules and vesicles forming erythematous, 1- to 10-cm diameter, coin-shaped (i.e., nummular) plaques with overlying vesicles and erosions on a background of dry skin (Fig. 8.5). Plaques may develop central clearing mimicking tinea corporis. Nummular dermatitis plaques are intensely pruritic, occurring most often on the lower legs in a symmetric bilateral fashion. Lesions may reoccur in the same locations. The upper extremities and trunk are involved less frequently.

25. How is nummular dermatitis treated?

Mid-potent to super-potent topical corticosteroids are the primary treatment. Limiting baths and soap exposure, avoiding irritants, frequent use of moisturizers, minimizing scratching, and avoiding dry environments all have a role in treatment. Monitoring for secondary impetiginization with *Staphylococcus aureus* or Group A beta-hemolytic *Streptococcus* is warranted in unresponsive disease. Infection should be treated with antistaphylococcal and streptococcal antimicrobials. Maintenance skin decolonization with dilute sodium hypochlorite (bleach) washes/baths can be a very effective management tool. Topical antibiotics should be used with caution due to increased risk of allergic contact dermatitis in this population. Systemic steroids are infrequently used in the management of nummular dermatitis. Prolonged flares may require steroid-sparing systemic therapy. Severe chronic cases may also benefit from phototherapy.

26. How does seborrheic dermatitis present in children?

Scalp seborrheic dermatitis is the most common manifestation in the infant, typically presenting in early infancy (Fig. 8.6A). The primary scalp lesions are round to oval patches of dry scales or yellowish-brown, greasy crusts with variable erythema. Napkin dermatitis or seborrheic dermatitis of the diaper area presents with dull salmon-colored, greasy scaled patches in the genital area, often with involvement of the inguinal crease. Seborrheic dermatitis presents in infants 2 to 10 weeks of age and generally clears by 8 to 12 months of age before reappearing at puberty. Seborrheic dermatitis occurs in areas of increased sebum production and at developmental stages of increased androgen production.

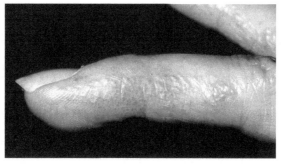

Fig. 8.4 Acute palmoplantar eczema. Characteristic "tapioca" vesicles on the sides of the fingers.

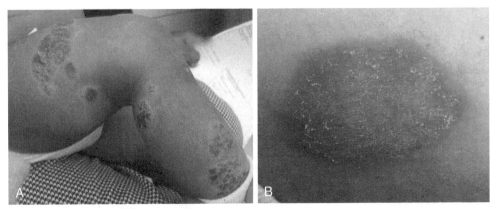

Fig. 8.5 Nummular dermatitis. **A,** Lower extremity circular-shaped lesions in a young child. **B,** Close-up of coin-shaped lesions of nummular dermatitis, also known as discoid eczema.

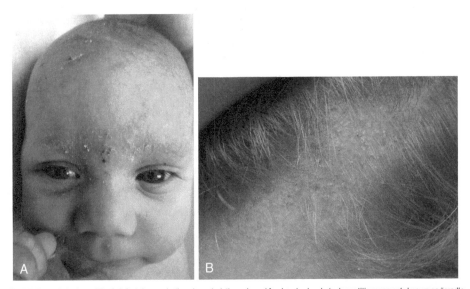

Fig. 8.6 Seborrheic dermatitis. **A,** Infant demonstrating characteristic scalp and forehead seborrheic dermatitis commonly known as "cradle cap." **B,** Adolescent scalp seborrheic dermatitis with diffuse greasy scale.

27. How does seborrheic dermatitis present in adults?

Dandruff—visible scalp desquamation—is the precursor lesion. The scalp may become inflamed and covered with greasy scale (Fig. 8.6B). Dull or yellowish-red, sharply marginated, nonpruritic lesions, covered with greasy scales are seen in areas with a rich supply of sebaceous glands. Characteristically, the medial eyebrows, glabella, melolabial folds, nasofacial sulci, and eyelid margins (blepharitis) are involved. Preauricular cheeks, postauricular sulci, and external auditory canal lesions are also commonly affected sites. The trunk may demonstrate presternal or interscapular involvement. Intertriginous areas, such as the inframammary creases, umbilicus, and genitocrural folds, are occasionally involved. Seborrheic dermatitis is one of the most common causes of chronic dermatitis of the anogenital area.

28. What is the etiology of seborrheic dermatitis?

It is believed that seborrheic dermatitis is due to an exuberant immune response to the commensal lipophilic yeast *Malassezia* (which lives in hair follicles) and/or sebum.

29. Is seborrheic dermatitis associated with other disease states?

An increased incidence and severity of seborrheic dermatitis are seen in persons with central nervous system (CNS) diseases such as Parkinson's disease, facial paralysis, poliomyelitis, syringomyelia, and quadriplegia. The CNS may stimulate increased rates of sebum production. HIV-infected individuals frequently demonstrate severe seborrheic dermatitis.

30. Discuss the treatment approaches to seborrheic dermatitis

- Goal of treatment is maintenance, as cure is not possible.
- Wash hair and scalp three to four times weekly with anti-*Malassezia* shampoos containing ketoconazole, selenium sulfide, or zinc pyrithione.
- For scalp with moderate scale, use scale-debriding shampoos containing keratolytics, such as tar or salicylic acid.
- For extremely thick scalp scale, massage Baker's P&S Liquid or fluocinolone oil into the scalp at bedtime, cover scalp with a swimming/shower cap overnight, then gently remove scale by combing out debris the following morning. Follow with antifungal shampoo. A loop of pantyhose or burn netting placed over the scalp cap will help keep the cap in place during sleep.
- Apply medium- to superpotent corticosteroid scalp lotions or foams (e.g., clobetasol, betamethasone, fluocinonide, fluocinolone, etc.) to the scalp after shampooing for inflammation reduction.
- For blepharitis, use warm water compresses, gentle cleansing with diluted nonirritating shampoo (such as baby shampoo), and topical sodium sulfacetamide ointment.
- Treat the face and trunk with mild topical steroids, TCIs, or antiyeast products.

31. Define the "id reaction."

Autosensitization dermatitis, commonly known as an id reaction, is an immunologically mediated cutaneous eruption in the absence of local infection or inciting agent. It presents as acute, monomorphous, papulovesicular dermatitis distant to an area of primary dermatitis. It usually erupts symmetrically on the hands, forearms, flexor aspects of the arms, extensor aspects of the arms and thighs, and, less commonly, on the face and trunk. In dermatologic usage, "id" derives from a Greek suffix for "offspring of" or "resemblance."

32. What are the most common settings for an id reaction and how should you treat it?

Chronic allergic contact dermatitis, stasis dermatitis, scabies, and dermatophyte infections (Fig. 8.7) are the most common settings. Nickel-based allergic contact dermatitis is a common cause in the pediatric population. The morphology of id reaction lesions is similar to that of primary dermatitis. Treatment of the underlying cause of the autosensitization reaction is primary. Many id reactions require symptomatic treatment with antipruritics, acetic acid soaks, potent topical corticosteroids, and, frequently, systemic corticosteroids.

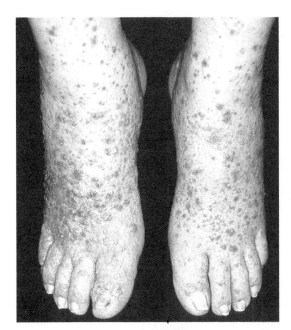

Fig. 8.7 Severe papulosquamous id reaction of the lower legs secondary to a severe dermatophyte infection. (Courtesy James E. Fitzpatrick, MD.)

33. What is a generalized eczematous dermatitis?

Exfoliative dermatitis or *erythroderma* is a generalized erythematous dermatitis that involves over 90% of the body surface. Erythrodermic patients may be ill-appearing, with systemic symptoms including hypo/hyperthermia, chills, pruritus, malaise, arthralgias, and anorexia, and in severe cases, cardiovascular compromise (Fig. 8.8).

34. What is the etiology of exfoliative dermatitis?

Erythroderma can be due to a multitude of causes including exacerbation of existing known dermatoses. Unfortunately, many times, the etiology of this serious skin eruption remains unknown. History and skin biopsy are helpful aids in making a diagnosis. Exfoliative dermatitis is most common in adults over age 40 but can occur in infants and children due to staphylococcal scalded skin syndrome, congenital ichthyoses, AD, and drug reaction (see Tables 8.3 and 8.4).

35. What general treatment measures are used to treat patients with exfoliative dermatitis?
- Treat the underlying disorder, if identified.
- Wet-wrap dressings with triamcinolone 0.1% cream often rapidly improve most cases of exfoliative dermatitis.
- Address systemic comorbidities: hypothermia, dehydration, high-output cardiac failure, and hypotension.
- Identify potential causative drugs. Stop all nonessential medications.
- Systemic corticosteroids may be of benefit but should be used with caution, as they may exacerbate the underlying etiology, for example, psoriasis and staphylococcal scalded skin syndrome.
- Phototherapy may be helpful in some cases, for example, psoriasis or AD.
- Treat secondary infection.

KEY POINTS: DERMATITIS

- The terms *atopic dermatitis* and *eczema* are used interchangeably.
- Skin barrier dysfunction is a basic component of AD pathophysiology.
- Barrier repair/skin moisturization and topical corticosteroid application are the mainstays of atopic dermatitis treatment.
- Wet-wrap dressings with topical corticosteroids are rapid, effective therapy for moderate-to-severe forms of dermatitis.
- Null filaggrin mutation is seen in over half of moderate and severe atopic dermatitis.
- Systemic nonsedating antihistamines have not been shown to be of benefit in AD management.
- New targeted therapies to inflammatory cascade molecules, e.g., IL-4 and IL-13, show great promise for severe atopic dermatitis.

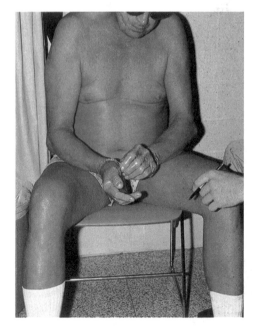

Fig. 8.8 Exfoliative dermatitis. Patient with full-body erythroderma of unknown cause. Note the normal hand for comparison. (Courtesy Fitzsimons Army Medical Center teaching files.)

Table 8.3 Adult erythroderma etiologies

1. Common
   a. Exacerbation of underlying dermatoses—psoriasis, atopic dermatitis, seborrheic dermatitis
   b. Drug reaction—antibiotics, aromatic ring anticonvulsants, allopurinol, etc.
   c. Idiopathic—typically elderly men
2. Uncommon
   a. Cutaneous T-cell lymphoma (CTCL)
   b. Paraneoplastic
   c. Pityriasis rubra pilaris
   d. Autoimmune bullous disease—bullous pemphigoid, pemphigus vulgaris, paraneoplastic pemphigus
   e. Dermatitis—allergic contact, actinic, stasis
   f. Id reaction—dermatophyte infection, allergic contact
3. Rare
   a. Immunodeficiencies, graft vs. host disease (GVHD), connective tissue disease, hypereosinophilic syndrome, papuloerythroderma of Ofuji, congenital ichthyoses

Table 8.4 Child and infant erythroderma etiologies

1. Genodermatoses
   a. Chondrodysplasia punctata
   b. Netherton's syndrome
   c. Epidermolytic hyperkeratosis
   d. Congenital ichthyosiform erythroderma
   e. Sjögren-Larsson syndrome
   f. Autosomal recessive congenital ichthyoses
2. Infection
   a. Staphylococcal scaled skin syndrome
   b. Herpes simplex
   c. Candida/other fungal
   d. Syphilis
3. Inflammatory dermatoses
   a. Atopic dermatitis
   b. Seborrheic dermatitis
   c. Psoriasis
   d. Diffuse cutaneous mastocytosis
   e. Pityriasis rubra pilaris
   f. Acute generalized exanthematous pustulosis (AGEP)
4. 4. Metabolic disease/nutritional deficiency
5. 5. Immunodeficiency
   a. Severe combined immunodeficiency (SCID)
   b. DiGeorge syndrome
   c. Wiskott-Aldrich syndrome
   d. Chronic granulomatous disease
   e. Hyperimmunoglobulin E syndrome
   f. Dock-8 deficiency

BIBLIOGRAPHY

Blattner CM, Murase JE. A practice gap in pediatric dermatology: does breast-feeding prevent the development of infantile atopic dermatitis? *J Am Acad Dermatol.* 2014;71:405–406.

Du Toit G, Roberts G, Sayre PH, et al. Randomized trial of peanut consumption in infants at risk for peanut allergy. *N Engl J Med.* 2015;372 (9):803–813.

Eichenfield LF, Tom WL, Chamlin SL, et al. AAD Work Group. Guidelines of care for the management of atopic dermatitis: section 1. Diagnosis and assessment of atopic dermatitis. *J Am Acad Dermatol.* 2014;70:338–351.

Eichenfield LF, Tom WL, Berger TG, et al. Guidelines of care for the management of atopic dermatitis. Section 2. Management and treatment of atopic dermatitis with topical therapies. *J Am Acad Dermatol.* 2014;71:116–132.

Flohr C, Yeo L. Atopic dermatitis and the hygiene hypothesis revisited. *Curr Prob Dermatol.* 2011;41:1–34.

Lloyd-Lavery A, Rogers N, Davies E, et al. What's new in atopic eczema? An analysis of systematic reviews published in 2015. Part 2: prevention and treatment. *Clin Exp Dermatol.* 2018;43:653–658.

Mayba J, Gooderham M. Review of atopic dermatitis and topical therapies. *J Cutan Med Surg.* 2017;21(3):227–236.

Pavlis J, Yosipovitch G. Management of itch in atopic dermatitis. *Am J Clin Dermatol.* 2018;19:319–332.

Seger E, Wechter T, Stowd L, Feldman S. Relative efficacy of systemic treatments for atopic dermatitis. *J Am Acad Dermatol.* 2019;80:411–416.

Sidbury R, Davis DM, Cohen DE, et al. Guidelines of care for the management of atopic dermatitis. Section 3. Management and treatment with phototherapy and systemic agents. *J Am Acad Dermatol.* 2014;71:327–349.

Sidbury R, Kodama S. Atopic dermatitis guidelines: diagnosis, systemic therapy, and adjunctive care. *Clin Dermatol.* 2018;36:648–652.

Silverberg J. Public health burden and epidemiology of atopic dermatitis. *Dermatol Clin.* 2017;35:283–289.

Simpson E, Irvine A, Eichenfield L, Freidlander S. Update on epidemiology, diagnosis, and disease course of atopic dermatitis. *Semin Cutan Med Surg.* 2016;35(suppl 5):S84–S88.

Spergel JM. From atopic dermatitis to asthma: the atopic march. *Ann Allergy Asthma Immunol.* 2010;105(2):99–106.

Yang E, Sekhon S, Sanchez I, et al. Recent developments in atopic dermatitis. *Pediatrics.* 2018;142:1–12.

CHAPTER 9

CONTACT DERMATITIS

Leslie A. Stewart

1. **Name the two pathogenic types of contact dermatitis.**
   Contact dermatitis refers to cutaneous inflammation resulting from the interaction of an external agent and the skin. These reactions occur through one of two mechanisms: a nonimmunologic irritant contact dermatitis (ICD) or an immunologic allergic contact dermatitis (ACD). ICD accounts for 80% of all reactions, while ACD is responsible for approximately 20%. Although over 3700 substances have been identified as contact allergens, almost any substance, under the right circumstances, can act as an irritant. It is important to note that irritating compounds can be allergenic, and allergenic compounds can be irritating.

2. **Name the two subtypes of ICD and describe them.**
   ICD can be divided into acute toxic and cumulative insult subtypes. Acute toxic eruptions occur from a single exposure to a strong toxic chemical, such as an acid or alkali, inducing erythema, vesicles, bullae, or skin sloughing. Reactions occur within minutes to hours after exposure, localize to the areas of maximal contact, and have sharp borders. In most cases, healing occurs soon after exposure. Chronic cumulative insult reactions are the more common type of ICD. These are due to multiple exposures of many low-level irritants, such as soaps and shampoos, over time. This dermatitis may take weeks, months, or even years to appear. It is characterized by erythema, scaling, fissuring, pruritus, lichenification, and poor demarcation from the surrounding skin.

3. **Explain the pathogenesis of ACD.**
   ACD is a type IV, delayed, cell-mediated, hypersensitivity reaction. Initially, a low-molecular-weight antigen hapten (<500 Da) contacts the skin and forms a hapten–carrier protein complex. This complex then associates itself with an epidermal Langerhans cell, which presents the complete antigen to a T-helper cell, causing the release of various mediators. Subsequently, T-cell expansion occurs in regional lymph nodes, producing specific memory and T-effector lymphocytes, which circulate in the general bloodstream. T_H1 was thought to be the main ACD mediator, but recent evidence suggests specific haptens such as fragrances can activate the T_H2 pathway. This whole process of sensitization occurs in approximately 5 to 21 days.

   Upon re-exposure to the specific antigen, there is proliferation of activated T cells, mediator release, and migration of cytotoxic T cells, resulting in cutaneous eczematous inflammation at the site of contact. This elicitation phase occurs within 48 to 72 hours after exposure. Because many allergens are irritants, preceding irritation is common and may enhance allergen absorption. In contrast to irritant reactions, relatively small concentrations of an allergen can be enough to elicit an inflammatory reaction. Acute ACD may have erythema, edema, and vesicle formation. Chronic ACD reactions are scaly, erythematous, and possibly lichenified and can mimic chronic ICD. Table 9.1 compares ACD and ICD.

Smith JS, Rajagopal S, Atwater AR. Chemokine signaling in allergic contact dermatitis: toward targeted therapies. *Dermatitis*. 2018; 29:179–186.
Kaplan DH, Igyártó BZ, Gaspari AA. Early immune events in the induction of allergic contact dermatitis. *Nat Rev Immunol*. 2012;12: 114–124.

4. **Can urticarial reactions occur from contact with a substance?**
   Occasionally, urticarial reactions may occur with certain exposures, instead of the eczematous changes seen with ACD and ICD (Fig. 9.1A). Allergic contact urticaria involves a specific IgE–mast cell interaction, resulting in the release of vasoactive compounds. While urticaria occurs at the site of contact, more generalized symptoms can appear, including angioedema, anaphylaxis, rhinoconjunctivitis, and widespread urticaria. A good example is the latex glove immediate reaction seen in health care professionals. Nonimmunologic contact urticaria occurs secondary to a non–antibody-mediated release of vasoactive mediators or due to a direct effect on the cutaneous vasculature. Many agents found in cosmetic products can cause a nonimmunologic contact urticaria. These include sorbic acid, benzoic acid, and cinnamic acid. This may explain the facial burning and stinging that some patients experience using cosmetics. To diagnose contact urticaria, a prick test is usually performed. In this test, a small amount of the allergen is placed on the skin, and a needle is used to prick the skin. An urticarial wheal of appropriate size constitutes a positive test, usually developing within 15 to 20 minutes after allergen administration (Fig. 9.1B).

Table 9.1 Comparison of irritant and allergic contact dermatitis

	IRRITANT	ALLERGIC
Examples	Water, soap	Nickel, fragrance, hair dye
Number of compounds	Many	Fewer
Distribution of reaction	Localized	May spread beyond area of maximal contact and become generalized
Concentration of agent needed to elicit reaction	High	Can be minute
Time course	Immediate to late	Sensitization in 2 weeks; elicitation takes 24–72 hours
Immunology	Nonspecific	Specific type IV delayed hypersensitivity reaction
Diagnostic test	None	Patch test

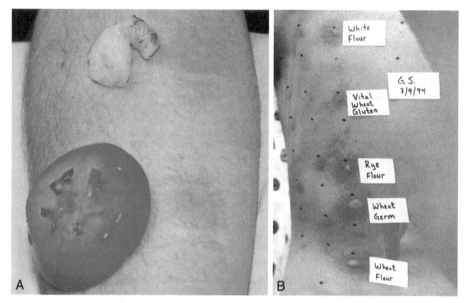

Fig. 9.1 A, Contact urticaria to shrimp and tomato. **B,** Prick test for the diagnosis of contact urticaria. The patient was a baker, allergic to flours and wheat.

5. Why is the distribution of a contact dermatitis rash important?

The location and distribution of the dermatitis are vital clues to the underlying culprit (Table 9.2), and the dermatitis is often most pronounced at the site of contact. For example, an eczematous dermatitis on the dorsal feet should alert the clinician to the possibility of shoe dermatitis (Fig. 9.2A). Hands are the most frequent site of ACD, followed closely by the face and a generalized patchy involvement.

6. List four common misperceptions regarding the location of a contact dermatitis.

1. Dermatitis must be bilateral if the exposure is bilateral, as, for example, with a shoe or glove allergy. In most cases, contact reactions tend to be patchy and do not have the same intensity at all sites of exposure.
2. The rash of contact dermatitis occurs only at the site of maximal contact. Allergic reactions frequently spread beyond the site of greatest contact and can even become generalized. Transfer dermatitis can also occur where an allergen can be spread to distant sites of contact. The classic example is when nail polish is spread to the eyelid, inducing dermatitis when a sensitized patient rubs her eyelids with her fingernails.
3. Contact dermatitis does not affect the palms and soles because of their thick stratum corneum. Although it is true that other, more sensitive areas such as the eyelids, face, and genitalia are more likely to be reactive, contact dermatitis should be considered when dealing with an eczematous dermatitis of the palms or soles.

Table 9.2 Location of contact dermatitis and suspicious agents

LOCATION	SUSPICIOUS AGENT
Eyelids	Nail polish, eye makeup, antiaging creams, airborne allergens
Earlobes or neck	Metal jewelry
Forehead, scalp margins	Hair dyes, shampoos
Face	Cosmetic fragrances and preservatives, airborne allergens
Axilla	Deodorants
Hands	Gloves, occupational contacts
Waistband	Elastic
Dorsal feet	Shoes

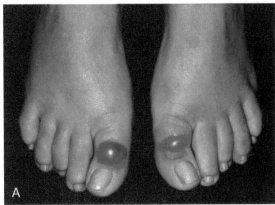

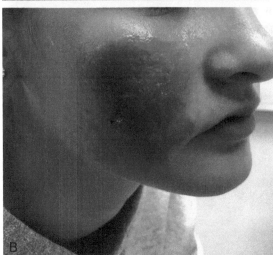

Fig. 9.2 A, Bullous allergic contact dermatitis on the dorsal surface of the big toes due to the rubber in the patient's footwear. *(Courtesy Fitzsimons Army Medical Center teaching files.)* **B,** Acute irritant contact dermatitis due to contact with caustic paint on the cheek and scrubbing with a washcloth.

4.   Patients must be using a new product in order for it to be suspicious for ACD. In reality, many people touch a substance for years before an allergy develops. Environmental factors can also play a role. With preceding irritation or sweating over time, the allergen absorption into the skin is enhanced.

7. How is patch testing done?

Because ICD and ACD can be indistinguishable both clinically and histologically, epicutaneous patch testing is the only method available to diagnose ACD and differentiate it from ICD. Two patch test methods are currently in widespread use: the chamber (Finn) method (Fig. 9.3A) and True Test systems (Fig. 9.3B). With the chamber method, a small amount of the allergen, usually in a petrolatum vehicle, is placed into individual polyethylene plastic or polypropylene-coated aluminum wells affixed to a strip of paper tape. With the True Test method, no advance preparation is necessary, as the allergens have already been commercially incorporated into the back of the paper tape strips. Only 35 "screening" allergens are currently available with the True Test, while hundreds are available with the chamber method. These strips are applied to the patient's upper back, which is the preferred testing site. After 48 hours, the patches are removed and the initial reading is recorded. Because these allergic reactions are delayed, a second interpretation must be performed optimally at 96 hours, or even at 1 week after the initial test application. Additional readings beyond 48 hours increase the positive patch test yield by 34%. The classic positive allergic patch test reaction shows spreading erythema, edema, and closely set vesicles that persist after removal of the patch or that appear after 2 to 7 days. Irritant reactions may have a glazed, scalded, follicular, or pustular appearance that usually fades after the patch is removed. It is important to delay patch testing until any acute inflammation has subsided in areas of patch test application. Otherwise, an "Angry Back" phenomenon can occur where the dermatitis flares, inducing many false-positive reactions to manifest. Topical steroids should not be used on the back 1 to 2 weeks prior to testing, as it may suppress positive reactions. A suntan can also decrease a patch test response. Immunomodulators are not an absolute contraindication for patch testing. However, the lowest possible dose of the drug should be used. Many theorize that the high dose per unit of allergen in patch testing is strong enough to exceed the threshold to elicit a delayed hypersensitivity reaction and overcome the immunosuppressive effect of the immunomodulator drug.

Davis MD, Bhate K, Rholinger Al, et al. Delayed patch test reading after 5 days: the Mayo Clinic experience. *J Am Acad Dermatol.* 2008; 59:225–233.
Rosmarin D, Gottlieb A, Aarch A, Scheinman P. Patch testing on systemic immunosuppressants. *Dermatitis.* 2009;20:265–270.

8. What substances are tested in the standard "screening" patch test?

Because of its convenience, most patients with a suspected ACD are patch tested with the True Test "standard" panel of 35 allergens (Table 9.3). However, this panel only detects anywhere from 28% to 50% of the most common allergens. The American Contact Dermatitis Society's Core Allergen Series tray of 80 allergens, which utilizes the chamber method, is a more efficacious screening series than more limited patch test series. The series contains suggested allergen groups that can be logically scaled up or down depending on the individual case. In comparisons of

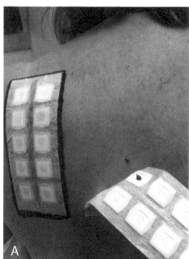
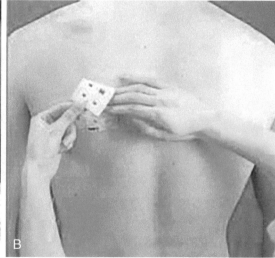

Fig. 9.3 A, Finn chamber method. **B,** True Test method.

Table 9.3 Allergens evaluated by the True Test

ALLERGEN	SOURCES
Nickel sulfate	Metal jewelry
Wool alcohols	Topical skin care products
Neomycin sulfate	Topical antibiotics
Potassium dichromate	Leather, cement
Caine mix	Topical anesthetic
Fragrance mix	Perfume, flavors
Colophony (rosin)	Adhesives, solder flux
Paraben mix	Cosmetic preservative
Balsam of Peru	Perfume, flavors, medications
Ethylenediamine dihydrochloride	Topical medications
Cobalt dichloride	Metal jewelry, paint
p-tert-Butylphenol formaldehyde resin	Glues
Epoxy resin	Glues, plastics
Carba mix	Rubber, fungicide
Black rubber mix	Black rubber
$Cl^+ Me^-$ isothiazoline (MCI/MI)	Cosmetic and industrial preservative
Quaternium 15	Cosmetic and industrial preservative
Methyldibromoglutaronitrile	Cosmetic and industrial preservative
p-Phenylenediamine	Hair dye
Formaldehyde	Preservative, fabric finishes
Mercapto mix	Rubber, fungicide
Thimerosal	Cosmetic and medicament preservative
Thiuram mix	Rubber, fungicide
Diazolidinyl urea	Cosmetic preservative
Quinoline mix	Topical antibacterial medicaments
Tixocortol 21-pivalate	Topical corticosteroid
Gold sodium thiosulfate	Gold jewelry, dental gold
Imidazolidinyl urea	Cosmetic preservative
Budesonide	Topical corticosteroid
Hydrocortisone-17-butyrate	Topical corticosteroid
Mercaptobenzothiazole	Rubber
Bacitracin	Topical antibiotics
Parthenolide	Plants (feverfew), herbal creams or tablets
Disperse Blue 106	Dark blue textile dye
2-Bromo-2-nitropropane-1,3-diol (Bronopol)	Cosmetic preservative

"standard trays" with fewer than 30 allergens and more than 60 allergens, the smaller series only completely evaluated 28% of those tested. Additional testing with more specialized allergen panels is frequently warranted to enhance allergen detection. Using supplemental allergen screening trays can increase diagnostic accuracy by 34%. Testing should only be done with known materials in accepted concentrations. Therefore, a negative patch test session does not necessarily mean the patient does not have ACD. Additional, patch testing may be warranted.

Schalock PC, Dunnick CA, Nedorost S, et al. American Contact Dermatitis Society Core Allergen Series. *Dermatitis.* 2013;24:7–9.
DeKoven JG, Warshaw EM, Zug KA, et al. North American Contact Dermatitis Group Patch Test results 2015–2016. *Dermatitis.* 2018; 29:297–309.

KEY POINTS: CONTACT DERMATITIS

1. Eighty percent of contact dermatitis reactions are due to irritation and 20% are due to allergic causes.
2. The location of the dermatitis can help identify the causative agent.
3. Patch testing is the only way to distinguish between allergic and irritant contact dermatitis.
4. Allergic contact dermatitis is frequently patchy and can spread beyond the site of maximal contact.
5. Allergen and irritant avoidance, moisturization, and topical medications are the keys to therapy.

9. **An astute physician should not need to patch test. Right?**
   Many clinicians believe that a thorough history and physical exam are sufficient for an accurate diagnosis of ACD. They believe that patch testing is unnecessary because they can tell whether a reaction is ICD or ACD simply by evaluating the dermatitis. The results of several studies, however, show that clinicians are often wrong when guessing whether contact dermatitis is irritant or allergic. In fact, experienced dermatologists may only suspect the true allergen in 50% of cases. Patch testing is the only way to differentiate between the two conditions because clinically and histologically, ICD and ACD cannot be reliably differentiated.

   Podmore P, Burrows D, Bingham EA. Prediction of patch test results. *Contact Dermatitis.* 1984;11:283–284.

10. **What is a repeated open application test (ROAT)?**
    The ROAT, or usage test, is used when patch testing is negative and yet there remains a strong clinical suspicion for ACD. Remember, patch testing is a one-time occlusive test that does not always duplicate low-level chronic daily exposure. With the ROAT, patients apply the suspected product to a quarter-sized area on the forearm twice a day for 2 weeks. If the patient is allergic, a localized dermatitis will occur, confirming the suspected allergy (Fig. 9.4).

11. **What is the differential diagnosis of contact dermatitis?**
    Contact dermatitis, with its scaling, erythema, lichenification, and/or vesicles, belongs in the group of eczematous disorders. Other such conditions—atopic dermatitis, nummular eczema, neurodermatitis, stasis dermatitis, seborrheic dermatitis, photodermatoses, dermatophyte infections, drug eruptions, cutaneous T-cell lymphoma, and dyshidrotic eczema (pompholyx)—should always be considered when evaluating a prospective patient for contact dermatitis. A complete history including previous skin diseases, drug and exposure histories, location and course of the eruption, patch testing, and potassium hydroxide tests should help point to the diagnosis of contact dermatitis.

12. **Which are some of the most common allergens on the standard tray?**
    Nickel, a metal found commonly in costume jewelry, is the most common allergen on the standard tray. Approximately 5.8% of the general population in the United States is sensitized, while patch test clinics around the country note a prevalence rate of 17.5% in their dermatitis populations (Fig. 9.5). The high rate of sensitization is felt to be secondary to ear piercing, which is why this allergy is more common in females. In men, nickel dermatitis is predominantly of occupational origin. Newer exposures are coming from technology, including phones, laptops, and tablets. The rest of

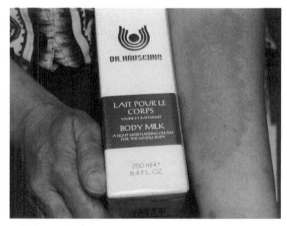

Fig. 9.4 Positive repeated open application test from a moisturizing cream.

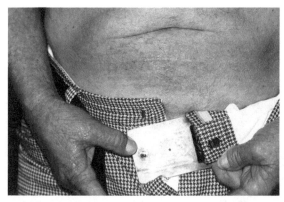

Fig. 9.5 Nickel allergic contact dermatitis on the patient's abdomen due to the presence of nickel in the metal buckle on his pants. The rash had been previously misdiagnosed as a nummular eczema.

the top 15 most frequent allergens include two topical antibiotics (neomycin and bacitracin), another metal (cobalt), three fragrances (fragrance mixes I and II and balsam of Peru) (Fig. 9.6), four preservatives found in cosmetics and toiletries (methylisothiazolinone, formaldehyde, methylchloroisothiazolinone/methylisothiazolinone, and iodopropynyl buylcarbamate), propylene glycol (emollient and emulsifier found in cosmetics, food and medications), lanolin alcohol (emollient), carba mix (rubber accelerator), and hair dye (paraphenylenediamine).

DeKoven JG, Warshaw EM, Zug KA, et al. North American Contact Dermatitis Group Patch Test results 2015–2016. *Dermatitis*. 2018; 29:297–309.

13. Is nickel the most common allergen overall?
    Poison ivy is the most common type IV allergen, with approximately 50% to 70% of the general population being sensitized.

14. What is the "allergen of the year"?
    The American Contact Dermatitis Society has an annual vote to draw attention to an allergen that physicians and patients need to be aware of. The allergen may be one that is increasing in importance, one that is underrecognized, or one that is very common (Table 9.4). However, in 2019 parabens was chosen as the "non allergen" of the year to highlight its excellent safety record and very low rate of sensitization. In 2020, isobornyl acrylate was chosen to recognize its importance as an adhesive allergen used in glucose sensors and insulin pumps.

15. If a change in a skin care product does not lead to clearing of a patient's rash, does this mean that the original product was not the culprit?
    Not necessarily. Many consumer cosmetic and toiletry products contain the same allergens (usually fragrances and preservatives). Moreover, many products contain cross-reacting agents that can exacerbate the original problem. For example, patients who are allergic to the hair dye allergen paraphenylenediamine will need to avoid the over-the-counter topical anesthetic benzocaine. Both compounds belong to the para-amino group and can cross-react with one another.

16. How is contact dermatitis managed?
    If the patient has ACD, the allergen should be detected by patch testing, and subsequently, it should be thoroughly avoided. Sources of the allergen as well as cross-reacting agents should be explained to the patient. An acceptable nonsensitizing substitute should be offered. The American Contact Dermatitis Society's Contact Allergen Management Program (CAMP) is a database that generates lists of personal care products that are free of the patient's individualized ingredients causing ACD. For ICD, avoidance of as many irritants as possible is crucial. Frequent water exposure, which desiccates and chaps the skin, should be kept to a minimum. Frequent moisturization and hand protection with gloves, if indicated, are important. With contact dermatitis, systemic steroids should be used only in acute situations. Compresses may be helpful if vesicles are present. When the condition is chronic, topical steroids of appropriate strength and moisturizers are the mainstay of therapy. Nonsteroidal topical macrolide immunosuppressive agents, tacrolimus and pimecrolimus, have been used increasingly, with good results. Lastly, phototherapy, systemic immunosuppressants, and Grenz ray therapy have also been used in difficult cases.

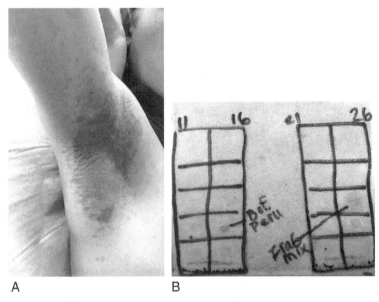

Fig. 9.6 A. Allergic contact dermatitis of the axilla due to fragrance in the patient's antiperspirant. **B,** Positive patch test reactions in this patient to fragrance screening agents, Balsam of Peru and Fragrance Mix.

Table 9.4 American Contact Dermatitis Society allergens of the year	
2000	Disperse blue dyes
2001	Gold
2002	Thimerosal
2003	Bacitracin
2004	Cocamidopropyl betaine
2005	Corticosteroids
2006	p-Phenylenediamine
2007	Fragrance
2008	Nickel
2009	Mixed dialkyl thioureas
2010	Neomycin
2011	Dimethylfumarate
2012	Acrylate
2013	Methylisothiazolinone
2014	Benzophenones
2015	Formaldehyde
2016	Cobalt
2017	Alkyl glucosides
2018	Propylene glycol
2019	"Non-allergen" parabens
2020	Isobornyl acrylate

VESICULOBULLOUS DISORDERS

Whitney A. High

CHAPTER 10

1. **What is the difference between a vesicle and a bulla?**
   Size. If a blister is less than 5 mm in diameter, it is referred to as a vesicle. If a blister is 5 mm or larger, it is called a bulla. Some dermatologists require bulla be 1 cm or larger. The term "vesiculobullous" may be used for blistering disorders, as it encompasses blisters of varying size.

2. **How are the bullous diseases defined?**
   Bullous diseases are characterized by blisters (skin lesions that contain fluid) that may arise at various depths in the epidermis and dermis. Often, the depth at which a blister forms can be used to classify the disorder. "Intraepidermal" refers to blisters that arise within the epidermis, while "subepidermal" refers to blisters that arise beneath the epidermis (Table 10.1). Some blistering disorders develop because of autoantibodies directed against a component of the epidermis or basement membrane zone ("autoimmune bullous conditions"), while others develop because of structural defects of skin components ("congenital blistering disorders"). Refer to Fig. 10.1 for the location of these components in normal skin, as they are discussed in the following questions.

3. **What things cause vesicles and bullae?**
   Blisters of the skin may be caused by a wide variety of external agents and/or diseases, including trauma, infections, metabolic disorders, genetic deficiencies, and inflammatory diseases, to name a few. Blisters caused by infections are discussed in Chapters 25 (viral) and 27 (bacterial).

4. **How do you approach a patient who presents with an acute onset of a vesiculobullous eruption?**
   History is important in the evaluation of a blistering skin disorder. Acute onset of blisters may suggest an exposure to a contact allergen, arthropod bites, phototoxic agents, or other drugs or chemicals, trauma, or infectious agents. Some chronic vesiculobullous diseases may have an acute onset, but then may persist or recur (Table 10.2).

5. **Which skin findings are helpful in evaluating a patient with blisters?**
   Important features of a blistering disorder include the skin distribution, assessment of symmetry, involvement of mucosal surfaces, and associated lesions (such as erosions, ulcers, and crusts). Other types of skin lesions, such as urticaria, should be sought. For example, in bullous pemphigoid (BP), urticarial lesions often precede the development of blisters. In some vesiculobullous diseases, such as dermatitis herpetiformis (DH), only excoriations may be present, without intact blisters.
   Characteristics of the blister may be important. Flaccid blisters may indicate a more superficial blistering process than is seen with tense blisters, but the anatomic site must also be considered. Blisters on acral skin, with a thick stratum corneum, may appear tense, even if superficial. In some other diseases, like toxic epidermal necrolysis, full-thickness sloughing of the skin can make it challenging to recognize vesiculation.

6. **Do particular vesiculobullous diseases occur in characteristic distributions?**
   DH is a disorder that affects chiefly the knees, elbow, buttock, and posterior scalp. Table 10.3 details some classic patterns of distribution.

Table 10.1 Intraepidermal versus subepidermal blisters

INTRAEPIDERMAL BLISTERS	SUBEPIDERMAL BLISTERS
Allergic contact dermatitis (spongiotic)	Porphyria cutanea tarda
Bullous dermatophyte infection (spongiotic)	Bullous pemphigoid
Herpes simplex (intraepidermal acantholytic)	Cicatricial pemphigoid
Herpes zoster/varicella (intraepidermal acantholytic)	Dermatitis herpetiformis
Bullous impetigo (subcorneal)	Linear IgA bullous dermatosis
Miliaria crystallina (subcorneal)	Bullous systemic lupus erythematosus (SLE)
Epidermolysis bullosa simplex (mechanobullous)	Epidermolysis bullosa acquisita
Pemphigus vulgaris (suprabasilar acantholytic)	Dystrophic epidermolysis bullosa
Pemphigus foliaceus (subcorneal acantholytic)	Junctional epidermolysis bullosa
Paraneoplastic pemphigus	Anti–p200 pemphigoid
Hailey-Hailey disease (intraepidermal acantholytic)	Anti–p105 pemphigoid
Incontinentia pigmenti (spongiotic)	
Epidermolytic ichthyosis (mechanobullous)	

STRUCTURAL COMPONENTS OF THE BASEMENT MEMBRANE ZONE

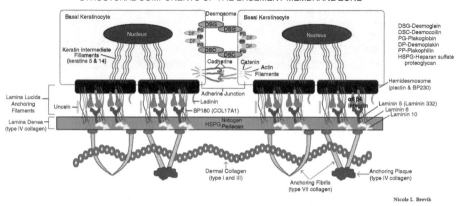

Fig. 10.1 Structural components of the basement membrane zone. *(Courtesy Nicole Fasano.)*

Table 10.2 Acute versus chronic onset of vesiculobullous eruption

ACUTE	CHRONIC
Allergic contact dermatitis	Bullous pemphigoid
Arthropod bites	Bullous systemic lupus erythematosus
Drug eruptions (may become chronic if drug is not withdrawn)	Cicatricial pemphigoid
Erythema multiforme (may recur, especially with herpes simplex)	Dermatitis herpetiformis
Hand, foot, and mouth disease	Epidermolysis bullosa acquisita
Herpes simplex	Linear immunoglobulin A bullous dermatosis
Varicella-zoster virus	Pemphigus foliaceus
Impetigo	Pemphigus vulgaris
Miliaria crystallina	Genetic blistering diseases
Physical-, thermal-, or chemical-induced blisters	
Toxic epidermal necrolysis	
Stevens-Johnson syndrome	

Table 10.3 Characteristic distribution of vesiculobullous diseases

DISEASE	CHARACTERISTIC DISTRIBUTION
Acrodermatitis enteropathica	Acral, periorificial
Allergic contact dermatitis	Reflects pattern of contact; often linear
Bullous dermatophyte infection	Feet, hands
Bullous diabeticorum	Distal extremities
Bullous pemphigoid	Flexural areas, lower extremities
Cicatricial pemphigoid	Eyes, mucous membranes
Dermatitis herpetiformis	Elbows, knees, buttocks
Erythema multiforme	Acral areas, palms, soles, mucosa
Hailey-Hailey disease	Intertriginous areas, neck
Hand, foot, and mouth disease	Mouth, palms, fingers, soles
Herpes zoster	Dermatomal distribution
Linear immunoglobulin A bullous dermatosis (childhood type)	Groin, buttocks, perineum
Pemphigus vulgaris	Oral mucosa, head, trunk, other sites
Pemphigus foliaceus	Head, neck, trunk

7. Which tests are most useful in evaluating vesiculobullous diseases?

Diagnostic tests for vesiculobullous eruptions are often performed on the blister itself. When infectious causes are considered, appropriate cultures (aerobic bacteria, viruses, fungi) may be obtained. Provider-performed microscopy, such as a Tzanck smear, can reveal multinucleate keratinocytes in *Herpes viridae* family infections. For noninfectious vesiculobullous diseases, a skin biopsy is often a useful test.

8. How should a skin biopsy of a vesiculobullous eruption be performed?

An early lesion should be biopsied to avoid secondary changes that can confound histologic examination. A small, intact blister is ideal, as the entire lesion and some of the surrounding skin can be removed intact, using a saucerization or excision technique. If a punch technique is employed, it is best to sample from the edge of the blister overlapping onto normal skin. The specimen should be placed in 10% neutral-buffered formalin (NBF) unless direct immunofluorescence studies are desired (see below). Appropriate clinical information, including the age/sex of the patient, a clinical description of the appearance and distribution of lesions, associated symptoms, exacerbating factors or relieving treatments, and a solid clinical differential diagnosis should be provided with the specimen.

9. When are special tests necessary to diagnose blistering diseases of the skin?

A skin biopsy for direct immunofluorescence may be helpful in including or excluding immunobullous diseases (Table 10.4). Direct immunofluorescent (DIF) technique uses special fluorescent antibodies directed against immunoglobulin G (IgG), IgA, IgM, C3, and fibrin that are detected in tissue with a special fluorescent microscope (Fig. 10.2). Immunofluorescent mapping, electron microscopy, or genetic studies may be necessary to diagnose some blistering conditions. Other tests to consider in special circumstances may include urine, serum, or stool porphyrin tests when porphyria is being considered or zinc levels, glucagon levels, or hepatitis panels when necrolytic erythemas are suspected.

van Beek N, Zillikens D, Schmidt E. Diagnosis of autoimmune bullous diseases. *J Dtsch Dermatol Ges.* 2018;16:1077–1091. https://doi.org/10.1111/ddg.13637.

Table 10.4 Direct immunofluorescence findings of vesiculobullous diseases

DISEASE	TARGET ANTIGEN	DIRECT IMMUNOFLUORESCENCE FINDINGS
Bullous pemphigoid	BP180, BP230	Linear C3, IgG at DEJ
Bullous SLE	COL7A1	Linear/granular IgG, other Igs at DEJ
Cicatricial pemphigoid	BP180, LAM5, and others	Linear C3, IgG, IgA at DEJ
Dermatitis herpetiformis	eTG	Granular IgA, C3 in upper dermis (see Fig. 10.1)
Epidermolysis bullosa acquisita	COL7A1	Linear IgG, IgA, other Igs at DEJ
Herpes gestationis	BP180	Linear C3, IgG at DEJ
Linear IgA bullous dermatosis	BP180, COL7A1, LAD	Linear IgA, C3 at DEJ
Pemphigus foliaceus	DSG1	IgG, C3 in intercellular spaces
Pemphigus vulgaris	DSG3 (mucous membrane only) DSG3 and DSG1 (mucous membrane and skin)	IgG, C3 in intercellular spaces
IgA pemphigus	DSC1, DSG1, DSG3	IgA in intercellular spaces
Paraneoplastic pemphigus	DSG1, DSG3, DP1, DP2, BP180, BP230, EP, PP, γ-catenin (PG), plectin, 170 kDa, DSC2, DSC3	IgG, C3 in intercellular spaces, DEJ
Porphyria cutanea tarda	None (not antibody mediated)	Homogeneous IgG at DEJ and around vessels
Anti–p200 pemphigoid	200-kDa antigen	IgG, C3 at DEJ
Anti–p105 pemphigoid	105-kDa antigen	IgG, C3 at DEJ

BP, bullous pemphigoid; *C3,* Third complement component; *COL,* collagen; *DEJ,* dermopidermal junction; *DP,* desmoplakin; *DSC,* desmocollin; *DSG,* desmoglein; *EP,* envoplakin; *eTG,* epidermal transglutaminase; *Ig,* immunoglobulin; *LAM,* laminin; *PG,* plakoglobin; *PP,* periplakin; *SLE,* systemic lupus erythematosus.

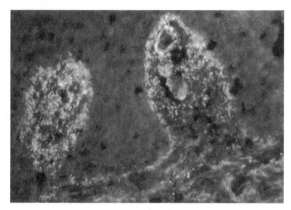

Fig. 10.2 Direct immunofluorescence of skin demonstrating linear granular immunoglobulin A along the basement membrane zone and in the papillary dermis in a patient with dermatitis herpetiformis. *(Courtesy Fitzsimons Army Medical Center teaching files.)*

10. How are specimens obtained for direct immunofluorescence (DIF)?

Specimens for DIF testing are obtained from "perilesional" skin (uninvolved skin next to a blister). Specimens for DIF should be placed in normal saline, in Michel transport media, or snap-frozen in liquid nitrogen. Placement of skin specimens in 10% NBF for as little as 2 minutes may ruin any attempt at DIF testing, and such specimens will often be refused by the lab. While DIF is a rapid and sensitive means to screen for some diseases, like BP, other, rarer diseases, such as cicatricial pemphigoid (CP) and epidermolysis bullosa acquisita (EBA), may appear essentially identical to BP by DIF alone (see below).

11. For which vesiculobullous diseases are indirect immunofluorescence (IIF) helpful?

IIF uses patient antibodies (from a blood draw) and laboratory substrate. This modality is often used to diagnose paraneoplastic pemphigus and pemphigus vulgaris (PV) or to discriminate between BP, EBA, and CP. Because IIF measures antibodies in patient serum (separated from blood), titers may be used to gauge disease activity. Only a few laboratories perform IIF testing, so availability must be verified before ordering. Enzyme-linked immunosorbent assay (ELISA) testing for these same serum antibodies is also commercially available and is both sensitive and specific. ELISA testing has replaced IIF studies at many institutions for determining antibody titers and for detecting certain antibodies in autoimmune blistering disorders, such as BP180, BP230, desmoglein 1, and desmoglein 3.

12. List the most common blistering diseases due to external agents.

- **Allergic contact dermatitis:** Direct contact with allergens may cause an acute, pruritic vesicular eruption (Fig. 10.3). When it is due to plants, such as poison ivy, the pattern is often linear, corresponding to areas where the skin brushes the plant. Appropriate history and clinical findings usually establish the diagnosis. Skin biopsy for routine histologic examination may be helpful in difficult cases (see Chapter 9).

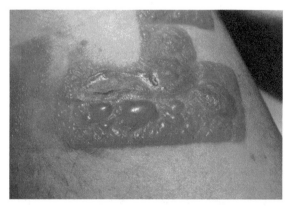

Fig. 10.3 Acute bullous allergic contact dermatitis on the arm. *(Courtesy Fitzsimons Army Medical Center teaching files.)*

- **Bullous drug eruptions:** Some drugs can produce vesiculobullous eruptions through toxic, immunologic, idiopathic, or phototoxic/photoallergic mechanisms (see Chapter 14).
- **Miliaria crystallina:** Obstruction of eccrine sweat ducts can lead to small, shallow blisters filled with sweat. Predisposing factors include high temperature ("prickly heat"), high fever occlusion, and sunburn. The diagnosis is usually established on clinical grounds, but sometimes cases require a skin biopsy.
- **Blisters caused by physical agents:** Heat, cold, chemicals, friction, pressure, and radiation (including ultraviolet radiation of a second-degree sunburn) can induce blisters. Such causes are usually identified readily by history and physical examination.
- **Bullous arthropod bites:** Small blisters around ankles, a distribution otherwise limited to exposed skin or delimited by tight clothing, pet ownership, or travel/outdoor activities, may suggest this cause.
- **Bullous impetigo:** Fragile blisters, often with collarete of scale, and a positive culture for *Staphylococcus* or *Streptococcus* may suggest this cause.

13. Name examples of drugs that can cause vesiculobullous eruptions.
    See Table 10.5.

14. What is epidermolysis bullosa (EB)?
    EB is a group of genetic diseases caused by inherited defects in skin proteins that yield blisters, either spontaneously or with minor trauma. Subtypes of EB exist (Table 10.6):
    - **Epidermolysis bullosa simplex** is an autosomal dominant genetic disease. Blisters develop at birth or in childhood, due to minor skin trauma, and heal without scarring.
    - **Junctional epidermolysis bullosa (JEB)** is an autosomal recessive disease. Blisters typically begin at birth, and the disorder presents as generalized blistering, or as periorificial erosions. The upper airway may be involved in JEB. Blisters are caused by defective skin proteins that anchor the epidermis to the dermis.
    - **Dystrophic epidermolysis bullosa (DEB)** may be an autosomal dominant or autosomal recessive disorder. Blistering may be mild, or it may be so severe that it is disfiguring. DEB is due to defects in anchoring fibrils (type VII collagen) of the dermis.
      For all types of EB, the diagnosis is usually established based upon skin biopsy, immunomapping with immunofluorescence microscopy, electron microscopy, or genetic analysis. Referral to a center specializing in EB care is ideal. Further information may be found at National Institute of Arthritis and Musculoskeletal and Skin Diseases: www.niams.nih.gov. Mechanobullous skin diseases are covered in Chapter 6.

15. Describe other genetic blistering diseases.
    - **Acrodermatitis enteropathica:** A blistering disorder caused either by acquired zinc deficiency (e.g., premature infants, alcoholics, or those on long-term parenteral nutrition) or by autosomal recessive genetic defects in a zinc-specific transporter (SLC39A4). Periorificial and acral distribution of scaling and blistering is common and may be associated with alopecia. Diarrhea is often present. Skin biopsy and serum zinc levels are useful to establish the diagnosis. Deficiencies of essential fatty acids and amino acids may also cause acrodermatitis enteropathica. Maternal SLC30A2 mutations cause reduced zinc levels in breast milk, and a transient zinc deficiency in neonates, with early-onset acrodermatitis enteropathica that resolves upon weaning.
    - **Bullous congenital ichthyosiform erythroderma (epidermolytic ichthyosis):** An autosomal dominant condition that presents with diffuse erythema at birth, later flaccid bullae, and still later, with furrowed hyperkeratosis. It is caused by defects in keratins 1 and 10. The diagnosis is made by clinical observation, skin biopsy, and family history. Ichthyosis bullosa of Siemens (keratin 2e defect) may present in a similar fashion but with a less severe clinical course. Some inherited palmoplantar keratodermas caused by defects in keratin 1 and 9 may present with acral blisters.

Table 10.5 Drugs that can cause vesiculobullous eruptions

ERUPTION	OFFENDING DRUG(s)
Bullous pemphigoid	Erlotinib, furosemide, ibuprofen, and other nonsteroidal anti-inflammatory drugs (NSAIDs), captopril, penicillamine, anti-PD1/anti-PD1L therapy, other antibiotics
Erythema multiforme	Anticonvulsants, barbiturates, sulfonamides, NSAIDs, antibiotics
Linear IgA bullous dermatosis	Vancomycin, lithium, captopril, antibiotics
Phototoxic drug eruption	Psoralens, thiazides, furosemide, fluoroquinolones, doxycycline (and other TCNs), sulfonamides
Porphyria-like drug eruption	Furosemide, tetracycline, naproxen, other NSAIDs
Toxic epidermal necrolysis and Stevens-Johnson syndrome	Anticonvulsants, sulfonamides, NSAIDs, allopurinol, antiretrovirals

IgA, Immunoglobulin A; *TCNs*, tetracyclines.

Table 10.6 Subtypes of epidermolysis bullosa

LEVEL OF SPLIT	DISEASE	DEFECT
Suprabasal	Acral peeling skin syndrome (APSS)	Transglutaminase 5 (TGM5)
	EBS superficialis (EBSS)	Unknown
	EBS, acantholytic (EBS-acanth)	Desmoplakin (DSP); plakoglobin (JUP)
	Skin Fragility Syndromes	
	Skin fragility-woolly hair syndrome (EBS—desmoplakin)	Desmoplakin (DSP)
	Skin fragility-plakoglobin deficiency (EBS—plakoglobin)	Plakoglobin (JUP)
	Skin fragility-ectodermal dysplasia syndrome (EBS—Plakophilin)	Plakophilin-1 (PKP1)
Basal	EBS, localized (Weber-Cockayne) (EBS-loc)	Keratins 5 and 14 (KRT5 and KRT14)
	EBS, generalized severe (Dowling-Meara) (EBS-gen sev)	
	EBS, generalized, intermediate (Koebner, non-DM)(EBS-gen intermed)	
	EBS, mottled pigmentation (EBS-MP)	Keratin 5 (KRT5)
	EBS, migratory circinate (EBS-migr)	Keratin 5 (KRT5)
	EBS, autosomal recessive K14 (EBS-AR K14)	Keratin 14 (KRT14)
	EBS, autosomal recessive-exophilin 5 deficiency (EBS-AR exophilin 5)	Exophilin 5 (Slac2-b) (EXPH5)
	EBS with muscular dystrophy (EBS-MD)	Plectin (PLEC1)
	EBS with pyloric atresia (EBS-PA)	Plectin (PLEC1); $\alpha6\beta4$ integrin
	EBS, Ogna type (EBS-Og)	Plectin (PLEC1)
	EBS, autosomal recessive-BP230 deficiency (EBS-AR BP230)	Bullous pemphigoid antigen-1 (BPAG1; BP230) (DST)
Intra-lamina lucida	JEB, generalized severe (Herlitz) (JEB-gen sev)	Laminin-332 ($\alpha3$, $\beta3$, $\gamma2$) (LAMA3, LAMB3, LAMC2)
	JEB, generalized intermediate (non-Herlitz; GABEB) (JEB-gen intermed)	Laminin-332 ($\alpha3$, $\beta3$, $\gamma2$) (LAMA3, LAMB3, LAMC2); BP180/collagen XVII (COL17A1)
	JEB with pyloric atresia (JEB-PA)	Integrins $\alpha6$, $\beta4$ (ITGA6, ITGB4)
	JEB, late onset (JEB-LO)	BP180/collagen XVII (COL17A1)
	JEB with respiratory and renal involvement (JEB-RR)	integrin $\alpha3$ (ITGA3)
	JEB, localized (JEB-loc)	Laminin-332 ($\alpha3$, $\beta3$, $\gamma2$) (LAMA3, LAMB3, LAMC2); BP180/Collagen XVII (COL17A1); Integrins $\alpha6$, $\beta4$ (ITGA6, ITGB4)
	JEB, inversa (JEB-inv; JEB-I)	Laminin-332 ($\alpha3$, $\beta3$, $\gamma2$) (LAMA3, LAMB3, LAMC2)
	JEB-LOC syndrome (no blistering)	Laminin $\alpha3$ (LAMA3)

Table 10.6 Subtypes of epidermolysis bullosa (*Continued*)

LEVEL OF SPLIT	DISEASE	DEFECT
Sublamina densa	Dystrophic epidermolysis bullosa (DEB)	Type VII collagen (COL7A1)
	Dominant dystrophic epidermolysis bullosa (DDEB)	
	Recessive dystrophic epidermolysis bullosa (RDEB)	
Mixed	Kindler syndrome	Kindlin-1 (KIND1/FERMT1)

DEB, Dystrophic epidermolysis bullosa; *EBS*, epidermolysis bullosa simplex; *JEB*, junctional epidermolysis bullosa.
From Fine JD, Bruckner-Tuderman L, Eady RA, et al. Inherited epidermolysis bullosa: updated recommendations on diagnosis and classification, *J Am Acad Dermatol*. 2014;70(6):1103–1126.

- **Hailey-Hailey disease (benign familial pemphigus):** Is an autosomal dominant disorder that presents with blisters, erosions, and crusts in intertriginous areas. Blisters are caused by a loss of cohesion between keratinocytes (acantholysis) due to mutations in the *ATP2C* gene, which encodes a calcium pump. Secondary bacterial infections are common. A diagnosis is established by clinical exam and routine skin biopsy.
- **Incontinentia pigmenti (IP):** This X-linked disease, caused by mutation in the IKK-gamma/NEMO gene, and the disease is seen nearly exclusively in females (affected males usually die in utero). The condition begins in neonatal life, with vesicles in a linear or whorled pattern, followed by verrucous lesions, and followed later as hyperpigmented and hypopigmented patches. Skin biopsy is a helpful diagnostic test for IP.

16. List the vesiculobullous diseases caused by metabolic disorders.
    - Bullous diabeticorum (bullous eruption of diabetes mellitus)
    - Pellagra (see question 18)
    - Porphyria cutanea tarda (the most common of all porphyrias)
    - Necrolytic erythemas (necrolytic acral erythema—hepatitis C associated; migratory necrolytic erythema—glucagonoma)
    - Acrodermatitis enteropathica (zinc deficiency—may be inherited or acquired)

17. Describe the clinical findings in bullous diabeticorum.
    Bullous diabeticorum presents as tense bullae that arise spontaneously on the distal extremities in patients with both insulin-dependent and non–insulin-dependent diabetes (Fig. 10.4). The condition is chronic. The diagnosis is made by clinical findings and skin biopsy, and while the histologic findings are nonspecific, the biopsy helps to exclude other bullous conditions.

18. What is the cause of pellagra?
    Pellagra is a nutritional disorder caused by a deficiency of niacin (vitamin B_3) or tryptophan (niacin precursor). The classic triad caused is dermatitis, diarrhea, and dementia. The dermatitis is often photodistributed (particularly upon the neck—"Casal necklace"—and forearms) and consists of vesicles, papules, erosions, and hyperpigmentation. In developed countries, alcoholics and those on isoniazid therapy are most likely to develop pellagra. Clinical findings and laboratory tests are used to make the diagnosis.

KEY POINTS: VESICULOBULLOUS DISORDERS

1. Vesiculobullous disorders can often be distinguished by the clinical history, distribution, and location of the split (superficial versus deep blister formation).
2. Vesiculobullous disorders often require biopsies of intact blisters for optimal diagnosis.
3. Direct immunofluorescence (DIF) of perilesional skin is useful to diagnose autoimmune bullous diseases.
4. Drug eruptions may mimic many of the vesiculobullous disorders or cause some bullous disorders (e.g., anti-PD1/PD1L therapy used in melanoma can cause BP).

19. What is the difference between porphyria cutanea tarda and pseudoporphyria?
    Porphyria cutaneous tarda (PCT) occurs chiefly on sun-exposed skin and is characterized by skin fragility, tense blisters, scarring, and milia. The dorsal hands are often affected (Fig. 10.5). Patients have decreased levels of the enzyme uroporphyrinogen decarboxylase, and the condition is often unmasked or exacerbated by alcoholic liver disease or drugs such as estrogen and iron. Hypertrichosis may develop on the face. The diagnosis is suggested by skin biopsy and established by porphyrin studies, including a 24-hour urine collection for uroporphyrins. Variegate porphyria and hereditary coproporphyria may present with similar cutaneous findings but can be distinguished by complete porphyrin

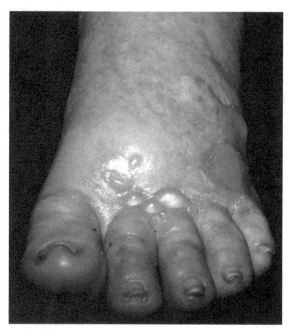

Fig. 10.4 Bullous diabeticorum. Tense bullae and erosions on the feet of a patient with diabetes mellitus. *(Courtesy Fitzsimons Army Medical Center teaching files.)*

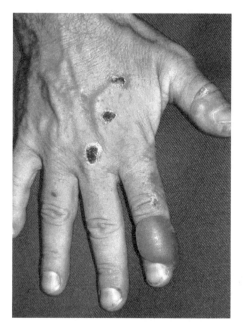

Fig. 10.5 Porphyria cutanea tarda. Tense bullae and increased skin fragility manifesting hemorrhagic crusts on the back of a hand. *(Courtesy Fitzsimons Army Medical Center teaching files.)*

studies. DIF may show perivascular deposition of IgG and IgM but is not specific for only PCT. Pseudoporphyria demonstrates similar cutaneous findings, but porphyrin studies are normal. Pseudoporphyria is associated with uremia, hemodialysis, and some drugs, especially nonsteroidal antiinflammatory drugs, such as naproxen. Histology and DIF findings in pseudoporphyria are identical to PCT.

Green JJ, Mander SL. Pseudoporphyria. *J Am Acad Dermatol.* 2001;44:100–108.

20. What are the necrolytic erythemas?

   Necrolytic erythemas are a group of cutaneous diseases of diverse origin that share certain histopathologic features. Such conditions include acrodermatitis enteropathica, necrolytic migratory erythema ("glucagonoma syndrome"), necrolytic acral erythema (associated with hepatitis C), and Hartnup's disease, among others.

21. What is the difference between bullous pemphigoid and cicatricial pemphigoid?

   BP is an autoimmune bullous disease that most often affects older adults and it is caused by the antibodies BP180 and BP230. It is the most common of all autoimmune bullous conditions, and its incidence has increased threefold in the last decade. Primary lesions range from urticarial plaques to tense bullae (Fig. 10.6). BP lesions often occur on flexural surfaces but can be widespread. Blisters usually heal without scarring. The oral mucosa is affected in about 20% of cases, and the lesions are usually minor. CP is a chronic autoimmune blistering disorder, chiefly affecting the elderly, that causes scarring of mucosal surfaces, and it is also called mucous membrane pemphigoid. CP is caused by antibodies directed against multiple antigens at the basement membrane zone, including BP180. The diagnosis of BP and CP is established by correlating clinical findings with routine histologic examination of lesional skin, direct immunofluorescence of perilesional skin, and IIF or ELISA testing of serum. Drug-induced cases of BP/CP should always be considered.

Kridin K. Subepidermal autoimmune bullous diseases: overview, epidemiology, and associations. *Immunol Res.* 2018;66:6–17. https://doi.org/10.1007/s12026-017-8975-2.

22. How do pemphigus vulgaris and pemphigus foliaceus differ?

   PV is a chronic blistering disease caused by antibodies to DG1 and DG3. PV usually affects adults and often begins in the oral mucosa. Flaccid vesicles and bullae develop on the face, scalp, neck, chest, groin, and intertriginous areas. The lesions are often painful rather than pruritic. PV can be generalized and life-threatening. Pemphigus foliaceus (PF) is caused by antibodies to DSG1 only and is more superficial, and generally not as severe, as PV. Patients with PV develop superficial vesicles and bullae, typically on the scalp, face, upper chest, and back, which often rupture and manifest only as erosions with scale and crust. The diagnosis of PF/PV is made by routine histologic exam of an early blister, as well as by DIF of perilesional skin, and IIF or ELISA testing of serum. In June 2018, rituximab, an anti-CD20 monoclonal antibody, received Food and Drug Administration approval for use in PV, representing the first major advancement in the treatment of the disease in ~60 years.

Kirdin K, Ahn C, Huagn WC, et al. Treatment update of autoimmune blistering diseases. *Dermatol Clin.* 2019;3:215–228. https://doi.org/10.1016/j.det.2018.12.003.

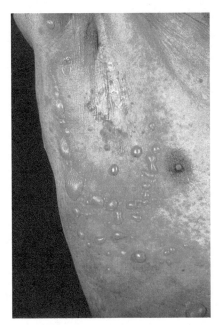

Fig. 10.6 Bullous pemphigoid. Erythematous, urticarial plaques with multiple vesicles and bullae are seen. Many of the blisters are tense.

23. Linear IgA bullous dermatosis occurs in two different clinical situations. What are they?

Linear IgA bullous dermatosis (LABD) in childhood is classically referred to as **chronic bullous disease of childhood.** Pruritic, urticarial blisters, often sausage-shaped or like a string of pearls, develop on the buttocks and perineal areas, as well as the trunk and extremities (Fig. 10.7). Mucosal lesions are common. In adults, LABD may occur spontaneously, but it is also often associated with drugs, particularly vancomycin. Skin lesions in LABD can resemble BP or DH. Diagnosis of LABD is made by routine histologic exam of an early blister, by DIF of perilesional skin, or IIF to detect IgA antibodies directed at components of the basement membrane zone.

Lammer J, Hein R, Roenneberg S, et al. Drug-induced linear IgA bullous dermatosis: a case report and review of the literature. *Acta Derm Venereol.* 2019;99:508–515.

24. Describe the clinical findings in dermatitis herpetiformis.

DH is an autoimmune disease caused by IgA autoantibodies directed against tissue transglutaminase-3 (TGM3). DH is an extremely pruritic condition, and the itching has been so intense that it has led to suicide. DH classically begins in early adulthood and it is characterized by symmetrically distributed papules and vesicles that develop on the elbows, knees, buttocks, extensor forearms, scalp, and, sometimes, face and palms (Fig. 10.8). It is now thought that most patients with DH have an associated gluten-sensitive enteropathy, even if it is subclinical. The diagnosis of DH is established by routine histologic exam of an early blister and by DIF of perilesions or even nonlesional skin (IgA deposited in dermal papillae) (see Fig. 10.2). Scratching may destroy all intact blisters in DH and so DIF studies may be a particularly helpful test. Serologic testing for antibodies directed against TGM3 can also be utilized.

Collin P, Salmi TT, Hervonen K, et al. Dermatitis herpetiformis: a cutaneous manifestation of coeliac disease. *Ann Med.* 2017;49:23–31. https://doi.org/10.1080/07853890.2016.1222450.

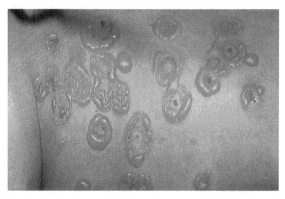

Fig. 10.7 Linear immunoglobulin A bullous dermatosis. Tense, circular, sausage-shaped bullae in a child.

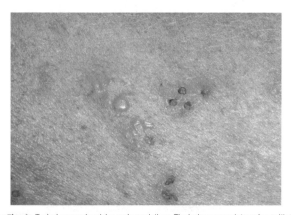

Fig. 10.8 Dermatitis herpetiformis. Typical grouped vesicles and excoriations. The lesions are so intensely pruritic that in some patients only excoriations are seen. *(Courtesy Fitzsimons Army Medical Center teaching files.)*

25. Does herpes gestationis have anything to do with herpesviruses?

No. Herpes gestationis, also called gestational pemphigoid, is a form of BP seen in pregnant women, usually in the second trimester. Lesions often begin in the periumbilical area and may first be urticarial. Later, tense vesicles and bullae develop. The disease may flare after delivery and may recur in subsequent pregnancies. Premature birth or small-for-gestational-age infants have occurred in some patients. The diagnosis is made from clinical findings, routine histology of an early blister or urticarial lesion, and by direct immunofluorescence and IIF studies.

26. What is bullous systemic lupus erythematosus (SLE)?

Bullous SLE is a rare blistering eruption that occurs chiefly in patients with established SLE. In most cases, autoantibodies are directed against type VII collagen located deep in the basement membrane zone. Vesicles and bullae may develop on inflamed or noninflamed skin. Sometimes, lesions may resemble BP or EBA. The diagnosis is made via clinical findings, routine histologic exam (which may show a subepidermal split with neutrophils similar to DH or LABD), and with direct and IIF studies, including the latter performed on salt-split skin.

Contestable JJ, Edhegard KD, Meyerle JH. Bullous systemic lupus erythematosus: a review and update to diagnosis and treatment. *Am J Clin Dermatol.* 2014;15:517–524. https://doi.org/10.1007/s40257-014-0098-0.

27. What is epidermolysis bullosa acquisita?

EBA is an autoimmune bullous disease with autoantibodies directed against type VII collagen located deep in the basement membrane zone. In this disease, vesicles and bullae follow trauma and tend to occur on areas with minor trauma, such as the fingers, knees, and elbows. Mucosal lesions are common. As with bullous SLE, the diagnosis is made via clinical findings, routine histology, and direct immunofluorescence and IIF studies, with the latter performed salt-split skin.

Cobos G, Mu E, Cohen J, et al. Epidermolysis bullosa acquisita. *Dermatol Online J.* 2017;3(12).

28. What is anti–p200 pemphigoid?

Anti–p200 pemphigoid is a rare subepidermal blistering skin disease with autoantibodies directed against a 200-kDa protein located on the dermal side of salt-split skin. It is characterized by tense blisters and vesicles, erosions, and urticarial plaques on the trunk and extremities, similar to BP. Histology reveals a subepidermal split with neutrophils. Autoantibodies to laminin γ1 have been identified in the sera of up to 90% of patients with anti–p200 pemphigoid, but additional details of the disease, including the mechanism of pathologeneis, are still being discovered.

Goletz S, Hashimoto T, Zillikens D, et al. Anti-p200 pemphigoid. *J Am Acad Dermatol.* 2014;71:185–191.

CHAPTER 11

PUSTULAR ERUPTIONS

James E. Fitzpatrick

1. **How does a pustule differ from a vesicle or bulla?**

   A pustule is a purulent vesicle or bulla. Whereas a vesicle contains clear or translucent fluid, a pustule is filled with neutrophils or, less commonly, eosinophils. Pustules are one of the primary lesions in skin. Most pustular eruptions begin as pustules, but others may pass through a transitory stage in which they appear vesicular (vesiculopustules).

2. **How are pustules classified?**

   Pustules may be classified on the basis of where the acute inflammatory cells accumulate (e.g., subcorneal, follicular, sweat duct), pathogenesis (e.g., infectious, autoimmune), predominant inflammatory cells (e.g., neutrophils, eosinophils), and clinical presentation (Table 11.1). Pustules may be unilocular or multilocular.

3. **What is the most common pustular skin eruption?**

   Acne vulgaris, although not all lesions in this condition are pustular (Fig. 11.1). The infectious pustular eruptions are also common (see Chapter 27).

4. **Name the different types of pustular psoriasis. How do they differ?**

   Pustular psoriasis may be broadly subdivided into localized and generalized forms. Localized pustular psoriasis may occur on any site and may also occur within plaques of classic psoriasis. Distinctive variants include acrodermatitis continua of Hallopeau (Fig. 11.2A), which is characterized by pustules and crusting of the distal fingers and toes and localized pustular psoriasis of the palms and soles (Fig. 11.2B). It is unclear whether pustular eruptions confined to the palms and soles represent a form of localized psoriasis or a different disease called pustular bacterid. Variants of generalized pustular psoriasis include generalized pustular psoriasis of von Zumbusch, exanthematic generalized pustular psoriasis, and impetigo herpetiformis. The von Zumbusch variant presents as generalized pustules in patients with preexisting plaque-type psoriasis or erythrodermic psoriasis. Exanthematic generalized pustular psoriasis arises suddenly without preceding psoriasis (Fig. 11.2C). Impetigo herpetiformis is associated with pregnancy. Hypocalcemia is also frequently present (see Chapter 59).

5. **Do any factors precipitate generalized pustular psoriasis?**

   The most important inciting factor is the administration of systemic corticosteroids. In a study of 104 patients, corticosteroids were implicated as the precipitating factor in 37 patients (36%). This association is one of the primary reasons that psoriasis is not treated with systemic corticosteroids. Less common precipitating factors included infection (13%), hypocalcemia (9%), pregnancy (3%), and other drugs (e.g., terbinafine, lithium).

   Baker H, Ryan TJ. Generalized pustular psoriasis: a clinical and epidemiologic study of 104 cases. *Br J Dermatol.* 1968;80:771–793.

6. **Is pustular psoriasis treated differently than classic plaque-type psoriasis?**

   Most treatments that are used on classic plaque-type psoriasis can also be used for the management of pustular psoriasis. The National Psoriasis Board reviewed the literature and concluded that the quality of literature was weak but did make recommendations to divide treatment into first-line and second-line treatments. First-line treatments include acitretin, cyclosporine, methotrexate, and infliximab. Second-line treatments include adalimumab, etanercept, and psoralen plus ultraviolet light (PUVA). Patients whose symptoms may have been induced or exacerbated by medications should have these withdrawn.

   Robinson A, Van Voorhees AS, Hsu S, et al. Treatment of pustular psoriasis: from the Medical Board of the National Psoriasis Foundation. *J Am Acad Dermatol.* 2012;67:279–288.

7. **What is pustular bacterid?**

   Pustular bacterid (of Andrews) is a controversial clinical eruption. While many dermatologists consider it to be a form of pustular psoriasis localized to the palms and soles, new cases continue to be reported in the literature. As originally defined by Andrews, pustular bacterid is a pustular eruption of the palms and soles in which the patient has no history or other clinical signs of psoriasis. Rarely, the lesions may spread to other parts of the body. The lesions are induced by low-grade bacterial infection in occult or evident foci, such as the teeth, tonsils, or gallbladder. The pustular eruption totally resolves with eradication of the infection. A later study has noted that injected *Candida* antigen aggravated up to

Table 11.1 Classification of Pustules

PATHOGENESIS	SITE OF ACCUMULATION
Autoimmune	
IgA pemphigus	Subcorneal
Infectious	Variable
Candidiasis	Subcorneal
Furuncle/carbuncle	Follicular
Impetigo	Subcorneal
Hot tub (pseudomonal) folliculitis	Follicular
Kerion (tinea capitis)	Follicular
Pityrosporum folliculitis	Follicular
Vaccinia infection/vaccination	Intraepidermal
Inherited	
Pustular psoriasis	Subcorneal, intraepidermal
Reiter's syndrome	Subcorneal, intraepidermal
Drug Eruptions	
Acneiform drug-induced eruptions	Follicular
Acute generalized exanthematous pustulosis	Subcorneal
Halogenodermas	Intraepidermal
Miscellaneous	
Acne necrotica miliaris	Follicular
Acne vulgaris	Follicular
Arthropod reactions	Intraepidermal
Erythema toxicum neonatorum	Follicular
Eosinophilic pustular folliculitis	Follicular
Folliculitis decalvans	Follicular
Infantile acropustulosis	Subcorneal, intraepidermal
Miliaria pustulosa	Sweat duct
Pustular bacterid	Intraepidermal
Rosacea	Follicular
Subcorneal pustular dermatosis	Subcorneal
Transient neonatal pustular dermatosis	Subcorneal

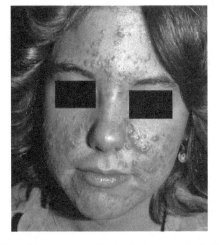

Fig. 11.1 Gram-negative pustular acne vulgaris. (Courtesy Fitzsimons Army Medical Center teaching files.)

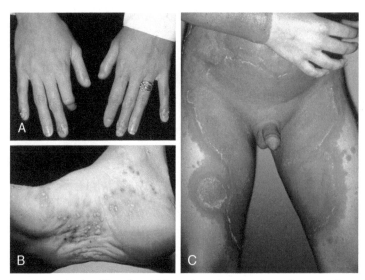

Fig. 11.2 Pustular psoriasis. **A,** Acrodermatitis continua of Hallopeau demonstrating extensive crusting and nail dystrophy. **B,** Chronic pustular eruption of the sole of the foot. **C,** Generalized pustular psoriasis demonstrating marked erythema with numerous pustules. (Courtesy Fitzsimons Army Medical Center teaching files.)

37% of patients with this disorder, suggesting that this phenomenon may not be restricted to bacterial infections. The recent recognition of bacterial "superantigens" provides a possible immunologic mechanism for induction of this disorder.

Kamiya K, Ohtsuki M. Acute generalized pustular bacterid. *J Gen Fam Med.* 2018;19:32–33.

8. Why do some consider pustular bacterid a form of localized pustular psoriasis of the palms and soles?

   The argument is based on the observation that some patients with pustular eruptions of the palms and soles also have typical psoriasis elsewhere. The clinical appearance and histologic findings of the palmar lesions are identical to those of pustular bacterid. Some dermatologists prefer the term *palmar and plantar pustulosis* as a noncommittal name for this entity.

9. What is subcorneal pustular dermatosis (Sneddon-Wilkinson disease)?

   Subcorneal pustular dermatosis is a rare, benign, chronic, relapsing dermatosis that was described by Sneddon and Wilkinson in 1956. It most commonly affects middle-aged women, although any age group, including children, may be affected. The lesions typically occur on the trunk, with accentuation in the flexural and intertriginous areas, where they present as superficial vesiculopustules or pustules that often assume annular or gyrate patterns. The lesions may demonstrate peripheral extension and resolve with variable crusting and scaling. The lesions may be asymptomatic or they may be pruritic. Typically, patients are otherwise healthy, but there are isolated case reports of an associated seronegative rheumatoid-like arthritis.

Von dem Borne PA, Jonkman MF, van Doorn R. Complete remission of skin lesions in patient with subcorneal pustular dermatosis (Sneddon-Wilkinson disease) treated with antimyeloma therapy: association with disappearance of M-protein. *Br J Dermatol.* 2017;176:1341–1344.

10. Discuss the pathogenesis of subcorneal pustular dermatosis.

    The pathogenesis of subcorneal pustular dermatosis is unknown, although some cases have been associated with plasma cell dyscrasias. Even the nosology is controversial. While many authors accept this condition as a distinct entity, a few consider it to be synonymous with, or a variant of, pustular psoriasis. Histologically, both entities demonstrate a subcorneal vesicle filled with neutrophils. The strongest points against the relationship of subcorneal pustular dermatosis and psoriasis are that the former has a distinct clinical presentation, patients do not have preceding plaque-type psoriasis, and they are not likely to develop classic psoriasis during the course of their disease. Some drugs such as lithium carbonate may exacerbate subcorneal pustular dermatosis by increasing neutrophil migration into lesions.

11. How is subcorneal pustular dermatosis treated?

Subcorneal pustular dermatosis cannot be cured, but it can be managed. The disease is uncommon enough that good therapeutic studies comparing different treatment modalities are not available. Anecdotal reports have described excellent therapeutic results with dapsone and acitretin. Less frequently used therapies include oral prednisone, topical corticosteroids, sulfapyridine, cyclosporine, vitamin E, and phototherapy with broadband ultraviolet B (UVB) light therapy, narrowband UVB, infliximab or PUVA.

Cheng S, Edmonds E, Beh-Gashir M, et al. Subcorneal pustular dermatosis: 50 years on. *Clin Exp Dermatol.* 2008;33:229–233.

12. What is superficial IgA pemphigus?

Recently, it has been demonstrated that some cases of what were formerly classified as subcorneal pustular dermatosis may demonstrate intraepidermal IgA between the keratinocytes. Most authorities feel that cases with intraepidermal IgA on direct immunofluorescence or by enzyme-linked immunosorbent assay should be reclassified as superficial IgA pemphigus (Fig. 11.3). It has been demonstrated that the IgA autoantibodies are directed against desmocollin 1 and possibly desmocollins 2 and 3, which are molecules that are important for normal adhesion between keratinocytes.

13. What are the cutaneous findings in reactive arthritis (Reiter's disease)?

The classic triad of reactive arthritis (formerly Reiter's disease) consists of nongonococcal urethritis, conjunctivitis, and arthritis. However, this triad is present in only 40% of the cases at the time of presentation, and the mucocutaneous findings are helpful in establishing the diagnosis. The mucocutaneous findings include a nonspecific stomatitis, nail changes (subungual hyperkeratosis and onycholysis), circinate balanitis, and keratoderma blennorrhagicum. Keratoderma blennorrhagicum is present in about one-third of cases and presents as pinpoint erythematous papules that progress to pustules (Fig. 11.4) and hyperkeratotic papules and plaques. These are most commonly seen on the bottom of the feet but may also occur on the scalp, elbows, knees, buttocks, and genitalia. Histologically, the findings are identical to the pustules seen in pustular psoriasis.

14. Which drugs are commonly associated with pustular drug eruptions?

Drugs may produce different patterns of pustular drug eruptions, including aggravation of preexisting pustular eruptions such as psoriasis or subcorneal pustular dermatosis. Primary pustular drug eruptions can be classified as acneiform, halogenodermas, and acute generalized exanthematous pustulosis.

- Acneiform drug eruptions: Systemic corticosteroids (steroid acne), phenytoin, lithium, iodides, bromides, isoniazid (Fig. 11.5).
- Halogenodermas: Iodides, bromides, and fluorides may produce both acneiform drug eruptions and nonfollicular pustules (Fig. 11.6).
- Acute generalized exanthematous pustulosis: A drug eruption that presents as fever, malaise, and diffuse erythema studded with small pustules; caused by numerous medications including cotrimoxazole, erythromycin, hydroxychloroquine, streptomycin, terbinafine, clindamycin, and cephalosporins.

Alniemi DT, Wetter DA, Bridges AG, et al. Acute generalized exanthematous pustulosis: clinical characteristics, etiologic associations, treatments, and outcomes in a series of 28 patients at Mayo Clinic, 1996–2013. *Int J Dermatol.* 2017;56:404–414.

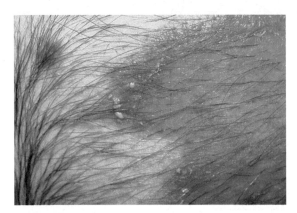

Fig. 11.3 Isolated pustule and annular lesions demonstrating scale-crust superficial pustules in a patient with IgA pemphigus. In the past, this would have been considered to be subcorneal pustular dermatosis.

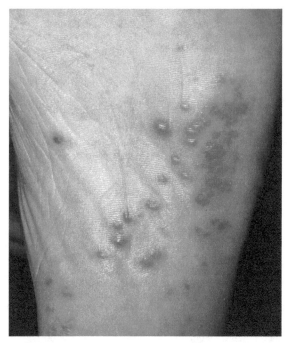

Fig. 11.4 Acute keratoderma blennorrhagicum in a patient with reactive arthritis demonstrated erythematous papules with early pustule formation. (Courtesy Fitzsimons Army Medical Center teaching files.)

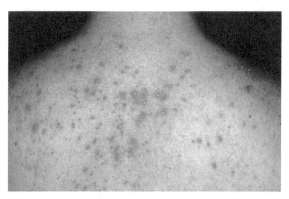

Fig. 11.5 Corticosteroid-induced acne manifesting as the explosive onset of numerous follicular-based papules and pustules.

15. What is folliculitis decalvans?

Folliculitis decalvans (Quinquaud's disease) is a rare, scarring alopecia of unknown etiology. Clinically, it presents as follicular-based pustules that may assume annular or circinate configurations. The pustules rapidly form crusts; in many patients, the crusts may predominate. The hairs are permanently lost, leaving patches of atrophic hairless skin (Fig. 11.7). Treatment is generally unsatisfactory; topical or intralesional corticosteroids and oral antibiotics (rifampin, clindamycin, and tetracyclines) are typically used.

Miguel-Gómez L, Rodrigues Barata AR, Molina-Ruiz A, et al. Folliculitis decalvans: effectiveness of therapies and prognostic factors in a multicenter series of 60 patients with long-term follow-up, *J Am Acad Dermatol.* 2018;79:878–883.

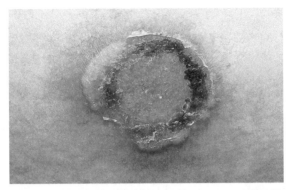

Fig. 11.6 Annular pustular eruption of the back secondary to oral potassium iodide (iododerma).

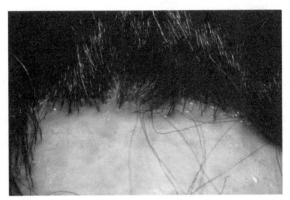

Fig. 11.7 Folliculitis decalvans. Characteristic perifollicular erythema and follicular pustules associated with atrophic scarring alopecia. (Courtesy Fitzsimons Army Medical Center teaching files.)

16. Discuss the pathogenesis of miliaria pustulosa.

All forms of miliaria result from the retention of sweat secondary to occlusion of the sweat ducts. The pathogenesis of miliaria pustulosa is not entirely understood, but it is believed that heat and occlusion result in the proliferation of surface bacteria that produce toxins that damage the acrosyringium (intraepidermal portion of the eccrine sweat duct). Clinically, it presents as superficial pustules associated with surrounding macular erythema.

17. How is miliaria pustulosa treated?

Once miliaria pustulosa has developed, there is no satisfactory treatment except removing the patient from the hot and humid environment. Occlusive wear that may have aggravated the condition should also be eliminated. Anecdotally, some dermatologists have tried weak solutions of salicylic acid to produce exfoliation or tape stripping of the stratum corneum to remove the obstruction to sweating, but there are no studies to document the efficacy of these treatments. Some patients may require weeks or even months to establish normal sweating after severe attacks.

18. What is Ofuji's disease?

Ofuji's disease is the eponymic name for eosinophilic folliculitis that was initially described in Japan. It is a very rare, chronic dermatosis that may occur in any ethnic group. It is characterized by recurrent superficial papules and pustules that are often arranged in circinate plaques with central clearing. While most of the pustules are centered on hair follicles, they can also arise within the epidermis. The cause of eosinophilic folliculitis is unknown; however, there are other disorders such as some fungal infections, some drug eruptions, immunosuppression, and HIV-associated eosinophilic folliculitis that are histologically similar. The pathogenesis of this disorder is unknown.

19. What is the differential diagnosis of a pustular eruption in a neonate?
- Erythema toxicum neonatorum (ETN)
- Transient neonatal pustular melanosis (TNPM)
- Incontinentia pigmenti (more commonly vesicular)
- Neonatal acne

- Miliaria pustulosa
- Staphylococcal infection
- Herpes simplex (more commonly vesicular)
- Candidiasis
- Congenital syphilis

KEY POINTS: NEONATAL PUSTULAR ERUPTIONS

1. Neonates are frequently born with pustular lesions, with the majority of them being transient.
2. The pathogenesis of neonatal pustular eruptions includes hormonal (neonatal acne), infectious (herpes simplex infection, candidiasis, staphylococcal infection, congenital syphilis), occlusive (miliaria rubra), or idiopathic (transient neonatal pustular melanosis, erythema toxicum neonatorum).
3. Most cases can be clinically differentiated based on the clinical distribution.
4. Problematic cases should be evaluated by diagnostic studies to include examining the blister contents with Wright's stain to look for the primary inflammatory cell type (neutrophils vs. eosinophils) and balloon cells to exclude herpes virus infection and Gram stains to rule out bacteria and *Candida* infection.

20. How do ETN and TNPM differ?

ETN and TNPM are both benign vesiculopustular disorders of unknown etiology that present during the first few days of life. ETN does not demonstrate a racial predilection and is very common, with up to 20% of neonates being affected. Clinically, it usually presents as macular erythema that usually affects the face initially; approximately 10% to 20% of cases develop pustules within the center of the areas of macular erythema (Fig. 11.8). Biopsies of the pustules demonstrate an acute superficial folliculitis composed primarily of eosinophils. Peripheral eosinophilia may be present in 20% of cases. The lesions resolve without permanent sequelae in 7 to 10 days. Epidemiologically, TNPM differs from ETN in that it occurs in about 5% of black neonates but in less than 1% of white neonates. Clinically, it presents as vesiculopustules that are not associated with surrounding erythema. The vesiculopustules resolve within 48 hours and are followed by hyperpigmented macules that may take 3 months to resolve. In contrast to ETN, biopsies demonstrate subcorneal pustules that are not follicular based, and the primary inflammatory cells are neutrophils. Peripheral eosinophilia is absent. Both conditions are benign and self-limited. Treatment is not recommended.

Reginatto FP, Muller FM, Peruzzo J, Cestari TF. Epidemiology and predisposing factors for erythema toxicum neonatorum and transient neonatal pustular: a multicenter study. *Pediatr Dermatol.* 2017;34:422–426.

21. What is infantile acropustulosis?

Infantile acropustulosis, also referred to as acropustulosis of infancy, is an inflammatory disease first described in 1979. Most case reports have been in black infants from the southern United States, but it has also been reported in other racial groups and countries including Scandinavia. Clinically, the condition is characterized by recurrent crops of 1- to 2-mm intensely pruritic vesiculopustules on the extremities (Fig. 11.9). Histologically, there are

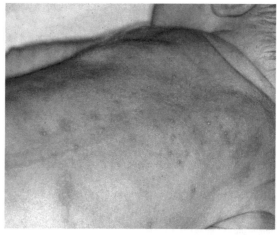

Fig. 11.8 Erythema toxicum neonatorum. Newborn with macular erythema and scattered pustules of on the back, neck and face. (Courtesy of the William Weston Collection.)

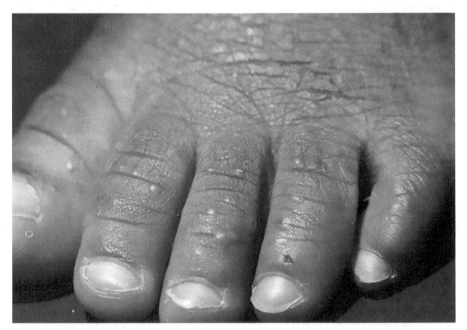

Fig. 11.9 Infantile acropustulosis demonstrating typical, pruritic acral pustules in a black child.

well-circumscribed intraepidermal pustules filled with neutrophils. Most cases spontaneously resolve by 2 years of age. The pathogenesis is not understood, but it has been postulated that it may be a nonspecific host response to arthropod bites.

22. What is the best treatment of infantile acropustulosis?
Nothing works very well. The disease is self-limited; it usually disappears spontaneously by age 2 years. Patients with severe pruritus can be treated with high doses of antihistamines. Some patients respond to potent topical corticosteroids, while rare patients may require treatment with oral dapsone.

Mancini AJ, Frieden IJ, Paller AS. Infantile acropustulosis revisited: history of scabies and response to topical corticosteroids. *Pediatr Dermatol.* 1998;15:337–341.

CHAPTER 12

LICHENOID SKIN ERUPTIONS

Whitney A. High

1. How do lichenoid eruptions differ from other papulosquamous conditions?

   Lichenoid skin eruptions are a subcategory of papulosquamous skin disease. While most papulosquamous eruptions present with scaling papules, lichenoid eruptions differ in that the scale is often subtle, and the papules tend to remain small and discrete. On occasion, confluent plaques may form.

2. What does "lichenoid" mean?

   The term *lichenoid* has at least three commonly accepted applications/definitions:
   - Originally, "lichenoid" referred to a clinical resemblance of such eruptions to lichens (the latter a composite organism of algae or cyanobacteria living among filaments of fungus).
   - Lichen planus (LP) is the prototypical disease in this category, and eruptions sharing clinical features with LP may be described as "lichenoid."
   - "Lichenoid" also refers to a histologic reaction pattern with as a "bandlike" infiltrate of mononuclear inflammatory cells (chiefly lymphocytes) subjacent to the dermoepidermal junction.

3. What is the most common lichenoid skin disease?

   LP is a relatively common disorder, accounting for about 1% of all patient visits to dermatology clinics. The disease most often affects middle-aged adults. Although LP is thought to have no consistent gender predilection, some studies have found women to be more often affected. A recent meta-analysis regarding the incidence of oral LP found an overall age-standardized prevalence of 1.27% (0.96% in men and 1.57% in women).

Gorouhi F, Davari P, Fzel N. Cutaneous and mucosal lichen planus: a comprehensive review of clinical subtypes, risk factors, diagnosis, and prognosis. *ScientificWorldJournal.* 2014;30:742826. (free text online.)

4. What anatomic locations are most often affected by LP?

   LP may affect both the skin and mucosa. Examination of both areas is essential when the diagnosis of LP is suspected. The frequency of involvement for these areas is somewhat controversial. In general, patients with mucosal disease may not demonstrate skin lesions, but 50% or more of patients with cutaneous disease will demonstrate mucosal lesions. Flexural areas, such as the wrists and ankles, are often involved. Other sites of preferential involvement include the neck, buttocks, sacrum, anogenital region, penis, and buccal or vaginal mucosa.

5. Describe the characteristic primary skin lesions of LP.

   LP is a disease characterized by "P-words":
   - *P*lentiful
   - *P*ruritic
   - *P*olished
   - *P*urple
   - *P*olygonal
   - *P*lanar
   - *P*apules and *p*laques

   Primary lesions of the skin are 1- to 5-mm, flat-topped, violaceous, shiny papules (Fig. 12.1). While papules are often clustered, individual lesions tend to be discrete, with angulated (polygonal) borders. Wickham's stria, a lacy white network present on the surface of the papules, is often of great diagnostic value.

6. What are the characteristic oral findings of LP?

   Mucosal lesions of LP differ from cutaneous lesions through demonstration of Wickham's stria in the absence of a papular component. A white, reticulated, "netlike" pattern is often present upon the buccal mucosa, the tongue, or other mucosal surfaces (Fig. 12.2). Other forms of mucosal LP may be ulcerative. Some experts believe that some cases of oral LP may be associated with mercury-containing dental amalgams, but the evidence is not conclusive. Still, others believe such cases represent a separate category of disease, more aptly termed a mercury-associated lichenoid stomatitis. The rate of malignant transformation in oral LP is low (<2%).

Giuliani M, Troiano G, Cordaro M, et al. Rate of malignant transformation of oral lichen planus: a systematic review. *Oral Dis.* 2019;25:693–709. https://doi.org/10.1111/odi.12885.

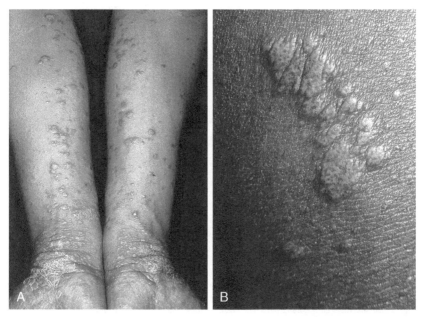

Fig. 12.1 Lichen planus. **A,** Typical violaceous, flat-topped, polygonal papules. The location on the volar wrist is characteristic. **B,** Note the Wickham's striae. (Courtesy James E. Fitzpatrick, MD.)

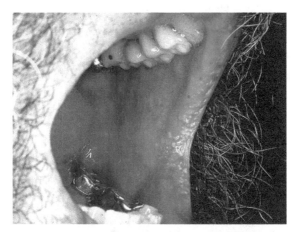

Fig. 12.2 Lichen planus, showing reticulated leukoplakia of the buccal mucosa. (Courtesy James E. Fitzpatrick, MD.)

7. Describe the isomorphic response of LP.
   The isomorphic response (Koebner phenomenon) refers to the development of new lesions at sites of external trauma. This phenomenon is characteristic of both LP and psoriasis, among other rarer conditions. In LP, linear aggregates of papules may be induced by scratching or rubbing (Fig. 12.3).

8. What causes LP?
   The cause of LP is unknown. Etiologic hypotheses include hypersensitivity reactions, viral infection (particularly hepatitis C), or autoimmune mechanisms. Case reports have linked LP to viral hepatitis, neurologic disease, and severe psychic trauma. Other autoimmune diseases such as vitiligo, inflammatory bowel disease, and autoimmune thyroiditis are seen with increased frequency in those with LP. Lichenoid eruptions (otherwise identical to idiopathic LP) may be

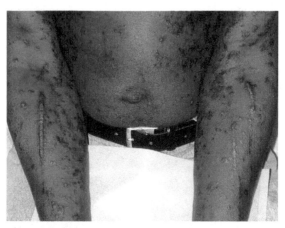

Fig. 12.3 Lichen planus with Koebner phenomenon. Note the linear distribution of secondary lesions that develop in sites of excoriation. (Courtesy Whitney A. High, MD.)

a reaction to drugs or as a manifestation of graft-versus-host disease (GVHD) following allogeneic bone marrow transplantation. Oral disease and, to a lesser degree, cutaneous LP have been associated with hypersensitivity to dental amalgams. Most LP occurs in otherwise healthy people without an identifiable cause.

Tziotzios C, Lee JYW, Brier T, et al. Lichen planus and lichenoid dermatoses: clinical overview and molecular basis. *J Am Acad Dermatol.* 2018;79(5):789–804. https://doi.org/10.1016/j.jaad.2018.02.010.

9. What are the less common presentations of LP?

Nail changes occur in about 10% to 15% of patients and include longitudinal ridging, irregular pitting, nail plate splitting, nail loss, and pterygium formation with severe onychodystrophy, including "20-nail dystrophy" (Fig. 12.4). Desquamative vaginitis may occur. Clinical and histologic variants of LP include annular (Fig. 12.5), atrophic (Fig. 12.6), hypertrophic, ulcerative, vesiculobullous, follicular, and actinic induced. LP may also involve the scalp, yielding a scarring alopecia known as lichen planopilaris. Many authorities consider frontal fibrosing alopecia to be a variant of lichen planopilaris.

Weston G, Payette M. Update on lichen planus and its clinical variants. *Int J Womens Dermatol.* 2015;1:140–149. https://doi.org/10.1016/j.ijwd.2015.04.001.

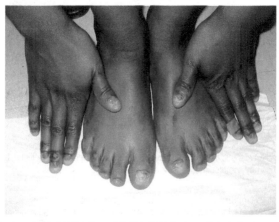

Fig. 12.4 Twenty-nail dystrophy secondary to lichen planus. Note that all 20 nails demonstrate varying degrees of nail dystrophy. (Courtesy Whitney A. High, MD.)

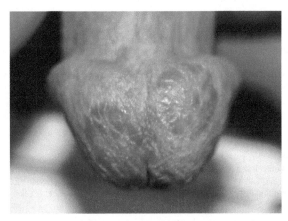

Fig. 12.5 Annular lichen planus on the glans was originally misdiagnosed as squamous cell carcinoma until its annular quality was noted by the dermatologist. (Courtesy Whitney A. High, MD.)

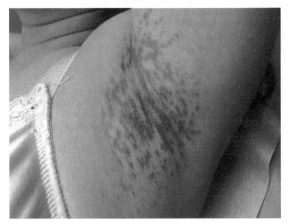

Fig. 12.6 Hyperpigmented atrophic lichen planus of the axillae. This clinical variant is called axillary "lichen planus pigmentosus-inversus." (Courtesy James E. Fitzpatrick, MD.)

10. How is trachyonychia (20-nail dystrophy) related to LP?

The etiology of trachyonychia is controversial. This destructive nail disorder affects mostly children, and it is not commonly associated with cutaneous lesions. Typically, any number of nails show excessive longitudinal ridging, with thin, brittle, opalescent nails. While some experts consider LP to be a possible etiology, other studies utilizing nail biopsy have demonstrated a spongiotic pattern of inflammation rather than a lichenoid process.

Shehgal VN. Twenty nail dystrophy trachyonychia: an overview. *J Dermatol.* 2007;34:361–366.

11. Is LP associated with systemic diseases?

LP has been associated with numerous disorders, but such relationships often engender controversy. Associated conditions include viral hepatitis, chronic active hepatitis, primary biliary cirrhosis, diabetes mellitus, internal malignancy, and autoimmune or connective tissue disease. The relationship to infection with hepatitis C virus (HCV) is controversial and not fully understood. Most studies conclude that LP may be a result of the host immune response to the HCV, but it is not a direct result of the virus on skin cells. At present, it is recommended that patients with LP be queried about major risk factors (intravenous [IV] drug use or sex with IV drug users) or minor risk factors (history of blood transfusion, male sex, and age 30 to 49 years) and that those with significant risk be screened for HCV antibodies.

Georgescu SR, Tampa M, Mitran MI, et al. Potential pathogenic mechanisms involved in the association between lichen planus and hepatitis C virus infection. *Exp Ther Med.* 2019;17:1045–1051. https://doi.org/10.3892/etm.2018.6987.

12. What is the prognosis of LP?

The duration of disease activity is related to the site of involvement. Isolated mucosal involvement portends a more chronic course, perhaps lasting decades. Additionally, patients with oral LP are at increased risk of squamous cell carcinoma arising within chronic lesions. Conversely, isolated cutaneous involvement typically resolves spontaneously within 1 to 2 years. Patients with both mucosal and cutaneous lesions typically have an intermediate prognosis. Certain clinical subtypes, such as ulcerative, palmoplantar, and actinic LP, are more persistent and recalcitrant to treatment. Twenty percent of patients may relapse after an initial clearing.

Carbone M, Arduino PG, Carrozzo M, et al. Course of oral lichen planus: a retrospective study of 808 northern Italian patients. *Oral Dis.* 2009;15:235–243.

13. What is the primary symptom of LP?

The pruritus of LP is often intense. Nearly all patients report some itching. Interestingly, the pruritus of LP often maintains a special quality that will induce rubbing, rather than scratching, for relief. Such rubbing may account for the polished appearance of the lesions. If excoriation occurs, new lesions are likely to develop within wounds (Koebnerization).

14. Describe the characteristic histopathologic features of classic LP.

- The stratum corneum is thickened (hyperkeratotic) but is largely devoid of retained keratinocytic nuclei (essentially no parakeratosis).
- The granular layer is focally accentuated ("wedge-shaped" hypergranulosis).
- The malpighian layer (stratum spinosum and stratum granulosum) is irregularly thickened, demonstrating a "sawtooth" acanthosis, with occasional necrotic keratinocytes in the superficial dermis (Civatte bodies).
- The basal layer is disrupted and appears lost or flattened ("interface reaction").
- The dermal-epidermal junction is vacuolated and obscured by a "bandlike" lymphocytic inflammatory infiltrate. This pattern of infiltration is so typical of LP, it is referred to as a "lichenoid infiltrate."

15. How is LP treated?

Topical corticosteroids and oral antihistamines are used to ameliorate the pruritus in mild cases. Hypertrophic lesions may not respond to topical treatment and instead may require intralesional corticosteroids. The optimal treatment of severe disease is difficult to determine, since the studies regarding treatment have been primarily anecdotal or consist of small series. The most commonly used treatment is systemic corticosteroids, but variable degrees of success have also been reported with topical calcineurin inhibitors (tacrolimus and pimecrolimus), psoralen plus ultraviolet A (PUVA) light therapy, narrowband ultraviolet B light therapy, oral retinoids (isotretinoin and acitretin), griseofulvin, methotrexate, cyclosporine, sulfasalazine, and thalidomide.

Tziotzios C, Brier T, Lee JYW, et al. Lichen planus and lichenoid dermatoses: conventional and emerging therapeutic strategies. *J Am Acad Dermatol.* 2018;79:807–818. https://doi.org/10.1016/j.jaad.2018.02.013.

16. What conditions enter the differential diagnosis of a "LP-like" eruption?

Lichenoid drug eruptions may be indistinguishable from idiopathic LP. Any exogenous ingestant, or rarely a topical chemical, may be causative. Common etiologic agents are listed in Table 12.1. Anti-PD1/PD1L therapy, which has

Table 12.1 Common etiologic drug classes in LP-like drug eruptions

Antihypertensives
Beta-blockers
ACE inhibitors
Thiazides
Furosemide
Methyldopa

Antimicrobials
Acyclovir
Isoniazid
Tetracyclines

Antiinflammatory agents
Nonsteroidal antiinflammatory drugs
Gold salts
Sulfones

Table 12.1 Common etiologic drug classes in LP-like drug eruptions (*Continued*)

Antimalarials
Chloroquine
Quinacrine
Anticonvulsants
Carbamazepine
Phenytoin

Neurologic agents
Benzodiazepines
Phenothiazines

Lipid-lowering agents
Lovastatin
Fluvastatin

Biologic response modifiers
Tumor necrosis factor–α antagonists (infliximab, etanercept, adalimumab)
Imatinib mesylate
Anti-PD1/PD1L (programmed death protein 1/programmed death protein ligand 1) therapy

Miscellaneous
Sulfonylureas
Chlorpropamide
Allopurinol
Penicillamine
Sildenafil
Misoprostol

ACE, Angiotensin-converting-enzyme; *LP,* lichen planus.

revolutionized the care of advanced melanoma, represents a new class of medication that can yield a lichenoid dermatitis. Other potables, such as alcoholic liqueurs containing gold particles, have been implicated in lichenoid eruptions. Contact with certain chemicals, particularly those involved with photo developing, may result in a lichenoid contact dermatitis. Clues suggesting a lichenoid drug eruption include an atypical distribution or lack of mucosal involvement. Histopathologic clues to a drug-induced eruption may include significant parakeratosis, an increased number of dyskeratotic cells (particularly in the upper epidermis), as well as increased eosinophils and plasma cells within the dermal inflammatory infiltrate.

Sibaud V. Dermatologic reactions to immune checkpoint inhibitors: skin toxicities and immunotherapy. *Am J Clin Dermatol.* 2018;19:345–361. https://doi.org/10.1007/s40257-017-0336-3.

Lage D, Juliano PB, Metze K, et al. Lichen planus and lichenoid drug-induced eruption: a histological and immunohistochemical study. *Int J Dermatol.* 2012;51:1199–1205.

17. Are LP and systemic lupus erythematosus related?
    Systemic lupus erythematosus (SLE) has been diagnosed in patients with LP, and an "LP-SLE overlap" syndrome has been described. Papulosquamous lesions of SLE, particularly those of acral areas, may resemble LP, but other features of SLE are usually present, allowing for discrimination.

Nagao K, Chen KR. A case of lupus erythematosus/lichen planus overlap syndrome. *J Dermatol.* 2006;33:187–190.

18. Are LP and bullous pemphigoid related?
    LP pemphigoides is a rare skin disease that presents with overlapping features of LP and bullous pemphigoid. It is characterized by bullous lesions arising on LP-like papules and also upon uninvolved skin. While the condition may arise de novo, particularly in children, it may also be induced by medications including cinnarizine, captopril, ramipril, simvastatin, PUVA, antituberculous medications, and some Chinese herbs.

Zaraa I, Mahfoudh A, Sellami MK, et al. Lichen planus pemphigoides: four new cases and a review of the literature. *Int J Dermatol.* 2013;52:406–412.

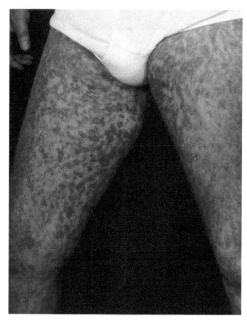

Fig. 12.7 Lichenoid graft-versus-host disease in a patient with myelogenous leukemia after an allogeneic bone marrow transplant. (Courtesy Fitzsimons Army Medical Center teaching files.)

19. Why is GVHD a consideration in LP-like eruptions?

GVHD is a complication of allogeneic bone marrow transplantation. In GVHD, the immune effector cells of the donor bone marrow (the "graft") react against antigens of the recipient tissues (the "host"). The resultant eruption may be indistinguishable, both clinically and histopathologically, from that of LP (Fig. 12.7). Lichenoid GVHD reaction is often more generalized than is classic LP, and the history would certainly be suggestive. GVHD resulting from solid-organ transplantation is exquisitely rare.

Wu PA, Cowen EW. Cutaneous graft-versus-host disease—clinical considerations and management. *Curr Probl Dermatol.* 2012;43:101–115.

KEY POINTS: LICHEN PLANUS

1. The primary lesion of lichen planus is a flat-topped, pruritic, purple, polygonal papule.
2. Lichen planus, in addition to affecting skin, can also affect the oral or vaginal mucosal surface, nails, or hair.
3. Lichen planus frequently demonstrates the isomorphic response (Koebner phenomenon), which refers to the development of new lesions in sites of minor trauma.
4. Lichen planus may be clinically and histologically mimicked by numerous drugs (lichenoid drug eruptions).

20. Describe the primary lesion of lichen nitidus.

Lichen nitidus (LN) manifests as innumerable, 1- to 2-mm, round or polygonal, flat-topped, shiny, flesh-colored papules occurring in well-circumscribed areas upon the extremities, abdomen, or penis (Fig. 12.8). Rarely, mucosal or nail changes are present.

Al-Mutairi N, Hassanein A, Nour-Eldin O, et al. Generalized lichen nitidus. *Pediatr Dermatol.* 2005;22:158–160.

21. What are the other clinical features of LN?

LN is uncommon relative to LP. It too has no gender, age, or race predilection. It may affect any age, but it is more common in children and young adults. The eruption is typically idiopathic, chronic, and, fortunately, asymptomatic. An isomorphic response may be demonstrated. The disease is most often self-limited and resolves spontaneously over months to years. There are no well-recognized disease associations.

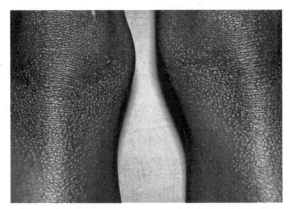

Fig. 12.8 Lichen nitidus, with numerous characteristic 1- to 2-mm, shiny, flat-topped papules. (Courtesy Walter Reed Army Medical Center teaching files.)

22. Does LN demonstrate a lichenoid infiltrate upon biopsy?

No. While LN appears "lichenoid" clinically, the histopathologic findings are granulomatous in nature. Typically, the epidermis demonstrates central atrophy, while peripheral epidermal rete ridges extend into the papillary dermis in "clawlike" fashion, surrounding a granulomatous aggregate of lymphocytes and histiocytes.

23. What is lichen striatus?

Lichen striatus is an uncommon idiopathic dermatosis that presents as a linear plaque, most often on the extremity or neck of a child or, less commonly, an adult. The condition consists of a coalescent group of flesh or rose-colored lichenoid papules (Fig. 12.9). The resultant linear plaque may form a band several centimeters wide and may course the entire length of the extremity. It may even involve the nail. Histologically, lichen striatus not only has lichenoid

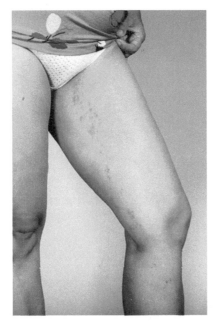

Fig. 12.9 Lichen striatus. Linear plaque composed of violaceous, slightly hyperpigmented papules confined to the lower extremity of a young adult. Most cases occur in children. (Courtesy Fitzsimons Army Medical Center teaching files.)

inflammation in the shallow dermis, but often a deeper perieccrine inflammatory infiltrate, and this is a distinguishing feature in comparison to most other lichenoid dermatoses.

Kim M, Jung HY, Eun YS, et al. Nail lichen striatus: report of seven cases and review of the literature. *Int J Dermatol*. 2015;54:1255–1260. https://doi.org/10.1111/ijd.12643.

Patrizi A, Neri I, Fiorentini C, et al. Lichen striatus: clinical and laboratory features of 115 children. *Pediatr Dermatol*. 2004;21:197–204.

24. **Discuss the natural history and prognosis of lichen striatus.**

    Lichen striatus develops rapidly over a period of weeks. Pruritus is common but may be minimal. Spontaneous resolution within a few years is characteristic. Patients with minimal pruritus require only reassurance. Recalcitrant or intensely pruritic cases may respond to topical corticosteroids.

25. **What is lichen simplex chronicus?**

    Lichen simplex chronicus (LSC) is not a disease but rather a reaction of the skin to chronic friction from rubbing or scratching. LSC may be superimposed upon normal skin, but it is often a secondary condition of chronically inflamed skin. The clinical appearance, termed *lichenification*, is characteristic, regardless of the underlying etiology. Relative thickening of the skin, with accentuation of the normal skin lines, is typical. Closely set lichenoid papules may be discerned at the periphery. Frequently, the lichenified plaque maintains a dusky violaceous hue.

26. **How is LSC treated?**

    LSC is a self-perpetuating dermatosis, and it will persist until the initiating stimulus is eliminated. Interruption of the "itch-scratch cycle" is requisite to resolution. A short course of medium- or high-potency topical corticosteroids is typically employed. Covering the plaque is often important, as this acts as a physical barrier to continued frictional trauma and also acts as an occlusive adjunct for the topical preparation. Patients who express insight into the cause of their condition fare better. Resultant postinflammatory dyspigmentation may last for years, even after the changes of lichenification have resolved.

27. **What is lichen spinulosis?**

    Lichen spinulosis is an uncommon dermatosis, but this may be due, in part, to underreporting. The condition presents most often in children and young adults, usually as a plaque or plaques, 2.5 to 5.0 cm in diameter, in which there is perifollicular keratosis and prominence. The lesions may appear similar to keratosis pilaris but exist in a circumscribed, plaque-like form. The neck, buttocks, abdomen, elbows, knees, and extensor surfaces of the arms are often affected. The etiology of the condition is unknown. Some authors have suggested that lichen spinulosus is part of atopy and/or xerosis. Clustered cases in families may suggest a genetic predisposition. The disorder is largely of cosmetic significance and is treated with moisturizers and keratolytics, in a manner akin to keratosis pilaris.

CHAPTER 13

GRANULOMATOUS DISEASES OF THE SKIN

Grant Plost and Lori D. Prok

1. **What is meant by "granulomatous diseases of the skin"?**

   Granulomatous disorders of the skin comprise a broad category of diseases that are characterized by the accumulation of activated macrophages with an epithelioid appearance in the dermis or subcutaneous tissue. A granuloma is a distinct aggregate composed of epithelioid macrophages with or without multinucleated giant cells. These aggregates are typically surrounded by a rim of lymphocytes with plasma cells being variably present. Macrophages develop from bone marrow–derived monocytes that leave the circulation and enter the skin.

2. **What is a "histiocyte"?**

   A histiocyte is a bone marrow–derived cell that is part of the mononuclear phagocytic system. Examples of histiocytes include tissue macrophages, Langerhans cells, and dermal dendritic cells. Histiocytes play an important role in the immune system, particularly with phagocytosis and antigen presentation.

3. **What is the difference between an immune granuloma and a foreign body granuloma?**

   Immune granuloma formation is a local tissue response to a poorly soluble substance that can induce a cell-mediated immune response (e.g., cutaneous tuberculosis). The persistent presence of a poorly soluble substance in the skin causes the activation of T cells, which secrete various cytokines that activate additional T cells, which transform macrophages into epithelioid macrophages and multinucleated giant cells. In contrast, foreign body granulomas typically are the result of larger aggregates of inert foreign material that cannot be phagocytized by a single macrophage (e.g., wood splinter). In general, granulomas are produced by infectious agents, foreign bodies, or alterations in the host immune system.

4. **List some common granulomatous diseases that affect the skin.**

   See Table 13.1.

5. **Can granulomas be recognized clinically?**

   Sometimes. Granulomas usually present as dermal and/or subcutaneous nodules, although epidermal changes can be present. Foreign body granulomas may demonstrate a central erosion or ulceration secondary to an attempt by the body to extrude the foreign material. Granulomas often present as nonspecific erythematous nodules; however, they also may present as dermal nodules with an "apple-jelly hue" that is highly suggestive of an underlying granulomatous process. This apple-jelly hue can frequently be appreciated by using diascopy (applying pressure to the lesion with a glass slide).

6. **How do endogenous "foreign" bodies cause granulomas?**

   Endogenous substances produce a granulomatous reaction when they come in contact with the dermis or subcutaneous fat. For example, one of the most common foreign body reactions occurs when an epidermal inclusion cyst wall ruptures and its keratin contents come in contact with the dermis. Normally, the keratin within the cyst is protected from the dermis by the cyst's epithelial lining. However, when a cyst ruptures, the keratin is exposed to the dermis, and being a poorly soluble substance, it produces a granulomatous response.

   A second mechanism occurs when endogenous substances that are normally soluble crystallize into large aggregates, which then provoke a granulomatous foreign body reaction (e.g., uric acid crystals in gouty tophi and calcium in calcinosis cutis).

7. **What are the sources of the exogenous foreign body agents?**

   See Table 13.2 and Fig. 13.1.

8. **Do cosmetic fillers ever produce foreign body granulomas?**

   Yes. Numerous cosmetic fillers, including products made from collagen (Fig. 13.2), silicone, hyaluronic acid, poly-L-lactic acid, calcium hydroxylapatite, and polymethylmethacrylate, have been reported to produce foreign body granulomas. Granulomas due to biodegradable cosmetic fillers may disappear spontaneously, while granulomas due to nonbiodegradable fillers may be permanent. As the use of cosmetic fillers for wrinkle reduction and soft tissue augmentation becomes more common, the number of reported cases of filler-induced foreign body granulomas is increasing.

Parada MB, Michalany NS, Hassun KM, et al. A histologic study of adverse effects of different cosmetic skin fillers. *Skinmed*. 2015;4: 345–346.

Requena L, Requena C, Christensen L, et al. Adverse reactions to injectable soft tissue fillers, *J Am Acad Dermatol*. 2011;64:1–34.

Table 13.1 Agents and diseases that can produce granulomas

Infectious agents

FUNGI	BACTERIA	MISCELLANEOUS INFECTIONS
Blastomycosis	Actinomycosis	Leishmaniasis
Candidiasis	Cat scratch fever	Prototheosis (algae infection)
Chromomycosis	Granuloma inguinale (donovanosis)	
Coccidioidomycosis	Mycobacterial infections	
Cryptococcosis	Nocardiosis	
Histoplasmosis	Syphilis	
Sporotrichosis	Tularemia	

Foreign body agents

Exogenous	Endogenous	Miscellaneous Diseases
Aluminum	Bone	Actinic granuloma
Cosmetic fillers	Calcium	Crohn's disease
Hair	Cholesterol	Granuloma annulare
Insect parts	Keratin	Granulomatous cheilitis
Paraffin	Hair	Granulomatous rosacea
Silica	Sebum	Lupus miliaris disseminatus faciei
Splinters	Urate crystals	Necrobiosis lipoidica
Starch		Rheumatoid nodule
Sutures		Sarcoidosis
Talc		
Tattoo pigment		

Table 13.2 Sources of foreign bodies

AGENT	SOURCE
Silicone	Breast implants, joint prostheses, soft tissue injections, hemodialysis tubing
Silica	Soil and rock (very abundant), glass
Paraffin (oils)	Cosmetic injection (historically), factitial injection, grease gun injury
Starch	Surgical gloves contaminating wounds
Graphite	Pencil lead (see Fig. 13.1A)
Thorns	Roses, cactus, yucca (see Fig. 13.1B)
Hair	Barbers, dog groomers, sheep shearers
Talc	IV drug use, wound contamination
Aluminum	Adjuvant in diphtheria, pertussis, and tetanus immunizations
Zirconium	Deodorant sticks
Beryllium	Metal, ceramic, and electronic industries; fluorescent lamp workers (historically, as this ceased in 1951)

9. Can the cause of a foreign body reaction be diagnosed histologically?
   Sometimes. A tattoo granuloma may retain some color or pigment that can help with the diagnosis. Silicone, paraffin, and other oils are often accompanied by fibrosis and a characteristic "Swiss cheese" appearance. The Swiss cheese–like holes are cavities formerly filled with the oily material that is lost during tissue processing. Also, some foreign bodies are birefringent under polarized light (e.g., talc, starch, silica, and some types of sutures).

10. What is sarcoidosis?
   Sarcoidosis is a systemic granulomatous disease characterized by the formation of noncaseating granulomas. The most commonly involved organs are the lungs, lymph nodes, and skin. The cause of sarcoidosis is unknown, but certain individuals may have a genetic predisposition. Sarcoidosis is more common in African Americans and women. The course is unpredictable, as the granulomas in sarcoidosis may resolve or progress to fibrosis.

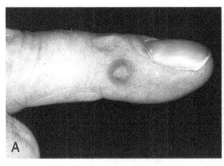 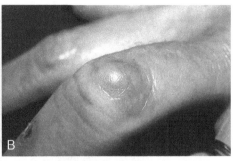

Fig. 13.1 A, Typical graphite granuloma due to pencil lead injury. **B,** Skin-colored nodule due to yucca thorn embedded in the skin for several years.

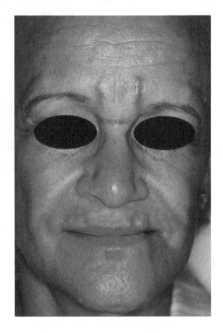

Fig. 13.2 Patient with foreign body reaction to cosmetic filler demonstrating erythematous papules and linear lesions at the site of bovine collagen injection. (Courtesy Fitzsimons Army Medical Center teaching files.)

11. How often is the skin involved in sarcoidosis?

The skin is involved in at least 20% of patients and may be the first manifestation of the disease. The skin findings are divided into specific and nonspecific lesions. Specific lesions demonstrate noncaseating granulomas on histology, while nonspecific lesions demonstrate reactive changes.

12. Describe the specific cutaneous findings in sarcoidosis.

The most common specific cutaneous findings are papules that are smooth and red-brown in color. Papules are typically found around eyelids and nasolabial folds (Fig. 13.3). Papules are associated with a good prognosis and usually heal without scarring.

The second most common specific skin lesions are plaques that are located on the back, buttocks, face, and extensor surfaces. Sometimes, plaques assume an annular configuration. Plaques are associated with chronic disease and may heal with scarring.

Less common types of specific cutaneous findings include subcutaneous, psoriasiform, verrucous, erythroderma, lichenoid, involvement of scars and tattoos, nail dystrophy, and alopecia.

13. What is lupus pernio?

This distinct form of cutaneous sarcoidosis presents as violaceous, indurated plaques on the nose and cheeks (Fig. 13.4). Lupus pernio is an insidious process that is challenging to treat and often results in scarring, fibrosis, and deformity. It is associated with multisystemic disease with intrathoracic, upper respiratory tract, bone, and lymph node involvement.

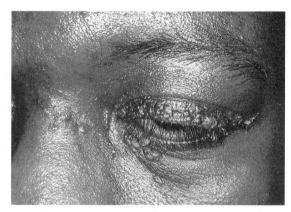

Fig. 13.3 Typical numerous periocular papules in a patient with sarcoidosis.

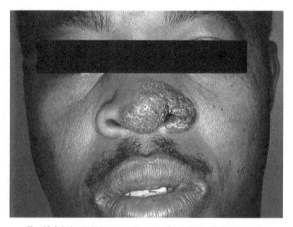

Fig. 13.4 Indurated plaque on the nose of a patient with lupus pernio.

14. Describe the nonspecific cutaneous lesions of sarcoidosis.

The most common nonspecific cutaneous lesion is erythema nodosum, which may be present in up to 25% of patients. Clinically and histologically, it is identical to erythema nodosum associated with other conditions. Less common nonspecific cutaneous lesions include acquired ichthyosis (Fig. 13.5A), calcinosis cutis, erythema multiforme, and nail clubbing.

15. Does sarcoidosis ever present in the skin without extracutaneous involvement?

Yes. Even though sarcoidosis is defined as a multisystem disorder, some patients present with cutaneous lesions without any evidence of involvement of other organ systems. It is possible that some of these patients have minimal or asymptomatic involvement of other organ systems. In other cases, the skin lesions precede the discovery of multisystem involvement.

16. What is Löfgren syndrome?

This is the classic acute presentation of sarcoidosis. It consists of the erythema nodosum, arthritis, bilateral hilar adenopathy, uveitis, and fever (Fig. 13.5B). Sarcoidosis that presents in this manner has an 80% chance of resolving within 2 years.

17. What is Heerfordt syndrome?

Heerfordt syndrome or uveoparotid fever is a variant of sarcoidosis presenting as uveitis, facial nerve palsy, fever, and parotid gland swelling.

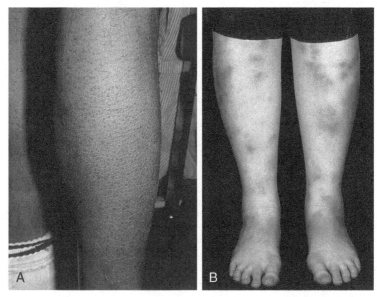

Fig. 13.5 A, Acquired ichthyosis in a patient with sarcoidosis. **B,** Patient with Löfgren syndrome demonstrating tender red subcutaneous lesions characteristic of erythema nodosum.

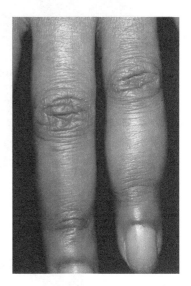

Fig. 13.6 Subcutaneous sarcoidosis (Darier-Roussy disease) demonstrating skin-colored subcutaneous swelling. (Courtesy Walter Reed Army Medical Center teaching files.)

18. What is Darier-Roussy disease?

    Darier-Roussy disease is the subcutaneous variant of sarcoidosis. The clinical lesions often present as skin-colored subcutaneous nodules or areas of induration (Fig. 13.6).

19. How should cutaneous sarcoidosis be treated?

    Treatment is recommended for patients with symptomatic or disfiguring cutaneous sarcoidosis. For patients with localized and mild skin involvement, high-potency topical corticosteroids or intralesional corticosteroids are the treatment of choice. For patients with extensive or disfiguring skin involvement, systemic corticosteroids, hydroxychloroquine, methotrexate, and tetracyclines are reasonable treatment options. Refractory patients may benefit from tumor necrosis factor-α antagonists such as adalimumab and infliximab.

Haimovic A, Sanchez M, Judson MA, et al. Sarcoidosis: a comprehensive review and update for the dermatologist: part 1. Cutaneous disease. *J Am Acad Dermatol.* 2012;66:699.

Haimovic A, Sanchez M, Judson MA, et al. Sarcoidosis: a comprehensive review and update for the dermatologist: part 2. Extracutaneous disease. *J Am Acad Dermatol.* 2012;66(5):719.

KEY POINTS: CUTANEOUS SARCOIDOSIS

1. Cutaneous sarcoidosis occurs in at least 20% of patients with sarcoidosis.
2. Cutaneous sarcoidosis may be the first sign of sarcoidosis.
3. Lupus pernio is a variant of cutaneous sarcoidosis associated with multisystem involvement that presents as violaceous, indurated plaques on the nose and cheeks.
4. Löfgren syndrome consists of erythema nodosum, arthritis, bilateral hilar adenopathy, uveitis, and fever.
5. Heerfordt syndrome, or uveoparotid fever, is a variant of sarcoidosis presenting as uveitis, facial nerve palsy, fever, and parotid gland swelling.

20. What is the typical presentation of granuloma annulare?

Localized granuloma annulare is the most common variant. It typically presents with flesh-colored to pink, dermal papules or plaques arranged in an annular configuration on the dorsal hands and feet (Fig. 13.7A). Generalized granuloma annulare manifests with more extensive involvement of the trunk and extremities. Subcutaneous granuloma annulare (Fig. 13.7B) presents as subcutaneous nodules on the lower extremities in children.

21. What is annular elastolytic giant cell granuloma?

Annular elastolytic giant cell granuloma, also known as actinic granuloma, is a variant of granuloma annulare that presents with annular plaques with central atrophy in a sun-exposed distribution (Fig. 13.8).

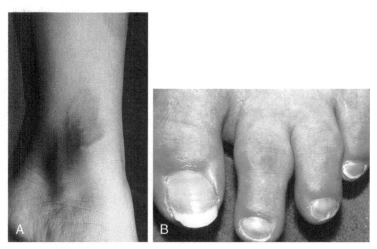

Fig. 13.7 **A,** Typical lesion of granuloma annulare demonstrating raised annular lesions without scale. **B,** Subcutaneous granuloma annulare of proximal second toe.

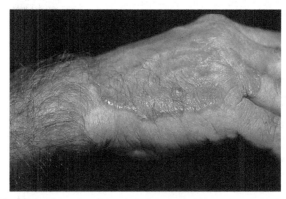

Fig. 13.8 Actinic granuloma demonstrating large annular lesion on sun-exposed skin.

22. Do any systemic associations occur with granuloma annulare?

Granuloma annulare generally occurs in isolation without any associated systemic process. Some studies show that generalized granuloma annulare may be associated with diabetes and hyperlipidemia.

23. What is the typical course of granuloma annulare?

Approximately 50% of patients with localized granuloma annulare will have spontaneous resolution within 2 years. Recurrence, however, is common. Generalized granuloma annulare tends to have a much more protracted course and is frequently less responsive to therapy.

24. How is granuloma annulare treated?

Given the chance for spontaneous resolution, observation is an acceptable treatment option for granuloma annulare. For patients with symptomatic or disfiguring granuloma annulare, there are several proposed treatments. For localized granuloma annulare, intralesional corticosteroids can be effective. For generalized granuloma annulare, hydroxychloroquine and phototherapy have been reported to be helpful.

Piette EW, Rosenbach M. Granuloma annulare: Clinical and histologic variants, epidemiology, and genetics. *J Am Acad Dermatol*. 2016; 75(3):457–465.
Piette EW, Rosenbach M. Granuloma annulare: pathogenesis, disease associations and triggers, and therapeutic options. *J Am Acad Dermatol*. 2016;75(3):467–479.

25. What is the most common extra-articular manifestation of rheumatoid arthritis?

Rheumatoid nodules

26. What is the typical presentation of rheumatoid nodules?

Rheumatoid nodules present as firm, subcutaneous nodules on extensor surfaces adjacent to joints and in areas of pressure. Common locations include the elbow (Fig. 13.9) and dorsal hands. Rheumatoid nodules are present in up to 35% of individuals with rheumatoid arthritis.

27. What are the treatment options for rheumatoid nodules?

Rheumatoid nodules that are asymptomatic and do not impair function can be observed without treatment. For symptomatic rheumatoid nodules, intralesional corticosteroids may provide relief. Surgical excision is another treatment option.

28. What is accelerated nodulosis?

Accelerated nodulosis is the paradoxical onset of rheumatoid nodules in a small subset of patients with rheumatoid arthritis who are treated with methotrexate.

Tilstra JS, Lienesch DW. Rheumatoid nodules. *Dermatol Clin*. 2015;33(3):361–371.

29. Do patients with lupus miliaris disseminatus faciei have lupus erythematosus?

No. Lupus miliaris disseminatus faciei is a misnomer. It is a chronic granulomatous disorder of unknown etiology. It presents as monomorphic, flesh-colored to yellow-brown papules of the face (Fig. 13.10). Extrafacial lesions involving the axillae and genitalia have also been reported. Some dermatologists consider lupus miliaris disseminatus faciei to be a variant of granulomatous rosacea or granulomatous periorificial dermatitis.

Free R, Pflederer RT, et al. Flesh-colored papules and nodules on the face. *JAAD Case Rep*. 2018;4(6):512–514.

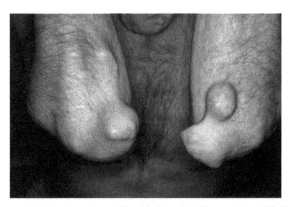

Fig. 13.9 Unusually large dermal and subcutaneous rheumatoid nodules in a patient with severe rheumatoid arthritis. (Courtesy Fitzsimons Army Medical Center teaching files.)

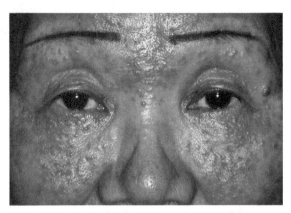

Fig. 13.10 Lupus miliaris disseminatus faciei. Numerous red to reddish-brown papules of the central face. (Courtesy Walter Reed Army Medical Center teaching files.)

30. What is the typical presentation of necrobiosis lipoidica?

Necrobiosis lipoidica presents as yellow-brown, waxy, atrophic plaques that are most commonly on the bilateral lower extremities. These plaques often become ulcerated with minor trauma.

31. Which systemic disease is associated with necrobiosis lipoidica?

Diabetes mellitus. Approximately 16% of patients with necrobiosis lipoidica have diabetes at the time of diagnosis or will develop diabetes later in life. Less than 1% of patients with diabetes will develop necrobiosis lipoidica.

32. What is the first-line treatment for necrobiosis lipoidica?

Intralesional corticosteroids or high-potency topical steroids.

Reid SD, Ladizinski B, et al. Update on necrobiosis lipoidica: a review of etiology, diagnosis, and treatment options. *J Am Acad Dermatol.* 2013 Nov;69(5):783–791.

33. What are the cutaneous manifestations of Crohn disease?

Perianal fissures and fistulae are found in up to 33% of patients with Crohn disease. Genital lymphedema is another manifestation of Crohn disease. Orofacial granulomatosis is a less common cutaneous finding that presents with cobblestone-like papules of the oral mucosa and edema of the vermilion lips.

Hagen JW, Swoger JM, Grandinetti LM. Cutaneous manifestations of Crohn disease. *Dermatol Clin.* 2015;33(3):417–431.

CHAPTER 14

DRUG ERUPTIONS

Lori D. Prok

1. **A patient presents to your office with a 10-page typed-out medical history. She states that she is "allergic" to 20 different medicines. Is she likely to have drug allergies or drug intolerances to most of these drugs?**

   Drug intolerances account for 90% of adverse drug reactions. An adverse reaction to a drug is an undesirable and usually unanticipated response independent of the intended therapeutic purpose of the medication. An adverse drug reaction may be either immunologic (i.e., drug allergy) or nonimmunologic (i.e., drug intolerance).

2. **Name some nonimmunologic drug reactions.**
   - Nonimmunologic activation of effector pathways, such as direct release of histamine from mast cells and basophils by aspirin, nonsteroidal antiinflammatory drugs (NSAIDs), opiates, polymyxin B, d-tubocurarine, and radiocontrast media.
   - Overdosage.
   - Cumulative toxicity, such as the accumulation of drugs or metabolites in the skin (e.g., argyria with the use of silver nitrate spray).
   - Normal pharmacologic effects of the drug that are not the primary therapeutic objective (e.g., alopecia following chemotherapy).
   - Drug interactions (e.g., administration of ketoconazole may lead to higher levels of cyclosporine and increased toxicity).
   - Metabolic changes, such as warfarin producing a hypercoagulable state that results in warfarin necrosis.
   - Exacerbation of preexisting dermatologic diseases (e.g., lithium can exacerbate acne, psoriasis, and subcorneal pustular dermatosis).
   - Ecologic changes, such as antibiotics that reduce the bacteriologic flora, predisposing the patient to candidal infections.
   - Inherited enzyme or protein deficiencies (e.g., the phenytoin hypersensitivity syndrome occurs in patients deficient in epoxide hydrolase, an enzyme required for metabolism of a toxic epoxide derived from phenytoin).
   - Jarisch-Herxheimer phenomenon secondary to bacterial endotoxins and microbial antigens that are liberated from antimicrobial treatment (e.g., a patient with syphilis develops fever, tender lymphadenopathy, arthralgias, and urticaria while being treated with penicillin).

3. **What is the most common manifestation of an adverse drug reaction?**

   Cutaneous reactions are the most common adverse drug reaction and produce a wide range of manifestations: pruritus, maculopapular eruptions, urticaria, angioedema, phototoxic and photoallergic reactions, fixed drug reactions, erythema multiforme, vesiculobullous reactions, and exfoliative dermatitis. Drug-attributed skin reactions are seen in 2% to 5% of inpatients and greater than 1% of outpatients.

Hoetzenecker W, et al. Adverse cutaneous drug eruptions: current understanding. *Semin Immunopathol.* 2016 Jan;38(1):75–86.

4. **How does a cutaneous drug eruption typically present?**
   - Maculopapular or morbilliform exanthem: 46%
   - Urticaria and angioedema: 26%
   - Fixed drug eruptions: 10%
   - Erythema multiforme: 5%
   - Stevens-Johnson syndrome: 4%
   - Exfoliative dermatitis: 4%
   - Photosensitivity reactions: 3%
   - Anaphylaxis: 1.5%
   - Toxic epidermal necrolysis (TEN): 1.3%

KEY POINTS: DRUG ERUPTIONS

1. Consider a fixed drug eruption in a patient who presents with bullous or hyperpigmented lesions that are recurrent at the same site.
2. Consider a drug reaction in any patient who presents with an abrupt-onset, symmetrical, cutaneous reaction.
3. Consider a photoinduced drug reaction in a patient presenting with an erythematous, cutaneous reaction involving sun-exposed areas.
4. The clinical signs of a potentially life-threatening drug eruption include high fever, dyspnea or hypotension, angioedema and tongue swelling, palpable purpura, skin necrosis, blistering, mucous membrane erosions, confluent erythema, and lymphadenopathy.

5. How should a suspected drug reaction be evaluated?
Six variables should be evaluated:
- Previous experience or relative reaction rates of a given drug.
- Rule out alternative etiologies, such as exacerbation of a previous dermatosis or a new skin disease unrelated to the drug.
- Timing of events (most drug reactions occur within 1 to 2 weeks of initiation of therapy).
- Drug levels.
- Reaction to dechallenge (most drug reactions clear within 2 weeks of discontinuing drug).
- Response to rechallenge is most definitive.

6. Which commonly used drugs are most likely to produce a cutaneous reaction?
See Table 14.1.

7. Can preexisting diseases enhance the chance of getting a maculopapular skin eruption when using amoxicillin or ampicillin?
Amoxicillin or ampicillin produces a maculopapular eruption in about 5% of patients taking these drugs (Fig. 14.1). In patients with infectious mononucleosis, the risk of developing a maculopapular eruption increases to 69% to 100%. In chronic lymphocytic leukemia, the incidence is 60% to 70%. Some studies report that maculopapular eruptions are more common in patients who are also taking allopurinol, but this is not accepted by all authorities. The pathogenesis for this phenomenon is unknown.

8. What infectious disease increases the chance of a cutaneous adverse reaction to trimethoprim-sulfamethoxazole?
Acquired immunodeficiency syndrome (AIDS). The normal incidence of cutaneous reactions to trimethoprim-sulfamethoxazole is 3%, but this increases to 29% to 70% in patients with AIDS. The incidence of morbilliform drug reactions is 10-fold higher in human immunodeficiency virus–infected persons.

9. Which feared drug eruption results in sloughing of the entire skin surface and mucous membranes?
TEN is one of the most severe cutaneous drug eruptions. The skin is initially erythematous and tender but quickly sloughs off in large sheets like "wet wallpaper" (Fig. 14.2). The condition can progress very rapidly, with one of seven patients losing their entire epidermis in 24 hours. Without an epidermis, the body has difficulty keeping fluids in and bacteria out. Despite aggressive supportive care, the mortality rate ranges from 11% to 35%, with the majority of deaths being attributed to sepsis.

   The best therapy is to discontinue all likely drugs if possible, make sure the patient is well hydrated, and continually assess the patient for signs of secondary infection. Severe cases are best handled in burn units. The use of systemic corticosteroids, tumor necrosis factor-α inhibitors, and intravenous immunoglobulin has been investigated but remains controversial.

Egren EN, Hughey LC. Stevens-Johnson syndrome and toxic epidermal necrolysis. *JAMA Dermatol.* 2017 Dec 1;153(12):1344.

Table 14.1 Drugs most likely to produce a cutaneous reaction	
DRUG	**REACTIONS PER 1000 PATIENTS**
Amoxicillin	51.4
Trimethoprim-sulfamethoxazole	47
Ampicillin	42
Ipodate sodium	27.8
Whole blood	28
Cephalosporins	13

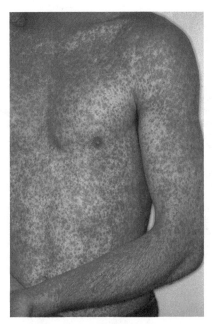

Fig. 14.1 Amoxicillin-induced maculopapular (morbilliform) drug eruption in a patient with infectious mononucleosis. In most studies, morbilliform drug eruptions are the most common cutaneous side effect. (Courtesy Scott D. Bennion, MD.)

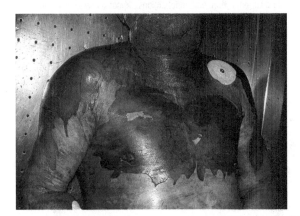

Fig. 14.2 Fatal case of toxic epidermal necrolysis secondary to captopril. The skin characteristically sloughs off in large sheets. (Courtesy James E. Fitzpatrick, MD.)

10. Why do some patients get TEN?

The etiology is not completely understood, but recent evidence has found a genetic predisposition in at least some classes of drugs (e.g., association of aromatic antiepileptic drugs and HLA-B*1502 in the Han Chinese). It is likely that continued research will uncover more ties to a genetic predisposition. The molecular and immunologic events are still not fully elucidated; however, the recent demonstration of very high levels of soluble FasL interacting with Fas, which is expressed on the keratinocytes in TEN, may provide insight into the pathophysiology of this life-threatening disorder. In one series, 77% of cases were clearly established as drug induced. Since the average patient with TEN is on 4.4 drugs, identifying the offending drug can be problematic. Frequent offenders include allopurinol, ampicillin, amoxicillin, carbamazepine, NSAIDs, phenobarbital, phenytoin, and sulfonamides.

Oussalah A, Yip V, Mayorga C, et al. Genetic variants associated with T-cell mediated cutaneous adverse drug reactions: a PRISMA-compliant systematic review—an EAACI Position Paper. Task Force "Genetic predictors of drug hypersensitivity" of the European Network on Drug Allergy (ENDA), European Academy of Allergy, Clinical Immunology (EAACI). *Allergy.* 2020;75:1069–1098.

11. What is the difference between erythema multiforme, Stevens-Johnson syndrome, and TEN?
    This is a critical and important question that is difficult to answer because this nosological nightmare continues to be controversial. The short version of these distinctions is as follows:
    - **Erythema multiforme** is best defined as presentation with targetoid skin lesions in the absence of systemic illness or severe mucosal disease (Fig. 14.3). While this variant can be drug-induced, it is more commonly induced by infections such as herpes simplex and *Mycoplasma*. Microscopically, the keratinocytes are being damaged by lymphocytes (satellite cell necrosis).
    - **Stevens-Johnson syndrome** is most commonly defined as presentation with widespread targetoid lesions that are flat and atypical when compared to the more defined lesions of erythema multiforme. Lesions are also more frequently purpuric. Patients may have fever and systemic symptoms. The lesions are more likely to become confluent and develop large areas of blisters and detachment of the epidermis. While some cases are idiopathic or induced by infections, the majority are drug induced. Histologically, the findings are identical to erythema multiforme in that the keratinocytes demonstrate satellite cell necrosis. Some dermatologists arbitrarily define this condition as affecting less than 30% of the body surface, and some authorities even recognize a Stevens-Johnson syndrome/toxic epidermal necrosis overlap syndrome.
    - **TEN** is best defined as a blistering disorder with extensive detachment of the skin that is almost always drug induced, although there are exceptions. Many of the drugs that produce classic Stevens-Johnson syndrome also produce TEN. Targetoid lesions are not usually present, but if present, are atypical. Microscopically, biopsies are cell poor, and keratinocytes become necrotic without evidence of satellite cell necrosis, suggesting a soluble factor. Some dermatologists arbitrarily differentiate this from Stevens-Johnson syndrome if more than 30% of the cutaneous surface is involved, and many dermatologists feel that TEN and Stevens-Johnson syndrome represent a spectrum of disease.

Yager JA. Erythema multiforme, Stevens-Johnson syndrome and toxic epidermal necrolysis: a comparative review. *Vet Dermatol.* 2014 Oct;25(5):406.

12. What drugs are typically associated with Stevens-Johnson syndrome?
    Commonly implicated drugs include allopurinol, amoxicillin, ampicillin, anticonvulsants, barbiturates, carbamazepine, gold, NSAIDs, phenobarbital, phenytoin, and sulfonamides. *Mycoplasma pneumoniae* and other infections are also well documented to produce Stevens-Johnson syndrome.

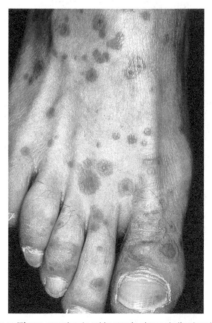

Fig. 14.3 Classic lesions of erythema multiforme secondary to cotrimoxazole, demonstrating targetoid appearance. (Courtesy James E. Fitzpatrick, MD.)

13. Which type of drug reaction can result in a quick death?
    Systemic anaphylaxis, which is IgE mediated, may present with variable findings, including mild pruritus, erythema, urticaria, asthma, circulatory collapse, laryngeal edema, and death. When a patient gives a history of reaction to a drug, the health care provider must ask for details about the previous reaction, particularly seeking a history of urticaria, breathing problems, collapse, and hospitalization.

14. What class of drugs is the most common cause of anaphylaxis?
    Beta-lactam antibiotics. Anaphylactic reactions occur in 1 to 5 per 10,000 administrations of penicillin. Most allergic reactions to beta-lactam antibiotics produce urticaria and angioedema, but 10% may result in life-threatening hypotension, bronchospasm, or laryngeal edema. Approximately 1% of all anaphylactic reactions are fatal. Fatal reactions may occur within minutes of parenteral administration of these drugs.

15. Name the drugs most likely to induce urticaria.
    Angiotensin-converting enzyme (ACE) inhibitors, gamma-globulin, NSAIDs, penicillins, and sulfonamides. Urticaria produced by drugs is clinically indistinguishable from urticaria produced by other allergens. Aspirin can exacerbate a preexisting urticaria. If possible, aspirin should be discontinued and not utilized in patients with active urticaria.

16. How is drug-induced urticaria mediated?
    Urticaria may be produced by both nonimmunologic and immunologic mechanisms. Drugs such as codeine, morphine, amphetamine, hydralazine, quinine, vancomycin, and x-ray contrast media produce urticaria by the nonimmunologic release of histamine by mast cells. Allergic urticaria may be due to a type I (Coombs and Gell) reaction mediated by IgE, causing the release of histamine. This usually develops within minutes to hours (usually within 1 hour) after giving the offending drug and may precede or be associated with anaphylaxis. Urticaria may also be produced by a type III reaction mediated by antigen-antibody complexes. In contrast to type I reactions, which occur within hours, type III urticaria usually develops 1 to 3 weeks after beginning the drug. The clinical appearance of urticaria is often mistaken for erythema multiforme.

17. A 45-year-old white man comes to the emergency room with large areas of nonpitting edema over the face, eyelids, neck, tongue, and mucous membranes, which developed 6 hours ago. Ten days earlier, he started a new drug for hypertension. What is the most likely cause of his reaction?
    The clinical description is that of a patient who has angioedema. An ACE inhibitor, such as captopril, enalapril, or lisinopril, is the most likely antihypertensive drug to produce this reaction. A recent study reported that 35% of 17 patients seen for angioedema during a 5-year period were on ACE inhibitors. In another study, 77% of patients experienced the reaction within 3 weeks of starting treatment.

18. A patient is evaluated for a several-day history of fever, malaise, urticaria, arthralgias, lymphadenopathy, and a peculiar erythema along the sides of his palms and soles. He has been started on several new medications in the last few weeks. What is the most likely diagnosis?
    The patient most likely has a serum sickness–like drug eruption caused by immune complexes and complement activation. The diagnostic cutaneous finding is the characteristic erythema on the sides of the palms and soles, a finding seen in 75% of cases of serum sickness–like drug eruptions. Other typical findings include fever and malaise (100%), urticaria (90%), arthralgias (50% to 67%), and lymphadenopathy (13%). Glomerulonephritis is common in serum sickness reactions in animals but uncommon in humans. Reactions occur 7 to 21 days after the drug is given but may occur with the first administration of the drug. Commonly implicated drugs include beta-lactam antibiotics, sulfonamides, thiouracil, cholecystographic dyes, and hydantoin.

19. A man complains of a recurrent burning eruption on his penis. He develops a single blister over the glans penis that heals over 1 to 2 weeks with hyperpigmentation. This same pattern has happened on three occasions in the last 2 years. What does he have?
    The history is characteristic of a fixed drug eruption. Fixed drug eruptions are cutaneous reactions that recur at the same site with each administration of the drug, typically within 6 to 48 hours of initiation of the causative agent. Characteristically, it occurs on the face or genitalia but may occur anywhere (Fig. 14.4). It is a well-demarcated erythematous lesion that often blisters and heals with hyperpigmentation. Drugs commonly associated include phenolphthalein in laxatives, sulfonamides, beta-lactam antibiotics, tetracycline, barbiturates, gold, oral contraceptives, diazepam, and aspirin. Foods have also been implicated in fixed drug reactions.

Patel S, John AM, Handler MZ, Schwartz RA. Fixed drug eruptions: an update, emphasizing the potentially lethal generalized bullous fixed drug eruption [published online ahead of print January 30, 2020]. *Am J Clin Dermatol.*

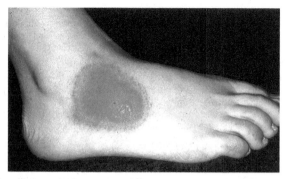

Fig. 14.4 Sulfonamide-induced fixed drug eruption of the ankle manifesting an erythematous plaque and focal blisters. (Courtesy James E. Fitzpatrick, MD.)

20. How does drug-induced lupus erythematosus (LE) differ from idiopathic systemic lupus erythematosus (SLE)?

Drug-induced LE is generally milder than idiopathic SLE. Drug-induced LE usually manifests as fever, malaise, pleuritis, pneumonitis, and arthralgias. Skin, mucous membrane, central nervous system findings, and renal disease are more commonly seen in idiopathic SLE. The antinuclear antibodies in drug-induced LE are usually antihistone and single-stranded DNA antibodies, whereas idiopathic SLE is associated with double-stranded DNA and Sm antibodies. Drug-induced LE usually resolves simply by stopping the drug. Drug-induced LE constitutes 5% to 10% of all cases of SLE. Less commonly patients may have drug-induced subacute cutaneous LE with anti-Ro/SSA antibodies or classic systemic lupus with drug-induced double-stranded DNA antibodies.

Borucki R, Werth VP. Cutaneous lupus erythematosus induced by drugs—novel insights. *Expert Rev Clin Pharmacol.* 2020 Jan;13(1):35–42.

21. What drugs are usually associated with drug-induced LE?

Of patients treated continuously with procainamide, 90% develop antinuclear antibodies after 2 years, and 10% to 20% develop symptoms of LE. Other commonly implicated drugs include hydralazine, isoniazid, chlorpromazine, procainamide, hydantoin, d-penicillamine, methyldopa, quinidine, and minocycline.

22. Which drug is usually associated with erythema nodosum?

Erythema nodosum, which is a form of panniculitis that characteristically presents as tender erythematous nodules over the shins, is most commonly associated with oral contraceptives. Sulfonamides, bromides, iodides, tetracycline, penicillin, and 13-cis retinoic acid have also been associated with erythema nodosum.

23. What drugs are associated with lichenoid drug eruptions?

Lichenoid drug eruptions clinically and histologically resemble lichen planus. The lesions are usually multiple, purple, discrete, flat-topped polygonal papules and plaques. As in the case of lichen planus, this reaction may also affect or even be limited to the oral mucosa. This differs from other drug reactions in that it may take weeks to years following administration of the drug to develop the lesions. Sulfonamides (especially thiazide diuretics), gold, captopril, propranolol, and antimalarials are the most common drugs that produce these reactions. It may take months for the rash to resolve following discontinuation of the drug.

Fessa C, Lim P, Kossard S, et al. Lichen planus-like drug eruptions due to β-blockers: a case report and literature review. *Am J Clin Dermatol.* 2012;13:417–421.

24. Name the drugs most likely to produce cutaneous hyperpigmentation and discoloration.

Drugs produce cutaneous hyperpigmentation and discoloration by different mechanisms. The two main mechanisms of hyperpigmentation and discoloration are drug deposition (e.g., heavy metals) and stimulation of melanocytic activity (Table 14.2; Fig. 14.5).

25. What drugs can produce subepidermal bullae and erosions on the dorsum of the hands?

This description is characteristic of the eruption seen in porphyria cutanea tarda and, less commonly, in variegate porphyria and hereditary coproporphyria but it can also be produced by drugs. This reaction is called pseudoporphyria, since the porphyrin levels are normal (Fig. 14.6). Tetracycline, nalidixic acid, oral contraceptives, cyclosporine, furosemide and other sulfonamides, dapsone, NSAIDs, 5-fluorouracil, isotretinoin, and pyridoxine are most likely to induce pseudoporphyria.

LaDuca JR, Bouman PH, Gaspari AA. Nonsteroidal anti-inflammatory drug-induced pseudoporphyria: a case series. *J Cutan Med Surg.* 2002;6:320–326.

Table 14.2 Drugs producing changes in skin pigmentation	
COLOR	**DRUG**
Slate-gray	Chloroquine Hydroxychloroquine (see Fig. 14.5A) Minocycline (see Fig. 14.5B) Phenothiazines
Slate-blue	Amiodarone
Blue-gray	Gold (chrysoderma)
Yellow	Beta-carotene Quinacrine
Red	Clofazimine
Brown (hyperpigmentation)	Adrenocorticotropic hormone (ACTH) Bleomycin Oral contraceptives Zidovudine

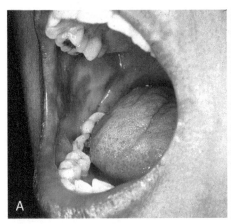 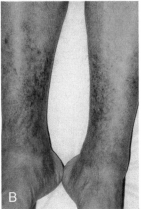

Fig. 14.5 A, Hydroxychloroquine-induced slate-gray pigmentation of the buccal mucosa. **B,** Minocycline-induced slate-gray pigment of lower legs. The minocycline is complexed with the extravascular hemosiderin from stasis dermatitis, which accounts for the distinctive distribution. (Courtesy Fitzsimons Army Medical Center teaching files.)

26. Name two drugs that commonly exacerbate porphyria cutanea tarda.
    Ethanol and estrogens.

27. A 30-year-old white woman is evaluated with a new case of "acne." Over the last few days, she has suddenly developed erythematous follicular papules and pustules over her upper trunk. She was admitted 3 weeks earlier with an acute exacerbation of SLE that is now improving. What is the most likely diagnosis?
    Steroid acne is the most likely diagnosis. Her history indicates a high probability that she was started on corticosteroids during the admission. Steroid acne typically presents with inflammatory papules and pustules, but comedones and cysts are typically absent. In contrast to acne vulgaris, steroid acne preferentially involves the trunk and demonstrates lesions in the same stage of development. Other drugs associated with similar eruptions include lithium, isoniazid, bromides, and iodides. Many chemotherapeutic agents have also been associated with acneiform reactions. These include cetuximab, dactinomycin, erlotinib, fluoxymesterone, gefitinib, medroxyprogesterone, and vinblastine.

Sibaud V. Dermatologic reactions to immune checkpoint inhibitors: skin toxicities and immunotherapy. *Am J Clin Dermatol.* 2018 Jun;19 (3):345–361.

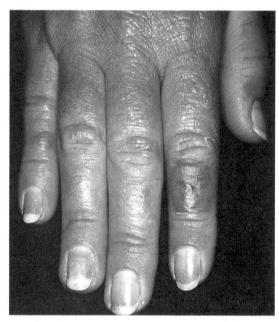

Fig. 14.6 Tetracycline-induced pseudoporphyria demonstrating hemorrhagic blisters and erosions over the back of the hand. (Courtesy James E. Fitzpatrick, MD.)

28. A middle-aged man who is a dialysis patient presents to your clinic with a "woody" appearance to his legs. He had magnetic resonance scan with gadolinium-containing contrast a few months prior. What might he be suffering from?

    Nephrogenic systemic fibrosis (formerly called nephrogenic fibrosing dermopathy). Nephrogenic systemic fibrosis is an uncommon disease with cutaneous manifestations that include induration, thickening, and hardening of the skin, most commonly on the extremities. The pathophysiology is related to the exposure of patients with renal insufficiency to gadolinium-based contrast agents.

High HA, Ayers RA, Cowper SE. Gadolinium is quantifiable within the tissue of patients with nephrogenic systemic fibrosis. *J Am Acad Dermatol.* 2007;56:710–712.

29. Describe a typical presentation of warfarin necrosis.

    The patient is typically a woman who has been given a loading dose of warfarin (Coumadin). Between 3 and 5 days after starting the drug, the patient develops one or more lesions over the thighs, buttocks, or breasts. Initially painful and red, the lesions rapidly become necrotic with hemorrhagic bullae and an erythematous edge (Fig. 14.7). A necrotic eschar rapidly develops.

    Rapid recognition of the characteristic lesions in the typical situation is the key to reducing tissue destruction. Therapy includes discontinuing warfarin, administering vitamin K to reverse the effect of warfarin, giving heparin as an anticoagulant, and administering monoclonal antibody-purified protein C concentrate. Therapy may also include debridement, grafting, and even amputation. Warfarin necrosis has frequently been associated with low levels of protein C. Most authorities recommend that the warfarin should be discontinued.

30. Name and describe the two types of photoinduced drug eruptions.

    Phototoxic drug reactions and photoallergic drug reactions. Phototoxic reactions occur within minutes to hours after exposure to both the drug and light and occur in all individuals given the specific drug and ultraviolet (UV) exposure. The rash clinically resembles a sunburn, and stinging is a prominent feature. Photoallergic drug reactions are mediated by type IV delayed hypersensitivity and occur 24 to 48 hours after UV exposure. Clinically, the lesions are on sun-exposed sites but are not as well demarcated as phototoxic reactions. They are also eczematous and pruritic.

31. What drugs commonly cause phototoxic drug reactions?

    Amiodarone, chlorpromazine, demeclocycline (Fig. 14.8), doxycycline, psoralens, and tetracycline.

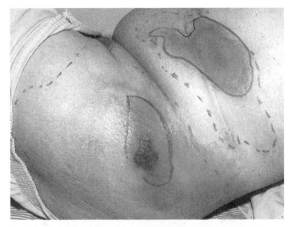

Fig. 14.7 Characteristic lesions of warfarin necrosis, demonstrating early necrosis and hemorrhagic bullae surrounded by a ring of erythema.

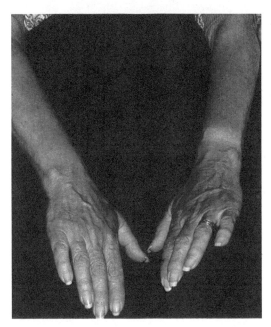

Fig. 14.8 Demeclocycline-induced phototoxic reaction on the dorsum of the hands. (Courtesy James E. Fitzpatrick, MD.)

32. What drugs commonly cause photoallergic drug reactions?
    Griseofulvin, quinine, quinolones, sulfonamides, phenothiazines, quinidine, hydrochlorothiazides, piroxicam, and pyridoxine.

33. What is AGEP? How does it present?
    AGEP is an acronym for **a**cute **g**eneralized **e**xanthematous **p**ustulosis. Patients present with an abrupt onset of a generalized, scarlatiniform, erythematous exanthem associated with numerous small, sterile, nonfollicular pustules (Fig. 14.9). There may be associated fever, prostration, and leukocytosis. In one study, 17% of patients had a personal history of psoriasis. The lesions typically occur within a few days of initiating the offending drug. Beta-lactam antibiotics are the most common culprits, followed by macrolides and mercury. The reaction is typically short lived. Resolution usually occurs within 1 to 2 weeks of discontinuing the offending agent and is accompanied by widespread skin desquamation.

Thienvibul C, Vachiramon V, Chanprapaph K. Five-year retrospective review of acute generalized exanthematous pustulosis. *Dermatol Res Pract.* Epub 2015, Dec. 10.

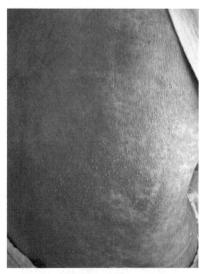

Fig. 14.9 Acute generalized exanthematous pustulosis due to amoxicillin, demonstrating typical small pustules on a background of erythema. (Courtesy James E. Fitzpatrick, MD.)

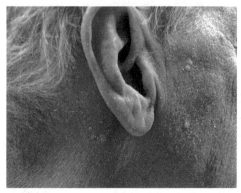

Fig. 14.10 Acute onset of numerous hyperkeratotic lesions in a patient with melanoma being treated with a BRAF inhibitor. (Courtesy James E. Fitzpatrick, MD.)

34. You have been treating a patient for severe, scarring acne with an oral medication for the last 3 months. Her acne looks great but now she is starting to lose hair. What drug are you most likely using?

    Isotretinion. Other, more common agents linked to alopecia are ACE inhibitors, allopurinol, anticoagulants, azathioprine, bromocriptine, beta-blockers, cyclophosphamide, didanosine, hormones, indinavir, NSAIDs, phenytoin, methotrexate, and valproate.

35. A patient presents with numerous eruptive hyperkeratotic lesions 1 month after starting treatment for metastatic melanoma. What type of drug is this patient likely to be using?

    This patient is most likely being treated with a BRAF inhibitor, such as vemurafenib or dabrafenib. These drugs have been associated with eruptive squamous cell carcinomas and keratoacanthomas, which typically occur within 2 to 14 weeks into treatment (Fig. 14.10). Cases of neutrophilic panniculitis have also been reported.

Chu EY, Wanat KA, Miller CJ, et al. Diverse cutaneous side effects associated with BRAF inhibitor therapy. A clinicopathologic study. *J Am Acad Dermatol.* 2012;67:1265–1272.

Choy B, Chou S, Anforth R, Fernández-Peñas P. Panniculitis in patients treated with BRAF inhibitors: a case series. *Am J Dermatopathol.* 2014 Jun;36(6):493–497.

CHAPTER 15

VASCULITIS

Curt P. Samlaska and James E. Fitzpatrick

1. How are vasculitic disorders defined and classified?

   Vasculitis is defined as inflammation of blood vessels. Vasculitis may be confined to the skin; however, the majority of cases of cutaneous vasculitis are part of multisystemic disorders that in addition to involving skin also involve other organ systems. Classification is problematic due to the lack of standardization and definition. The most accepted classification scheme for systemic vasculitis syndromes is based on the size of the involved blood vessels, as shown in Table 15.1. Subclassification of these syndromes is based on clinical and histologic criteria that have been determined to be suggestive of a specific disorder. The American College of Rheumatology Subcommittee on Classification of Vasculitis has determined classification criteria for many of these disorders (see Table 15.1). This classification system is excellent for systemic vasculitis, but it omits some forms of vasculitis that are confined to the skin. For example, it is now well accepted that cutaneous polyarteritis nodosa (PAN) is a distinct subtype of PAN.

   Jennette JC, Falk RJ, Andrassy K, et al. 2012 Revised International Chapel Hill consensus conference nomenclature of vasculitides. *Arthritis Rheum.* 2013;65:1–11.
   Caproni M, Verdelli. An update on the nomenclature for cutaneous vasculitis. *Curr Opin Rheumatol.* 2019;31:46–52.

2. Are there specific serologic markers for any of these vasculitic disorders?

   Yes. Antimyeloperoxidase antibodies directed against cytoplasmic components of neutrophils have been used to help identify patients with segmental necrotizing glomerulonephritis and some types of systemic vasculitis. Antibodies directed against serine proteinase 3 that is found in the cytoplasm of neutrophils (c-antineutrophilic cytoplasmic antibody [ANCA]) have been detected in 66% to 90% of patients with active granulomatosis with polyangiitis (GPA) (Wegener's granulomatosis). Patients with pulmonary-renal syndrome who have antibodies directed against cytoplasmic myeloperoxidase, in neutrophils that produce a peripheral antineutrophil cytoplasmic pattern (p-ANCA), are most likely to have microscopic polyangiitis (MPA) (Fig. 15.1).

   Kallenberg CGM. Anti-neutrophil cytoplasmic antibody (ANCA)–associated vasculitis: where to go? *Clin Exp Immunol.* 2011;164 (suppl 1):1–3.

3. What is a leukocytoclastic vasculitis?

   Patients with leukocytoclastic vasculitis, also referred to as leukocytoclastic angiitis and allergic or necrotizing vasculitis, present with characteristic purpuric papules, most frequently involving the extremities, known as palpable purpura (Fig. 15.2). It is classified as a single-organ vasculitis, involving the skin only. Biopsies of cutaneous leukocytoclastic vasculitis demonstrate an intense perivascular infiltrate composed of intact and fragmented neutrophils (nuclear dust) that focally infiltrate the vessel wall, producing fibrinoid changes and/or necrosis. These damaged vessels frequently demonstrate extravasation of erythrocytes and may also demonstrate thrombosis.

   Kluger N, Francès C. Cutaneous vasculitis and their differential diagnoses. *Clin Exp Rheumatol.* 2009; 27(1 suppl 52):S124–S138.

4. What are some important precipitating causes of small vessel leukocytoclastic vasculitis?

   - **Infections:** Bacterial (streptococcal infections, bacterial endocarditis), viral (parvovirus B19, human immunodeficiency virus [HIV], hepatitis to C), mycobacterial (Hansen's disease, tuberculosis), fungal (*Candida albicans*), protozoan (*Plasmodium malariae*), helminthic (*Schistosoma haematobium, S. mansoni, Onchocerca volvulus*)
   - **Drugs:** Aspirin, sulfonamides, penicillins, barbiturates, amphetamines, propylthiouracil
   - **Malignancies:** Lymphomas, colonic carcinoma, hairy cell leukemia, multiple myeloma, lung cancer, renal cell carcinoma, prostate cancer, breast cancer, head and neck cancer

   In the majority of cases of leukocytoclastic vasculitis, the precipitating antigen cannot be identified.

   Veraldi S, Mancuso R, Rizzitelli G, et al. Henoch-Schönlein syndrome associated with human parvovirus B19 primary infection. *Eur J Dermatol.* 1999;9:232–233.
   Goser MR, Laniosz V, Wetter DA. A practical approach to the diagnosis, evaluation, and management of cutaneous small-vessel vasculitis. *Am J Clin Dermatol.* 2014;15:299–306.

Table 15.1 Classification of systemic vasculitides with cutaneous findings

VESSEL SIZE	VASCULITIC SYNDROME
Large vessel vasculitis	Giant cell (temporal) arteritis
	Takayasu arteritis

Medium vessel vasculitis	Polyarteritis nodosa (classic PAN)
	    Benign cutaneous polyarteritis nodosa
	    Hepatitis B associated polyarteritis nodosa

	Kawasaki disease
Small vessel vasculitis ANCA positive	Granulomatosis with polyangiitis (Wegener's granulomatosis)
	Eosinophilic granulomatosis with polyangiitis (Churg-Strauss syndrome)
	Microscopic polyangiitis (polyarteritis)
Small vessel vasculitis ANCA negative	Henoch-Schönlein purpura
	Cryoglobulinemic vasculitis
	Cutaneous leukocytoclastic vasculitis

Adapted from Jennette JC. Overview of the 2012 revised International Chapel Hill Consensus Conference nomenclature of vasculitides. Clin Exp Nephrol. *2013;17:603–606.*

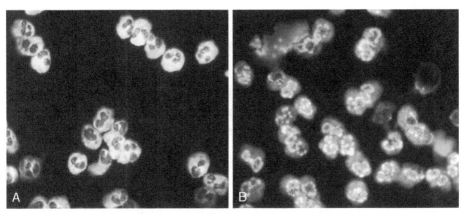

Fig. 15.1 A, c-ANCA demonstrating characteristic cytoplasmic location. **B,** p-ANCA demonstrating characteristic perinuclear localization. (Courtesy Fitzsimons Army Medical Center teaching files.)

5. **What is IgA vasculitis, formerly known as Henoch-Schönlein purpura?**
   Immunoglobulin A (IgA) vasculitis is a variant of leukocytoclastic vasculitis characterized by the deposition of immune complexes containing IgA in small vessels with the most commonly affected vessels being in the skin, kidney, and gastrointestinal (GI) tract. The precipitating antigen is not identifiable in all cases, but many are associated with respiratory viral infections or drugs. It is usually seen in young children, although any age can be affected. The classic four components of the syndrome include cutaneous palpable purpura, colicky abdominal pain, arthralgias and/or arthritis, and kidney involvement.

Calvo-Rio V, Loricera J, Mata C, et al. Henoch-Schonlein purpura in northern Spain: clinical spectrum of the disease in 417 patients from a single center. *Medicine (Baltimore).* 2014;93:106–113.

6. **What is the mnemonic that can help remember the clinical features of IgA vasculitis?**
   The mnemonic PAPAH (pä-pä) can be used to remember the clinical features of Henoch-Schönlein purpura (HSP): **p**urpura, **a**bdominal **p**ain, **a**rthralgias, **h**ematuria. Some patients with abdominal involvement demonstrate significant melena or less commonly develop intussusception of the bowel. While more than 40% of patients demonstrate at least some degree of renal involvement, primarily manifesting as hematuria and proteinuria, only 1% develop chronic renal impairment. Less commonly, other organs such as the brain or lungs can be involved.

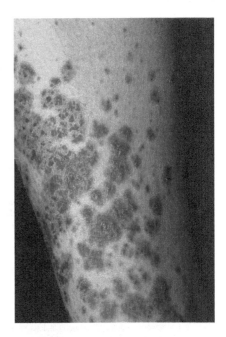

Fig. 15.2 Leukocytoclastic vasculitis demonstrating palpable purpura of the leg.

7. What is "acute hemorrhagic edema of infancy" and how does it differ from IgA vasculitis?

Acute hemorrhagic edema of infancy, also called "cockade purpura," is also an IgA-mediated immune complex leukocytoclastic vasculitis that affects small cutaneous vessels. This variant almost always affects young children (median age is 11 months), and like IgA vasculitis, it is usually associated with a preexisting upper respiratory infection. It differs in that the primary cutaneous clinical lesions are typically indurated, edematous plaques with variable hemorrhage that are less likely to ulcerate. The lesions frequently affect the head and neck region and extremities (Fig. 15.3). The children typically do not demonstrate significant involvement of the GI tract, joints, or kidneys and do not develop permanent sequelae.

Savino F, Lupica MM, Tarasco V, et al. Acute hemorrhagic edema of infancy: a troubling cutaneous presentation with a self-limiting course. *Pediatr Dermatol.* 2013; 30:149–152.

Serra E, Moura Garcia C, Sokolova A, et al. Acute hemorrhagic edema of infancy. *Eur Ann Allergy Clin Immunol.* 2015; 48:22–26.

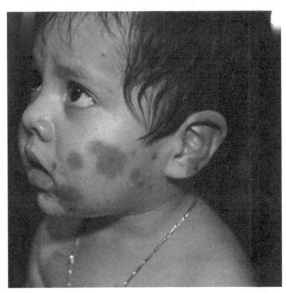

Fig. 15.3 Acute hemorrhagic edema of a young child demonstrating hemorrhagic indurated plaques of the head. As seen here, the ears and cheeks are frequently involved. (Courtesy Joanna Burch Collection.)

8. What are cryoglobulins?

Cryoglobulins are abnormal circulating IgG and IgM immunoglobulins that precipitate at low temperatures and redissolve at 37°C. Cryoglobulins are frequently found in patients with paraproteinemias, such as multiple myeloma and macroglobulinemia. Mixed cryoglobulinemia, with more than one antibody class involved, has been reported in systemic lupus erythematosus, rheumatoid arthritis, Sjögren's syndrome, and hepatitis B and C infection.

Retamozo S, Brito-Zeron P, Bosch X, et al. Cryglobulinemic disease. *Oncology (Williston Park).* 2013;27:1098–1105.

9. Can cryoglobulins produce a vasculitis?

Yes. Some authorities consider cryoglobulinemic leukocytoclastic vasculitis to be a distinct subset of leukcytoclastic vasculitis, and it is often discussed separately. Cryoglobulinemic vasculitis is most commonly associated with type II cryoglobulins (monoclonal immunoglobulins, usually IgM, with rheumatoid factor binding activity to the Fc portion of polyclonal IgG) and type III cryoglobulins (mixed polyclonal immunoglobulins that usually bind to IgG). Type I immunoglobulins (monoclonal immunoglobulin, most commonly IgM) are more likely to present as occlusive infarctive lesions without an associated infiltrate, although rare cases of vasculitis have been reported. Hepatitis B and C are emerging as major causes of mixed cryoglobulinemia. Clinically, patients with cryoglobulinemic leukocytoclastic vasculitis resemble those having classic adult leukocytoclastic vasculitis, except that the lesions are more commonly associated with cold exposure and are more commonly confined to acral areas where the body temperature is lower.

10. What is eosinophilic granulomatosis with polyangiitis (Churg-Strauss syndrome)?

Formerly Churg-Strauss syndrome (allergic granulomatosis), eosinophilic granulomatosis with polyangiitis (EGPA) is an uncommon multisystemic vasculitis that is characterized with asthma, eosinophilia, extravascular granulomas, and positive ANCA titers. The main systemic features of EGPA are summarized in Table 15.2. Pulmonary involvement and eosinophilia help discriminate EGPA from PAN. The primary cutaneous lesions most commonly consist of palpable purpura involving the extremities, although some patients may also demonstrate fixed papules or plaques or even subcutaneous nodules. Cutaneous lesions have been reported in 45% to 70% of patients. Cutaneous involvement should be considered an important feature when present; biopsies, in addition to demonstrating vasculitis of small blood vessels, frequently demonstrate large numbers of eosinophils and, less commonly, may demonstrate extravascular granulomatous inflammation (Fig. 15.4).

Mouthon L, Dunogue B, Guillevin L. Diagnosis and classification of eosinophilic granulomatosis with polyangiitis (formerly named Churg-Strauss syndrome). *J Autoimmun.* 2014;48–49:99–103.

Saku A, Furuta S, Hiraguri M, et al. Long term outcomes of 188 Japanese patients with eosinophilic granulomatosis with polyangiitis. *J Rheumatol.* 2018;45:1159–1166.

11. What were those features again?

To recall the diagnostic criteria for EGPA, remember the mnemonic **BEAN SAP**: **b**lood **e**osinophilia, **a**sthma, **n**europathy, **s**inus abnormalities, **a**llergies, and **p**erivascular eosinophils. The American College of Rheumatology has established these six criteria for the diagnosis of EGPA, with the presence of four of these six criteria yielding a diagnostic sensitivity of 85% and a specificity of 99.7%.

12. What is granulomatosis with polyangiitis (Wegener's granulomatosis)?

Formerly Wegener's granulomatosis, GPA is an uncommon multisystem vasculitis that is characterized by vasculitis and necrotizing granulomatosis inflammation that most commonly affects the upper respiratory tract, lungs, and

Table 15.2 Clinical features of eosinophilic granulomatosis with polyangiitis (Churg-Strauss Syndrome)

FINDING	SENSITIVITY
Asthma	100%
Blood eosinophilia >10%	95%
Paranasal sinus abnormalities	86%
Mononeuropathy or polyneuropathy	75%
Pulmonary infiltrates	40%
Extravascular (perivascular) eosinophils	14%
History of seasonal allergies	–

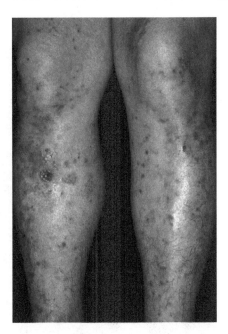

Fig. 15.4 Churg-Strauss syndrome (allergic granulomatosis) demonstrating both palpable purpura and ulcerated nodules of the lower extremity in a patient with asthma. (Courtesy Fitzsimons Army Medical Center teaching files.)

kidneys. Locations and forms of GPA are expanding and may also involve the musculoskeletal system, eyes, skin, and nervous system (neuropathy, mononeuritis multiplex, and meningitis). It has been estimated that the prevalence in the United States is approximately 3 per 100,000 individuals.

Genuis K, Pewarchuk J. Granulomatosis with polyangiitis (Wegener's) as a necrotizing gingivitis mimic: a case report. *J Med Case Rep.* 2014;8:297.

13. **What are the features needed to establish a diagnosis of GPA?**
   There are four criteria for establishing the diagnosis of GPA:
   - Abnormal urinary sediment (red cell casts or >5 red blood cells/high-power field)
   - Abnormal findings of chest radiographs (nodules, cavities, or fixed infiltrates)
   - Oral ulcers or nasal discharge
   - Granulomatous inflammation on biopsy.
     The presence of two or more of the four criteria gives a diagnostic sensitivity of 88% and a specificity of 92%. The majority of patients with active disease also demonstrate a positive c-ANCA; however, although supportive of this diagnosis, it is not specific because patients with EGPA, microscopic polyarteritis, and PAN may also demonstrate elevated c-ANCA titers.

de Groot K, Gross WL. Wegener's granulomatosis. *Lupus.* 1998;7:285–291.

14. **Is there an easy way to remember these diagnostic criteria?**
   Simply remember the mnemonic **ROUGH:**
   - Chest **R**adiograph
   - **O**ral ulcers
   - **U**rinary sediment
   - **G**ranulomas
   - **H**emoptysis

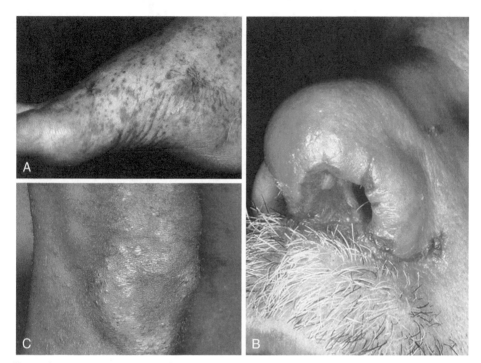

Fig. 15.5 Granulomatosis with polyangiitis (GPA). **A,** Fatal case demonstrating purpuric lesions. The patient was c-ANCA-positive. **B,** Nasal erosions and ulceration. **C,** Nonspecific papules on the knee in a patient with limited GPA involving the sinuses and the skin.

15. List the cutaneous findings in GPA
   - Leukocytoclastic vasculitis (Fig. 15.5A)
   - Papules (Fig. 15.5C)
   - Petechiae
   - Ulcerative lesions (Fig. 15.5B)
   - Urticaria
   - Erythema
   - Purpura
   - Pyoderma gangrenosum
      None of these cutaneous findings are *specific* for GPA.

16. Are ANCA titers part of the criteria used to categorize small vessel vasculitis?
   Yes. The 2012 Chapel Hill Consensus Conference acknowledges the importance of ANCA titers in small vessel vasculitis, dividing the entities into ANCA-associated vasculitis and immune complex small vessel vasculitis. Mounting evidence indicates that ANCA specificity identifies distinct categories of disease. ANCA-associated vasculitis is divided into MPA, GPA, and EGPA. Immune complex small vessel vasculitis (ANCA–) results from immunoglobulin deposition and complement activation—glomerulonephritis is a frequent finding. Specific disorders include IgA vasculitis Henoch-Shonlein purpura [HSP], cryoglobulinemic vasculitis, and hypocomplementemic vasculitis (see Table 15.1). Cutaneous leukocytoclastic vasculitis is considered a single-organ disease localized to the skin.

17. GPA and EGPA seem very similar. How do you distinguish between them?
   It is often difficult to distinguish between GPA and EGPA due to the presence of nasal, sinus, and pulmonary involvement in both diseases and the fact that all the classic features are rarely found in a single patient. There are many situations in which the features of systemic vasculitides overlap, and these are referred to as overlap vasculitis syndromes, similar to the overlap syndromes reported for other rheumatologic conditions.
   c-ANCA are usually present in high titers in GPA but not in EGPA. The presence or absence of other features should confirm the diagnosis in most cases (Table 15.3).

Table 15.3 Granulomatosis with polyangiitis (GPA) versus eosinophilic granulomatosis with polyangiitis (EGPA)

	GPA	EGPA
Asthma	−	+
Blood eosinophilia	−	+
Perivascular eosinophils on biopsy	−	+
Hemoptysis	+	−
Microhematuria	+	−

KEY POINTS: ANTINEUTROPHIL CYTOPLASMIC ANTIBODIES

1. Antineutrophilic cytoplasmic antibodies directed against serine proteinase 3 produce a distinct granular cytoplasmic staining pattern (c-ANCA).
2. c-ANCA is found in up to 90% of patients with GPA. High titers often correlate with increased disease activity.
3. Antineutrophilic cytoplasmic antibodies directed against myeloperoxidase produces a distinct perinuclear cytoplasmic pattern (p-ANCA).
4. p-ANCA is found in up to 70% of patients with microscopic polyarteritis nodosa and up to 50% of patients with EGPA.
5. EGPA patients found positive for p-ANCA are more likely to develop glomerulonephritis, mononeuritis multiplex, and alveolar hemorrhage, whereas p-ANCA–negative EGPA patients are more likely to develop heart disease.

18. **What forms of treatment are available for GPA and EGPA?**
Systemic corticosteroids are the mainstay for treatment of most forms of systemic vasculitis and represent the most common treatment used in EGPA. Corticosteroids alone are often not effective in GPA, and most patients require cyclophosphamide in combination with corticosteroids for effective control. However, in severe cases, rituximab in combination with systemic steroids is replacing cyclophosphamide and is becoming the treatment combination of choice for new cases.

Clain JM, Cartin-Ceba R, Fervenza FC, et al. Experience with rituximab in the treatment of antineutrophil cytoplasmic antibody associated vasculitis. *Ther Adv Musculoskelet Dis.* 2014;6:58–74.

19. **What are the major organs involved in classic (systemic) PAN?**
Kidneys, heart, liver, GI tract, and peripheral nerves. PAN, in its classic form, is a multisystem, segmented necrotizing inflammation of small- and medium-sized muscular arteries. Signs and symptoms are nonspecific and constitutional, reflecting the organ involvement. Pulmonary arteries are typically not involved. The mean age of onset is 48 years, with a male:female ratio of about 4:1. Diagnosis is established by demonstrating vasculitic changes on biopsy of involved organs or by demonstrating typical aneurysms of medium-sized vessels on angiography.

Ishiguro N, Kawashima M. Cutaneous polyarteritis nodosa: a report of 16 cases with clinical and histopathological analysis and a review of the published work. *J Dermatol.* 2010;37:85–93.

20. **How is classic PAN different from Kawasaki disease?**
Both disorders affect medium-sized vessels. PAN produces a necrotizing inflammation of medium-sized and/or small arteries without producing glomerulonephritis or vasculitis in arterioles, capillaries, or venules. Patients with Kawasaki disease are most often children with mucocutaneous lymph node syndrome (adenopathy, glossitis, cheilitis, conjunctivitis, polymorphous cutaneous eruption, edema of the palms and soles evolving into peeling in convalescent stage) with arteritis involving large (often resulting in coronary arteritis, coronary artery aneurysms, and myocardial infarctions), medium-sized, and small arteries. An infectious etiology is likely.

Marchesi A, Tarissi de Jacobis I, Rigante D, et al. Kawasaki disease: guidelines of the Italian society of pediatrics, part I—definition, epidemiology, etiopathogenesis, clinical expression and management of the acute phase. *Ital J Pediatr.* 2018;30:102.

21. **What is primary cutaneous PAN?**
As the name implies, this is PAN that is essentially confined to the skin, although it is not uncommon for patients to experience fever, arthralgias, and myositis. The cutaneous lesions are most commonly located on the lower extremity and manifest as painful subcutaneous nodules that may resemble erythema nodosum or demonstrate a characteristic "starburst" appearance (Fig. 15.6). This diagnostic appearance is due to the arteritis following the bifurcations of the

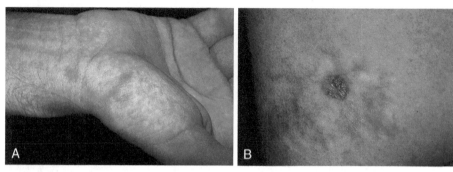

Fig. 15.6 Cutaneous polyarteritis nodosa. **A,** Characteristic linear erythematous lesion. Note the Y-shaped bifurcation. **B,** Reticulated hyperpigmented lesion with an associated ulceration.

small- and medium-sized arteries. Secondary changes that may be present include associated livedo reticularis and ulceration. In contrast to systemic PAN, peripheral gangrene is not seen. Laboratory studies are generally normal except for variable mild leukocytosis and an elevated erythrocyte sedimentation rate. Another distinct clinical variant is hepatitis B virus–associated PAN.

De Virgilio A, Magliulo G, Gallo A, et al. Polyarteritis nodosa: a contemporary overview. *Autoimmun Rev.* 2016;15:564–570.

22. What is the primary difference between MPA and PAN?

The distinguishing feature for these two systemic disorders is primarily based on the size of the vessel that is affected. Patients with MPA have involvement of small arterioles, whereas individuals with classic PAN have involvement of medium-sized arteries. MPA belongs to the ANCA-associated vasculitides, a majority of which are myeloperoxidase (MPO-ANCA) positive and a minority are proteinase (PR3-ANCA) positive. The major organs involved in MPA are the kidneys and the lungs; however, a surprisingly high percentage of patients also have ear, nose, and throat manifestations.

Kallenberg CG. The diagnosis and classification of microscopic polyangiitis. *J Autoimmun.* 2014;48–49:90–93.
Greco A, De Virgilio A, Rizzo MI, et al. Microscopic polyangiitis: advances in diagnostic and therapeutic approaches. *Autoimmun Rev.* 2015;14:837–844.

23. What is the difference between giant cell (temporal) arteritis (GCA) and Takayasu's arteritis?

Both disorders affect large vessels. Takayasu's arteritis manifests with a progressive granulomatous inflammation of the aorta and its major branches and most frequently afflicts patients less than 50 years old. GCA usually affects patients greater than 50 years old with a granulomatous vasculitis that can also involve the aorta and its major branches. However, GCA shows a predilection for the extracranial branches of the carotid artery, particularly the temporal artery, which can progress to visual loss and blindness if not treated with systemic steroids. The most common symptoms of GCA are severe headaches (75%) and jaw claudication (50%), while visual loss, either temporary or permanent, occurs 20% of the time. GCA may rarely demonstrate unilateral alopecia, cutaneous ulceration, or atrophy of the scalp due to loss of the blood supply to the skin.

Guida A, Tufano A, Perna P, et al. The thromboembolic risk in giant cell arteritis: a critical review of the literature. *Int J Rheumatol.* 2014;2014:806402.
Russo RAG, Katsicas MM. Takayasu arteritis. *Front Pediatr.* 2018;24:265.

24. What is erythema elevatum diutinum?

Erythema elevatum diutinum is a rare form of small vessel vasculitis that is confined to the skin. This chronic disorder is characterized by persistent, elevated, erythematous plaques, and/or nodules, with a predilection for overlying joint spaces, such as the fingers, wrists, elbows, knees, ankles, and toes (Fig. 15.7). The lesions are usually painful. Biopsies of developed lesions demonstrate a chronic leukocytoclastic vasculitis with extensive tissue fibrosis. There may be an associated IgA or, less commonly, an IgG monoclonal gammopathy (immune complex disease) and an association with inflammatory bowel disease, rheumatoid arthritis, systemic lupus erythematosus, streptococcal infection, IgA monoclonal gammopathy, multiple myeloma, myelodysplasia, celiac disease, relapsing polychondritis, and HIV infection. Initial treatment should target the underlying systemic disease. Many patients have shown a dramatic response to dapsone.

Momen SE, Jorizzo J, Al-Niaimi F. Erythema elevatum diutinum: a review of presentation and treatment. *J Eur Acad Dermatol Venereol.* 2014;28(12):1594–1602. https://doi.org/10.1111/jdv.12566.
Doktor V, Hadi A, Hadi A, et al. Erythema elevatum diutinum: a case report and review of literature. *Int J Dermatol.* 2019;58(4):408–415. https://doi.org/10.1111/ijd.14169.

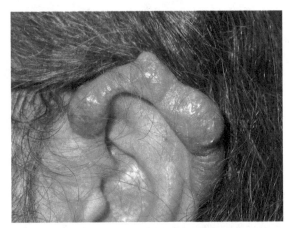

Fig. 15.7 Erythema elevatum diutinum of the ears demonstrating nodular lesions on the ears of an HIV-positive patient.

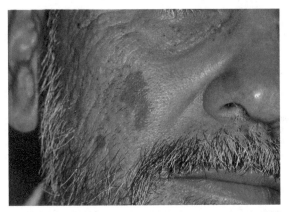

Fig. 15.8 Granuloma faciale demonstrating purplish indurated plaques of the nose and cheeks. (Courtesy Joanna Burch Collection.)

25. Are there any other obscure disorders known to dermatologists, but little known to other subspecialties, that could be classified as vasculitis?

Yes—granuloma faciale, which is an uncommon, chronic, benign, small vessel vasculitis that most commonly affects middle-aged adults. While sun-exposed skin on the face is the area most commonly affected, it has also been reported to appear on extrafacial sites including the trunk and upper and lower extremities. The lesions are characteristically solitary but can be multiple. The primary lesion is a papule, nodule, or plaque that varies in size from millimeters to several centimeters (Fig. 15.8). The overlying epidermis is characteristically smooth with the follicular orifices being accentuated, producing a characteristic "peau d'orange" appearance. The color is highly variable and varies from yellowish to amber to brown to red to violaceous. Most lesions are asymptomatic, although occasional patients may complain of mild pruritus or burning. Once present, the lesions typically persist for years or decades, and progressive enlargement of lesions is not uncommon. The disease is notoriously resistant to therapy. The pathogenesis of this peculiar form of cutaneous vasculitis is unknown, but recent evidence suggests that it may be part of the spectrum of IgG4-related sclerosing diseases.

Lindhaus C, Elsner P. Granuloma faciale treatment: a systematic review. *Acta Derm Venereol.* 2018;98:14–18.
Cesinaro AM, Lonardi S, Facchetti F. Granuloma faciale: a cutaneous lesion sharing features with IgG4-associated sclerosing diseases. *Am J Surg Pathol.* 2013;37:66–73, 2013.

CHAPTER 16

DEPOSITION DISORDERS

Lori D. Prok

KEY POINTS: CUTANEOUS DEPOSITION DISORDERS

1. Amyloid deposition can result in both localized and systemic disease.
2. Pretibial myxedema is associated with Graves' disease.
3. The porphyrias are a group of diseases caused by defects in heme biosynthesis–related enzymes.
4. Lesions of lichen myxedematosus result from an increase in both dermal mucin and fibroblasts.
5. Immunoglobulin G lambda paraproteinemia is the most common serum abnormality associated with scleromyxedema.
6. Lesions of gout result from uric acid deposition in the skin and soft tissues.
7. Calciphylaxis usually occurs in the setting of renal disease.

1. How is "deposition disorder" defined?

Deposition disorders comprise a diverse group of conditions or diseases in which there is accumulation, deposition, or production of substances in the skin. Typically, these substances are products of abnormal metabolism or degenerative phenomena occurring locally or systemically. The major cutaneous deposits may be subdivided into the hyalinoses, mucinoses, and mineral salts.

Molina-Ruiz AM, Cerroni L, Kutzer H, Requena L. Cutaneous deposits. *Am J Dermatopathol.* 2014;36:1–48.

2. What is amyloid?

Amyloid is a protein with distinct tinctorial and ultrastructural properties found as extracellular deposits. It is composed of a nonfibrillary protein known as the amyloid P component and a fibrillary component that is derived from various sources. The amyloid fibril has an antiparallel, β-pleated sheet configuration. Ultrastructurally, amyloid is composed of rigid, nonbranching fibrils measuring 6 to 10 nm in diameter.

3. How is amyloid identified?

With light microscopy, amyloid appears as amorphous, hyaline-like, eosinophilic deposits. Amyloid demonstrates green birefringence with the alkaline Congo red stain, reddish metachromasia with crystal violet, and yellow-green fluorescence with thioflavin-T stain (Fig. 16.1). These stains are not absolutely specific for amyloid, as false-positive results may occur with the other hyaline-like deposition disorders.

4. Name the various types of amyloidosis.

Amyloidosis may be classified according to clinical presentation and type of amyloid fibril protein deposition (Table 16.1). The amyloid in the macular and lichenoid variants is derived from degenerated tonofilaments of keratinocytes. Nodular amyloidosis is formed from light-chain–derived AL protein produced locally by plasma cells. It cannot be distinguished from primary systemic amyloidosis, and therefore systemic disease should be excluded in all patients with nodular amyloidosis. There are also rare forms of hereditary systemic amyloidoses that have less frequent skin manifestations.

5. What are the cutaneous manifestations of primary or myeloma-associated systemic amyloidosis? How often do they occur?

Cutaneous lesions are seen in about 30% of cases of primary or myeloma-related systemic amyloidosis. The most common skin lesions are petechiae or ecchymoses due to amyloid deposition within blood vessel walls with subsequent fragility and dermal hemorrhage. These are often seen at sites predisposed to trauma, such as the hands or intertriginous areas. Pinching the skin gives characteristic purpuric lesions known as "pinch purpura." Purpura around the eyes may occur spontaneously but is also seen following proctoscopy ("postproctoscopic purpura") or vomiting (Fig. 16.2). Waxy papules, nodules, or plaques may be present. Less common manifestations include sclerodermoid plaques, bullae, alopecia, and nail dystrophy.

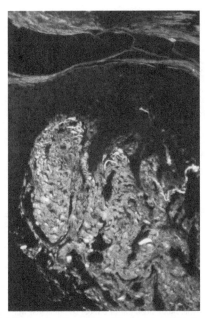

Fig. 16.1 Lichen amyloidosis. Thioflavin-T demonstrates strong staining of fluorescent amyloid in the papillary dermis. (Courtesy James E. Fitzpatrick, MD.)

Table 16.1 Classification of amyloidosis

CLINICAL DISORDER	AMYLOID PROTEIN PRECURSOR	AMYLOID PROTEIN
Systemic Amyloidosis		
Primary systemic amyloidosis	Immunoglobulin light chain	AL
Myeloma-associated amyloidosis	Immunoglobulin light chain	AL
Secondary systemic amyloidosis	Serum amyloid A lipoprotein	AA
Primary Localized Cutaneous Amyloidosis		
Macular amyloidosis	Keratinocyte tonofilaments	—
Lichen amyloidosis	Keratinocyte tonofilaments	—
Nodular amyloidosis	Immunoglobulin light chain (produced locally by plasma cells)	AL

6. Name the other organ systems that may be involved in primary or myeloma-associated amyloidosis.

Mucous membrane involvement with macroglossia occurs in 20% of cases. Hepatomegaly is found in about 50% of cases. Cardiac involvement may manifest as a restrictive cardiomyopathy or constrictive pericarditis. Peripheral nerve involvement results in paresthesias, peripheral neuropathy, and median nerve entrapment (carpal tunnel syndrome). Proteinuria is found in 80% to 90% of patients at some time during their course. Renal failure usually develops late in the disease course but may be a cause of death.

Prokaeva T, Spencer B, Kaut M, et al. Soft tissue, joint, and bone manifestations of AL amyloidosis: clinical presentation, molecular features, and survival. *Arthritis Rheum.* 2007;56:3858–3868.

Silverstein SR. Primary, systemic amyloidosis and the dermatologist: where classic skin lesions may provide the clue for early diagnosis. *Dermatol Online J.* 2005;11:5.

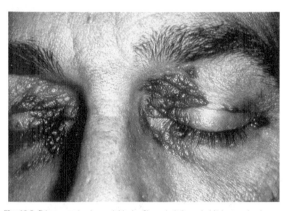

Fig. 16.2 Primary systemic amyloidosis. Characteristic periorbital purpuric plaques.

7. Compare lichen amyloidosis and macular amyloidosis.

In lichen amyloidosis lesions are pruritic, flesh-colored to brown papules, often with overlying scale (Fig. 16.3A). Papules may coalesce into verrucous plaques. The shins are the most common site of involvement. In macular amyloidosis, pruritic macular hyperpigmentation occurs most commonly in the interscapular area. The chest or extremities are less commonly involved. The lesions have a characteristic reticulate or rippled appearance. Both of these variants of primary localized cutaneous amyloidosis occur more frequently in patients from the Middle East, Asia, and Central and South America. The etiology of both lichen and macular amyloidosis is unclear but thought to be related to chronic scratching or frictional exposure. An autosomal dominant family history may be found in up to 10% of patients with lichen amyloidosis. Lichen amyloidosis is occasionally associated with multiple endocrine neoplasia type 2A.

Tanaka A, Arita K, Lai-Cheong JE, Palisson F, Hide M, McGrath JA. New insight into mechanisms of pruritus from molecular studies on familial primary localized cutaneous amyloidosis. *Br J Dermatol.* 2009;161:1217–1224.
Verga U, Fugazzola L, Cambiaghi S, et al. Frequent association between MEN 2A and cutaneous lichen amyloidosis. *Clin Endocrinol (Oxf).* 2003;59:156–161.

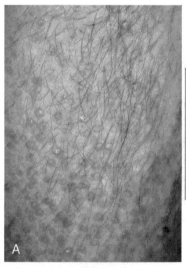

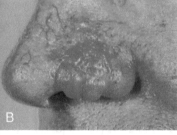

Fig. 16.3 A, Lichen amyloidosis. Numerous pruritic, scaly papules on the anterior shin. (Courtesy Fitzsimons Army Medical Center teaching files.) **B,** Nodular amyloidosis demonstrating large waxy nodule on the nose.

8. How does primary localized cutaneous nodular amyloidosis present? With what is it associated?

Primary localized cutaneous nodular amyloidosis typically presents as solitary or multiple waxy nodules (Fig. 16.3B). Common sites of involvement include the face, scalp, lower extremities, and genitalia. It may be associated with the subsequent development of systemic amyloidosis in up to 15% of cases. Rarely, it is found in association with Sjögren's syndrome.

Kalajian AH, Waldman M, Knable AL. Nodular primary localized cutaneous amyloidosis after trauma: a case report and discussion of the rate of progression to systemic amyloidosis. *J Am Acad Dermatol.* 2007;57(suppl 2):S26–S29.
Yoneyama K, Tochigi N, Oikawa A, Shinkai H, Utani A. Primary localized cutaneous nodular amyloidosis in a patient with Sjögren's syndrome: a review of the literature. *J Dermatol.* 2005;32:120–123.

9. What is secondary systemic amyloidosis and what are its systemic manifestations?

Secondary systemic amyloidosis is associated with chronic systemic disease, such as infection, connective tissue disease, or neoplasm. Organs commonly involved in secondary systemic amyloidosis include the liver, spleen, and kidneys, resulting in hepatosplenomegaly and nephrotic syndrome, respectively. Although skin lesions are generally lacking, biopsy of subcutaneous abdominal fat may demonstrate amyloid deposition.

Hazenberg BP, Bijzet J, Limburg PC, et al. Diagnostic performance of amyloid A protein quantification in fat tissue of patients with clinical AA amyloidosis. *Amyloid.* 2007;14:133–140.
Lachmann HJ, Goodman HJ, Gilbertson JA, et al. Natural history and outcome in systemic AA amyloidosis. *N Engl J Med.* 2007;356:2361–2371.

10. What is lipoid proteinosis?

Lipoid proteinosis, also known as hyalinosis cutis et mucosae and Urbach-Wiethe disease, is a rare autosomal recessive genodermatosis in which skin and mucous membranes are infiltrated with a hyaline scleroprotein. The presenting symptom, hoarseness, develops in infancy due to involvement of the vocal cords with hyaline deposits. Bullae, pustules, and crusts, followed by acneiform scars, are seen on the face and extremities. Waxy papules develop along the eyelids, producing a characteristic "string of beads" appearance. Later, verrucous plaques occur on the elbows and knees. Lipoid proteinosis is caused by loss-of-function mutations in the extracellular matrix protein 1 gene (*ECM1*).

Bahhady R, Abbas O, Ghosn S, Kurban M, Salman S. Erosions and scars over the face, trunk, and extremities. *Pediatr Dermatol.* 2009;26:91–92.

11. What is colloid milium?

Colloid milium is a cutaneous eruption characterized by flesh-colored to yellow-brown translucent papules that may coalesce into plaques (Fig. 16.4). The eruption is most commonly found in adults in areas of chronic sun exposure, but

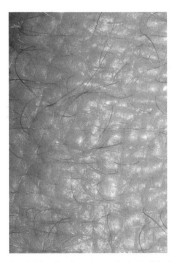

Fig. 16.4 Colloid milium. Numerous dome-shaped skin-colored papules on the back of the hand of a man with history of extensive sun exposure. (Courtesy Fitzsimons Army Medical Center teaching files.)

a rare juvenile form is also recognized. Amorphous fissured eosinophilic material in the papillary dermis is seen on histopathology. Excessive sun exposure is a likely etiologic factor in adult colloid milium.

Pourrabbani S, Marra DE, Iwasaki J, Fincher EF, Ronald LM. Colloid milium: a review and update. *J Drugs Dermatol.* 2007;6:293–296.

12. Which histologic feature or "deposit" is common to all porphyrias?
    The porphyrias are a group of diseases resulting from defects in the enzymes that regulate heme biosynthesis. The biochemical and clinical features are different for each type of porphyria, yet all demonstrate similar cutaneous histology with deposits of eosinophilic, hyaline material around blood vessels. This material stains positively with the periodic acid–Schiff stain and represents reduplicated basal lamina or type IV collagen.

13. Which porphyria classically demonstrates the largest deposits? What are its cutaneous features?
    Erythropoietic protoporphyria, also termed protoporphyria, has the largest eosinophilic deposits in cutaneous lesions. This autosomal dominant disorder of porphyrin metabolism is caused by a deficiency of the enzyme ferrochelatase (heme synthetase). Symptoms begin in early childhood and include photosensitivity, pruritus, burning, erythema, and edema. Chronic changes include a waxy, "cobblestone" thickening of the skin and shallow scars or pits. Increased protoporphyrin may be identified in the feces and blood, although urinary porphyrins are usually normal.

Lecha M, Puy H, Deybach JC. Erythropoietic protoporphyria. *Orphanet J Rare Dis.* 2009;4:19.

14. Name some of the cutaneous mucinoses.
    The mucinoses are a heterogeneous group of disorders characterized by dermal mucin deposition. This mucin is largely hyaluronic acid, an acid mucopolysaccharide, with smaller amounts of chondroitin sulfate and heparin. Disorders resulting in diffuse mucin deposition include generalized myxedema, pretibial myxedema, lichen myxedematosus, scleredema, reticular erythematous mucinosis, and the mucopolysaccharidoses (storage diseases). Mucin deposition may also be focal or localized, as with follicular mucinosis (alopecia mucinosa), cutaneous focal mucinosis, and digital mucous cyst.

Jackson EM, English JC III. Diffuse cutaneous mucinoses. *Dermatol Clin.* 2002;20:493–501.

15. Describe the clinical lesions seen in pretibial myxedema and its disease associations.
    Patients with pretibial myxedema develop nodules or diffuse plaques usually on the anterior lower legs, although involvement of other sites has been rarely reported (Fig. 16.5A). The lesions result from large amounts of dermal mucin deposition. Pretibial myxedema is seen in 1% to 4% of patients with Graves' disease and, less commonly, in patients with autoimmune thyroiditis.

Fatourechi V. Pretibial myxedema: pathophysiology and treatment options. *Am J Clin Dermatol.* 2005;6(5):295–309.

16. Describe the clinical lesions seen in lichen myxedematosus.
    In localized lichen myxedematosus, also known as papular mucinosis, numerous flesh-colored to erythematous, grouped waxy papules are found primarily on the trunk and extremities. Rare cases have been reported in association with human immunodeficiency virus or hepatitis C infection. In the scleromyxedema variant, lesions coalesce into indurated plaques resulting in diffuse skin thickening. It often involves the face, neck, upper extremities, trunk, and thighs. Scleromyxedema can involve internal organs resulting in neurologic, musculoskeletal, gastrointestinal, pulmonary, renal, and cardiovascular sequelae. Lesions of localized lichen myxedematosus/scleromyxedema result from an increase in both dermal mucin and fibroblasts. In scleromyxedema, there is also an increase in collagen.

17. What serum abnormality has been associated with scleromyxedema?
    Scleromyxedema is nearly always associated with serum paraproteinemia, usually IgG with lambda light chains. Rare cases with kappa light chains have been reported. Waldenström's macroglobulinemia or multiple myeloma may be rarely associated.

Rongioletti F, Rebora A. Updated classification of papular mucinosis, lichen myxedematosus, and scleromyxedema. *J Am Acad Dermatol.* 2001;44:273–281.

18. Describe the clinical lesions in scleredema and its disease associations.
    Scleredema presents as a firm, woody induration of the skin typically involving the upper trunk, posterior neck, and shoulders. Histologically, it is characterized by an accumulation of dermal mucin and increased sclerosis of dermal

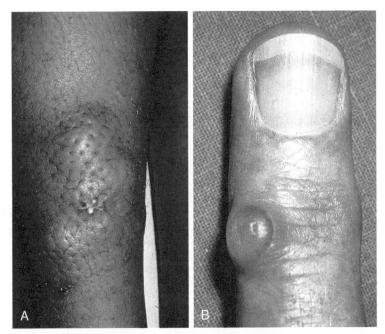

Fig. 16.5 **A,** Pretibial myxedema. Thick plaques on anterior lower legs with peau d'orange change secondary to dermal mucin. **B,** Digital mucous cyst. Dome-shaped cystic nodule overlying the distal interphalangeal joint.

collagen. Scleredema may be seen in several different clinical settings, including postinfection, in association with diabetes mellitus, and in the setting of paraproteinemia.

Boin F, Hummers LK. Scleroderma-like fibrosing disorders. *Rheum Dis Clin North Am.* 2008;34:199–220.

19. What is a digital mucous (myxoid) cyst?
    A digital mucous cyst is a common solitary, asymptomatic, semitranslucent, dome-shaped nodule that typically presents in adults and elderly patients on the dorsal finger near the proximal nail fold or distal interphalangeal joint (Fig. 16.5B). It may distort the nail matrix, resulting in a groove in the nail plate. Clear, gelatinous mucoid material can be expressed from the cyst. The pathogenesis is controversial; however, it is often attributed to degenerative changes in the distal interphalangeal joints.

Lin YC, Wu YH, Scher RK. Nail changes and association of osteoarthritis in digital myxoid cyst. *Dermatol Surg.* 2008;34:364–369.

20. What substance is elevated in gout?
    Gout is a heterogeneous group of disorders of purine metabolism resulting in elevated levels of uric acid (monosodium urate). Patients have either increased uric acid production or decreased renal excretion. Some risk factors for hyperuricemia include alcohol use, obesity, high purine diets, diabetes, myeloproliferative disorders, renal disease, and/or diuretic therapy.

21. Where is the uric acid deposited in gout? What are the resulting clinical manifestations?
    Uric acid crystals in gout are most commonly deposited in the synovium, soft tissues, and skin. The most common site is the synovium of joints, producing acute gouty arthritis. The metatarsophalangeal joint of the great toe is classically involved. Uric acid deposition in the skin and soft tissues results in gouty tophi, which are seen in 20% to 50% of patients. Common sites of involvement include the helix of the ear, elbows, and digits (Fig. 16.6A). These gouty tophi may ulcerate and discharge monosodium urate crystals that appear as a thick chalky material. Under light microscopy, these crystals are needle-shaped and birefringent (Fig. 16.6B).

Thissen CA, Frank J, Lucker GP. Tophi as first clinical sign of gout. *Int J Dermatol.* 2008;47(suppl 1):49–51.

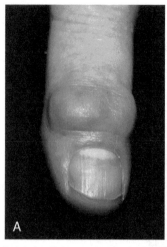 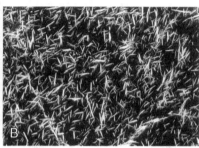

Fig. 16.6 **A,** Gouty tophus. Tophaceous deposits of gout overlying a digit. **B,** Aspirate from gouty tophus demonstrating diagnostic birefringent gout crystals with polarization. (Courtesy Fitzsimons Army Medical Center teaching files.)

22. Describe the types of calcinosis cutis.
    - **Dystrophic calcinosis cutis:** Occurs when there is deposition of calcium salts within inflamed or damaged tissue. Calcium and phosphorus metabolism is normal. It may be localized, such as within acne scars or epidermoid cysts, or widespread. Widespread dystrophic calcinosis cutis most often occurs in association with connective tissue disease, such as dermatomyositis or scleroderma.
    - **Metastatic calcinosis cutis:** Is seen with aberrations in calcium or phosphorus metabolism. It usually occurs when the serum calcium-phosphorus product exceeds 60.
    - **Idiopathic calcinosis cutis:** Is the term used when no obvious underlying cause can be identified for tissue calcification. Examples include subepidermal calcified nodules, tumoral calcinosis, and scrotal calcinosis.
    - **Iatrogenic calcinosis cutis:** Deposition of calcium due to medical agents such as intravenous calcium gluconate, intravenous calcium chloride, calcium alginate dressings, and calcium chloride electrode paste.

Reiter N, El-Shabrawi L, Leinweber B, Berghold A, Aberer E. Calcinosis cutis: part I. Diagnostic pathway. *J Am Acad Dermatol.* 2011;65:1–12.

23. What underlying medical conditions have been associated with metastatic calcinosis cutis?
    - Hyperparathyroidism
    - Pseudohypoparathyroidism
    - Vitamin D toxicity
    - Milk-alkali syndrome
    - Sarcoidosis
    - Destructive bone disease
    - Malignancies
    - Chronic renal failure

24. What is calciphylaxis and who develops it?
    Calciphylaxis is a type of metastatic calcification in which there is calcification of the walls of small- and medium-sized blood vessels in the dermis and subcutis, resulting in infarction of the overlying skin. Clinically, patients develop livedo reticularis—like mottling, painful hard plaques, and necrotic ulcers. It is usually seen in the setting of chronic renal failure and secondary hyperparathyroidism (Fig. 16.7). Calciphylaxis, however, has uncommonly been reported with normal levels of calcium and phosphate and in the absence of renal disease.

Daudén E, Oñate MJ. Calciphylaxis. *Dermatol Clin.* 2008;26:557–568.

25. What is osteoma cutis?
    Osteoma cutis is the deposition of bone within cutaneous tissues. Primary osteoma cutis involves normal skin and can be associated with several syndromes including Albright hereditary osteodystrophy, fibrodysplasia ossificans

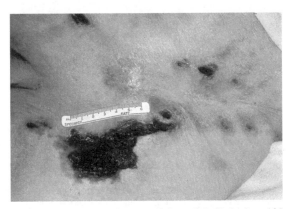

Fig. 16.7 Calciphylaxis. Necrosis of overlying skin in a patient with chronic renal failure.

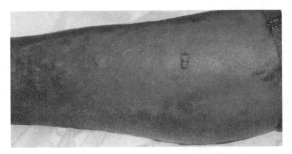

Fig. 16.8 Nephrogenic fibrosing dermopathy. Erythematous to brawny sclerotic plaque with a cobblestone surface on the lower extremity. (Courtesy Johann Gudjonsson, MD.)

progressiva, and congenital platelike osteomatosis. Secondary osteoma cutis or metaplastic ossification occurs in association with or secondary to trauma, inflammatory skin conditions, or neoplasia. Miliary osteoma cutis of the face presents as multiple, small, firm papules on the face, typically in women afflicted with acne, although it may also arise on normal skin.

26. **What is nephrogenic systemic fibrosis and in what setting do patients develop this condition?**
Nephrogenic systemic fibrosis, also known as nephrogenic fibrosing dermopathy, is a systemic fibrosing disorder that involves the skin and internal organs. It is seen almost exclusively in those patients with renal insufficiency or renal failure who have had imaging studies with gadolinium as a contrast agent. Patients with this condition develop large areas of indurated, brawny plaques and bound down skin, often with a peau d'orange or cobblestone surface. The extremities are most commonly involved (Fig. 16.8). Flexion contractures may develop in severe cases.

27. **What are histologic features of nephrogenic systemic fibrosis? What condition does it most resemble?**
Nephrogenic systemic fibrosis is characterized by a diffuse proliferation of fibroblasts, dermal dendrocytes, thickened collagen bundles, and mucin deposition. It resembles scleromyxedema histologically.

Girardi M, Kay J, Elston DM, Leboit PE, Abu-Alfa A, Cowper SE. Nephrogenic systemic fibrosis: clinicopathological definition and workup recommendation. *J Am Acad Dermatol.* 2011;65:1095–1106.e7.
Daftari Besheli L, Aran S, Shaqdan K, Kay J, Abujudeh H. Current status of nephrogenic systemic fibrosis. *Clin Radiol.* 2014;69:661–668.

Acknowledgments
The author wishes to acknowledge the contributions of the previous authors, Lisa E. Maier, MD, and Lori Lowe, MD.

CHAPTER 17

PHOTOSENSITIVE DERMATITIS

Whitney A. High

1. What is "photosensitivity"?

   Photosensitivity is defined as development or exacerbation of a skin eruption and/or skin symptoms (such as pruritus or pain) after exposure to light (particularly to sunlight, but possibly due to an artificial light source of similar wavelength). Admittedly, the patient may not always directly relate an eruption to light exposure, and there may also be a delay in the onset of signs or symptoms following light exposure. Ergot, when a skin eruption is "photodistributed" (see below), even without a definite history of exacerbation after light exposure, many dermatologists classify it as a probable "photodermatosis." Some photosensitivity reactions may simply appear as a "sunburn," but the reactions occur with lesser light exposure than would normally be required to induce a sunburn.

   Santoro FA, Lim HW. Update on photodermatoses. *Semin Cutan Med Surg.* 2011; 30:229–238.

2. What is the clinical appearance of a "photodistributed" eruption?

   A "photodistributed" eruption affects the skin of the sun-exposed face, the distal/lateral forearms, the dorsal hands, a V-shaped area of the upper chest (where collars open), the lateral and posterior neck, and any other area exposed to visible light (typically the sun). Such eruptions usually spare the upper eyelid, the skin beneath (in the shadow of) the nose and lower lip, the neck beneath the chin (in shadow), and inner arms, the upper thigh, and other clothing-protected sites. In "photocontact processes" the reaction appears in a similar distribution, but it is due to both exposure to a photoactive chemical and light, together.

3. What is the difference between a phototoxic reaction and a photoallergic reaction?

   A "phototoxic" reaction (Fig. 17.1) is an exaggerated sunburn-type reaction, where skin cells are damaged directly by light/ultraviolet light through the production of free radicals, toxic metabolites, heat, or by direct damage to DNA, augmented by external chemicals. Phototoxic reactions occur within minutes to hours of exposure, although on occasion, the reaction is delayed for a day or two. A phototoxic reaction does not involve an immune hypersensitivity, and it can be produced in anyone with the appropriate dose of a chemical and light/ultraviolet light. It can happen on first exposure without prior sensitization. Phototoxic reactions are well demarcated.

   A photoallergic reaction occurs only in previously sensitized individuals light/ultraviolet light, interacts with an endogenous (Fig. 17.2A) or exogenous (Fig. 17.2B) chemical, converting it to an allergen that the immune system recognizes, prompting a further immune-mediated response. Photoallergic reactions usually occur 1–3 days after exposure (with the exception of solar urticaria, which is nearly immediate). Photoallergic reactions are photodistributed, but may extend to covered areas or even distant sites due to "autoeczematous (id)" phenomenon. Sometimes, chemicals may produce both a phototoxic and photoallergic reaction.

4. Name some common topical phototoxic and photoallergic agents and the action spectra.

   Almost all topical phototoxic and photoallergic reactions are caused by ultraviolet A (UVA) light and, less often, ultraviolet B (UVB) or visible light. Some of the most common topical agents are listed in Table 17.1.

5. Name common systemic phototoxic and photoallergic agents and their action spectra.

   As in the case of the topical agents, the action spectrum for almost all systemic phototoxic and photoallergic reactions is UVA, rarely UVB or visible light. Some of the most common systemic agents are listed in Table 17.2.

   Stein KR, Scheinfeld NS. Drug-induced photoallergic and phototoxic reactions. *Expert Opin Drug Saf.* 2007; 6:431–443.

6. Give some examples of unique phototoxic/photoallergic reactions.
   - Pseudoporphyria (nonsteroidal antiinflammatory drugs [NSAIDs], especially naproxen).
   - Photo-onycholysis (tetracyclines, fluoroquinolones, diuretics, NSAIDs, and psoralens).
   - Hyperpigmentation (amiodarone, tricyclics, diltiazem, minocycline, hydroxychloroquine, gold, silver).
   - Lichenoid eruptions (quinine, quinidine, gold, hydrochlorothiazide, calcium channel blockers).
   - Phytophotodermatitis (furocoumarins in lime juice, parsley, celery, parsnips, some grasses).
   - Radiation recall reaction (methotrexate given after radiation or sunburn, which reproduces or exaggerates the original burn reaction).

7. What are some scenarios in which the skin may be more sensitive to ultraviolet radiation?
   - Isotretinoin and retinoids (due to thinning of the stratum corneum).

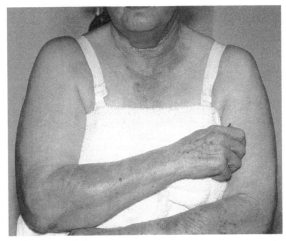

Fig. 17.1 Phototoxic drug eruption. Sunburn-like erythema on the cheeks, neck, v-area of the chest, and dorsal forearms.

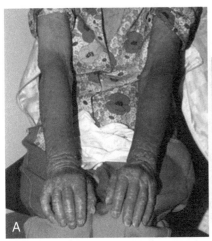 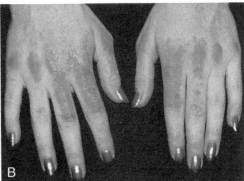

Fig. 17.2 A, Photoallergic drug eruption due to oral compazine demonstrating marked erythema and swelling of the dorsum of the hands, arms, and v of the chest. *(Courtesy Fitzsimons Army Medical Center teaching files.)* **B,** Photoallergic contact dermatitis. Erythema of the dorsal hands and fingers due to a sunscreen containing para-aminobenzoic acid.

- 5-Fluorouracil (due to the antimetabolite affecting DNA repair).
- Methotrexate (due to antimetabolite affecting enzymatic recovery after UV damage).

8. What are important questions to ask a patient with a suspected photosensitivity reaction?
   - How long does it take for the skin reaction to develop following light exposure? Some reactions (solar urticaria) occur within minutes of sun exposure, while others may take days, hours, or weeks to develop.
   - Have you ever had a similar skin reaction to light? Some light-induced conditions, such as polymorphous light reaction (PMLE), tend to be recurrent and seasonal, while others may be one-time events.
   - Is there a family history of skin reactions to light? Some photosensitivity disorders are familial (erythropoietic protoporphyria) or occur more often in certain ethnic groups (actinic prurigo of Native Americans).
   - What skin products do you use? Numerous products (soaps, perfumes, sunscreens) may produce a photoallergic contact dermatitis in certain individuals.
   - What oral medications do you use? Numerous drugs, prescription and nonprescription, can produce photosensitive reactions.
   - Do you have itching or pain? Pruritus is common with some conditions, such as photoallergic contact dermatitis, while pain or burning is more often associated with phototoxic disorders and some porphyrias.
   - Do you have any other symptoms? Some photosensitive dermatoses are limited to the skin, but others, such as systemic lupus, may be associated with internal involvement.

Table 17.1 Topical agents causing phototoxic and photoallergic reactions

PHOTOTOXIC CHEMICALS	PHOTOALLERGIC CHEMICALS
Benzocaine	Sunscreens: oxybenzone, benzophenone, para-aminobenzoic acid (PABA) derivatives, cinnamates, salicylates, etc.
Benzoyl peroxide (UVB)	
Coal tar	Fragrances: methylcoumarin, musk ambrette, sandalwood oil
Halogenated salicylanilides	NSAIDs
Hydrocortisone	Oxicams: ampiroxicam, droxicam, meloxicam, piroxicam, tenoxicam
Ketoprofen	Priopionic acid derivatives: benzophenone, dexketoprofen, ketoprofen, piketoprofen, suprofen (UVA and UVB), tiaprofenic acid, diclofenac
Porphyrins (visible light and UVB)	Antimicrobials: bithionol, chlorhexidine, fenticlor, hexachlorophene
Psoralens	Phenothiazines: chlorpromazine, promethazine
Furocoumarins	Pesticides
Fluorescein	Acyclovir
Tar	Dibucaine
Aminolevulinic acid	Halogenated salicylanilides (UVA and UVB)
Photofrin	Hydrocortisone

NSAID, Nonsteroidal antiinflammatory drug; *UVA*, ultraviolet A; *UVB*, ultraviolet B.

Table 17.2 Systemic agents causing phototoxic and photoallergic reactions

PHOTOTOXIC	PHOTOALLERGIC
Antimicrobials	**NSAIDs:** piroxicam, celecoxib, ketoprofen
Tetracyclines: demeclocycline, dimethylchlortetracycline, doxycycline, lymecycline, minocycline, tetracycline	**Sulfur-containing medications:** hydrochlorothiazide, sulfacetamide (UVB), sulfadiazine (UVB), sulfapyridine (UVB), sulfonamides (UVB), sulfonylureas
Quinolones: ciprofloxacin, enoxacin, fleroxacin, levofloxacin, lomefloxacin (UVA and UVB), nalidixic acid, pefloxacin, sparfloxacin	**Antimalarials:** chloroquine, hydroxychloroquine (UVB), quinidine, quinine
Erythromycin	**Antimicrobials:** chloramphenicol unknown, enoxacin, lomefloxacin (UVA and UVB), sulfonamides, griseofulvin
Griseofulvin, voriconazole	
Efavirenz	**Phenothiazines:** chlorpromazine, dioxopromethazine, perphenazine, thioridazine
Sulfur-containing medications: bumetanide, furosemide, hydrochlorothiazide, sulfonamides (UVB), sulfonylureas	**Miscellaneous:** amantadine, dapsone unknown, diphenhydramine (UVB), flutamide (UVA and UVB), pilocarpine, pyridoxine, ranitidine
NSAIDs: propionic acid derivatives: benzophenone, carprofen, ketoprofen, nabumetone, naproxen, suprofen (UVA and UVB), tiaprofenic acid	
Antimalarials: chloroquine unknown, hydroxychloroquine (UVB), quinidine, quinine	
Miscellaneous: amiodarone, atorvastatin (UVB), calcium-channel blockers, chlorpromazine, prochlorperazine, porphyrins (UVB and visible), psoralens, retinoids (UVA and UVB), St. John's wort (hypericin)	
Multikinase inhibitors, EGFR inhibitors, *BRAF* inhibitors: imatinib, sunitinib, erlotinib, vemurafenib, dabrafenib	

EGFR, epidermal growth factor receptor; *NSAID*, nonsteroidal antiinflammatory drug; *UVA*, ultraviolet A; *UVB*, ultraviolet B.

9. **What are the most common causes of photosensitive dermatoses?**
   Medications, both systemic and topical, can cause photosensitivity. Polymorphous light eruption is the most common photodermatitis, and it appears to have a hereditary element.

10. **What is persistent light reactivity?**
    In persistent light reactivity, a photodermatitis, originally triggered by topical or systemic drugs, persists long after the causative agent has been discontinued. Affected patients may be sensitive to a broad range of light, even visible light. The disease may be incapacitating. Chronic actinic dermatitis (actinic reticuloid) is a severe photodermatitis that occurs chiefly in older men (Fig. 17.3). Some experts believe chronic actinic dermatitis/actinic reticuloid begins as a photoallergic condition that becomes chronic and severely debilitating.

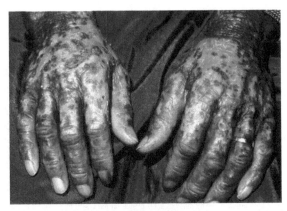

Fig. 17.3 Actinic reticuloid. Elderly man with chronic, highly pruritic photosensitivity with erythema, scale, pigmentary changes, and lichenification of the skin. (Courtesy Fitzsimons Army Medical Center teaching files.)

KEY POINTS: PHOTOSENSITIVE DERMATITIS

1. In general, phototoxic reactions resemble sunburn reactions (erythema, burning pain), while photoallergic reactions resemble dermatitis (erythema, pruritus).
2. Over 350 drugs have been reported to produce photosensitive reactions.
3. Photosensitive drug reactions may be triggered by UVA or UVB light. Because UVA passes through window glass, photosensitive drug reactions can occur in persons inside their homes or cars.
4. Photosensitivity is a component of some genetic disorders characterized by defective DNA repair (xeroderma pigmentosum) or enzymatic deficiencies (phototoxic porphyrias).

11. What is PMLE?

PMLE is a common, immunologically mediated photo-eruption that usually begins at some point in the first three decade of life. There may be a family history of photosensitivity in PMLE patients. The disease usually begins in spring or early summer. Patients sometimes demonstrate "hardening," or a gradual improvement with continuing sun through the summer. Typically, PMLE begins at least 4–6 hours after light exposure begins, and it resolves 2–3 days after light exposure ends. The skin lesions of PMLE can take on different forms (i.e., "polymorphous"), but the most common presentations include erythematous macules, patches, papules, plaques (Fig. 17.4), and vesicles and bullae, upon sun-exposed skin. The etiology of the condition is unknown, but most patients with PMLE do **not** have antinuclear antibodies. Actinic prurigo, hydroa aestivale, and hydroa vacciniforme are also considered by some experts to be variants of PMLE.

Guarrera M. Polymorphous light eruption. *Adv Exp Med Biol*. 2017; 996:61–70.

12. How is PMLE diagnosed?

PMLE is diagnosed clinically, based upon a history of a recurrent photoeruption, usually occurring each spring or early summer, and with a compatible time course, which is different from solar urticaria. A biopsy may support the diagnosis, demonstrating a perivascular dermatitis with papillary dermal edema, but there is no laboratory finding that can establish the diagnosis of PMLE. Other causes of photosensitivity, such as lupus erythematosus, porphyria, and a drug-induced process, should be excluded. In this regard, a skin biopsy, a biopsy for direct immunofluorescence testing of lesional skin, serologic testing for antinuclear antibodies, a porphyrin screen, and patch/photopatch testing could be useful to exclude other diseases. Phototesting may demonstrate a lowered minimal erythema dose that is less than one would predict on the basis of skin type (Fig. 17.5).

13. How is PMLE treated?

PMLE is managed with sun avoidance, sunscreens, and other photoprotective measures. If these measures are not effective, topical steroids, extracts of the fern plant *Polypodium leucotomos*, antimalarials, and hardening with psoralen plus UVA or narrow-band ultraviolet B (NB-UVB) are alternatives that may prove successful in some cases of PMLE.

14. What is actinic prurigo?

While controversial, actinic prurigo (PMLE of Native Americans) may be a variant of classic PMLE. In this population, the family history is usually positive, although sporadic cases do occur. Actinic prurigo can occur in other ethnicities (Fig. 17.6). Patients with actinic prurigo often demonstrate involvement of the lips (cheilitis).

Ross G, Foley P, Baker C. Actinic prurigo. *Photodermal Photoimmunol Photomed*. 2008; 24:272–275.

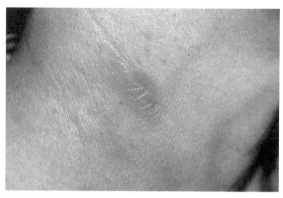

Fig. 17.4 Polymorphous light eruption. Erythematous, scaly plaque on the lateral neck, which tended to recur each spring.

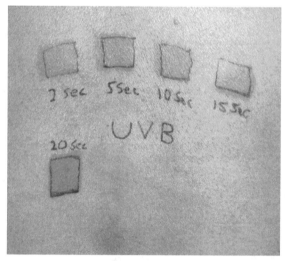

Fig. 17.5 Ultraviolet B *(UVB)* (290 to 320 nm) phototest sites in a patient with polymorphous light eruption demonstrating marked photosensitivity. These test sites were read at 48 hours. (Courtesy Fitzsimons Army Medical Center teaching files.)

15. What is solar urticaria?

Solar urticaria is urticaria (hives) that is triggered by light exposure. UVA wavelengths are the most common trigger; UVB and even visible light can cause disease. Urticarial papules or plaques develop within minutes of light exposure. Pruritus or pain may be perceived. Rarely, systemic reactions, such as anaphylactic shock, occur. Solar urticaria is a photoallergic reaction (type I hypersensitivity response) that is probably IgE-mediated, although direct degranulation of mast cells is another proposed mechanism. Erythropoietic protoporphyria may present in similar fashion but can be excluded with appropriate porphyrin studies. Treatment includes light avoidance, photoprotection, antihistamines, and perhaps even omalizumab.

Photiou L, Foley P, Ross G. Solar urticaria—an Australian case series of 83 patients. *Autralas J Dermatol*. 2019; 60:110–117.

16. Discuss the differential diagnosis of photodermatoses in infants or young children.

Photodermatoses are uncommon in neonates and young children, probably due in part to a minimal degree sunlight exposure in this age group. However, cutaneous lesions of neonatal lupus erythematosus occur in early life and are

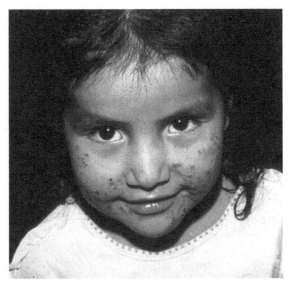

Fig. 17.6 Actinic prurigo. Native American child with pruritic photosensitive dermatitis of nose, cheeks, and chin. Note that she also has a low-grade cheilitis on her lower lip. (Courtesy Fitzsimons Army Medical Center teaching files.)

photoexacerbated. These patients develop erythematous, often annular plaques, usually distributed on the face and scalp ("raccoon eyes"). Cardiac conduction defects may be present. Nearly all affected infants, and their mothers, have circulating anti–Ro/SS-A antibodies. Photosensitivity in pediatric patients may be related to a genodermatoses (Table 17.3). The differential diagnosis of photosensitivity in this age group also includes PMLE (including juvenile springtime eruption, hydroa aestivale, and hydroa vacciniforme), photodrug eruptions, photocontact dermatitis, erythropoietic protoporphyria, and cutaneous lupus.

17. **How do hydroa aestivale and hydroa vacciniforme differ?**
Hydroa aestivale and hydroa vacciniforme are rare vesiculopapular photoeruptions of unknown etiology that occur in childhood. The conditions involve the face, particularly the ears, nose, and cheeks, and the chest and dorsal hands. Hydroa aestivale occurs more often in girls and does not leave scarring. Hydroa vacciniforme is more common in boys, and it heals with shallow scars. Epstein-Barr virus may be associated with hydroa vacciniforme. Some experts consider both diseases to be variants of PMLE.

Table 17.3 Genodermatoses associated with photosensitivity

DISEASE	SKIN FINDINGS	INHERITANCE	OTHER
Xeroderma pigmentosum	Lentigines, skin cancers, photoaging	Autosomal recessive	Photophobia, keratitis, corneal opacification and vascularization, neurologic abnormalities: hyporeflexia, deafness, seizures (most common in groups A and D; do not usually occur in XP variant). XP variant patients usually have no neurologic problems. Complementation groups A to G: defective global genomic nucleotide excision repair (GG-NER) of UVR-induced DNA damage (e.g., pyrimidine dimers) from any part of the genome
Cockayne syndrome	Photosensitivity without pigmentary changes or	Autosomal recessive	Loss of adipose tissue, prominent ears, dental caries, thinning of

Continued on following page

Table 17.3 Genodermatoses associated with photosensitivity (*Continued*)

DISEASE	SKIN FINDINGS	INHERITANCE	OTHER
	increased risk of skin cancer. Scaly facial photodermatitis		skin and hair. Hypogonadism, stooped posture, joint contractures, short stature with extremely thin body habitus ("cachectic dwarfism"), microcephaly, mental retardation, deafness. Calcification of basal ganglia, demyelination, pigmentary retinal degeneration, osteoporosis. Cockayne's syndrome (CS) cells are defective in the repair of pyrimidine dimer photoproducts and oxidative DNA base modifications typically induced by UVB and UVA, respectively. CS also has significantly defective RNA synthesis recovery after UV irradiation (defect in transcription-coupled nucleotide excision repair [TC-NER]).Two complementation groups: CS-A (mutations in *ERCC8*) and CS-B (mutations in *ERCC6*); identical phenotypes. Mutations in *XPB*, *XPD*, and *XPG* genes have been associated with combined XP/CS phenotypes
Trichothiodystrophy	Ichthyosis, brittle hair. Hair shaft: alternating light and dark bands ("tiger tail banding"), trichoschisis, trichorrhexis nodosa	Autosomal recessive	PIBI(D)S: photosensitivity, ichthyosis, brittle hair, intellectual impairment, decreased fertility, short stature. Other features: microcephaly, receding chin, protruding ears. Mutations in *XPD*, *XPB*, general transcription factor IIH polypeptide 5 (*GTF2H5* or *TFB5*), and *C7orf11*
UV-sensitive syndrome (UVsS)	Photosensitivity, ephelides (freckling)	Autosomal recessive	Similar to CS: defective TC-NER, normal GG-NER; however, unlike CS, patients with UVsS only are defective in repair of UVB-induced photoproducts (not repair of oxidative damage), and they do not have neurologic or skeletal abnormalities. Three complementation groups: mutations in *ERCC6*, *ERCC8*, and *UVSSA* genes.
Bloom syndrome		Autosomal recessive	Elongated face with malar hypoplasia and prominent

Table 17.3 Genodermatoses associated with photosensitivity (*Continued*)

DISEASE	SKIN FINDINGS	INHERITANCE	OTHER
	Malar erythema and telangiectasias, café-au-lait macules, hypopigmentation		nose, short stature, diabetes mellitus, recurrent infections. Small at birth, severe growth retardation, respiratory infections, malignancy. Increased frequency of leukemia, lymphoma, gastrointestinal adenocarcinoma. Men: sterile; women: reduced fertility. Normal intelligence. Decreased IgA, IgM, sometimes IgG. Mutations in BLM *(RECQL3)*, resulting in chromosomal instability (increased sister chromatid exchanges, chromosomal breakage and rearrangement). Quadriradial configurations in lymphocytes and fibroblasts are diagnostic.
Rothmund-Thomson syndrome	Erythema, edema, and vesicles on the cheeks and face during the first few months of life, followed by poikiloderma that also typically affects the dorsal aspect of the hands/forearms and the buttocks. Sparse hair (scalp, eyebrows, eyelashes), hypoplastic nails, acral keratoses (in adolescents and adults)	Autosomal recessive syndrome	Cataracts, usually normal intelligence, and cerebellar ataxia. Short stature, skeletal (e.g., radial ray defects, osteoporosis) and dental abnormalities, juvenile cataracts, chronic diarrhea/vomiting during infancy, pituitary hypogonadism (may be associated with midface hypoplasia/"saddle nose"). Osteosarcoma (10%–30%), squamous cell carcinoma (5%; often acral). Normal immune function, intelligence, and life span (in the absence of malignancy). Mutations in *RECQL4*; protein product is a DNA helicase. Genomic instability may account for propensity for malignancies.
Hartnup disease	Pellagra-like eruption	Autosomal recessive	Intermittent ataxia, which may be accompanied by nystagmus and tremors. Psychiatric disturbances and other nonspecific neurologic abnormalities have been reported in some patients, but significant mental retardation is not a feature. Defective renal and intestinal neutral amino acid transport. Marked aminoaciduria and tryptophan deficiency.
Kindler syndrome		Autosomal recessive	Subtype of epidermolysis bullosa (EB). Loss-of-function

Continued on following page

Table 17.3 Genodermatoses associated with photosensitivity (*Continued*)

DISEASE	SKIN FINDINGS	INHERITANCE	OTHER
	Poikiloderma, trauma-induced skin blistering, mucosal inflammation		mutations in the *FERMT1* (KIND1) gene. Clinical overlap between Kindler syndrome and dystrophic EB. Unlike other forms of EB, Kindler syndrome is characterized by impaired actin cytoskeleton–extracellular matrix interactions and a variable plane of blister formation at or close to the dermal–epidermal junction.

IgA, Immunoglobulin A; *IgG*, immunoglobulin G; *IgM*, immunoglobulin M; *UV*, ultraviolet; *UVA*, ultraviolet A; *UVB*, ultraviolet B; *UVR*, ultraviolet radiation.

Data from Online Mendelian Inheritance in Man (OMIM). McKusick-Nathans Institute of Genetic Medicine, Johns Hopkins University (Baltimore, MD) and National Center for Biotechnology Information, National Library of Medicine (Bethesda, MD). Available at: www.ncbi.nlm.nih.gov/omim/.

18. Which porphyrias are associated with photodermatoses?

Porphyria cutanea tarda (PCT) is the most common porphyria that yields skin findings. Lesions, which often include blisters, develop hours or days after sun exposure, and many patients do not recognize the condition as a photosensitivity disorder. Cutaneous changes similar to PCT may be seen in other porphyrias, including variegate porphyria (VP) and hereditary coproporphyria, or in pseudoporphyria caused by hemodialysis or certain medications (furosemide, nalidixic acid, mefenamic acid, tetracyclines, quinolones, hydrochlorothiazide, and naproxen). More acute photosensitivity can be seen with erythropoietic protoporphyria, congenital erythropoietic porphyria, and erythropoietic coproporphyria, and in these conditions, there are often burning and stinging within minutes of exposure, followed by erythema, blistering, and possible scarring.

19. Describe the cutaneous changes in PCT.

In PCT, tense vesicles and bullae develop on the dorsal hands, fingers, and feet and sometimes on the face and upper trunk. The skin may be perceived to be "fragile." Lesions heal with erosions, scarring, atrophy, milia, and pigmentary changes (Fig. 17.7). Hypertrichosis and thickened, sclerotic plaques can develop on the face or chest. Patients may not recognize the association with sun exposure, but upon questioning, often the condition is worsened during summer or following periods of intense sun exposure.

20. What causes PCT?

Porphyrias are caused by enzymatic deficiencies in heme. Porphyrins that accumulate due to these inherent errors of metabolism absorb light in the 400 to 410 nm wavelength ("Soret band"). This absorbed light energy is then transferred to cellular structures or to molecular oxygen, resulting in damage to tissues.

PCT is due to a deficiency of the enzyme uroporphyrinogen decarboxylase. The disease may be acquired or hereditary. Patients with acquired PCT have the enzyme deficiency in the liver only, and attacks may be triggered by alcohol, estrogen, hexachlorobenzene, and iron. PCT may also develop in patients with HIV or chronic liver disease (hepatitis C infection or hemochromatosis). In hereditary PCT, uroporphyrinogen decarboxylase is deficient in tissue beyond the liver. Heterozygous and homozygous enzyme deficiencies can occur, and more severe disease is observed with homozygous loss.

21. How is PCT diagnosed?

Fluorescent spectrophotometric analysis of plasma is a rapid screen for porphyria. Plasma is exposed to light with a wavelength of 400 to 410 nm, and the emission peaks are measured. A sharp emission peak at 619 nm confirms porphryia. To differentiate among the various porphyrias, a 24-hour urine specimen is submitted for study. In PCT, uroporphyrin I and 7-carboxylporphyrin III are elevated in the urine. Similarly, in PCT, patients' stool samples have normal levels of protoporphyrins but increased isocoproporphyrins.

22. How is VP distinguished from PCT?

VP can cause skin lesions that are indistinguishable from those of PCT (Fig. 17.8), but patients with VP have increased protoporphyrins in their stool and only moderately increased urine porphyrins. Unlike PCT patients, persons with VP typically have acute attacks, with skin lesions, but also with gastrointestinal pain and neurologic deficits, similar to those seen in patients with acute intermittent porphyria. Ergot, it is important to distinguish VP from PCT.

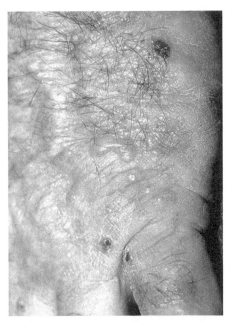

Fig. 17.7 Porphyria cutanea tarda (PCT). Vesicles, crusts, and milia on the hand of a patient with alcohol-triggered PCT.

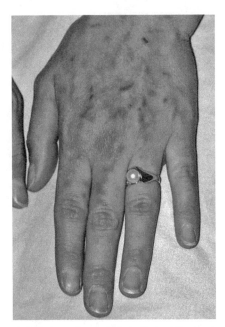

Fig. 17.8 Variegate porphyria. Erosions and scar on the back of the hand. (Courtesy James E. Fitzpatrick, MD.)

23. What treatments are used in PCT?
    - Eliminate agents that may trigger PCT, such as alcohol.
    - Protect from both ultraviolet and visible light.
    - Phlebotomy may improve PCT by decreasing excessive iron stores. Removal of about 500 mL of whole blood is done at periodic intervals, as tolerated, until the hemoglobin level is about 10 to 11 g/dL, or until side effects of anemia are experienced.

- Low-dose chloroquine or hydroxychloroquine therapy is an alternate treatment that requires very close monitoring for hepatotoxicity. High doses of these agents can be fatal.

24. What are the cutaneous findings in erythropoietic protoporphyria?

Erythropoietic protoporphyria usually begins in childhood, although some cases may present in adult life. Photosensitivity in this disease can be severe, with immediate burning and stinging of the sun-exposed skin. Erythema, edema, vesicles, and purpura may develop, particularly on the nose, cheeks, and dorsal hands (Fig. 17.9A). Over time, these areas scar from repeated eruptions. The skin over the knuckles may become thickened, wrinkled, and shiny, giving the appearance of "aged hands."

25. How is a diagnosis of erythropoietic protoporphyria made?

Erythropoietic protoporphyria is caused by deficiency of the enzyme, ferrochelatase. Red blood cells (RBCs) and feces show increased protoporphyrins. Additionally, RBCs of affected patients fluoresce a "coral red" when examined under a fluorescent microscope (Fig. 17.9B). This fluorescence is transient, and RBCs should be examined quickly after collection. In October 2019, the Food and Drug Administration approved use of afamelanotide, a synthetic analogue of α-melanocyte stimulating hormone, to ameliorated skin damage from the sun in people with erythropoietic protoporphyria. This drug may be used in addition to photoprotection.

Lane AM, McKay JT, Bonkovsky HL. Advances in the management of erythropoietic protoporphyria—role of afamelanotide. *Appl Clin Genet.* 2016; 2;9:179–189.

26. Do any other medical problems occur in patients with erythropoietic protoporphyria?

About 11% of patients with erythropoietic protoporphyria have a mild anemia of unknown cause. Cholelithiasis is seen at an early age. Liver disease is common but only rarely leads to fatal hepatic failure.

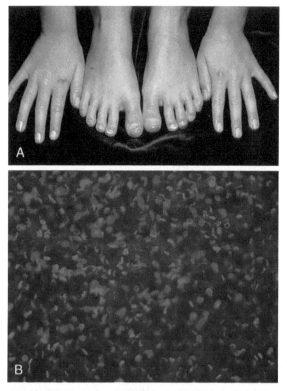

Fig. 17.9 Erythropoietic protoporphyria (EPP). **A,** Young child with intense photosensitivity of hands and feet (associated with wearing sandals) manifesting as tense blisters, crusting, and very early thickening of the skin. (Courtesy Fitzsimons Army Medical Center teaching files) **B,** Fluorescent red blood cells in a child with EPP. (Courtesy James E. Fitzpatrick, MD.)

27. What forms of cutaneous lupus result in photosensitivity?

    Subacute cutaneous lupus and neonatal lupus (both anti–Ro/SS-A positive conditions) result in photosensitivity that is induced and/or exacerbated by UV light. Acute cutaneous lupus ("butterfly" malar rash) and chronic cutaneous lupus ("discoid lupus") are also triggered or exacerbated by UV light. Drug-induced subacute systemic lupus erythematosus can result from tumor necrosis factor-α blockers, hydrochlorothiazide, terbinafine, omeprazole, calcium channel blockers, nonsteroidal antiinflammatory drugs (e.g., naproxen), griseofulvin, and antihistamines. Lesions of drug-induced lupus may or may not clear after the offending medication is discontinued.

28. Name some other conditions associated with cutaneous photoexposure.

    Sunburn (UVB), immediate pigment darkening (photo-oxidation of melanin with UVA), tanning (melanin synthesis with UVB > UVA exposure), cutaneous and some systemic immunosuppression (UVB > UVA), vitamin D_3 synthesis, actinic keratoses, skin cancers, photoaging, solar elastosis, solar lentigines, ephelides, poikiloderma of Civatte, Favre-Racouchot syndrome, colloid milium, erosive pustular dermatosis of the scalp, mid-dermal elastolysis, actinic granuloma (annular elastolytic granuloma), giant cell arteritis, and brachioradial pruritus, among others.

CHAPTER 18

DISORDERS OF PIGMENTATION

Andrew Fischer and Lori D. Prok

1. **Are some disorders of pigmentation markers for systemic disease?**
   Yes. Examples include the following:
   - Generalized depigmentation: Albinism.
   - Generalized hyperpigmentation: Addison's disease.
   - Ash-leaf hypopigmented macules: Tuberous sclerosis.
   - Axillary and inguinal freckles: Neurofibromatosis.
   - Lentigines: Peutz-Jeghers syndrome.

2. **How do you diagnose a pigmentation disorder?**
   The clinical history is the most important aspect when considering a pigmentation disorder. It should focus on the time of onset (such as at birth, during childhood, or later in life), if there has been progression or spread, and a detailed family and personal medical history. Other facts to elucidate include any associated illness or symptoms, drug ingestion, chemical exposure, occupation, and exposure to sunlight, artificial ultraviolet light, heat, or ionizing radiation. Finally, a careful review of systems should be performed, followed by a skin examination with a keen eye toward color, morphology, and distribution, and occasionally additional labs or a biopsy may be needed.

3. **What are the important elements of a skin examination of a patient with a pigmentation disorder?**
   The entire skin surface should be evaluated with attention to the color, shape, and distribution of the lesion(s). Lesion **color** (e.g., depigmented, hypopigmented, hyperpigmented, mixed) helps place the disorder into a specific category and narrow the diagnostic possibilities. The **shape** (e.g., oval, linear, reticulate) of a lesion is sometimes diagnostic, such as ash-leaf–shaped hypopigmented macules in tuberous sclerosis, or reticulate hyperpigmentation in erythema ab igne. The **distribution** (e.g., localized, diffuse) of pigmentation also aids diagnosis. Symmetrical depigmentation on the arms, legs, and/or torso suggests vitiligo, whereas hypopigmentation localized to an area of prior inflammation would represent postinflammatory hypopigmentation. Increased pigmentation of the oral mucosa, axillae, and palmar creases is associated with Addison's disease, whereas hyperpigmentation of the central face may represent melasma.
   Other diagnostic tests: Wood's lamp examination can often be helpful. Skin biopsy, with or without special stains for melanocytes (e.g., tyrosinase, MART-1, Melan-A) and melanin (e.g., silver nitrate, Fontana-Masson stain), determines the number of epidermal melanocytes and the extent and location of epidermal and dermal pigmentation.

4. **What is a Wood's lamp?**
   It is a handheld black light. A Wood's lamp emits light in a narrow spectrum of long-wave ultraviolet to short-wave visible light with a peak emission at 365 nm. Hypopigmented areas appear lighter than surrounding skin, and depigmented areas appear pure white and are sharply demarcated. Furthermore, epidermal hyperpigmentation is enhanced (appears darker), whereas dermal hyperpigmentation is not. The Wood's lamp can be especially helpful in distinguishing between hypo- and depigmented lesions and in identifying these lesions in fair-skinned individuals.

LEUKODERMA: PARTIAL OR COMPLETE LOSS OF SKIN PIGMENTATION

5. **Name some heritable forms of leukoderma**
   - **Albinism** is a group of autosomal recessive disorders characterized by generalized pigmentary dilution, decreased visual acuity, and nystagmus secondary to alterations in the formation of melanin.
   - **Piebaldism** is a rare, autosomal dominant condition characterized by a white forelock and patchy areas of depigmentation on the midline ventral surface or symmetrically on the mid-extremities due to defective melanocyte development and migration.
   - **Waardenburg's syndrome** is a group of inherited conditions that may include findings of congenital deafness, heterochromia irides, amelanotic skin macules, white forelock, laterally displaced medial canthi, and widening of the nasal root due to the abnormal distribution of melanocytes during development.
   - **Hermansky-Pudlak syndrome** is a rare autosomal recessive disorder in which affected individuals suffer from generalized hypopigmentation, excessive bleeding due to platelet abnormalities, and lysosomal defects leading to ceroid lipofuscin accumulation in most body tissues secondary to impaired lysosome (including melanosome) formation and trafficking.

Dessinioti C, Stratigos AJ, Rigopoulous D, et al. A review of genetic disorders of hypopigmentation: lessons learned from the biology of melanocytes. *Exp Dermatol*. 2009;18:741–749.

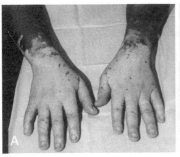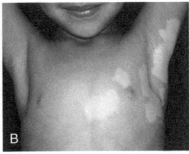

Fig. 18.1 Vitiligo. **A,** African-American man with vitiligo. Note the complete loss of skin pigmentation of the hands and wrists. **B,** Segmental vitiligo. (Courtesy James E. Fitzpatrick, MD.)

6. Name the skin disorder that manifests with complete loss of skin pigmentation

Vitiligo is an acquired depigmenting disorder due to loss of epidermal melanocytes. The overall incidence is 0.5%–2% worldwide, and all races and both sexes are affected equally. There is strong genetic influence. Vitiligo has been reported to be associated with autoimmune disorders, including thyroid disease and diabetes mellitus type 1. The pathogenesis is not totally understood but likely involves intrinsic defects within melanocytes and autoimmunity that target these cells. Patients with vitiligo have an increased number of autoreactive, melanocyte-specific, cytotoxic T lymphocytes, which can be seen infiltrating affected skin. The IFN-γ–induced chemokines seems to play an important role in selectively recruiting these cells to the skin.

Rodrigues M, Ezzedine K, Hamzavi I, et al. New discoveries in the pathogenesis and classification of vitiligo. *J Am Acad Dermatol.* 2017; 77(1):1–13.

7. Describe the clinical appearance of the skin lesions in vitiligo

Typically, lesions of vitiligo are flat and stark white and have a well-demarcated border without other skin changes. Sometimes, the border is hyperpigmented, or rarely erythematous. Commonly affected areas include the periorbital, perioral, and anogenital areas, as well as the elbows, knees, axillae, inguinal folds, and forearms. Frequently, lesions of vitiligo develop symmetrically on the trunk and extremities (Fig. 18.1A) and less commonly as focal or segmental (Fig. 18.1B). Vitiligo also causes depigmentation of hair (poliosis).

8. When does vitiligo have its onset?

The peak incidence occurs in the second and third decades of life, with 50% of cases occurring before age 20. Vitiligo has been reported in all age groups with onset as early as 6 weeks after birth and as late as 81 years.

9. Do any factors influence the onset of vitiligo?

Patients presenting with vitiligo usually describe asymptomatic areas of skin that have rapidly lost all pigment. Rarely do patients recall an associated illness, but they may report a particularly stressful event around the time of onset, and skin trauma is commonly reported to cause vitiligo lesions. The appearance of vitiligo lesions in areas of trauma, in a predisposed individual, is called the Koebner phenomenon.

10. Is vitiligo treatable?

Yes. Vitiligo repigments partially from the border, but mostly from the hair follicle. Localized vitiligo may be treated with high-potency topical steroids, topical calcineurin inhibitors, as well as with excimer laser (308 nm). For more generalized vitiligo, narrowband ultraviolet light B (UVB, 311 nm) is the treatment of choice. It must be administered two to three times weekly for many months. All patients with vitiligo should use sunscreen to protect their depigmented skin from sun damage. Further, a quality-of-life assessment should be done to help guide treatment.

Ezzedine K, Eleftheriadou V, Whitton M, van Geel N. Vitiligo. *Lancet.* 2015;386:74.

KEY POINTS: NORMAL SKIN PIGMENTATION: A COMBINATION OF FOUR PIGMENTS IN THE EPIDERMIS AND DERMIS

1. Oxygenated hemoglobin (red) in the arterioles and capillaries.
2. Deoxygenated hemoglobin (blue) in the venules.
3. Any ingested carotenoids or incompletely metabolized bile (yellow).
4. Epidermal melanin (brown), which is synthesized by epidermal melanocytes. Melanin is the most important pigment in determining skin color.

1. Pigmentation is determined by the type of melanin synthesized and how it is distributed to the surrounding keratinocytes.
2. There are two types of melanin: red-yellow pheomelanin and brown-black eumelanin.
3. Individuals with red hair produce an abundance of red-yellow pheomelanin and a lesser amount of the brown-black eumelanin.
4. Individuals with blonde, brown, and black hair primarily produce the brown-black eumelanin and a lesser amount of pheomelanin.
5. Differences in skin color between fair and dark-complected individuals are due to the variations in the number of melanosomes produced, size of the melanosomes, efficiency in transferring melanosome to keratinocytes, and variability in degradation. There is no difference in the overall number of melanocytes.

1. Most patients, over a lifetime, will suffer from a pigmentation disorder.
2. Fortunately, the most common pigmentation disorders are benign, self-limited, and reversible. For example, one of the most common develops following a cutaneous inflammatory reaction, when the skin is either more darkly pigmented (postinflammatory hyperpigmentation) or less pigmented (postinflammatory hypopigmentation) than surrounding normal skin, sometimes referred to collectively as postinflammatory dyspigmentation.
3. Postinflammatory changes in pigmentation slowly revert to normal over several months.
4. The two major types of cutaneous dyspigmentation are leukoderma and melanoderma. Patients with leukoderma present with areas of skin that appear lighter than surrounding normal skin, whereas patients with melanoderma have skin that appears darker than normal.
5. The major forms of cutaneous dyspigmentation can be broken down into subtypes, depending on whether there is alteration in the melanocyte number or pigment content of the skin.

1. Sunlight stimulates epidermal melanocytes to increase melanin synthesis inside melanosomes and stimulates melanocytes to transfer these melanosomes to keratinocytes. This melanocyte response to sunlight is called *tanning.*
2. The action spectrum of sunlight that causes tanning is the ultraviolet spectrum (wavelengths 290 to 400 nm).
3. Excess sunlight exposure causes abnormal melanocyte function, resulting in areas of melanocyte overproduction of melanin and increased melanocyte proliferation.
4. Sunlight-induced overproduction of melanin in a localized area causes the development of light brown macules called *freckles*, seen in fair-skinned individuals.
5. Similarly, *solar lentigines* are pigmented macules that develop on sun-damaged skin and are made up of increased numbers of keratinocytes and melanocytes with increased melanin synthesis.

11. What is piebaldism?

    Piebaldism is an uncommon autosomal dominant depigmentation disorder that is characterized by a white scalp forelock and hyperpigmented macules within larger depigmented patches on the skin. Piebaldism is due to mutations in the *KIT* proto-oncogene, which is located on chromosome 4. A functional KIT receptor is required for normal development and migration of melanocytes. Melanocytes typically migrate during embryologic development in a dorsal-to-ventral direction, but melanocytes in piebaldism fail to properly migrate to the ventral skin surfaces, such as the forehead, abdomen, and volar arms and legs. For this reason, depigmented areas in piebaldism predominate on the ventral skin surfaces. Patients are otherwise healthy. There is no treatment available for piebaldism.

12. What is albinism?

    Albinism is a group of inherited disorders of the melanin pigment system. All forms are autosomal recessive. In oculocutaneous albinism type 1 (OCA1), there is a defect in the enzyme tyrosinase with an absence in melanin synthesis. Generally, albinism presents with depigmented or hypopigmented skin and hair, nystagmus, photophobia, and decreased visual acuity (Fig. 18.2). Some forms affect the skin, hair, and eyes (oculocutaneous albinism); other forms primarily affect the eyes (ocular albinism). There are seven different forms of oculocutaneous albinism and two forms of ocular albinism. There is no treatment available for albinism.

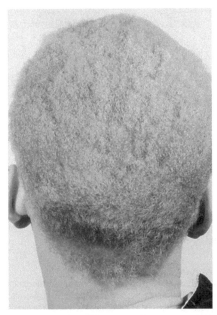

Fig. 18.2 Albino African-American boy with generalized hypopigmentation.

13. **How does albinism differ from the other inherited leukodermas?**
    The common feature of vitiligo, piebaldism, and the rarer leukoderma syndromes is a decrease or total absence of epidermal melanocytes. By comparison, patients with albinism have a normal number of epidermal melanocytes, but the melanocytes are unable to synthesize melanin appropriately.

14. **Can disorders of amino acid metabolism cause leukoderma?**
    Yes. This is typically due to a disruption of melanin synthesis or stimulation. For example, in phenylkenoturia, patients are lacking the enzyme need to convert phenylalanine to tyrosine, and therefore cannot build melanin.
    See Table 18.1.

Majid I. Metabolic disorders of pigmentation. In: Koushik L, et al, eds. *Pigmentary disorders: a comprehensive compendium.* New Delhi, India: Jaypee Brothers Medical Publishers; 2014:53–58.

15. **How do chemicals cause skin depigmentation or skin hypopigmentation?**
    Monobenzyl ether of hydroquinone (MBEH) and para–substituted phenols (PSPs) cause skin depigmentation by destroying melanocytes. It is believed that both MBEH and PSP are taken up by melanocytes and metabolized into toxic products that then kill the melanocytes. Hydroquinone, a commonly used skin-lightening agent, causes decreased melanin synthesis by competing with tyrosine and dihydroxyphenylalanine for the enzyme tyrosinase. With hydroquinone bound to its active site, tyrosinase is unable to synthesize melanin. Other chemicals, such as arsenic, mercaptoethyl amines, chloroquine, hydroxychloroquine, and corticosteroids, act to metabolically suppress melanocytes, resulting in decreased melanin synthesis and skin lightening. With the exception of MBEH, in most cases, the effects of these chemicals are reversible.

16. **Can patients with nutritional disorders suffer from leukoderma?**
    Yes. Patients suffering from protein loss or deficiency diseases, including kwashiorkor, intestinal malabsorption, and nephrotic syndrome, often manifest with facial, truncal, and extremity hypopigmentation. This is thought to be due to faulty melanogenesis secondary to a lack of tyrosine or other elements required for normal melanin synthesis, such as copper and selenium. Normal pigmentation returns following treatment of the nutritional disorder.

17. **What disorders should the clinician consider in a patient with hypopigmented macules and patches?**
    Tuberous sclerosis, nevus depigmentosus, Blaschkoid hypomelanosis, sarcoidosis, discoid lupus erythematosus, cutaneous T-cell lymphoma, eczema, psoriasis, secondary syphilis, leprosy, and tinea versicolor.

18. **What is tuberous sclerosis?**
    Tuberous sclerosis is a multifaceted, autosomal dominant disorder, with an incidence of 1:5–10,000 births, which causes tumors to form in nearly every organ in the body. See Chapter 5, Neurocutaneous Disorders.

Table 18.1 Inherited disorders of amino acid metabolism with related leukoderma

DISORDER	AFFECTED AMINO ACID	INCIDENCE	INHERITANCE	MANIFESTATIONS
Phenylketonuria	Phenylalanine	1:10,000 to 1:20,000	AR	Hypopigmentation of hair, eyes, and skin; mental retardation if not treated early
Histidinemia	Histidine	1:12,000	AR	Often asymptomatic, but may have hypopigmentation, loss of terminal hairs, and mental retardation
Homocystinuria	Methionine	1:58,000 to 1:1,000,000 depending on geographic region	AR	Hypopigmentation of skin, hair, and eyes; CNS abnormalities; skeletal abnormalities (Marfan's syndrome–like); thromboembolic disease

AR, Autosomal recessive; *CNS*, central nervous system.

19. What is nevus depigmentosus?

Nevus depigmentosus consists of single or multiple hypopigmented (not depigmented as the name implies) macules or patches that grow proportionally with the patient. The trunk is the most commonly affected body area. However, nevus depigmentosus has been reported to occur on the extremities, buttocks, and face. Most lesions present by age 3 years, with the remainder (about 7%) presenting later in childhood. The lesions are localized, circumscribed, irregular, oval, round, or rectangular macules or patches. It is thought to be caused by an abnormal clone of melanocytes, which have a reduced ability to produce melanin. Lesional skin has normal melanocyte number, but reduced numbers of melanosomes in the melanocytes and surrounding keratinocytes.

20. How does nevus depigmentosus compare to Blaschkoid hypomelanosis?

The skin lesions of Blaschkoid hypomelanosis (the more commonly used terminology is "hypomelanosis of Ito") very closely resemble those of nevus depigmentosus, and a dysfunctional clone of melanocytes seems to be central to both disorders. However, Blaschkoid hypomelanosis lesions are larger, whorled, and more widespread (Fig. 18.3). Moreover, a small proportion of patients with Blaschkoid hypomelanosis will suffer from disorders of the central nervous system, eyes, hair, teeth, and musculoskeletal system, which is not the case with nevus depigmentosus.

21. Which infectious disorders can have associated leukoderma?

Secondary syphilis, pinta, yaws, onchocerciasis, and leprosy. The inflammatory reaction associated with these diseases alters melanocyte homeostasis, with a resultant decrease in melanin synthesis and subsequent transfer to keratinocytes.

22. Describe the pigmentation changes seen with the treponematoses

- **Secondary syphilis:** Hypopigmented macules can be found on the neck, shoulders, upper chest, and axillae in patients with secondary syphilis (due to *Treponema pallidum*). The hypopigmented neck lesions have been termed the "necklace of Venus."
- **Pinta:** Pinta is a chronic nonvenereal disease caused by *T. carateum* that is endemic in Central and South America. The primary lesion, at the site of inoculation, is a hypopigmented patch or plaque on the arm, leg, or torso. Secondary pinta lesions (pintides) are at first erythematous then become hyper- and hypopigmented. Later in the disease, pinta lesions become more uniformly hypopigmented.
- **Yaws:** Yaws is a nonvenereal disease caused by *T. pallidum* subspecies *pertenue* that is common in children in impoverished, very warm, tropical areas of Africa. It may also be seen in Southeast Asia, the Pacific Islands, and tropical America. The primary lesion heals as an atrophic hypopigmented scar. Secondary yaws often heals without dyspigmentation, but the gummatous tertiary yaws lesions localized to the lower extremities, volar wrists, and dorsal hands are depigmented.

23. What cutaneous lesions are seen with Hansen's disease?

Hansen's disease, or leprosy, is a chronic infectious disease caused by *Mycobacterium leprae*, which infects the skin and peripheral nerves and in some patients may produce anesthetic, hypopigmented patches, plaques, or nodules. Patients with indeterminate and tuberculoid leprosy have one or few lesions, whereas patients with lepromatous leprosy have many lesions. Lesions may repigment following antibiotic cure. The reason for hypopigmentation is unknown.

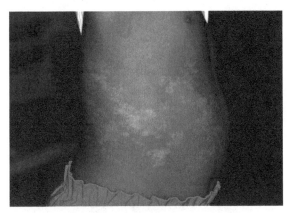

Fig. 18.3 Blaschkoid hypomelanosis. (Courtesy William L. Weston, MD collection.)

24. Why is lesional skin of tinea versicolor frequently hypopigmented?

Tinea (pityriasis) versicolor is caused by overgrowth of the normal skin flora of several species of yeast in the genus *Malassezia (Pityrosporum)*, including *M. globosa, M. sympodialis, M. furfur, M. obtusa,* and *M. slooffiae.* In its pathogenic hyphal form, *Malassezia* secretes an enzyme that breaks down epidermal unsaturated fatty acids to azelaic acid, which inhibits melanocyte tyrosinase, leading to hypopigmentation. Tinea versicolor is most common in tropical climates but may be found worldwide in all races and age groups. The typical lesion is a slightly scaly macule or patch located on the proximal anterior and posterior torso (Fig. 18.4), which may be hypopigmented, hyperpigmented, or slightly erythematous.

Prohic A, Ozegovic L. *Malassezia* species isolated from lesional and non-lesional skin in patients with pityriasis versicolor. *Mycoses.* 2007; 50:58–63.

MELANODERMA: ABNORMAL DARKENING OF THE SKIN

25. What are lentigines? What heritable disorders manifest these?

Lentigines are homogenous, brown to dark brown, 1- to 5-mm macules that may occur on any cutaneous surface, including non–sun-exposed areas. They resemble freckles, but on biopsy, these lesions have increased numbers of melanocytes and increased melanocyte and basal keratinocyte pigmentation.

A benign condition characterized by the rapid development of hundreds of lentigines widespread over the skin surface in adolescents or young adults has been described. However, the presence of multiple lentigines at a young age is suggestive of autosomal dominant disorders, especially LEOPARD syndrome or Peutz-Jeghers syndrome (Fig. 18.5).

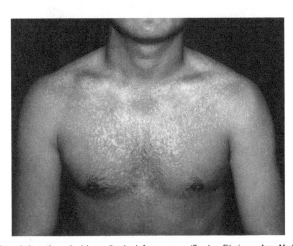

Fig. 18.4 Multiple hypopigmented macules and patches on the chest of a young man. (Courtesy Fitzsimons Army Medical Center teaching files.)

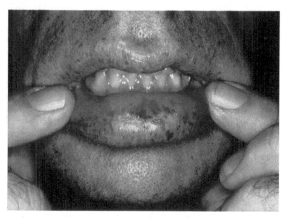

Fig. 18.5 A 45-year-old man with numerous hyperpigmented macules of Peutz-Jeghers syndrome.

26. Why is it important to identify patients with Peutz-Jeghers syndrome?

Patients with Peutz-Jeghers syndrome have widespread mucocutaneous lentigines that involve, most commonly, the lips and perioral region, buccal mucosa, palms, and soles. In addition, they suffer from gastrointestinal (GI) polyps, usually in the small bowel, which, by the second decade of life, can become symptomatic with diarrhea, hemorrhage, obstruction, or intussusception. Malignant degeneration of GI polyps has been reported, and these patients are at a significantly increase risk of developing GI cancers, most commonly in the large intestine, but also in the small intestine and stomach.

27. Describe the clinical manifestations of LEOPARD syndrome

Patients with LEOPARD syndrome (Noonan syndrome with multiple lentigines) have hundreds of lentigines on the face, trunk, and extremities. Half of these patients may also demonstrate café-au-lait macules (CALMs) (Fig. 18.6). The mnemonic **LEOPARD** has been applied to the clinical symptoms associated with this syndrome:

- **L**entigines
- **E**lectrocardiographic conduction defects
- **O**cular hypertelorism
- **P**ulmonic stenosis

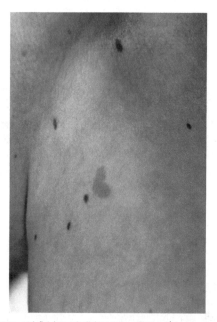

Fig. 18.6 LEOPARD syndrome. Numerous oval, flat, brown lentigines and a solitary café-au-lait macule. (Courtesy William L. Weston, MD collection.)

- **A**bnormal genitalia
- Growth **R**etardation
- Sensorineural **D**eafness

28. Are there pigmentation disorders associated with neurofibromatosis?

Yes. Common pigmented lesions of neurofibromatosis 1 (NF1, von Recklinghausen's disease) are CALMs and freckling. CALMs are, as the name would imply, flat, tan to light brown lesions resembling the color of "coffee with milk." They can be located anywhere on the body and range from a few millimeters to several centimeters in diameter. Greater than 90% of CALMs in NF1 are present at birth or appear within the first year of life. CALMs are relatively common, and a patient must have six or more for the diagnosis of NF1 to be considered. The freckling is not present at birth but appears by age 3 to 5 years. It has a predilection for the intertriginous areas, specifically the inguinal and axillary areas. NF1 is a relatively common autosomal dominant disorder that occurs in 1:3000 live births.

29. Do any other disorders manifest with CALMs?

Yes. McCune-Albright syndrome is associated with polyostotic fibrous dysplasia, endocrine dysfunction with precocious puberty in females, and CALMs. The CALMs of McCune-Albright syndrome differ from those of NF1 by being larger and occurring predominantly on the forehead, posterior neck, sacrum, and buttocks. The CALMs of McCune-Albright syndrome tend to be unilateral, do not cross the midline, and have an irregular, jagged border (so-called "coast of Maine"), whereas the CALMs of NF1 exist in a random, generalized pattern and have a smooth border. The CALMs of McCune-Albright syndrome appear at or soon after birth.

30. What is Becker's melanosis?

Becker's melanosis (also known as Becker's pigmentary hamartoma or Becker's nevus) is a benign pigmented lesion that can be present at birth but often develops around puberty with a historical male:female ratio of 5:1. There is no predominance of race, and one large study reported a prevalence of 0.52% in males between ages 17 and 26 years. Greater than 80% of lesions occur on the trunk, specifically on the scapula or chest, appearing as a tan to dark brown patch or thin plaque with an irregular border, often larger than 10 cm in diameter. There may be an underlying smooth muscle hamartoma, and excess hair growth has been reported in 56% of cases. When onset is around puberty, Becker's melanosis can be easily differentiated from a congenital nevus or CALM, which are present at or soon after birth. Once fully developed, Becker's melanosis remains stable for the life of the patient.

Tymen R, Forestier JF, Boutet B, Colomb D. Late Becker's nevus. One hundred cases. *Ann Dermatol Venereol.* 1981;108:41.

31. What is a nevus spilus?

Nevus spilus (also known as a speckled lentiginous nevus) is a CALM that contains darkly pigmented, 1- to 3-mm–diameter macules or papules. The background CALM is present at birth, and the darkly pigmented lesions, which are junctional or compound nevi, appear over time. Any cutaneous surface can be involved and there is a small increased risk of developing melanoma.

32. Do any natural factors stimulate human epidermal pigmentation?

Yes. The following factors have been reported to enhance melanocyte growth and pigmentation:

- Adrenocorticotropic hormone (ACTH)
- Basic fibroblast growth factor
- Endothelin-1
- Granulocyte-macrophage colony–stimulating factor
- KIT ligand (formerly steel factor)
- Leukotriene C4 and B4
- Melanocyte-stimulating hormone (MSH)
- Nerve growth factor
- Prostaglandin E2 and F2 α
- Stem cell factor

Videira IF, Moura DF, Magina S. Mechanisms regulating melanogenesis. *An Bras Dermatol.* 2013; 88(1):76–83.

33. What drugs are used to stimulate skin pigmentation? How do they work?

Psoralens (of the furocoumarin family) are potent, plant-derived, photosensitizing compounds, which have been used for thousands of years to stimulate skin pigmentation. The most commonly used agent in dermatology for skin photosensitization is 8-methoxypsoralen (8-MOP). The exact mechanism of skin photosensitization is not known, but 8-MOP is preferentially taken up by epidermal cells, where it intercalates between cellular DNA in the nucleus. Upon photoactivation, 8-MOP causes alterations in cell membrane signaling and forms covalent bonds with DNA that lead to the formation of psoralen-DNA adducts. Together, the altered cell membrane signaling and psoralen-DNA adducts incite a cascade of events that stimulate melanin synthesis and transfer to keratinocytes, resulting in increased skin pigmentation.

34. Can other drugs cause increased skin pigmentation?

    Yes. Many drugs can cause increased skin pigmentation, including most commonly arsenicals, busulfan, 5-fluorouracil, cyclophosphamide, topical nitrogen mustard (mechlorethamine), and bleomycin. The mechanisms by which these drugs cause hyperpigmentation are largely unknown, but it is possible that the drug or a metabolite either directly stimulates epidermal melanocytes to increase melanin synthesis or indirectly stimulates metabolic pathways that cause increased epidermal melanization.

    _____

    Litt J, ed. *Litt's drug eruption and reaction manual*. 25th ed. New York: CRC Press; 2019.

35. Can endocrine and metabolic disorders cause altered skin pigmentation?

    Yes, there are many disorders that can influence skin pigmentation. Addison's disease is the prototypical disorder presenting with diffuse hypermelanosis and associated pigment accentuation in mucous membranes, skin folds, palmar creases, and pressure points (elbows, knees, knuckles, and coccyx) in response to elevated ACTH and MSH, which stimulate melanogenesis. Similarly, ACTH- and MSH-producing tumors or systemic administration of ACTH and MSH may cause skin hyperpigmentation. Additionally, hyperthyroidism and hereditary hemochromatosis can lead to generalized hyperpigmentation.

    Pregnancy and estrogen therapy can cause hyperpigmentation, usually of the nipples and anogenital skin. Moreover, a mask-like hyperpigmentation, called melasma, can develop on the forehead, temples, cheeks, nose, and upper lip in women who are pregnant or receiving estrogen therapy.

    Patients with porphyria cutanea tarda can have profound hyperpigmentation of sun-exposed skin associated with facial hirsutism. Nutritional disorders, such as kwashiorkor, pellagra, and intestinal malabsorption, can cause skin hyperpigmentation along with areas of hypopigmentation.

36. Can forms of radiation other than ultraviolet radiation cause increased skin pigmentation?

    Yes. Thermal (infrared) and ionizing radiation skin injury can result in hyperpigmentation, probably due to melanocyte-stimulating inflammatory mediators and immune cytokines released in response to injury from these different forms of radiation.

BLUE-GRAY DYSPIGMENTATION

37. Are there other types of dyspigmentation besides leukoderma and melanoderma?

    Yes. Blue-gray skin discoloration can develop from melanin in dermal melanocytes, dermal melanin deposition, or nonmelanin dermal dyspigmentation (Table 18.2).

38. Name the different types of hyperpigmentation due to excess numbers of dermal melanocytes

    Mongolian spot, nevus of Ota, and nevus of Ito. Some providers prefer the descriptive term "dermal melanocytosis," as these are all characterized by sparse, dendritic melanocytes scattered among collage bundles in the dermis but differing in their anatomical location.

39. Differentiate a nevus of Ota from a nevus of Ito.

    Nevus of Ota (oculodermal melanocytosis) is an acquired disorder of dermal melanocytosis with an age of onset in early childhood or young adulthood. Less than 1% of Asiatic individuals are affected, and non-Asiatic races are affected even less frequently. Females are affected five times more frequently than males, with color hues ranging from dark brown, to purplish-brown, to blue-black. In its most common form, it involves the periorbital skin of one eye, although bilateral forms can occur, and pigmentation can extend to involve the temple, forehead, periorbital cheek, nose, and ocular structures (Fig. 18.7).

    A variant of nevus of Ota, called nevus of Ito, can occur over the shoulder and neck region and has the same natural history as nevus of Ota.

40. What types of hyperpigmentation are due to dermal melanin deposition?

    - **Macular amyloidosis:** Rippled, brownish-gray, thin papules and plaques on the torso or extremities.
    - **Fixed drug eruption:** Reddish-brown to blue-gray macule or patch, with erythema (see Chapter 16), edema, scale, and sometimes blisters (see Chapter 14).
    - **Erythema ab igne:** Reticulated blue-gray patches, sometimes with erythema and scale.
    - **Erythema dyschromicum perstans:** Erythematous, ash-gray macules and patches on the trunk.
    - **Postinflammatory hyperpigmentation:** Brown to gray macules and patches in areas of prior inflammation (Fig. 18.8).

41. How does erythema ab igne occur?

    Erythema ab igne is a skin reaction to thermal injury. Chronic heating pad use is a common cause of this disorder. Usually, the affected area has a netlike pattern of blue-gray discoloration, sometimes with associated erythema and scale. Patients often complain that the affected area burns, stings, or itches. Treatment requires discontinuing heating pad use (or other cause of thermal injury), which allows the skin dyspigmentation to slowly resolve over several months to a year, although permanent dermal scarring and hyperpigmentation can result.

Table 18.2 Classification of dermal hyperpigmentation

INCREASED MELANOCYTE NUMBER	INCREASED MELANIN	NONMELANIN PIGMENTS
Genetic		
Mongolian spot	—	—
Nevus of Ota	—	—
Nevus of Ito	—	—
Chemical or Drug		
—	Fixed drug eruption	Silver
—	—	Mercury
—	—	Bismuth
—	—	Gold
—	—	Antimalarials
—	—	Phenothiazines
—	—	Minocycline
—	—	Amiodarone
Endocrine or Metabolic		
—	Chronic nutritional deficiency	Ochronosis
—	Melasma	—
Physical		
—	Erythema ab igne	—
Inflammation and Infection		
—	Macular amyloidosis	—
—	Erythema dyschromicum perstans	—
—	Postinflammatory hyperpigmentation	—

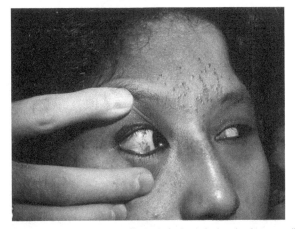

Fig. 18.7 Nevus of Ota. Unilateral macular blue-black pigment affecting the forehead, cheek, and ocular mucosa. (Courtesy Fitzsimons Army Medical Center teaching files.)

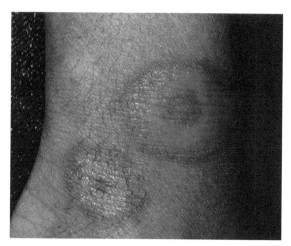

Fig. 18.8 Two target-shaped patches of postinflammatory hyperpigmentation on the dorsal wrist of a woman following resolution of erythema multiforme.

42. **Are there any metabolic disorders associated with nonmelanin skin dyspigmentation?**

   Yes. Ochronosis (alkaptonuria) is a rare autosomal recessive inherited deficiency of homogentisic acid oxidase that results in the accumulation of homogentisic acid in connective tissue, where it causes a dark brown to bluish-gray dyspigmentation. Commonly affected skin areas include the pinna, nasal tip, sclera, extensor tendons of the hands, fingernails, and tympanic membranes. Less commonly, blue macules develop on the central face, axillae, and genitalia.

   Homogentisic acid is also deposited in the bones and articular cartilage, causing ochronotic arthropathy that results in premature degenerative arthritis. Overall, the course of ochronosis is progressive dyspigmentation and articular degeneration with no successful treatment available.

43. **What pigmentation disorders are associated with heavy-metal deposition in the dermis?**

   Silver, mercury, bismuth, arsenic, and gold can all cause brown to blue-gray discoloration due to metal deposition in the dermis. Silver, mercury, and bismuth toxicity result in blue-gray discoloration of the skin, nails, and mucosa. Silver toxicity (argyria) is most prominent in sun-exposed areas. Chrysoderma is an uncommon brown skin pigmentation that develops following parenteral gold administration and is most prominent in sun-exposed areas.

44. **What drugs can deposit in the dermis and cause pigmentary changes?**

   Amiodarone (Fig. 18.9), bleomycin, busulfan, chloroquine, chlorpromazine, clofazimine, minocycline, ifluoperazine, thioridazine, and zidovudine cause blue-gray pigmentation of the skin and mucosa.

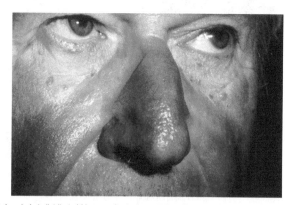

Fig. 18.9 Amiodarone-induced photodistributed blue-gray hyperpigmentation. (Courtesy Fitzsimons Army Medical Center teaching files.)

CHAPTER 19

PANNICULITIS

Lori D. Prok

KEY POINTS: PANNICULITIS

1. Given the similar clinical appearance among panniculitides, histopathologic characterization is often critical for a correct diagnosis.
2. An incisional biopsy with a wide base in the fat is far more likely to be diagnostic than a deep shave or punch biopsy.
3. The biopsy should be taken from the most indurated lesion; if that lesion has an ulcer, the biopsy should avoid the ulcer base.
4. If the lesions are ulcerated or suppurated, consider tissue culture at the time of the biopsy.

KEY POINTS: ERYTHEMA NODOSUM

1. Erythema nodosum is the most common cause of panniculitis.
2. Erythema nodosum lesions typically last 3 to 6 weeks but frequently recur.
3. Erythema nodosum can occur at any age and can be located at any site on the body; classically, however, it is a disease most frequently found in women in their 20s to 40s and is mainly located on the anterior shins.
4. Spontaneous ulceration does not occur in erythema nodosum; if present, suspect another diagnosis such as erythema induratum, thrombophlebitis, polyarteritis nodosa, alpha-1 antitrypsin deficiency, necrobiosis lipoidica, pancreatic panniculitis, ulcerative sarcoidosis, or infection.
5. One should always consider the possibility that the presence of erythema nodosum reflects a reaction to a drug, a remote focus of infection, pregnancy, inflammatory bowel disease, malignancy, or sarcoidosis.

KEY POINTS: LUPUS PANNICULITIS

1. Lupus panniculitis can be associated with systemic lupus erythematosus (SLE) in about 10% of cases and can occur before other systemic manifestations of SLE are clinically apparent. It is more commonly associated with discoid lupus erythematosus (30% to 33% of cases).
2. Lupus panniculitis often occurs in places where other forms of panniculitis would be very unusual: the head, neck, upper trunk, and upper proximal extremities.
3. There can be considerable overlap in histology between lupus panniculitis and subcutaneous panniculitis–like T-cell lymphoma; consider rebiopsy if cases diagnosed as lupus panniculitis fail to respond to traditional treatment or if there is rapid progression of lesions.

1. **What is panniculitis?**
   Panniculitis represents infiltration of subcutaneous tissue by inflammatory cells, neoplastic cells, or both. This condition presents clinically as a deep induration or swelling of the skin. Associated signs and symptoms may include erythema, ulceration, drainage, warmth, and pain. Under certain circumstances, induration or nodularity may be present without significant inflammation or may persist after the inflammation has largely subsided.

2. **Name the various types of panniculitis. How are they classified?**
   Although no single classification seems to be totally satisfactory, disorders tend to be grouped by a combination of histopathologic features and etiologies (Table 19.1). **Septal panniculitis** refers to a predominance of inflammation involving the connective tissue septa between fat lobules, whereas **lobular panniculitis** indicates predominant involvement of the fat lobules themselves. **Lipodystrophy** and **lipoatrophy** may be end-stage changes of the fat brought about by several different etiologies, including inflammation, trauma, metabolic, or hormonal alterations.

3. **What is erythema nodosum?**
   Erythema nodosum (Fig. 19.1) consists of an eruption of erythematous, tender nodules—typically over the pretibial areas but occasionally elsewhere—that are regarded as a hypersensitivity response to some antigenic challenge. It is typically an acute process lasting 3 to 6 weeks, but a more chronic form can occur. Some experts consider the

Table 19.1 Major forms of panniculitis

Septal Panniculitis	**Traumatic Panniculitis**
Erythema nodosum	**Infectious Panniculitis**
Subacute nodular migratory panniculitis	**Malignancy**
Scleroderma panniculitis	**Other Changes of the Fat**
Lobular and Mixed Panniculitis	**Lipodystrophy**
Nodular vasculitis (erythema induratum)	**Lipoatrophy**
Lupus panniculitis	**Lipohypertrophy**
Other types of connective tissue panniculitis	
Metabolic Derangements	
Altered melting/solidification points of fat	
Sclerema neonatorum	
Subcutaneous fat necrosis of the newborn	
Pancreatic (enzymatic) fat necrosis	
Alpha-1 antitrypsin deficiency panniculitis	

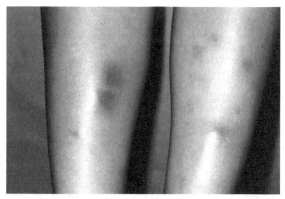

Fig. 19.1 Typical lesions of erythema nodosum on the legs. Erythema nodosum heals without scarring.

condition termed **subacute nodular migratory panniculitis** (Vilanova's disease or erythema nodosum migrans) to be a chronic variant of erythema nodosum.

Requena L, Yus ES. Panniculitis. Part I. Mostly septal panniculitis. *J Am Acad Dermatol.* 2001;45:163–183.

4. What is the pathogenesis of erythema nodosum?
Erythema nodosum is usually considered to represent a delayed hypersensitivity response that reflects a common reaction pattern to a wide variety of eliciting factors. The subcutaneous septa in well-developed lesions often contain granulomas, and research has shown a strong correlation between genetic polymorphisms of tumor necrosis factor-α (TNF-α) and erythema nodosum (TNF-α promotes granuloma formation). Reactive oxygen intermediates may be involved in the tissue damage and inflammation that accompany erythema nodosum.

McDougal KE, Fallin MD, Moller DR, et al. Variation in the lymphotoxin-alpha/tumor necrosis factor locus modified risk of erythema nodosum in sarcoidosis. *J Invest Dermatol.* 2009;129:1921–1926.

5. List some of the common underlying conditions associated with erythema nodosum.
Streptococcal infection of the upper respiratory tract and medications (especially oral contraceptives, sulfonamides, penicillins, bromides, and iodides) are among the most common known causes. Other triggers include deep fungal infections (such as coccidioidomycosis), *Yersinia* infection, pregnancy, sarcoidosis, inflammatory bowel disease, and leukemia. Many episodes are idiopathic: A cause is not identified in one-third to one-half of cases.

6. How should a biopsy of erythema nodosum be obtained?
The specimen should be obtained from the most fully developed (central) portion of the lesion (Fig. 19.2). It is absolutely critical that the biopsy be deep enough to incorporate subcutaneous fat. Incisional biopsies that include a generous horizontal expanse of subcutis are preferred to small punch biopsies.

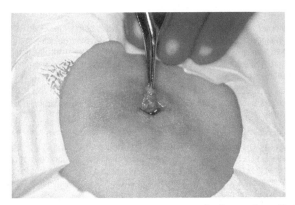

Fig. 19.2 Appropriate wedge biopsy technique for panniculitis as shown in a case of erythema nodosum. The biopsy extends from the epidermis to a wide base in the subcutaneous fat. (Courtesy Kenneth E. Greer, MD.)

7. What are the characteristic microscopic features of erythema nodosum?

    The typical histologic features include a predominantly septal panniculitis with a slight spillover of inflammatory cells into the fat lobules. Cell types may include lymphocytes, neutrophils, and eosinophils, especially in acute disease. In older lesions, small granulomas (Miescher's granulomas) are sometimes observed within connective tissue septa. Perivascular infiltrates are common, but true vasculitis with destruction of vessel walls is not observed.

8. How is erythema nodosum treated?

    Treatment of the underlying disorder, if known, is of primary importance. Salicylates or nonsteroidal antiinflammatory drugs, bed rest, and potassium iodide (particularly in chronic forms of the disease) are usually considered to be first-line therapies while colchicine, dapsone, hydroxychloroquine, and prednisone are second-line therapies used in recalcitrant cases.

9. What is nodular vasculitis?

    This form of panniculitis most commonly occurs on the posterior lower legs (Fig. 19.3), as opposed to the classically anterior location of erythema nodosum. Ulceration and drainage sometimes occur.

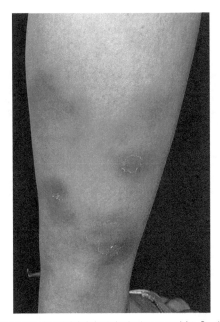

Fig. 19.3 Erythema induratum demonstrating characteristic indurated subcutaneous nodules. Spontaneous ulceration is common. (Courtesy James E. Fitzpatrick, MD.)

10. **What causes nodular vasculitis?**

    It was originally considered a hypersensitivity reaction to tuberculosis and termed **erythema induratum of Bazin.** Studies confirm that in many cases, *Mycobacterium tuberculosis* DNA can be detected in the lesions by polymerase chain reaction; however, nodular vasculitis can also be idiopathic or associated with other infectious agents (*Nocardia*, hepatitis C) or drugs (propylthiouracil). These cases with nontuberculous etiologies are sometimes termed **erythema induratum of Whitfield.**

    Chen S, Chen J, Chen L, Zhang Q, Luo X, Zhang. *Mycobacterium tuberculosis* infection is associated with the development of erythema nodosum and nodular vasculitis. *PLoS One.* 2013;8:e62653.

11. **Describe the microscopic features of nodular vasculitis.**

    Nodular vasculitis presents as a lobular panniculitis with a mixed infiltrate that may be granulomatous. Vasculitis of a medium-sized artery or vein is present deep in the fat. Caseous necrosis is present in up to 50% of cases. Although necrosis can occur in cases not associated with tuberculosis, it may be more common in lesions that are positive for *Mycobacterium tuberculosis*–complex DNA.

    Magalhães TS, Dammert VG, Samorano LP, Litvoc MN, Nico MM. Erythema induratum of Bazin: epidemiological, clinical and laboratorial profile of 54 patients. *J Dermatol.* 2018;45(5):628–629.

12. **What is the differential diagnosis of nodular vasculitis?**

    Clinical clues to an association with tuberculosis include constitutional symptoms, elevated erythrocyte sedimentation rate, an abnormal chest radiograph, or a positive tuberculin skin test. Both polyarteritis nodosa and superficial thrombophlebitis also show vasculitis involving medium-sized vessels in the subcutis. In both conditions, the inflammation is more specifically directed toward the vessel, and extensive lobular inflammation obscuring the vessel changes is uncommon. The clinical findings are also quite different in these two disorders (e.g., hypertension, renal, and central nervous system disease in systemic polyarteritis; association with internal malignancy in superficial migratory thrombophlebitis). In one author's experience (JWP), true examples of nodular vasculitis are seldom seen, but this might change with the recent rise in number of cases of tuberculosis associated with human immunodeficiency virus.

13. **How should nodular vasculitis be treated?**

    Treatment should be directed toward any underlying infection, especially tuberculosis. Studies have demonstrated the responsiveness of mycobacteria-associated lesions to multidrug antituberculous therapy. Symptomatic care includes bed rest, bandages, antiinflammatory agents, and avoidance of potential aggravating factors such as smoking. In more severe nontuberculous cases, potassium iodide, dapsone, colchicine, antimalarials, tetracyclines, and prednisone can be used.

    Mascaró Jr JM, Baselga E. Erythema induratum of Bazin. *Dermatol Clin.* 2008;26:439–445.

14. **What are the clinical features of lupus panniculitis?**

    Lupus panniculitis, also termed **lupus profundus**, consists of erythematous or flesh-colored subcutaneous nodules. The lesions occur on the face, upper outer arms, shoulders, and trunk, including the breasts. They sometimes show overlying follicular plugging, epidermal atrophy, and hyperpigmentation—changes associated with cutaneous (discoid) lupus erythematosus. The overlying skin can be "bound down" to the subcutaneous nodule or plaque, resulting in an obvious depression in the skin surface (Fig. 19.4).

15. **Describe the microscopic features of lupus panniculitis.**

    There is typically a mixed septal and lobular panniculitis with a predominance of lymphocytes in a patchy or diffuse and/or perivascular distribution. Nodular aggregates of lymphocytes surrounded by plasma cells may be present; there may even be formation of lymphoid follicles with germinal centers. Interstitial mucin deposition and hyalinization of the fat also occur. Overlying epidermal changes associated with cutaneous lupus erythematosus may be seen in close to one half of cases.

    Ng PP, Tan SH, Tan T. Lupus erythematosus panniculitis: a clinicopathologic study. *Int J Dermatol.* 2002;41:488–490.

16. **What is the significance of diagnosing lupus panniculitis?**

    Panniculitis may be a presenting finding of either cutaneous or systemic lupus erythematosus, or rarely of dermatomyositis or other autoimmune diseases. A small percentage of patients presenting with lupus panniculitis fulfill criteria for systemic lupus erythematosus, and other complications have been reported, such as the development of antiphospholipid antibody syndrome. Antinuclear antibodies are common, and occasionally other circulating

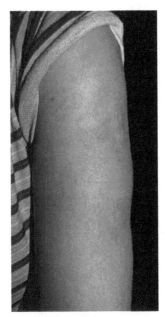

Fig. 19.4 Lupus panniculitis on the upper arm demonstrating focal erythema, focal hypopigmentation, and depression of the skin surface. (Courtesy Fitzsimons Army Medical Center teaching files.)

antibodies are detected, such as antineutrophil cytoplasmic antibodies. Because of the unusual clinical locations of lupus panniculitis, the true diagnosis may not be suspected for months or years. Early biopsy and direct immunofluorescence study of these lesions may provide the first clues to the diagnosis of lupus erythematosus and allow for early institution of appropriate therapy. Treatments for the panniculitis include intralesional corticosteroids, systemic antimalarials, and dapsone.

17. Are sclerema neonatorum and subcutaneous fat necrosis of the newborn the same thing?
   No, but in both conditions, there are varying degrees of sclerosis of the subcutaneous fat of newborns. **Sclerema neonatorum** is very rare and occurs in premature, hypothermic infants with underlying medical problems. It is characterized by diffusely cold, rigid, boardlike skin; neonatal death is common. In **subcutaneous fat necrosis of the newborn** (Fig. 19.5A), relatively discrete, firm subcutaneous nodules develop several weeks after birth in an otherwise healthy baby. Hypercalcemia may very rarely be present, causing seizures and nephrocalcinosis, but the overall prognosis for survival and resolution of the lesions is excellent.

Ladoyanni E, Moss C, Brown RM, Ogboli M. Subcutaneous fat necrosis in a newborn associated with asymptomatic and uncomplicated hypercalcemia. *Pediatr Dermatol.* 2009;26:217–219.

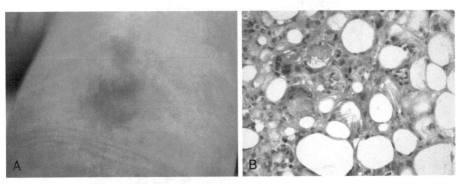

Fig. 19.5 A, Subcutaneous fat necrosis of the thigh of an otherwise healthy infant. **B,** Biopsy of subcutaneous fat necrosis demonstrating characteristic lobular panniculitis with needle-shaped clefts that induce a foreign body reaction consisting of macrophages and multinucleated giant cells.

18. **How similar are the microscopic features of sclerema neonatorum and subcutaneous fat necrosis of the newborn?**

Both conditions show needle-shaped clefts within lipocytes, presumably representing triglyceride crystals that have been dissolved during tissue processing. Sclerema neonatorum tends to show thickened fibrous septa and little inflammation, while subcutaneous fat necrosis shows a substantial lobular panniculitis with a foreign body reaction to the needle-shaped clefts (Fig. 19.5B).

19. **Why do these disorders occur in neonates and infants?**

Neonatal fat has an increased ratio of saturated to unsaturated fatty acids, which results in higher melting and solidification points for stored fat. This, plus other possible metabolic defects, leads to crystal formation, fat necrosis, and inflammation when the fat is subjected to stresses such as ischemia or trauma.

20. **What is pancreatic fat necrosis?**

Subcutaneous nodules occur on the legs (Fig. 19.6) or elsewhere associated with acute or chronic pancreatitis or pancreatic carcinoma. Visceral fat may also be involved. Although immune mechanisms may play a role in producing this form of fat necrosis, the weight of evidence favors the effects of circulating pancreatic lipase, amylase, and trypsin on subcutaneous fat. The frequent co-occurrence of arthritis with joint fluid analysis revealing free fatty acids is a clinical reminder of the systemic effects of these pancreatic enzymes. Treatment is directed toward the underlying pancreatic disease.

Preiss JC, Faiss S, Loddenkemper C, Zeitz M, Duchmann R. Pancreatic panniculitis in an 88-year-old man with neuroendocrine carcinoma. *Digestion.* 2002;66:193–196.

21. **Are there any characteristic histopathologic features of pancreatic fat necrosis?**

The changes are rather unique and include necrosis of the fat with formation of lipocyte remnants with thick, shadowy walls ("ghost cells") and pools of basophilic material that represent saponification of fat by calcium salts.

22. **What is the role of alpha-1 antitrypsin deficiency in the development of panniculitis?**

Since the mid-1970s, it has become apparent that patients with this inherited proteinase inhibitor deficiency, especially those most severely affected and having the homozygous PiZZ phenotype, are prone to develop painful hemorrhagic subcutaneous nodules (Fig. 19.7) that ulcerate and drain. Without alpha-1 antitrypsin, the activity of neutrophil elastase is unchecked. It is believed that in such individuals, a variety of triggering factors, such as trauma, may initiate a sequence of events that includes unchecked complement activation, inflammation, endothelial cell damage, and tissue injury. Microscopic clues to the diagnosis include diffuse neutrophilic infiltration of the reticular dermis and liquefactive necrosis of the dermis and the subcutaneous septa, with resultant separation of fat lobules. Treatment options include dapsone, systemic corticosteroids, plasma exchange therapy, and, more recently, parenteral administration of a proteinase inhibitor.

Chowdhury MM, Williams EJ, Morris JS, et al. Severe panniculitis caused by homozygous ZZ alpha-1-antitrypsin deficiency treated successfully with human purified enzyme (Prolastin). *Br J Dermatol.* 2004;147:1258–1261.

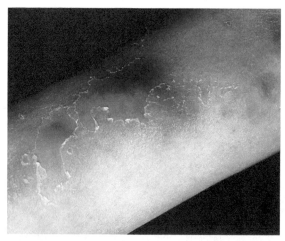

Fig. 19.6 Pancreatic fat necrosis, showing involvement of an arm. Note the desquamation of the lesions, suggesting that spontaneous discharge may occur.

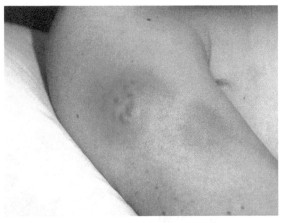

Fig. 19.7 Alpha-1 antitrypsin deficiency panniculitis showing foci of hemorrhage in the center of the lesion. (Courtesy Kenneth E. Greer, MD.)

23. Name some types of trauma that can produce panniculitis.

Numerous forms of trauma, either accidental or purposeful, can produce painful subcutaneous nodules or plaques. These include cold injury ("popsicle panniculitis" on the cheeks of children), injection of foreign substances such as oils or medications (Fig. 19.8), or blunt force trauma. There are some unique microscopic clues for each of these types of injury, so biopsy is particularly helpful when traumatic panniculitis is suspected. Polarization microscopy is one simple test for detecting the presence of refractile foreign material in tissue sections. The therapeutic challenge lies in finding and removing the source of the injury that has produced the panniculitis.

24. Which infectious organisms can produce panniculitis?

Panniculitis can result from localized or generalized infection caused by gram-positive and gram-negative bacteria, mycobacteria (Fig. 19.9A), *Nocardia*, *Cryptococcus* (Fig. 19.9B), *Candida,* and *Fusarium* species. Other organisms that have been associated with panniculitis include streptococci, *Toxocara, Trypanosoma*, and *Borrelia burgdorferi* (as a manifestation of Lyme disease). Immunosuppressed patients appear to be particularly at risk for infection-induced panniculitis. Microscopic features vary and can occasionally mimic other forms of panniculitis. However, findings that should suggest the possibility of infection include mixed septal-lobular involvement, neutrophilic infiltration, vascular proliferation, hemorrhage, and sweat gland necrosis. Special stains and cultures are crucial to making the correct diagnosis and instituting appropriate antimicrobial therapy.

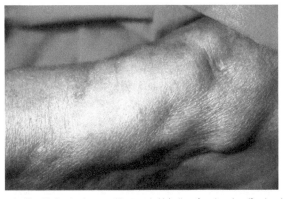

Fig. 19.8 Sclerosing panniculitis with lipoatrophy caused by repeated injection of pentazocine. (Courtesy Kenneth E. Greer, MD.)

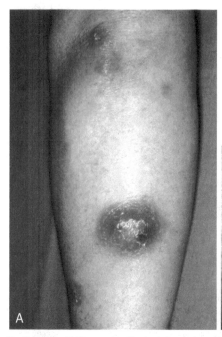
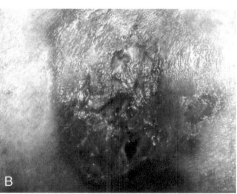

A

B

Fig. 19.9 A, Panniculitis caused by *Mycobacterium marinum*. The classic linear appearance of the lesions denotes local lymphangitic spread, common in cutaneous infections with this organism. **B,** Ulceronecrotic panniculitis secondary to *Cryptococcus neoformans*. Skin disease is most often due to hematogenous spread of primary pulmonary infection. (Courtesy Kenneth E. Greer, MD.)

25. Describe the role of malignancy in producing panniculitis.

   Malignant infiltrates can sometimes produce subcutaneous nodules that mimic other forms of panniculitis. Malignancies that are capable of producing panniculitis-like lesions include poorly differentiated carcinomas, lymphomas (Fig. 19.10), multiple myeloma, and leukemias. Microscopic clues to the recognition of malignant infiltrates include a monotonous cell population and/or cytologic atypia, "lining up" of atypical cells between collagen bundles, and minimal alteration of connective tissue in the presence of dense cellular infiltration. Also, forms of more traditional inflammatory panniculitis can accompany malignancy, including erythema nodosum, migratory thrombophlebitis, and pancreatic fat necrosis. Therefore, diagnosis again is heavily dependent on biopsy.

Cassis TB, Fearneyhough PK, Callen JP. Subcutaneous panniculitis-like T-cell lymphoma with vacuolar interface dermatitis resembling lupus erythematosus panniculitis. *J Am Acad Dermatol*. 2004;50:465–469.

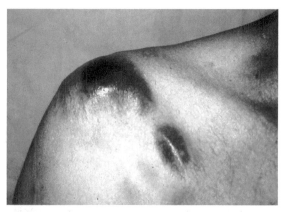

Fig. 19.10 B-cell lymphoma mimicking panniculitis. (Courtesy Kenneth E. Greer, MD.)

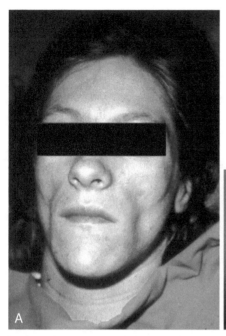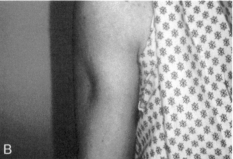

Fig. 19.11 **A,** Acquired partial lipodystrophy with associated C3 nephritic factor. Note the prominent wasting of the facial fat in this patient. **B,** Localized lipoatrophy associated with injection of medication. (Courtesy Kenneth E. Greer, MD.)

26. What is lipodystrophy?

Lipodystrophy generally refers to a paucity or complete absence of subcutaneous fat, sometimes due to redistribution. It can be generalized or localized, inherited or acquired. Lipodystrophy can be idiopathic, but is often associated with inherited syndromes, endocrine abnormalities such as insulin-resistant diabetes mellitus, complement abnormalities (Fig. 19.11A), or autoimmune disease. It is well recognized that antiretroviral therapy, particularly protease inhibitors, causes a distinctive redistribution of subcutaneous fat with accumulation of fat in abdominal and cervical areas and apparent wasting of the face and extremities.

Koutkia P, Grinspoon S. HIV-associated lipodystrophy: pathogenesis, prognosis, treatment, and controversies. *Annu Rev Med.* 2004;55:303–317.

27. What is lipoatrophy?

This term is sometimes used interchangeably with lipodystrophy, but it is more commonly used to describe a focal loss of subcutaneous fat. Probably the most common form of lipoatrophy is postinflammatory in nature and can occur following several types of panniculitis. Microscopically, lipoatrophy features "collapse" of fat lobules, with a reduced number of variably sized lipocytes and development of numerous capillaries in a mucinous background stroma. Localized lipoatrophy also occurs following injection of medications, especially corticosteroids (Fig. 19.11B). A variety of plastic surgical procedures has been used to improve or correct lipoatrophy.

28. What is lipohypertrophy?

Lipohypertrophy, which manifests as induration of involved skin, occurs in some individuals due to repeated injections of insulin. This effect is apparently independent of the source of insulin and can even occur with human recombinant insulin. Growth hormone injections have also resulted in lipohypertrophy. In lipohypertrophy, lipocytes are enlarged and appear to encroach upon the midportion of the dermis. Rotation of insulin injection sites is a key to management of lipohypertrophy, both to prevent or minimize the hypertrophic changes and to assure adequate insulin absorption.

Chernausek SD, Backeljauw PF, Frane J, et al. Long-term treatment with recombinant insulin-like growth factor (IGF)-I in children with severe IGF-I deficiency due to growth hormone insensitivity. *J Clin Endocrinol Metab.* 2007;92:902–910.

Chowdhury TA, Escudier V. Poor glycemic control caused by insulin-induced lipohypertrophy. *Br Med J.* 2003;327:383–384.

29. Discuss the approach to use when attempting to diagnose an "unknown" case of panniculitis.
    - Careful history and physical examination are of greatest importance, emphasizing the location of the eruption, as well as its timing in relation to any possible drug ingestion, infection, or trauma.
    - Laboratory studies should be guided by the clinical history but might include cultures of distant sites (e.g., for possible streptococcal pharyngitis in erythema nodosum), antinuclear antibody determination (to rule out lupus panniculitis), or measurement of alpha-1 antitrypsin levels (for evaluation of proteinase inhibitor–deficiency panniculitis).
    - Skin biopsy can be of tremendous benefit, and recognition of established microscopic patterns of disease can be complemented by special stains and polarization microscopy.
    - Immunohistochemistry can be useful in selected cases where malignancy is a possibility, and x-ray microanalysis is a specialized test that can be used to determine the identity of foreign material in cases of traumatic panniculitis.

Acknowledgments

The author wishes to acknowledge the contribution of prior authors, Melissa D. Darling, MD, and James W. Patterson, MD

ALOPECIA

Brittney DeClerck

CHAPTER 20

1. How is alopecia classified?

Alopecia (hair loss) can be divided into (1) disorders of the hair shaft and (2) all other forms of hair loss. Abnormalities of the hair shaft can produce alopecia because the shafts are fragile and "break off." The other forms of alopecia can be divided into cicatricial (scarring) and noncicatricial alopecia. In cicatricial alopecia, hair is lost permanently. In noncicatricial alopecia, hair follicles may return to growth either spontaneously or with treatment. Both cicatricial and noncicatricial alopecia can be divided into diffuse and patterned hair loss. In diffuse hair loss, hair thins evenly from all parts of the scalp, and discrete "bald spots" do not occur. In patterned alopecia, certain areas of the scalp are affected more than others.

Eudy G, Solomon AR. The histopathology of noncicatricial alopecia. *Semin Cutan Med Surg.* 2006;25:35–40.
Sperling LC, Cowper SE. The histopathology of primary cicatricial alopecia. *Semin Cutan Med Surg.* 2006;25:41–50.

2. What are some common types of patterned hair loss?

- **Patchy:** Multiple scattered lesions
- **Moth-eaten:** Myriad, diffusely distributed, small lesions
- **Ophiasis:** Hair loss around periphery of the scalp
- **Male pattern alopecia:** Symmetrical, progressive hair loss predominantly affecting the top (vertex) of the scalp possibly leading to complete baldness
- **Female pattern alopecia:** Partial hair loss on the frontal and vertex of the scalp with reduction of hairs, not leading to complete baldness

3. Can cicatricial and noncicatricial alopecia be differentiated clinically?

In the setting of alopecia, cicatricial means that there has been permanent destruction of hair follicles, and they have been replaced by fibrous tissue. Usually, an obvious scar, such as that seen after wounding, is not evident, but there is a loss of follicular openings that gives the scalp a smooth and shiny appearance (Fig. 20.1). The texture of the scalp may remain soft and supple, although sometimes induration or firmness is palpable.

4. What causes common hair loss?

People who become bald or develop thinning hair have hair follicles that are genetically programmed to miniaturize under the influence of postpubertal androgens. Probably, several genes (inherited from both mother and father) influence the severity of balding. Until very late in the balding process, the number of hairs does not decrease, but the hairs become progressively smaller until they are no longer visible to the naked eye. Except in very marked and long-standing balding, very fine, short hairs can be seen exiting from follicular orifices if a magnifying lens is used.

Randall VA. Androgens and hair growth. *Dermatol Ther.* 2008;21(5):314–328.
Yip L, Rufaut N, Sinclair R. Role of genetics and sex steroid hormones in male androgenetic alopecia and female pattern hair loss: an update of what we now know. *Australas J Dermatol.* 2011;52(2):81–88.

5. How effective are medical treatments for common hair loss?

About one-third of balding patients who use topical minoxidil solution experience significant (cosmetically obvious) hair regrowth. Any regrowth that occurs is only maintained while the drug is used. If therapy is stopped, hair density reverts to its pretreatment state. Oral finasteride, a 5α-reductase inhibitor, is somewhat more effective and can be used in combination with topical minoxidil in men and postmenopausal women. Other antiandrogen oral medications can also be used in refractory cases.

Rousso DE, Kim SW. A review of medical and surgical treatment options for androgenetic alopecia. *JAMA Facial Plast Surg.* 2014;16 (6):444–450.

6. Is common hair loss in women managed differently than in men?

Women whose hair loss is a manifestation of hyperandrogenism (excessive production of circulating androgens) may benefit from therapy directed at the cause of the hyperandrogenism. Polycystic ovarian syndrome, late-onset congenital adrenal hyperplasia, Cushing's syndrome, and adrenal and ovarian neoplasms are potential causes of

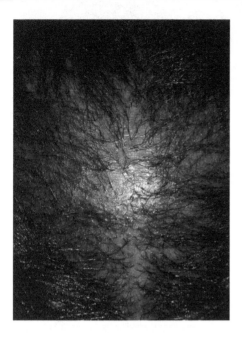

Fig. 20.1 Central, centrifugal, cicatricial alopecia, a common form of hair loss in the African-American population. In this patient, the smooth skin, devoid of most follicular openings, reflects light like a mirror.

hyperandrogenism. In the absence of elevated circulating androgens, nonspecific therapy directed at suppressing ovarian androgen production or blocking the peripheral effect of androgens can be effective. Oral contraceptive agents (to suppress ovarian androgen production) and spironolactone are most often utilized for this purpose. Topical minoxidil solution is also useful, but oral finasteride is seldom used in women unless postmenopausal.

7. What are the surgical options for treatment of balding?

Men, and occasionally women, can achieve permanent cosmetic improvement by undergoing a hair transplantation procedure. Hair follicles from the occipital area (donor site) are moved to the balding area (recipient site). The procedure is tedious and expensive, but the cosmetic results can be quite good. Various other surgical procedures, including scalp reductions (which involve excising the bald areas) and scalp flaps, are sometimes used in selected patients.

8. Discuss the common causes of circular bald spots.

Although many forms of alopecia can result in a circular bald patch, the most common causes are tinea capitis and alopecia areata. **Tinea capitis** is a superficial fungal infection with a predilection for children. The surface of the skin is scaly and sometimes inflamed, and small dark stubs of hair ("black dots") may be scattered within the affected area. In this condition, the hair shaft is invaded and replaced by myriad circular fungal spores. In the United States, *Trichophyton tonsurans* is usually the culprit. A circular, scaly, or crusted bald spot on the scalp of a child should be considered to be tinea capitis until proven otherwise (Fig. 20.2A).

   Alopecia areata also commonly affects children, but adults often develop the condition. In alopecia areata, the affected areas may be totally hairless, but the scalp surface looks otherwise normal, without scaling and minimal, if any, erythema. A few short hairs may be present in the bald spot; these diseased hairs tend to be much shorter, thinner, and less deeply pigmented than surrounding normal hairs (Fig. 20.2B).

9. What is alopecia totalis?

Alopecia areata may cause one or many bald spots. If it affects the entire scalp, it is called **alopecia totalis** (Fig. 20.3). If the entire body (all body hair) is affected, it is referred to as **alopecia universalis.**

10. How is alopecia areata treated?

When a solitary lesion of alopecia areata is small (<5 cm in diameter), no treatment may be needed. The prognosis for such a lesion is excellent, and spontaneous regrowth often occurs. Intralesional corticosteroids, and sometimes potent topical corticosteroids, may hasten regrowth. Larger or more numerous lesions carry a more guarded prognosis. Intralesional corticosteroid injections are often begun. For extensive hair loss involving 30% to 100% of the scalp surface, a short (e.g., 3-month and/or pulsed) course of systemic corticosteroids (usually prednisone or pulsed dexamethasone) may be tried. If hair regrowth does not resume or if hair loss recurs once corticosteroids are stopped, the prognosis is poor. The use of systemic corticosteroids to treat extensive alopecia areata is controversial. Appropriate risk-versus-benefit considerations must be carefully analyzed.

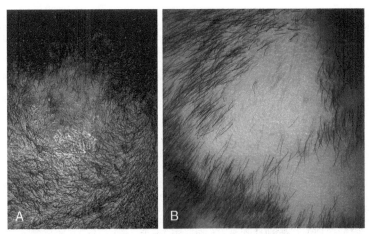

Fig. 20.2 A, Tinea capitis. A large bald patch studded with small inflammatory papules surrounded by smaller, similar lesions. Close examination may reveal "black dots" scattered within the bald area. **B,** A patch of alopecia areata showing shorter, thinner, and less deeply pigmented hairs growing within the bald zone.

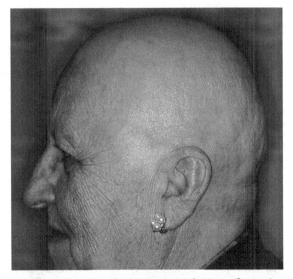

Fig. 20.3 Alopecia totalis demonstrating total loss of scalp hair and most of eyebrows. (Courtesy James E. Fitzpatrick, MD.)

Topical immunotherapy with chemicals causing allergic contact dermatitis (e.g., diphencyprone or squaric acid dibutyl ester) is also useful for treatment of severe disease. This mechanism of action appears to stem from altered local immunity. Recent studies have presented a new class of medications that help in the treatment of severe alopecia areata. The janus kinase (JAK) inhibitors, tofacitinib and ruxolitinib, show a beneficial effect on treatment of refractory disease. However, the JAK inhibitors carry an increased risk of infection and should be used cautiously.

Hordinsky M, Donati A. Alopecia areata: an evidence-based treatment update. *Am J Clin Dermatol.* 2014;15(3):231–246.
Liu LY, Craiglow BG, Dai F, King BA. Tofacitinib for the treatment of severe alopecia areata and variants: a study of 90 patients. *J Am Acad Dermatol.* 2017;76(1):22.

11. How is tinea capitis treated?

Although topical antifungal agents work well for tinea corporis, they are of little value in treating tinea capitis. Systemic antifungal agents are required to eradicate the spores that invade affected hair shafts. A course of treatment generally takes 1 to 3 months. **Griseofulvin** has historically been the treatment of choice because it is safe and effective, rarely causing significant side effects. Ultra-microsized formulations of griseofulvin can be given in half the dose required with microsized forms of the drug. Fungal resistance to griseofulvin is rare. Side effects of Griseofulvin include headache or gastrointestinal upset. Terbinafine is also now considered a first-line therapy for tinea capitis caused by *Trichophyton* sp. and leads to a slightly higher cure rate in a shorter time than Griseofulvin.

Gupta AK, Drummond-Main C. Meta-analysis of randomized, controlled trials comparing particular doses of griseofulvin and terbinafine for the treatment of tinea capitis. *Pediatr Dermatol.* 2013;30(1):1–6.
Chen X, Jiang X, Gonzalez U, et al. Systemic antifungal therapy for tinea capitis in children. *Cochrane Database Syst Rev.* 2016;(5): CD004685.

12. What is trichotillomania?
Trichotillomania (trichotillosis) is compulsive hair pulling or plucking.

13. Who is most likely to be affected by trichotillomania?
The typical patient is a child or adolescent, although the condition can affect adults as well. In trichotillomania, hairs are forcibly plucked out of the scalp by the patient, usually as a mechanism for relieving tension or stress and sometimes as a manifestation of psychosis or an obsessive-compulsive neurosis. Although the patient may deny plucking, the often-bizarre shape of the bald area, combined with the presence of short hairs of various lengths within the area of thinning, suggests the diagnosis (Fig. 20.4). The diagnosis may be confirmed by a scalp biopsy demonstrating diagnostic features, or by creating a "hair growth window." This test is performed by weekly shaving of an involved area to prevent plucking; the hair will recover and regain normal density within the shaved area, resembling a "five o'clock shadow."

Woods DW, Houghton DC. Diagnosis, evaluation, and management of trichotillomania. *Psychiatr Clin North Am.* 2014;37(3):301–317.

14. Why do cancer patients lose their hair?
Cancer patients are susceptible to two forms of diffuse hair loss. **Anagen effluvium** is a direct effect of anticancer treatment. Patients receiving radiation therapy to the scalp or systemic chemotherapy can shed all or most of their hair within a few weeks of starting treatment. This hair loss is a direct effect of the chemotherapy or radiotherapy on the hair follicle, whose rapidly dividing cells are very susceptible to injury. When the hair matrix (the epithelial root that produces the hair shaft) is exposed to radiation or chemical toxins, it can only produce a thinned hair shaft that eventually tapers to a point (Fig. 20.5A). This marked tapering makes the shaft extremely fragile, and the hair shaft can literally be combed away or broken off by minor trauma. Unless the dose of radiation or chemotherapy is very high, regrowth of hair occurs once therapy is stopped.

In **telogen effluvium**, the metabolic and emotional "stress" of severe, debilitating illness causes many of the actively growing (anagen) hairs to enter the shedding (telogen) phase of hair growth prematurely. The hairs remain in telogen for about 3 months before they are finally shed (Fig. 20.5B), so there is always a "lag" time between the onset of severe disease and actual hair loss. Seldom is more than 50% of the hair shed in telogen effluvium, so patients develop thin hair but do not become completely bald. If the patient recovers and is no longer debilitated, hairs reenter the actively growing phase and the hair regrows.

Kligman AM. Pathologic dynamics of human hair loss: I. Telogen effluvium. *Arch Dermatol.* 1961;83:175–198.

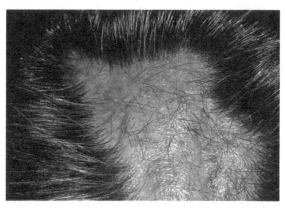

Fig. 20.4 Trichotillomania. The highly irregular shape, sharp circumscription, and presence of "broken off" hairs of various lengths are typical of this condition.

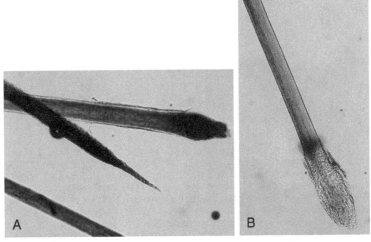

Fig. 20.5 Hair loss in cancer therapy. **A,** Anagen effluvium. The shaft tapers down to a pencil-like point and easily separates from the follicle. **B,** Normal telogen hair. About 50 to 100 telogen hairs such as these are normally shed during the course of the day. Much higher numbers are shed during a telogen effluvium.

15. **In what other clinical settings can a telogen effluvium occur?**

    Normally, about 10% of scalp hairs are in the telogen (preshedding) phase at any given time. Whenever an abnormally large number of hairs enter the telogen phase, a telogen effluvium occurs. There are several clinical situations in which a telogen effluvium is found, including severe illness such as metastatic cancer, but any serious illness or major surgical procedure can also result in a telogen effluvium. The most common form of telogen effluvium occurs in women about 3 months after giving birth. In addition, virtually all newborn infants develop a telogen effluvium during the first 6 months of life, which is why many babies have more hair at birth than at 3 to 4 months after birth. Many women also develop an unexplained, "chronic form of telogen effluvium" that is self-limited, but can last for years.

    Causes of telogen effluvium can be summarized as follows:
    - Physiologic effluvium of the newborn
    - Postpartum
    - Postfebrile (e.g., malaria)
    - Severe infection
    - Debilitating chronic illness
    - Postsurgical (major procedure or major trauma)
    - Hypothyroidism and other endocrinopathies
    - Crash or liquid protein diets; starvation
    - Drugs: Retinoids, anticoagulants, anticonvulsives, antithyroid, heavy metals

    Grover C, Khurana A. Telogen effluvium. *Indian J Dermatol Venereol Leprol.* 2013;79(5):591–603.

16. **To what forms of hair loss are black patients susceptible?**
    - Black children have a higher incidence of acquiring tinea capitis than other ethnicities.
    - Hair shaft fragility disorders are also common among African-American women because of certain hair grooming techniques using chemical hair "relaxers." These products are effective in straightening kinky or curly hair but are caustic, and with continued use, the hair shaft becomes frayed. The foci of fraying have a special appearance termed trichorrhexis nodosa, which looks like the bristles of two paint brushes that have been pushed together (Fig. 20.6). The hair shafts easily fracture at the points of trichorrhexis nodosa, leaving abnormally short hair shafts behind. Patients have scalp hair of very uneven length and may complain that their hair "falls out" with combing or "won't grow." In fact, the hair is growing but breaking off.
    - Central, centrifugal, cicatricial alopecia (CCCA) is also more common in black patients.

17. **What is central, centrifugal, cicatricial alopecia (CCCA)?**

    The most common form of cicatricial alopecia in black patients was once called "hot comb alopecia" but is now called *central, centrifugal, cicatricial alopecia* (CCCA). The condition more often affects adult women than men and typically causes hair loss that is most severe on the central crown of the scalp and slowly progresses centrifugally (see

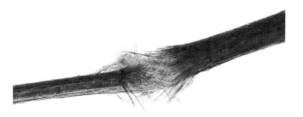

Fig. 20.6 Trichorrhexis nodosa fracture in a woman using chemical hair straighteners.

Fig. 20.1). When the bald patches are carefully examined, a few normal hairs may be found, but most follicular openings have been completely obliterated, suggesting a cicatricial process. Scattered inflammatory, perifollicular papules may be found in the peripheral zone where hair thinning has just begun. Scalp biopsy confirms that hair follicles are completely destroyed and replaced with fibrous tissue. "Hot combs" are rarely used nowadays for straightening hair, so hot comb alopecia is a misnomer. It is uncertain whether hair care products are primarily responsible for hair loss in these patients, but chemical relaxers and other cosmetics may exacerbate the condition. Hair styles exerting traction on the hair have also been implicated.

Gathers RC, Lim HW. Central centrifugal cicatricial alopecia: past, present, and future. *J Am Acad Dermatol.* 2009;60(4):660–668.

18. What are some medications that cause hair loss?

Anticancer (chemotherapeutic) medications, colchicine, thallium (rat poisons and insecticides), antiepileptic drugs (phenytoin, valproic acid, and carbamazepine), anticlotting drugs (heparin and warfarin [Coumadin]), and retinoids (acitretin).

Bergfeld W. Telogen effluvium. In: McMichael A, Hordinsky M, eds. *Hair and Scalp Diseases*. New York: Informa Healthcare; 2008: 119–135.
Brodin M. Drug-related alopecia. *Dermatol Clin.* 1987;5:571–579.

KEY POINTS: ALOPECIA

1. A circular, scaly, or crusted bald spot on the scalp of a child should be considered tinea capitis until proven otherwise.
2. Women whose balding is a manifestation of hyperandrogenism (excessive production of circulating androgens) may benefit from therapy directed at the cause of the hyperandrogenism.
3. When a solitary lesion of alopecia areata is small, no treatment may be needed. The prognosis for such a lesion is excellent, and spontaneous regrowth often occurs.
4. In trichotillomania, hairs are forcibly plucked out of the scalp by the patient, usually as a mechanism for relieving tension or stress.
5. The most common form of cicatricial alopecia in black patients is called *central, centrifugal, cicatricial alopecia*. It is not caused by cosmetic practices, but chemical relaxers or hair styles exerting traction may exacerbate the condition.

19. What is alopecia mucinosa?

This term actually refers to two entirely different causes of hair loss. The conditions have in common a similar histologic finding—**follicular mucinosis**, the accumulation of mucin (acid mucopolysaccharides) within the follicular epithelium, resulting in hair damage and hair loss.

The first form of alopecia mucinosa is a benign condition found in young and otherwise healthy individuals. One or more oval or circular hairless patches or plaques are present, which can be hypopigmented or erythematous and may be scaly, eczematous, or studded with minute papules. The condition usually involves the head, neck, upper arms, or upper torso. Spontaneous resolution usually occurs in months to years.

The second form of alopecia mucinosa occurs in patients with mycosis fungoides, a form of cutaneous T-cell lymphoma. Patients are usually elderly, and numerous, often large, hairless, erythematous, and indurated plaques are found (Fig. 20.7). Histologically, follicular mucinosis is present, but an atypical lymphocytic infiltrate that often invades the epidermis and follicles is also seen. This atypical cellular infiltrate allows for the diagnosis of mycosis fungoides. The hairless lesions and histologic follicular mucinosis are merely manifestations of the underlying lymphoma.

Gibson LE, Brown HA, Pittelkow MR, Pujol RM. Follicular mucinosis. *Arch Dermatol.* 2002;138(12):1615.

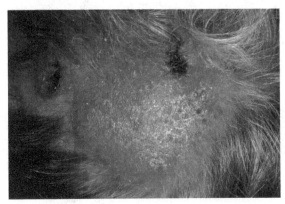

Fig. 20.7 Alopecia mucinosa occurring in a patient with mycosis fungoides. (Courtesy Fitzsimons Army Medical Center teaching files.)

20. **What is meant by the term "moth-eaten alopecia"?**

"Moth-eaten alopecia" is a form of noncicatricial, patterned hair loss in which there are myriad small foci of alopecia scattered over the scalp (Fig. 20.8). This pattern of alopecia is described as the classic form of alopecia seen in patients with secondary syphilis. However, other etiologies, such as alopecia areata and systemic lupus erythematosus, can result in the same pattern of hair loss. Furthermore, hair loss in syphilis can be diffuse as well as moth-eaten. Therefore, all sexually active patients with unexplained hair loss, particularly if the patients also have a rash, should be tested for syphilis.

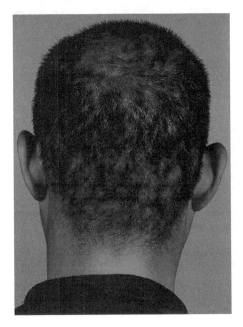

Fig. 20.8 Moth-eaten alopecia.

CHAPTER 21

ACNE AND ACNEIFORM ERUPTIONS

Joanna M. Burch and Lori D. Prok

KEY POINTS: ACNE

1. In acne, the pilosebaceous unit is the target of disease. The microcomedone is the earliest lesion.
2. Combination therapy including a retinoid plus benzoyl peroxide or an antimicrobial agent is the preferred approach for almost all patients with acne. A topical keratolytic (benzoyl peroxide or topical retinoids) should *always* be used with a topical or oral antibiotic in treating inflammatory acne.
3. Topical retinoids should be first-line agents in the maintenance therapy of acne.
4. Bacterial resistance to benzoyl peroxidase does not occur. Benzoyl peroxide used concomitantly with antimicrobial therapy for acne (as a leave-on or as a wash) is effective in limiting antibiotic resistance. Benzoyl peroxide used for 5 to 7 days between antibiotic courses may also reduce resistant organisms.
5. Drug-induced acne is caused most often by anabolic steroids and corticosteroids. It is differentiated from acne vulgaris by its sudden onset, distribution mainly on the upper trunk, and its monomorphous pustular appearance without comedones.

1. **How common is acne?**

Acne vulgaris is the most common dermatologic disorders, affecting between 40 million and 50 million individuals of all ages in the United States. Eighty-five percent of people between the ages of 12 and 24 years will have some acne. Moderate to severe acne affects around 20% of young people, and severity correlates with pubertal maturity. Acne persists into the 20s and 30s in around 64% and 43% of individuals, respectively. The heritability of acne is almost 80% in first-degree relatives. In the United States, the cost of acne is over $3 billion per year in terms of treatment and loss of productivity.

Bhate K, Williams HC. Epidemiology of acne vulgaris. *Br J Dermatol.* 2013;168:474–485.

2. **What is the pathophysiology of acne?**

The pilosebaceous unit, made up of a follicle (pore), sebaceous gland, and a hair, is the target organ affected in acne. The face, chest, and back are areas with the greatest concentration of pilosebaceous follicles and correspond to the areas most commonly affected by acne lesions. The primary lesion of acne is the microcomedo. This is the result of obstruction of the sebaceous follicles by sebum, deficiency of linolenic acid, excessive secretion of androgens, excess of free fatty acid, and abnormally differentiated and desquamated keratinocytes that may produce large comedones (Fig. 21.1). Proinflammatory cytokines including interleukin-1α (IL-1α) and tumor necrosis factor-α are, among others, considered to be responsible for furthering aberrant follicular hyperkeratinization.

The pathogenesis of acne vulgaris is multifactorial:
- Sebaceous gland hyperplasia with excess sebum production
- Excessive keratosis of excretory ducts and openings of sebaceous glands
- Inflammatory mediators in the skin
- *Propionibacterium acnes* colonization of the follicle

Bergler-Czop B. The aetiopathogenesis of acne vulgaris—what's new? *Int J Cosmet Sci.* 2014;36:187–194.
Contassot E, French LE. New insights into acne pathogenesis: *Propionibacterium acnes* activates the inflamasome. *J Invest Dermatol.* 2014;134:310–313.
Lee YB, Byun EJ, Kim HS. Potential role of the microbiome in acne: a comprehensive review. *J Clin Med.* 2019;8(7).

3. **What are the acne subtypes?**

Acne presents in many forms and variations. The most common form is acne vulgaris, which is classified according to the predominant lesion type as comedonal, papular, pustular, nodular, or cystic. It can be graded as mild, moderate, or severe (Fig. 21.2). Other clinical subtypes of acneiform skin lesions include:
- Acne conglobata
- Acne excoriée
- Acne fulminans
- Acne mechanica
- Acne rosacea

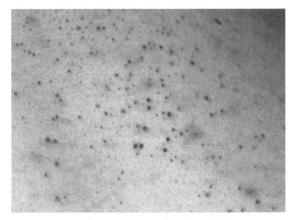

Fig. 21.1 Numerous microcomedones and comedones in patient with acne. (Courtesy William L. Weston, MD Collection.)

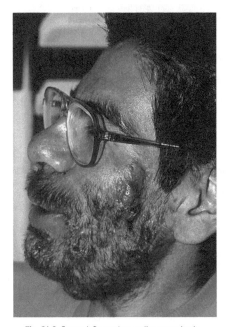

Fig. 21.2 Severe inflammatory cystic acne vulgaris.

- Drug-induced acne
- Favre-Racouchot syndrome
- Infantile acne
- Neonatal acne
- Perioral dermatitis
- Pyoderma faciale

4. How does the composition of sebum contribute to the formation of acne?

The major constituent of sebaceous lipid is triglyceride, which makes up over 50% of the lipid, wax esters account for 25%, squalene 15%, and there are small amounts of cholesterol esters and free cholesterol. Increased sebum production is characteristic of patients with acne, but the seborrhea itself is not sufficient to produce acne. Current evidence indicates that sebum composition (lipid quality) and not quantity plays a central role in the development of acne. Desaturation of the fatty acids in sebum may lead to the development of acne lesions. Lipoperoxidases characterize the sebum of acne patients, and this, along with other qualitative changes in the sebum lipids, induce alteration of keratinocyte differentiation and induce IL-1 secretion, leading to follicular hyperkeratinization.

Zouboulis CC, Jourdan E, Picardo M. Acne is an inflammatory disease and alterations of sebum composition initiate acne lesions. *J Eur Acad Dermatol Venereol.* 2014;28:527–532.

5. Does stress exacerbate acne?

Stress is a part of the modern routine; it affects individuals across their lifetime and may be correlated with acne. Studies demonstrate that a marked percentage of adults (50% to 71%) reported that the lesions worsened during stress periods. Sleep is one of the main regulators of the homeostasis of the body and is directly connected with well-being. Insufficient sleep represents an inherent stress condition in humans, increasing secretion of stress hormones, which may influence acne development. In one survey of 4576 consecutive patients with various dermatologic problems, 55% of those with acne reported that episodes of emotional stress were closely related to exacerbation of their acne. A prospective cohort study, published in 2003, of 22 university students with acne during exams showed increased acne severity that was significantly associated with increased stress levels. Another study in high school students also found that increased stress correlated with increased acne severity. There did not seem to be an increase in sebum production during times of stress in this study. The mechanisms underlying the triggering or aggravation of acne by stress remain unclear. Stress induces secretion of different neurotransmitters, cytokines, and hormones (corticotropin-releasing hormone, cortisol, glucocorticoids), which have skin receptors and can aggravate several skin diseases including acne. A recent study showed that skin diseases influence emotional status, through chemical mediators released by epidermal keratinocytes.

Albuquerque RG, Rocha MA, Bagatin E, et al. Could adult female acne be associated with modern life? *Arch Dermatol Res.* 2014;306:683–688.
Yosipovitch G, Tang M, Dawn AG, et al. Study of psychological stress, sebum production and acne vulgaris in adolescents. *Acta Derm Venereol.* 2007;87:35–39.

6. Does diet affect acne?

Historically, there was strong interest in the role of food (e.g., chocolate, sugar, iodine) in the exacerbation of acne; however, when several studies done in the late 1960s failed to demonstrate a link, this concept fell out of vogue with dermatologists. However, there has been renewed interest in a link between diet and acne as epidemiologic studies demonstrated that acne prevalence is low in rural, nonindustrialized societies and increases with the adoption of a Western diet. Milk and other dairy products have been implicated in three separate studies. There is some evidence to support the concept that milk products with low-fat content (e.g., skim milk) may be more important than other products with a low-fat content. It has been hypothesized that the hormonal content, not the fat in milk, may be responsible for the exacerbation of acne.

The role of glycemic load on exacerbation of acne has also received scrutiny, and several prospective trials have now been completed. One prospective randomized 12-week study done on teenage boys and young men demonstrated that subjects on a low–glycemic index diet lost significantly more weight and had significantly improved acne when compared to the subjects that had been on a high–glycemic index diet. The relative contribution of the high–glycemic load diet on acne pathogenesis versus the improvement in insulin and hormone levels with weight loss is unknown.

Adebamowo CA, Spiegelman D, Danby FW, et al. High school dietary intake and teenage acne. *J Am Acad Dermatol.* 2005;52:207–214.
Kumari R, Thappa DM. Role of insulin resistance and diet in acne. *Indian J Dermatol Venereol Leprol.* 2013;79:291–299.
Smith RN, Man NJ, Braue A, et al. The effect of a high-protein, low glycemic-load diet versus a conventional, high glycemic-load diet on biochemical parameters associated with acne vulgaris: a randomized, investigator-masked controlled trial. *J Am Acad Dermatol.* 2007;57:247–256.
Spencer EH, Ferdowsian HR, Barnard ND. Diet and acne: a review of the evidence. *Int J Dermatol.* 2009;48:339–347.

7. When can teenagers with acne expect their acne to resolve?

Acne persists into the 20s and 30s in around 64% and 43% of individuals, respectively. Most teenage boys can anticipate clearing of their acne between 20 and 25 years of age. For women, the news is not so good. The majority of patients with adult acne, including adult-onset acne, are women. A study of 2000 adults found that 3% of men and 5% of women still had a degree of acne between the ages of 40 to 49 years.

Bhate K, Williams HC. Epidemiology of acne vulgaris. *Br J Dermatol.* 2013;168:474–485.
Mwanthi M, Zaenglein AL. Update in the management of acne in adolescence. *Curr Opin Pediatr.* 2018;30(4):492–498.

8. Discuss the role of topical retinoid therapy in acne vulgaris

The single most important topical medications used to treat acne are retinoids. There are numerous topical preparations to choose from that are less irritating and decrease the most common complaint associated with this class of acne therapy. These include adapalene (Differin), tazarotene (Tazorac), and tretinoin (Avita, Retin-A, Retin-A Micro). Twelve weeks of use is required for maximum benefit. Retinoids are the only drugs that normalize keratinization within the follicular infundibulum and prevent comedo formation. *Propionibacterium acnes,* the anaerobic bacterium associated with acne pathogenesis, stimulates the innate immune response via Toll-like receptors (TLRs). This sets off an inflammatory cascade of cytokines. Retinoids are known to downregulate TLRs and inhibit downstream inflammatory transcription factors. Recent recommendations from a global alliance to improve outcomes in acne recommended that retinoid-based combination therapy (retinoid plus antimicrobial or benzoyl peroxide [BPO]) be the first-line treatment for most forms of acne vulgaris. Retinoids have been shown to maintain improvement achieved with this initial combination therapy.

Sevimli Dikicier B. Topical treatments of acne vulgaris: efficiency, side effects, and adherence rates. *J Int Med Res.* 2019;47:2987–2992.
Kolli SS, Pecone D, Pona A, Cline A, Feldman SR. Topical retinoids in acne vulgaris: a systematic review. *Am J Clin Dermatol.* 2019;20:345–365.

9. What is the role of topical antibiotics in the treatment of acne vulgaris?

It is important to understand that acne vulgaris is not an infection. In general, topical antibiotic monotherapy should be avoided, particularly for long periods of time because of the development of bacterial resistance. More than half of patients undergoing therapy with a single topical antibiotic will develop resistance. Topical antibiotics are useful, as they do reduce *Propionibacterium acnes* colonization on the skin and reduce the bacteria's proinflammatory effects.

In general, it is best to utilize topical antibiotics (erythromycin, clindamycin, and sodium sulfacetamide) in combination with BPO either as fixed-dose combination products or two separate medications. BPO has the added benefit of being modestly comedolytic and can minimize the risk for bacterial antibiotic resistance. Other topical treatments are α-hydroxy acids, salicylic acid, azelaic acid, dapsone, and taurine bromamine. Minocycline topical foam is currently being studied for the treatment of moderate to severe acne.

Bonati LM, Dover JS. Treating acne with topical antibiotics: current obstacles and the introduction of topical minocycline as a new treatment option. *J Drugs Dermatol.* 2019;18:240–244.
Dessinioti C, Katsambas A. Propionibacterium acnes and antimicrobial resistance in acne. *Clin Dermatol.* 2017;35:163–167.

10. Discuss oral antibiotic use in acne vulgaris.

Oral antibiotics are indicated in patients with inflammatory lesions (red papules, pustules, or nodules) of moderate to severe grade. There is a low evidence level that oral antibiotics are more effective than topical preparations for mild to moderate facial acne. Tetracyclines are the first-line oral antibiotic therapy in acne. Minocycline and doxycycline are most frequently used. Sarecycline, a novel tetracycline, has recently been FDA approved for the treatment of acne in patients 9 years of age and older. Overall, there is insufficient evidence to support one tetracycline over another in terms of efficacy. Antibiotics reduce the numbers of *P. acnes* in the follicles and also have numerous anti-inflammatory effects.

Oral antibiotics should *never* be used as monotherapy in acne because of a significant problem with antibiotic resistance, and only two of the four main pathophysiologic mechanisms of disease are being addressed. Oral antibiotics should be combined with a keratolytic such as a topical retinoid and topical BPO. Oral therapy will take 4 to 8 weeks to show significant improvement. After adequate clinical response in 3 to 6 months, the dose should be tapered in an attempt to provide maintenance with topical medications. Erythromycin is an alternative in patients who are intolerant or allergic to tetracyclines and may be used in pregnancy; however, because of worldwide resistance, the use of this antibiotic has waned. Alternative oral antibiotics such as clindamycin, azithromycin, cotrimoxazole, and quinolones should be used cautiously because of increased potential for severe adverse reactions.

Chien AL, Tsai J, Leung S, et al. Association of systemic antibiotic treatment of acne with skin microbiota characteristics. *JAMA Dermatol.* 2019;155:425–434.
Adler BL, Kornmehl H, Armstrong AW. Antibiotic resistance in acne treatment. *JAMA Dermatol.* 2017;153:810–811.
Kircik, L. What's new in the management of acne vulgaris. Cutis 2019;104(1).

11. Will the oral antibiotics used in acne interfere with the efficacy of oral contraceptives (OCs) to prevent pregnancy?

Probably not. Whether the contraceptive efficacy of OCs is adversely affected by antibiotics such as penicillins, sulfonamides, and tetracyclines is highly controversial. Tetracycline, doxycycline, ampicillin, and metronidazole have been shown in pharmacokinetic studies not to decrease contraceptive steroid levels. When contraceptive failure rates of dermatology patients on OCs and antibiotics were compared to patients who take OCs but not antibiotics, no difference was found. However, there is a theoretical risk, and this should be discussed with female patients taking both antibiotics and OCs.

Table 21.1 Combination oral contraceptives for acne

ESTROGEN	PROGESTIN	BRAND NAMES	OTHER INFORMATION
Ethinyl estradiol	Desogestrel	Apri, Cyclessa, Desogen, Ortho-Cept	Third-generation progestin
Ethinyl estradiol	Gestodene	N/A (not available in the United States)	Third-generation progestin
Ethinyl estradiol	Norgestimate	Mononessa, Ortho Cyclen, Orthotricyclen, Orthotricyclen Lo, Sprintec, Trinessa	Third-generation progestin
Ethinyl estradiol	Norethindrone	Brevicon, Estrostep, Junel, Modicon, Necon, Nelova, Norethin, OrthoNovum, Ovcon-35, TriNorinyl	Second-generation progestin
Ethinyl estradiol	Ethynodiol diacetate	Demulen, Ovulen, Zovia	Second-generation progestin
Ethinyl estradiol	Levonorgestrel	Alesse, Aviane, Empresse, Levlen, Levlite, Lovora, Nordette, Portia, TriLevlen, Triphasil, Trivora	Second-generation progestin
Ethinyl estradiol	Drospirenone	Yasmin, YAZ	New progestin that is an analog of spironolactone Has antiandrogenic and antimineralocorticoid properties

12. Discuss the use of OCs in the treatment of acne.

The OCs that are most often used today to treat acne are a combination of ethinyl estradiol and a progestin. The only OCs officially approved by the FDA for use in acne are Ortho-TriCyclen (Ortho-McNeil Pharmaceutical, Raritan, NJ), Estrostep (Warner-Chilcott, Rockaway, NJ), and, most recently, YAZ (Bayer Healthcare Pharmaceuticals, Montville, NJ). The second- and third-generation progestins, combined with an estrogen, are the most appropriate choices for the treatment of acne because they have the lowest androgenic activity (Table 21.1). Multiple studies suggest that OCs are significantly better than placebo in the treatment of mild to moderate acne. The trials comparing different OCs are somewhat conflicting. The estrogen inhibits luteinizing hormone and follicle-stimulating hormone, which suppress ovulation and ovarian androgen production. This subsequent reduction in androgens results in a decreased activation of androgen receptors at the level of the sebaceous gland. Estrogen also stimulates the production of steroid hormone-binding globulin in the liver, which decreases circulating levels of testosterone. The effect of progestin on acne is unclear. Some studies suggest that it can lower androgen effects by inhibiting 5α-reductase or competitively inhibiting androgen receptors. Patients should be screened for risk factors associated with OCs prior to beginning this therapy (see Table 21.1). The World Health Organization and the American College of Obstetricians and Gynecologists no longer require a pelvic exam before initiating OC therapy in most healthy female patients of childbearing age.

Lam C, Zaenglein AL. Contraceptive use in acne. *Clin Dermatol.* 2014;32:502–515.
Marson JW, Baldwin HE. An overview of acne therapy, part 2: hormonal therapy and isotretinoin. *Dermatol Clin.* 2019;37:195–203.

13. Can spironolactone be used to treat acne?

Yes. Spironolactone is typically used as an adjunctive therapy for acne in dermatology. It has been used for more than two decades to treat acne in women, although it is an off-label use. Spironolactone has antiandrogenic effects. It competes with testosterone and dihydrotestosterone (DHT) for androgen receptors on sebaceous glands and reduces sebocyte proliferation. Additionally, it has been shown to suppress cytochrome P450, inhibit steroidogenesis, and reduce 5α-reductase activity. In vitro studies demonstrate spironolactone can reduce sebum excretion by 30% to 50%.

14. When should a patient be started on isotretinoin therapy?

Isotretinoin is the mainstay of therapy for severe acne. It is indicated for patients with severe, scarring, nodulocystic acne, and those with moderate to severe acne who have failed an adequate trial (3 to 6 months) of conventional therapy (retinoid and/or BPO plus an oral antibiotic). Isotretinoin is also beneficial for patients with severe hidradenitis suppurativa (HS), acne rosacea, and gram-negative acne who are unresponsive to conventional therapy. However, it is not as effective in these diseases as it is in severe acne vulgaris, and relapses are more frequent. The recommended dose is 1.0 mg/kg/day for 20 to 24 weeks. Isotretinoin should be used as monotherapy for acne vulgaris.

Goldsmith LA, Bolognia JL, Callen JP, et al. American Academy of Dermatology Consensus Conference on the safe and optimal use of isotretinoin: summary and recommendations. *J Am Acad Dermatol.* 2004;50:900–906.
Zaenglein AL, Pathy AL, Schlosser BJ, et al. Guidelines of care for the management of acne vulgaris. *J Am Acad Dermatol.* 2016;74:945–973.e33.

15. What are the side effects of isotretinoin?

Isotretinoin is a potent teratogen. Of the pregnancies that have occurred in patients taking isotretinoin, one-third have resulted in spontaneous abortion, one-third ended in therapeutic abortion, and of the one-third that continued to term, 20% showed a major fetal malformation, including those of the brain, heart, and ears. Many of these patients, who had a pregnancy while taking isotretinoin were pregnant when the drug was started. When considering treatment with isotretinoin in females of childbearing age, the FDA requires documentation of two negative pregnancy tests. Contraceptive counseling must be done and documented on the patient's chart, and two forms of birth control are recommended for the duration of therapy plus 6 weeks post-therapy. Therapy should be started on the third day of the menstrual cycle, with a negative pregnancy test to ensure that the patient is not pregnant when therapy is initiated. Beginning in March 2006, the FDA requires all patients, prescribers, and dispensers of isotretinoin to be registered with the Internet-based iPLEDGE program (www.iPLEDGEprogram.com).

Other side effects of isotretinoin include dry skin, lips, and eyes, dry mucous membranes with nosebleeds, headache (including rare instances of pseudotumor cerebri), muscle and backaches, hypertriglyceridemia, increased liver function tests, and depression (see next question). These should be discussed in detail with the patient prior to starting therapy and documentation of the discussion made in the chart.

On SC, Zeichner J. Isotretinoin updates. *Dermatol Ther.* 2013;26:377–389.

16. What about depression and suicide with isotretinoin?

A number of case reports and case series appear in the literature that link depression, suicide, and suicidal ideation to isotretinoin use. In several of these cases, cessation of the drug resulted in improvement of the depressive symptoms and rechallenge caused recurrence of depression. Between 1982 and 2000, the FDA received reports of 394 cases of depression and 37 suicides occurring in patients exposed to isotretinoin. However, depression is more common in the age group affected by acne than in the general population. To complicate matters further, there is evidence that acne itself has significant psychological effects, and there are case reports of improvement in depression scores of acne patients during and after treatment with isotretinoin. Epidemiologic studies to date have not shown a causal relationship between isotretinoin and depression and suicide. Because depression and suicide are serious matters, careful monitoring of patients undergoing therapy with isotretinoin for signs/symptoms of depression and suicidal ideation is advisable. In November 2010, the American Academy of Dermatology issued a statement on the issue of isotretinoin and depression, as follows: "A correlation between isotretinoin use and depression/anxiety symptoms has been suggested but an evidence-based causal relationship has not been established."

Bray AP, Kravvas G, Skevington SM, Lovell CR. Is there an association between isotretinoin therapy and adverse mood changes? A prospective study in a cohort of acne patients. *J Dermatol Treat.* 2019;30:796–801.
Li C, Chen J, Wang W, et al. Use of isotretinoin and risk of depression in patients with acne: a systematic review and meta-analysis. *BMJ Open.* 2019;9:e021549.

17. Can isotretinoin trigger inflammatory bowel disease?

There are also several case reports of inflammatory bowel disease (IBD) being triggered by isotretinoin use. A review of adverse events reported to the U.S. FDA MedWatch scheme over a 5-year period (1997 to 2002) revealed 85 cases of IBD, of which the causal association with isotretinoin was considered probable or highly probable in 73% of cases. A 2013 study of 45,000 women of reproductive age on isotretinoin did not suggest an increase in the risk for IBD, either ulcerative colitis or Crohn's disease. Despite a lack of definitive evidence of a causal relationship, the FDA added IBD to the isotretinoin package insert in 2005 as a possible adverse effect. In 2010, the American Academy of Dermatology published a position statement addressing the issue of isotretinoin and IBD: "Current evidence is insufficient to prove either an association or a causal relationship between isotretinoin use and inflammatory bowel disease (IBD) in the general population."

Reddy D, Siegel CA, Sands BE, et al. Possible association between isotretinoin and inflammatory bowel disease. *Am J Gastroenterol.* 2006;101:1569–1573.
Lee SY, Jamal MM, Nguyen ET, Bechtold ML, Nguyen DL. Does exposure to isotretinoin increase the risk for the development of inflammatory bowel disease? A meta-analysis. *Eur J Gastroenterol Hepatol.* 2016;28:210–216.

18. Discuss optical treatments (laser therapy, light sources, and photodynamic therapy)

One of the important pathogenic mechanisms of acne is *Propionibacterium acnes* growth in the follicle. *P. acnes* produces porphyrins, which can be activated by visible light, inducing a photodynamic reaction that kills the bacteria. Several studies have shown improvement in acne utilizing visible light, especially in the blue light spectrum (400 to 420 nm), where these porphyrins are most strongly activated. Blue and red (660 nm) light combined has also been used, as well as light in the yellow and green spectrum (500 to 600 nm). Several studies have shown improvement in acne lesions with relatively few side effects. However, clearing seems to be variable among patients and relapse rates are high.

Photodynamic therapy utilizes a lower-power visible light source in which the effectiveness is amplified by the use of a topical photosensitizing agent, most often aminolevulinic acid. Photodynamic therapy tends to have more side effects, such as burning at the sites of treatment and postinflammatory hyperpigmentation. Existing studies suggest promise for this therapy, with sustained improvement in acne for up to 20 weeks after several treatments.

Several laser devices have been employed and studied in the treatment of acne. There are a few small studies evaluating the 1450-nm diode laser used to target and destroy sebaceous glands. Due to differences in treatment protocols and other allowed acne treatment, no comparisons can be made between studies.

The clinical development of optical therapies is also limited by adverse effects, including pain, erythema, edema, crusting, hyperpigmentation, and pustular eruptions. These therapies are not included among first-line treatments, especially with current high costs.

Barbieri JS, Spaccarelli N, Margolis DJ, James WD. Approaches to limit systemic antibiotic use in acne: systemic alternatives, emerging topical therapies, dietary modification, and laser and light-based treatments. *J Am Acad Dermatol.* 2019;80:538–549.
Posadzki P, Car J. Light therapies for acne. *JAMA Dermatol.* 2018;154:597–598.

19. What about complementary and alternative medications?

The use of complementary and alternative medications (CAMs) in acne is widespread, and there is a growing public demand for the application of CAMs to acne. Tea tree oil (TTO) is an essential oil and has a minimum content of terpinen-4-ol that exhibits strong antimicrobial and anti inflammatory properties. TTO has been reported to have broad-spectrum antimicrobial activity against bacterial, viral, fungal, and protozoal infections affecting skin and mucosa. When compared to 5% BPO, the effect of TTO was about the same but had slower onset of action. Several studies have suggested the uses of TTO for the treatment of acne vulgaris, seborrheic dermatitis, and chronic gingivitis. Other agents include spearmint herbal tea that has antiandrogenic properties in the management of polycystic ovarian syndrome; red reishi, which has been shown to reduce levels of 5-α reductase, the enzyme that facilitates conversion of testosterone to DHT; licorice, which has phytoestrogen effects and reduces testosterone levels; Chinese peony, which promotes the aromatization of testosterone into estrogen; and green tea, which contains epigallocatechins and also inhibits 5-α reductase, thereby reducing the conversion of normal testosterone into the more potent DHT. Zinc gluconate has been proven to be efficient at treating inflammatory dermatoses, such as acne vulgaris.

Cannabinoids are becoming increasingly available to patients, with reports of some using cannabinoid oils or creams for topical acne treatment. There are no strong data to suggest that these products are efficacious in acne treatment, although they may demonstrate in vitro antimicrobial and/or anti inflammatory properties.

Grant P. Spearmint herbal tea has significant anti-androgen effects in polycystic ovarian syndrome. A randomized controlled trial. *Phytother Res.* 2010;24:186–188.
Pazyar N, Yaghoobi R, Bagherani N, et al. A review of applications of tea tree oil in dermatology. *Int J Dermatol.* 2013;52:784–790.
Poiraud C, Quereux G, Knol AC, et al. Human β-defensin-2 and psoriasin, two new innate immunity targets of zinc gluconate. *Eur J Dermatol.* 2012;22:634–639.
Eagleston LRM, Kalani NK, Patel RR, et al. Cannabinoids in dermatology: a scoping review. *Dermatol Online J.* 2018;24(6).

20. What is SAPHO syndrome?

This is the acronym for a syndrome that includes **s**ynovitis, **a**cne, **p**ustulosis, **h**yperostosis, and **o**steitis. It is a disorder characterized by noninfectious osteoarticular inflammatory lesions and a variety of skin abnormalities demonstrating aseptic, neutrophil-rich pseudoabscesses. In adults, chronic multifocal osteomyelitis is a classic manifestation. Skin findings include palmoplantar or other forms of pustulosis, severe acne, or psoriasis. The acne associated with this syndrome is most often acne conglobata, with highly inflammatory comedones, nodules, abscesses, and draining sinuses located primarily on the trunk, which often heal with significant scarring. The etiology of this syndrome remains unclear but infectious, immunologic, and genetic factors are involved.

Kundu BK, Naik AK, Bhargava S, et al. Diagnosing the SAPHO syndrome: a report of three cases and review of the literature. *Clin Rheumatol.* 2013;32:1237–1243.

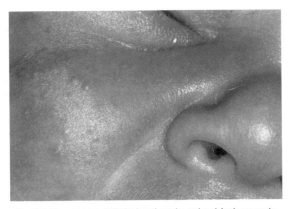

Fig. 21.3 Neonatal acne. Follicular-based papules and pustules in a neonate.

21. **Is there a difference between neonatal acne and infantile acne?**
Yes. Neonatal acne occurs in up to 20% of newborns; it usually develops during weeks 2 to 4 of life (Fig. 21.3). It is more common in males, is relatively mild, and regresses spontaneously in most infants by age 6 months. It is thought to be due to maternal androgens and is not associated with significant scarring or an increased incidence of acne in later life. Infantile acne usually begins between the third and sixth months of life and may persist to age 5 and rarely longer. It can be severe, with nodules, cysts, and significant residual scarring. Endocrine abnormalities and virilizing tumors can be associated. Some studies show an increased incidence of severe acne in later life.

22. **What is neonatal cephalic pustulosis?**
This is a recently recognized entity that may have been labeled in the past as neonatal acne. It appears during the first few days of life in both males and females with erythema, pustules, or papules mainly on the head and neck. It is thought to be an inflammatory reaction to *Malassezia* spp. The monomorphic appearance, absence of comedones, and the lack of a follicular distribution distinguish this entity from neonatal acne. It resolves spontaneously within 1 week.

23. **What is perioral dermatitis?**
This common distinctive acneiform skin eruption occurs mainly in women aged 15 to 25 years, but also occurs in children. Perioral dermatitis is characterized by erythema, scaling, and follicular papules that occur around the mouth, nose, and, less frequently, the eyes (Fig. 21.4). The etiology is unknown, but many patients have used mid- or high-potency topical steroids inappropriately. In one study, 20% of children with perioral dermatitis had a family history of rosacea. The treatment includes the cessation of all topical corticosteroids and an 8- to 10-week course of a tetracycline antibiotic. Tetracycline and derivatives should not be used in children under 8 years of age. Oral erythromycin and topical clindamycin are effective substitutes. Recurrences are rare.

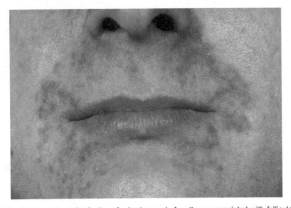

Fig. 21.4 Perioral dermatitis. Classic perioral distribution of a background of erythema associated with follicular-based papules and pustules. (Courtesy Fitzsimons Army Medical Center teaching files.)

Table 21.2 Drugs that cause or aggravate acne	
Steroid Hormones	Halogens
Topical corticosteroids	Iodides
Systemic corticosteroids	Bromides
Anabolic steroids	Halogenated hydrocarbons
Some progestins	Antituberculous Drugs
Testosterone	Isoniazid
Antidepressants	Miscellaneous Drugs
Lithium	Thiourea
Amineptine	Thiouracil
Antiepileptic drugs	PUVA
Phenytoin	
Trimethadione	

PUVA, Psoralen plus ultraviolet light, type A.

24. Do any drugs cause or aggravate acne?
    A wide range of drugs have been reported to cause or aggravate acne, although many of these associations are isolated case reports (Table 21.2).

25. How does steroid acne differ from acne vulgaris?
    Steroid acne has a sudden onset, the lesions are monomorphic (all lesions at the same stage of development), and comedones are absent. It occurs primarily on the upper trunk, less frequently on the face, and clears when the drug is withdrawn.

26. What is pyoderma faciale?
    This is an acute, ferocious skin disease of women aged 15 to 40. It strikes like a hurricane, often in patients with no previous history of acne. It most commonly involves the central face but may affect the upper trunk. It is characterized by severe pustules, nodules, cysts, and draining sinus tracts (Fig. 21.5). Many of the patients have a history of flushing, and some authors regard it as a severe variant of acne rosacea. It has been reported in some patients during pregnancy or immediately postpartum.

27. How do you treat pyoderma faciale?
    This is one of the few times that oral steroids should be used to treat acne. Prednisone in a dose of 40 to 60 mg daily tapered over 3 to 4 weeks is indicated. Isotretinoin should be started in a dose of 1 mg/kg/day in conjunction with the prednisone and continued for 4 to 6 months. Once the disease has been brought under control, it rarely, if ever, recurs.

Fender AB, Ignatovich Y, Mercurio MG. Pyoderma faciale. *Cutis.* 2008;81:488–490.

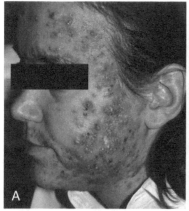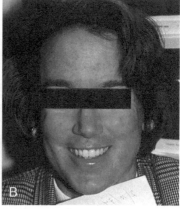

Fig. 21.5 Pyoderma faciale. **A,** This fulminant eruption developed when the patient was tapered off systemic corticosteroids. **B,** Same patient after treatment with a tapered course of prednisone and Accutane. The eruption did not recur.

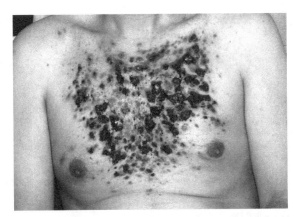

Fig. 21.6 Acne fulminans. Severe acne of the chest of a young male demonstrating the rapid onset of pustules, cysts, and hemorrhage. (Courtesy John L. Aeling, MD Collection.)

28. **What is acne fulminans?**
    This rare systemic disease is seen predominately in young men. Its clinical features include fever, polyarthritis, leukocytosis, malaise, weight loss, anorexia, and severe, acute cystic, and often ulcerative acne lesions. It occurs primarily on the upper trunk, but lesions may also be seen on the buttocks, proximal extremities, neck, and face (Fig. 21.6). The etiology is unknown, but it is thought to be immunologically mediated. It has been described in young men, particularly soldiers, who are introduced into a tropical environment where they are exposed to high humidity, temperature, and the friction of wearing a backpack. Like pyoderma faciale, it usually responds to treatment with isotretinoin and oral prednisone.

29. **What is hidradenitis suppurativa (HS)?**
    Hidradenitis is a chronic, suppurative, recurring inflammatory disease that affects apocrine gland–bearing sites. The axilla and groin are most frequently involved, but the disease is also seen on the perineum, buttocks, neck, and scalp (Fig. 21.7). It is more common in females and begins after puberty. Physical findings include inflammatory nodules, abscesses, scarring, and sinus tract formation. The Hurley classification system divides HS into three stages: stage I (abscess formation [single or multiple] without sinus tracts or cicatrization), stage II (recurrent abscesses with

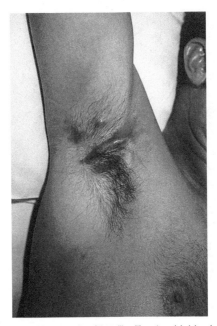

Fig. 21.7 Hidradenitis suppurativa of the axilla with cysts and draining sinus tracts.

track formation and cicatrization [single or multiple widely separated lesions]), or stage III (diffuse or near-diffuse involvement or multiple interconnected tracts and abscesses across the entire area).

30. **How do you treat HS?**

This frustrating chronic disease is treated by measures that reduce friction and moisture. Weight reduction, loose undergarments, topical antiseptic soaps, and topical aluminum chloride are helpful in some patients. There is fair evidence to support the use of both topical and systemic antibiotics in HS as first-line therapy. Topical clindamycin 1%, lotion or solution, for stage I is an excellent initial treatment in patients with early disease. Zinc gluconate (90 mg) once daily can be offered as an adjunctive treatment to patients. Systemic antibiotics are often used for stages II and III disease, with the combination of rifampicin and clindamycin being frequently used. Another study reported positive results with rifampicin-moxifloxacin-metronidazole combination therapy, but the long-term use of moxifloxacin is concerning. Dapsone has also been reported in two small series to be effective as a monotherapy at a dosage of 50 to 150 mg/day. There is fair evidence to support the use of biologic agents (such as infliximab or adalimumab) in the treatment of advanced HS (Hurley's stage II and III). Given the high cost of these therapies and potential adverse effect profile, they should be offered to patients with severe disease affecting their activities who have failed antibacterial therapy. It is appropriate to consider performing monthly therapy with neodymium:yttrium-aluminum-garnet (Nd:YAG) laser on the lesions. Carbon dioxide laser treatment is another viable option, showing some efficacy in clinical studies, that should be offered to patients.

Chronic inflammatory nodules can be treated with intralesional steroids. Systemic retinoids may help some patients but are not as effective as when used to treat severe acne vulgaris, and relapses are quite common.

Severe refractory hidradenitis is best treated by complete surgical excision of the involved area. Incision and drainage should be minimized because it often leads to chronic sinus tract formation.

Goldburg SR, Strober BE, Payette MJ. Part 1. Hidradenitis suppurativa: epidemiology, clinical presentation, and pathogenesis. *J Am Acad Dermatol.* 2019.
Goldburg SR, Strober BE, Payette MJ. Part 2. Current and emerging treatments for hidradenitis suppurativa. *J Am Acad Dermatol.* 2019.

31. **Discuss acne rosacea.**

Acne rosacea is a chronic skin disease that most commonly occurs between the ages of 30 and 50 years, although it can be seen in adolescents and elderly patients. The course is typically chronic with remissions and relapses. It is characterized by flushing, telangiectasia, papules, and pustules, and in severe late-stage disease, patients may develop chronic facial lymphedema and rhinophyma. It is usually symmetrical and is most commonly seen on the convex areas of the face, including the nose, cheeks, forehead, and chin (Fig. 21.8). Blepharitis, conjunctivitis, and keratitis are common associations.

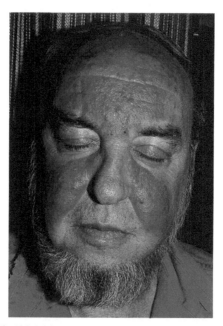

Fig. 21.8 Acne rosacea involving the convex surfaces of the face.

The etiology of rosacea is unknown. Genetic factors seem to play a role in that the disease is more common in persons of Celtic ancestry and less common in blacks. There are also factors that stimulate flushing, such as hot beverages, eating chocolate, nuts, spicy foods, and cheese, taking some medications, sun exposure, hot and cold weather, wind, humidity, indoor heat, certain cleansers, moisturizers, cosmetics, and physical and emotional stress. Menstruation and pregnancy can also exacerbate rosacea. It is thought to be due to hormonal fluctuations that increase cutaneous vascularity. A rosacea-like eruption can be induced by the topical application of fluorinated corticosteroids and tacrolimus ointment to the face. *Demodex* mites are found in very large numbers in the general population: with recent sensitive techniques the prevalence approaches almost 100% among rosacea patients. Proteins from this organism have the potential to induce an immune response in patients with rosacea.

Wang YA, James WD. Update on rosacea classification and its controversies. *Cutis.* 2019;104:70–73.

32. How is acne rosacea treated?

Trigger factors that produce flushing should be avoided. These triggers vary greatly from patient to patient. Avoiding sun exposure and sunscreens are of central importance to rosacea management. Both oral metronidazole and topical metronidazole are effective. Topical erythromycin, BPO, and clindamycin, azelaic acid cream, and sodium sulfacetamide have also been shown to be effective treatments. Other topical therapies include the calcineurin inhibitors tacrolimus and pimecrolimus for the papulopustular rosacea. Permethrin 5% may target *Demodex* mites. Recent case reports and small series have shown that the topical use of an alpha-1 agonist (oxymetazoline 0.05% solution) or an alpha-2 agonist (brimonidine tartrate) resulted in durable improvement in erytheam, flushing, and stinging. Tetracycline, doxycycline, minocycline, and erythromycin are effective systemic therapies for rosacea. Sub-antimicrobial doses of doxycycline (40-mg extended release tablet) have been shown to decrease papulopustules in rosacea via anti inflammatory effects. Combined with topical azelaic acid or metronidazole, there seems to be a synergistic effect. Oral isotretinoin is helpful for severe resistant cases, but the drug is not as effective as when used for severe cystic acne, and relapses are more common. It is effective both in erythematotelangiectatic and papulopustular rosacea. It is also the treatment of choice for granulomatous rosacea, rhinophyma, and rosacea fulminans. Oral antibiotics have little effect on flushing, telangiectasia, lymphedema, or rhinophyma (tetracyclines, macrolides, and metronidazole). Severe rhinophyma is best treated by surgical paring or electrosurgery. Vascular lasers and intense pulsed light sources prove to be highly effective treatments for ablation of telangiectasia and improving flushing and erythema.

33. What is Favre-Racouchot syndrome?

This describes the development of multiple open comedones located on the inferolateral aspect of the orbital rim in elderly patients. It is associated with marked solar elastosis of the surrounding skin.

CHAPTER 22

AUTOIMMUNE CONNECTIVE TISSUE DISEASES

Whitney A. High

1. Discuss the skin changes of lupus erythematosus.

Skin changes occur in about 855 of patients with lupus erythematosus (LE) and in this condition are second in frequency only to musculoskeletal complaints. Skin eruptions in LE may be categorized based upon diagnostic and prognostic significance. Skin lesions diagnostic of LE are called "lupus-specific eruptions." On biopsy, such lesions show characteristic histopathologic changes of cutaneous LE. In fact, it may be possible to subclassify the type of lupus present (discoid, tumid, subcutaneous, etc.) based upon the findings of a cutaneous biopsy.

However, lupus patients may also develop nonspecific skin changes (Table 22.1). These types of eruptions do not establish a diagnosis of LE but may have value in making an overall assessment of the connective tissue disease. For example, palpable purpura occurring in a patient with LE are not disease specific, as such lesions may occur in those without LE, yet the finding may point to concern for lupus-associated vasculitic disease of the kidney or central nervous system (CNS), and these data may be important in evaluation and management of the patient.

Kuhn A, Landmann A. The classification and diagnosis of cutaneous lupus erythematosus. *J Autoimmun.* 2014;49:14–19.

2. What is acute cutaneous lupus erythematosus (ACLE)?

ACLE presents as an acute malar rash or a more generalized photodistributed eruption. The term "butterfly rash" is used to characterize the malar rash because the rash upon the cheeks resembles the wings of a butterfly (Fig. 22.1). Nearly all patients presenting with ACLE will have systemic LE (SLE), often with an acute exacerbation. ACLE is typically transient, and it improves with the SLE improves, and it does not usually result in scarring.

3. Are there other common skin eruptions that can be confused with ACLE?

The differential diagnosis for erythematous conditions of the face includes rosacea, polymorphous light eruption, photoreactions to systemic medications or topical products, seborrheic dermatitis, tinea faciei, and certain types of porphyria (see Chapter 17). Rosacea can closely mimic ACLE, particularly for persons new to dermatology. Rosacea is both common and typically photoexacerbated. Additionally, nonspecific joint complaints are common, and 5% of the normal population will have a positive antinuclear antibody (ANA) test, and this can lead to misdiagnosis of ACLE. Remember, a patient with ACLE is most often experiencing an acute flare and will be "ill," whereas a rosacea patient will not typically be acute unwell. Also, seborrheic dermatitis is ubiquitous but often presents with waxy yellow scaling, erythema, and pruritus in the scalp, in the eyebrows, in the nasolabial folds, and the periauricular areas. Patients with seborrheic dermatitis are also not generally ill-appearing.

4. What is subacute cutaneous LE (SCLE)?

SCLE was first described and characterized in the late 1970s. Patients with SCLE have an eruption that is more persistent than that of ACLE, lasting weeks to months. The condition is most common in middle-aged white women. Lesions of SCLE consist of scaly, superficial, inflammatory macules, patches, papules, and plaques that are photodistributed, particularly on the upper chest and back, lateral neck, and dorsal arms and forearms. Several different morphologic types of SCLE have been described: annular, serpiginous, psoriasiform, and pityriasiform (Fig. 22.2). Some patients have lesions with more than one morphology. Nearly all patients with SCLE manifest anti-SSA (Ro) antibodies.

Many patients with SCLE will have four or more criteria for the classification of SLE, although most SCLE patients do not have serious renal or CNS LE. Typically, they have skin disease, photosensitivity, and musculoskeletal complaints. Dry eyes and dry mouth are also common. Some patients with SCLE experience severe manifestations of SLE, and thus, all SCLE patients should be monitored for systemic disease.

Alniemi DT, Gutierrez A, Drage LA, et al. Subacute cutaneous lupus erythematosus: clinical characteristics, disease associations, treatments, and outcomes in a series of 90 patients at Mayo Clinic, 1996–2011. *Mayo Clinic Proc.* 2017;92:406–414.

5. How do you make a diagnosis of SCLE?

SCLE is often diagnosed based upon a typical photodistributed eruption and a skin biopsy consistent with cutaneous LE. In further support of the diagnosis, nearly all patients with SCLE have anti-SSA (Ro) antibodies and less often

Table 22.1 Classification of cutaneous disease in lupus erythematosus

LUPUS-SPECIFIC ERUPTIONS	LUPUS-NONSPECIFIC ERUPTIONS
Acute cutaneous lupus erythematosus (ACLE)	Nonscarring alopecia
(Malar rash of lupus; macular or papular photodistributed eruption; lupus hairs)	Telangiectasia
Subacute cutaneous lupus erythematosus (SCLE)	Livedo reticularis and retiform
(Annular, serpiginous, psoriasiform, or pityriasiform)	purpura
Chronic cutaneous lupus erythematosus (CCLE)	Palpable purpura
(Discoid lupus erythematosus [DLE], hypertrophic DLE, tumid lupus	(leukocytoclastic vasculitis)
erythematosus [LE], chilblain LE, lupus mucinotic nodules)	Periungual erythema
Lupus panniculitis	Urticarial vasculitis
Bullous eruption of systemic lupus erythematosus (SLE)	Raynaud's syndrome
Neonatal lupus erythematosus (NLE)	Photosensitivity

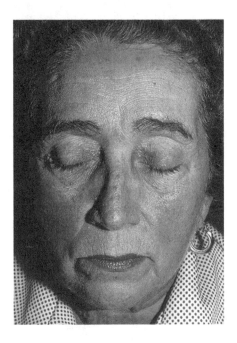

Fig. 22.1 Acute cutaneous lupus erythematosus. Note the classic malar erythema ("butterfly rash").

anti-SSB (La) antibodies. Direct immunofluorescence studies show granular deposition of immunoreactants at the dermoepidermal junction or particulate-like deposition in the lower epidermis. Such antibodies are not present in all patients with SCLE, and hence, the absence of these findings does not exclude this diagnosis. Additionally, a negative ANA does not exclude the diagnosis of SCLE, for some patients will have anti-SSA (Ro) in isolation.

6. What is the initial workup of SCLE?
   Once a diagnosis of SCLE is made, it is important to evaluate for the presence of SLE:
   - History and physical exam data should be culled to identify manifestations of SLE in other organ systems
   - Laboratory testing will often include a complete blood count with differential, urinalysis, basic serum chemistries (including renal function tests), liver function studies, and an ANA panel to include anti-SSA (Ro), anti-SSB (La), and anti-DNA antibodies. Complement determinations may be ordered, as some SCLE patients have partial or complete complement deficiencies
   - An increased risk of cancer has been associated with SCLE, so appropriate screening for various internal cancers such as breast cancer, lymphoma, respiratory cancer, and nonmelanoma skin cancer should be performed
   - A medication history is important, since SCLE may be triggered or worsened by a number of medications, especially thiazide diuretics, tumor necrosis factor-α blockers, terbinafine, angiotensin-converting enzyme inhibitors, proton pump inhibitors, and antiepileptics, among others (see Table 22.2).

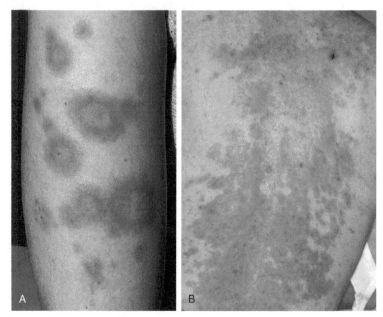

Fig. 22.2 Subacute cutaneous lupus erythematosus. **A,** Annular lesions on the upper arms. **B,** Erythematous papules and plaques on the back.

Table 22.2 Medications associated with subacute cutaneous lupus erythematosus
Adalimumab
Aldactone
Captopril
Cilazapril
Cinnarizine
Diltiazem
Docetaxel
Etanercept
Glyburide
Gold
Griseofulvin
Hydrochlorothiazide
Infliximab
Interferon-α, -β
Leflunomide
Naproxen
Nifedipine
Nitrendipine
Omeprazole
Oxprenolol
Penicillamine
Phenytoin
Piroxicam
Pravastatin
Procainamide
Ranitidine
Simvastatin
Spironolactone
Sulfonylureas
Taxotere
Terbinafine
Verapamil

7. How is SCLE managed?

Cutaneous complaints are often of most concern to patients with SCLE, and hence, dermatologists are often the physicians managing the disease. Because the disease is driven the sunlight exposure, photoprotective measures, such as broad-spectrum sunscreens, protective clothing, and lifestyle modification are important measures. Cutaneous lesions may respond to potent topical steroids or topical calcineurin inhibitors. Often, oral antimalarial therapy is the most beneficial, but it has a slow onset. Other treatments less frequently employed include dapsone, retinoids, systemic steroids, methotrexate, mycophenolate, azathioprine, and rarely thalidomide, clofazamine, intravenous immune globulin, and rituximab.

8. What is chronic cutaneous LE?

Several types of cutaneous LE that are persistent are termed *chronic cutaneous LE*. Discoid LE (DLE) is the most common of these chronic forms. DLE typically presents on the head and neck with thick keratotic scale and "triphasic" coloration. Scarring quickly results from DLE. Tumid LE has minimal scale and epidermal changes and consists chiefly of erythematous lesions caused by mucin accumulation in the underlying dermis. Lupus panniculitis and nodular cutaneous lupus mucinosis represent other forms of chronic cutaneous LE.

9. Describe the skin changes of DLE.

DLE consists of fixed, indurated, erythematous papules and plaques that are photodistributed and are particularly common on the head and neck, although any cutaneous region can be affected (Fig. 22.3A). Without intervention, DLE lesions can last for years and may produce extensive scarring. When DLE involves the scalp, permanent scarring alopecia may result. Pigmentary changes (both hyperpigmentation and hypopigmentation) are often seen with DLE. Epidermal changes, including scale, keratotic plugging of the hair follicles, and sometimes crusting, are typically present. The external ears, and particularly the conchal bowls, are often involved in DLE (Fig. 22.3B), and this area always be examined in patients with suspected DLE.

10. Do patients with DLE develop SLE?

If the initial workup of a patient with localized lesions of DLE does not reveal evidence of SLE, the risk of developing SLE is about 5%. If lesions are generalized, the risk of systemic disease may be slightly higher. However, DLE lesions are not uncommon in patients with a known diagnosis of SLE. About 25% of patients with SLE patients will develop DLE lesions in the course of their disease (Table 22.3).

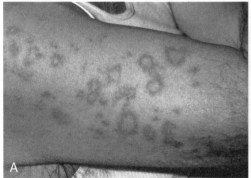 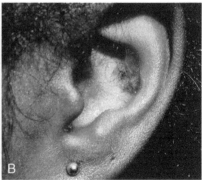

Fig. 22.3 Discoid lupus erythematosus (DLE). **A,** Fixed, erythematous, scaly discoid plaques of DLE with central atrophy on the upper arms. *(Courtesy John L. Aeling, MD Collection.)* **B,** DLE lesion in the concha of the ear. Hypopigmented and hyperpigmented areas, erythema, and scarring are present

Table 22.3 Comparison of lupus-specific eruptions

DISEASE	DURATION	% OF PATIENTS WITH SLE	PHOTOSENSITIVE
ACLE	Hours–weeks	99%	Yes
SCLE	Weeks–months	50%	Yes
CCLE	Months–years	5%	50%

ACLE, Acute cutaneous lupus erythematosus; *CCLE,* chronic cutaneous lupus erythematosus; *SCLE,* subacute cutaneous lupus erythematosus.

11. How is DLE treated?

As with other types of cutaneous LE, sunscreens and photoprotective measures are central to management. Potent topical steroids and intralesional corticosteroids are often helpful. Antimalarial drugs are often employed to attain disease control. Systemic therapy with other medications (see Question 8) is required for recalcitrant disease. Smoking cessation is important.

Garza-Mayers AC, McClurkin M, Smith GP. Review of treatment for discoid lupus erythematosus. *Dermatol Ther.* 2016;29:274–283.

12. What is minocycline-induced lupus?

This condition has been reported in patients taking minocycline for acne, usually for prolonged durations. Most patients are young women. The most common symptom of the disease is symmetric polyarthralgia, but fatigue, fever, elevated liver enzymes, pneumonitis, and anemia have also been reported. Other dermatological manifestation may include a malar rash, livedo reticularis, oral ulcerations, subcutaneous nodules, and alopecia. Nearly all patients will have a positive ANA serologic test, and many will have a positive perinuclear pattern of antineutrophil cytoplasmic antibodies, while antihistone antibodies are often negative. Once minocycline is discontinued, most patients have resolution of symptoms.

13. What is lupus panniculitis?

Lupus panniculitis is a rare variant of LE that may exist as a separate disease or it may coexist with SLE or DLE. When lupus panniculitis is accompanied by DLE, this may be referred to as lupus profundus. Regardless, as the inflammation of lupus panniculitis involves the subcutaneous tissue, the nodules are deeply situated, but may resolve as depressed scars. Lesions tend to favor the proximal extremities and trunk, and this is different from most other forms of panniculitis, which are more distal. About one-half of patients with lupus panniculitis have four or more criteria for the classification of SLE. The diagnosis is confirmed by a deep excisional biopsy, to include fat. Shallow biopsies will not be diagnostic. Subcutaneous panniculitis-like T-cell lymphoma has some clinical and histologic overlap with lupus panniculitis, and it may be difficult to discriminate between the entities. The treatment of choice for lupus panniculitis is antimalarial drugs or sometimes systemic steroids.

Morita TCAB, Trés GFS, García MSC, et al. Panniculitides of particular interest to the rheumatologist. *Adv Rheumatol.* 2019;59:35.

14. Describe the bullous eruption of SLE.

Bullous LE is a rare clinical presentation that occurs most often in patients with an already established diagnosis of SLE. The condition usually affects young women and it involves sun-exposed and nonexposed skin. Lesions appear as tense bullae on an erythematous base. There is predilection for face, upper trunk, and proximal extremities. Biopsies demonstrate subepidermal vesiculation with a neutrophil-rich inflammatory infiltrate. Antibodies to type VII collagen, a component of anchoring fibrils (see Chapter 1), are present in most patients with bullous SLE.

15. How is the bullous eruption of SLE treated?

Most reported cases of bullous SLE have respond rapidly to dapsone, and experts advocate use of this drug, unless it is contraindicated. Response to corticosteroids and other immunosuppressive drugs has been variable. Refractory cases have been treated with rituximab.

16. What is neonatal LE (NLE)?

In NLE, infants develop skin disease (50%), heart disease (50%), or both (10%). Skin lesions occur most often on the face and head, particularly around the eyes ("raccoon eyes") (Fig. 22.4). Skin lesions are transient, resolving over a few months, but rarely, atrophic scarring occurs. Heart disease usually manifests as isolated complete heart block, although lesser degrees of heart block have been reported, in addition to structural defects and cardiomyopathy. The heart block is often permanent and may require a pacemaker. About 10% to 20% of infants with NLE and heart disease die of cardiac complications. A few infants with NLE also have hematologic abnormalities and/or hepatobiliary disease. Nearly all infants with NLE, and their mothers, have anti-SSA (Ro) antibodies, and some have anti-SSB (La) antibodies. A few NLE patients/mothers may have anti-U1RNP antibodies instead. Cases caused by anti-U1RNP antibodies had typical cutaneous findings but did not develop heart block. NLE antibodies in babies are of maternal origin, transferred via the placenta, and are transient.

High WA, Costner MI. Persistent scarring, atrophy, and dyspigmentation in a preteen girl with neonatal lupus erythematosus. *J Am Acad Dermatol.* 2003;48:626–628.

17. Which tests should be done in an infant with suspected NLE?

When NLE is suspected, serologic testing for autoantibodies should be performed on the infant and mother. Specifically for anti-SSA (Ro), anti-SSB (La), and anti-U1RNP antibodies should be assayed. Skin biopsies for routine histology and direct immunofluorescence may be useful. Biopsies show histologic features and direct immunofluorescence features similar to SCLE.

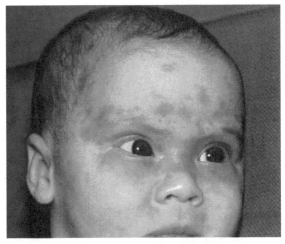

Fig. 22.4 Neonatal lupus erythematosus demonstrating sharply defined erythema of the scalp and face. Periocular involvement producing a "raccoon eyes" appearance is common and is strongly suggestive of the diagnosis. (Courtesy Fitzsimons Army Medical Center teaching files.)

18. **Once a diagnosis of NLE is made, what workup should be done?**

    A physical examination should be performed, but electrocardiogram testing and cardiac ultrasound are important. Because of possible involvement of the liver and decreased platelets, liver function tests and a platelet count should occur. Additional tests or procedures may be dictated based on the findings of physical exam and testing. Mothers of infants with NLE should be worked up as well, as some either have or will develop SCLE, SLE, or Sjögren's syndrome.

19. **What is a lupus band test?**

    Direct immunofluorescence testing performed on lesional skin or nonlesional (normal) skin may reveal deposits of immunoglobulins and complement is a bandlike pattern at the dermal–epidermal junction that is referred to as a "lupus band" (Fig. 22.5). When the pattern is seen in lesional skin, it supports a diagnosis of cutaneous LE. When found in nonlesional skin, it is suggestive of SLE. There are rare causes of a "false-positive" lupus band.

    Mehta V, Sarda A, Balachandran C. Lupus band test. *Indian J Dermatol Venereol Leprol.* 2010;76:298–300.

20. **What is scleroderma?**

    Scleroderma is a sclerosing disorder of the soft tissue yields thickened, nonpliable skin. It may be localized, as in morphea ("localized scleroderma"), or more limited, or even generalized, involving even visceral organs ("progressive systemic sclerosis"). In morphea, sclerotic, indurated plaques develop that may be solitary, multiple, linear, or

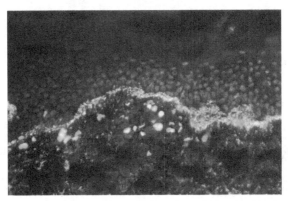

Fig. 22.5 Lupus band test. Linear granular bandlike deposition of C1q at the junction between the epidermis and dermis in a patient with discoid lupus erythematosus. (Courtesy Fitzsimons Army Medical Center teaching files.)

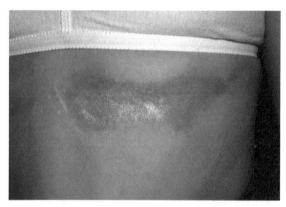

Fig. 22.6 Typical well-developed lesion of morphea demonstrating an indurated plaque with both lighter areas and brownish discoloration. This lesion was very firm to palpation. (Courtesy Fitzsimons Army Medical Center teaching files.)

generalized. The surface of morphea plaques is smooth, with the center of the lesion a whitish to brown color (Fig. 22.6), and in active lesions, the border is often violaceous ("lilac erythema"). Morphea usually involves the skin and subcutaneous tissues but may involve deeper structures, even bone. Patients with morphea **do not** develop visceral involvement, and for this reason, many dermatologists still prefer to use the term "morphea" over "localized scleroderma."

21. What is limited scleroderma (formerly CREST syndrome)?

What is referred to now as "limited scleroderma" was once referred to as CREST syndrome. One advantage of the older nosology was that it served as a mnemonic for recalling the major manifestations of the disease:
- **C**—calcinosis cutis
- **R**—Raynaud phenomenon
- **E**—esophageal dysfunction (or dysmotility)
- **S**—sclerodactyly
- **T**—telangiectasias

In addition to these findings, patients often develop hyperpigmentation, particularly in sun-exposed areas (Fig. 22.7). Anticentromere antibodies are also typically present in these patients.

22. Describe the early cutaneous findings in progressive systemic sclerosis (PSS).

Early cutaneous complaints of PSS are swelling of the hands and feet, often associated with Raynaud phenomenon. Telangiectasias may develop in the course of disease. The vasculature of the proximal nail fold is often affected, and

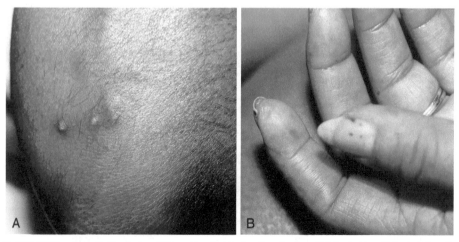

Fig. 22.7 CREST syndrome. **A,** Firm, tender, whitish papules of calcinosis cutis on the elbow. **B,** Sclerodactyly and telangiectasia on the fingers.

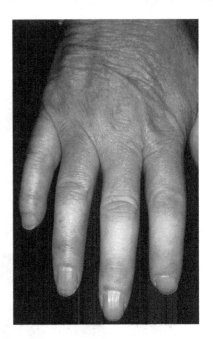

Fig. 22.8 Progressive systemic sclerosis. Characteristic sclerodactyly manifesting as tight, shiny, thickened skin. (Courtesy James E. Fitzpatrick, MD.)

this may include avascular areas (dropout) and marked dilatation of vessels. Over time, the skin of the digits becomes thickened and sclerotic ("sausage digits") (Fig. 22.8). It is increasingly difficult to "tent up" the skin on the dorsum of the digits. Sclerotic changes are often progressive, involving the face and extremities, and may eventually involve large areas of the body. Other later cutaneous manifestations include digital ulcers and necrosis of the digits.

23. **What is dermatomyositis?**
   Dermatomyositis is a disease of unknown etiology that causes inflammation of the skin and, often, skeletal muscles. Polymyositis is a term used for inflammation of skeletal muscles without cutaneous involvement. The muscle involvement usually presents as proximal muscle weakness, sometimes with pain, and later with muscle atrophy. Muscle involvement may precede, follow, or occur simultaneously with skin disease and, in some instances, may not be detectable. The latter is referred to as *amyopathic dermatomyositis*, and approximately 20% of cases present in this fashion. Cutaneous findings include a descending erythematous to violaceous rash, heliotrope (lilac-colored rash) of the eyelids, purpuric papules and plaques on overlying small joints of the hand ("Gottron papules), poikilodermatous changes, and calcinosis cutis.

Euwer RL, Sontheimer RD. Amyopathic dermatomyositis (dermatomyositis siné myositis): presentation of six new cases and review of the literature. *J Am Acad Dermatol.* 1991;24:959–966.

24. **Are there skin changes diagnostic of dermatomyositis?**
   There are three pathognomonic skin findings in dermatomyositis that are worthy of specific mention: heliotrope rash, Gottron papules, and Gottron sign. Heliotrope rash is a lilac-colored erythema of the eyelids, particularly the superior lid (Fig. 22.9A). Gottron papules are erythematous to purplish flat-topped papules on the skin overlying the interphalangeal joints of the hand. Gottron sign consists of symmetrical violaceous erythema, sometimes with edema, over the dorsal knuckles of the hands, elbows, knees, and medial ankles (Fig. 22.9B). Other skin findings seen in dermatomyositis are periungual telangiectasias with "ragged" cuticles and a photodistributed violaceous erythema of the forehead and sun-exposed areas of the neck, upper chest, shoulders, dorsal arms, forearms, and hands. In contrast to Gottron papules, lupus may cause erythema over the proximal dorsal phalanges, but typically, lupus spares the knuckles.

DeWane ME, Waldman R, Lu J. Dermatomyositis part I: clinical features and pathogenesis. *J Am Acad Dermatol.* 2019. doi:10.1016/j.jaad.2019.06.1309.

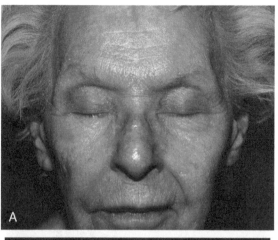

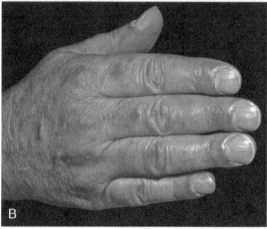

Fig. 22.9 Dermatomyositis. **A,** Characteristic heliotrope of the upper eyelids. *(Courtesy John L. Aeling, MD Collection.)* **B,** Gottron's papules over the knuckles. *(Courtesy Fitzsimons Army Medical Center teaching files.)*

KEY POINTS: DERMATOMYOSITIS

1. Gottron papules (erythematous to violaceous papules over the knuckles) are a cutaneous finding that is pathognomonic of dermatomyositis.
2. Patients with dermatomyositis frequently demonstrate lilac-tinged erythema of the upper eyelids that is referred to as heliotrope rash.
3. Amyopathic dermatomyositis is the presence of cutaneous findings of dermatomyositis without evidence of muscle involvement.
4. Between 10% and 50% of adult patients who present with dermatomyositis have an underlying malignancy.

25. What methods exist to assist in the diagnosis of dermatomyositis?
    - Skin biopsy may be helpful, although the findings in dermatomyositis overlap with other forms of connective tissue disease, such as cutaneous LE.
    - Muscle enzyme levels are often abnormal in dermatomyositis (except for amyopathic forms). An elevated creatine kinase is the most sensitive and specific muscle enzyme, but an aldolase test may also reveal abnormal results. Liver enzymes (aspartate aminotransferase and alanine transaminase) may be elevated but are nonspecific findings.

- Sometimes, elevation of muscle enzymes precedes clinically appreciable myositis. Ergo, if a patient who was previously without lab abnormalities develops elevation of muscle enzymes on repeat testing, the clinician should reassess for clinically apparent muscle disease.
- Other serologic abnormalities have been identified and may be subclassifying disease, but they are not used for routine diagnosis. These myositis-specific antibodies (MSAs) occur in about 30% of all patients with dermatomyositis or polymyositis (see below).
- Biopsy of an affected muscle may be useful, and magnetic resonance imaging (MRI) can prove useful in identifying muscle groups of high-yield for muscle biopsy. In fact, sometimes MRI findings may be so supportive of the diagnosis that a muscle biopsy is not necessary.

26. Are any other diseases associated with dermatomyositis?

In adults, up to 20% of dermatomyositis can be a paraneoplastic phenomenon, with the disease tracking to the clinical course of the cancer. This risk of paraneoplastic disease is highest in men and in those over 45 at the time of diagnosis. Screening with a careful history, physical examination, and age-appropriate laboratory screening tests is recommended in adult patients with dermatomyositis. Paraneoplastic DM is more common in adults with anti-TIF1 or anti-NXP2 antibodies (see below). The most common cancers associated with dermatomyositis include breast cancer, lung cancer, ovarian cancer, gastrointestinal cancer, nasopharyngeal cancer, pancreatic cancer, bladder cancer, and Hodgkin's lymphoma.

27. What is anti-synthetase syndrome?

Anti-synthetase syndrome is seen in polymyositis and dermatomyositis and it is associated with the anti-aminoacyl-tRNA synthetase autoantibodies: anti–Jo-1 antibody (most common), in addition to anti-PL7, -PL12, -OJ, -EJ, -KS, -Zo, and -Ha autoantibodies. In addition to typical skin and muscle involvement, patients with anti-synthetase syndrome may develop arthritis, Raynaud syndrome, and interstitial lung disease. **"Mechanic's hands"** is a finding often attributed to anti-synthetase syndrome, but perhaps not unique to only that disease. It refers to roughening and cracking of the skin of the fingers/fingertips that result in an irregular, dirty appearance, likened to the hands of a manual laborer.

Concha JSS, Merola JF, Fiorentino D, Werth VP. Re-examining mechanic's hands as a characteristic skin finding in dermatomyositis. J Am Acad Dermatol. 2018;78:769–775.

28. What are myositis-specific antibodies (MSAs)?

MSAs are antibodies associated with inflammatory myopathies, including dermatomyositis. These antibodies are not present in all cases of dermatomyositis, and even different clinically available testing modalities vary in sensitivity and specificity for these antibodies.

- **Anti-Mi-2**—antibodies against a nuclear DNA helicase. Patients with these antibodies often present with "classic" features of dermatomyositis and mild myopathy. These antibodies generally portend a favorable prognosis.
- **Anti-TIF1**—antibodies to a tumor suppressor protein. Adult patients with these antibodies have a higher rate of paraneoplastic dermatomyositis.
- **Anti-MDA5**—antibodies to a RNA-specific helicase. Patients with this antibody are more likely to have interstitial lung disease, which can be rapidly progressive.
- **Anti-NXP2**—antibodies to a protein involved in regulating transcription and RNA metabolism. Adults with anti-NXP2 have an elevated risk of paraneoplastic disease. Children with this antibody may have more severe disease and more calcinosis.
- **Anti-SAE**—antibodies to **S**mall ubiquitin-like modifier **A**ctivating **E**nzyme. Patients with this antibody present with more severe cutaneous disease but more minimal myopathy.

29. What is an overlap syndrome?

Many patients diagnosed with connective tissue disease maintain features that are difficult to fit into one clinical entity, such as SLE, dermatomyositis, or systemic sclerosis. "Overlap syndrome" is useful, for descriptive purposes, when a person has "overlapping" features of more than one clinically recognized connective tissue disease.

30. What is mixed connective tissue disease?

Contrary to the above, mixed connective tissue disease (MCTD) is a specific disorder characterized by a mixture of well-defined connective tissue disorders, such as SLE, PSS, dermatomyositis, and even Sjögren's syndrome, **BUT patients with MCTD have anti-U1RNP ribonuclear protein (U1RNP) antibodies**. Patients with MCTD present with Raynaud phenomenon, swollen digits (dactylitis), and arthritis. Patients may develop myositis, sclerodermoid lesions of the skin, and sclerodactyly. Interstitial lung disease and renal disease may also ensue.

Dima A, Jurcut C, Baicus C. The impact of anti-U1-RNP positivity: systemic lupus erythematosus versus mixed connective tissue disease. Rheumatol Int. 2018;38:1169–1178.

31. What is antiphospholipid antibody syndrome?

Antiphospholipid antibody syndrome (APS) is an autoimmune disease where antiphospholipid autoantibodies in the blood lead to a coagulopathy with dangerous clotting in arteries and veins. APS affects women five times more often than men, and it is typically diagnosed in the third and fourth decades of life. While up to 40% of patients with SLE have antiphospholipid autoantibodies, when tested, only half of these persons will develop thrombosis and/or miscarriages. Cutaneous findings include livedo reticularis, retiform purpura, ulcerations, deep venous thrombosis, or superficial thrombophlebitis. "Sneddon syndrome" is livedo reticularis/retiform purpura associated with cerebrovascular disease. Catastrophic APS (CAPS) is a severe form of disease with multiple organ systems involved over a short period. Typically, CAPS involves the CNS, lungs, kidneys, gastrointestinal tract, and skin, and it can be fatal.

32. What are some forms of connective tissue disease with cutaneous manifestations?

- **Autoimmune urticaria:** May affect up to 30% or more of chronic idiopathic urticaria patients (defined as >6 weeks of urticaria) with associated autoantibodies to the high-affinity IgE receptor or, less frequently, against IgE.
- **Juvenile idiopathic arthritis:** High episodic fever daily for 2 weeks with symmetrical polyarthritis or oligoarthritis, as well as one of the following: exanthem, generalized adenopathy, hepatosplenomegaly, serositis, elevated ferritin.
- **Adult-onset Still disease:** Recurrent episodes of high spiking fevers, frequently in the late afternoon, with quickly appearing and disappearing (evanescent) salmon-pink exanthem, arthritis with subsequent carpal ankylosis, and elevated ferritin.
- **Sjögren's syndrome:** Xerostomia and xerophthalmia, arthritis; petechiae and purpura, urticarial vasculitis, and annular erythema.
- **Relapsing polychondritis:** Inflammation of the cartilaginous portions of the ears and nose, that may lead to deformed ears or a saddle-nose. Acute involvement of the tracheal cartilage may airway collapse. Arthritis most often involves the costochondral joints. Other manifestations include audiovestibular damage, heart valve disease, and neurologic, ocular, and renal disease. Patients may die of rupture of the chordae tendineae of the heart valves.
- **Rheumatoid arthritis:** Patients present with arthritis. Cutaneous manifestations include rheumatoid nodules, rheumatoid neutrophilic dermatitis, palisaded neutrophilic and granulomatous dermatitis, leukocytoclastic vasculitis, and pyoderma gangrenosum.

33. What autoantibodies are associated with autoimmune connective tissue diseases?

See Tables 22.4, 22.5, and 22.6.

Sheldon J. Laboratory testing in autoimmune rheumatic diseases. *Best Pract Res Clin Rheumatol.* 2004;18:249–269.

Table 22.4 Autoantibodies associated with lupus erythematosus

AUTOANTIBODY	PREVALENCE	TARGET	CLINICAL ASSOCIATIONS
High Specificity for SLE			
dsDNA	50%–80%	Double-stranded (native) DNA	LE nephritis; useful in monitoring activity of SLE
Sm	15%–20%	Spliceosome	Highly specific for SLE
rRNP	30%–40%	Ribosomal P proteins	Neuropsychiatric LE
Low Specificity for SLE			
ANA	95%–98%		Most common IF patterns: homogeneous, peripheral
ssDNA	70%	Denatured DNA	Possible risk for SLE in DLE patients; also seen in RA, DM/PM, MCTD, SS, SjS, localized scleroderma
C1q	60%	C1q component of complement	Severe SLE, hypocomplementemic urticarial vasculitis
U1RNP	50%	Spliceosome RNP	Overlapping features with other CTD; MCTD (100%)

Table 22.4 Autoantibodies associated with lupus erythematosus (*continued*)

AUTOANTIBODY	PREVALENCE	TARGET	CLINICAL ASSOCIATIONS
Ro (SSA)	30%–90%	hYRNA/RNP complexes (targets misfolded RNA molecules for destruction)	SCLE (75%–90%), neonatal LE/congenital heart block (99%), SCLE-SjS overlap, SjS
Cardiolipin	50%	Cardiolipin, a negatively charged phospholipid	Arterial and venous thrombosis and recurrent spontaneous abortions, thrombocytopenia (cutaneous manifestations include livedo reticularis, retiform purpura, skin ulcers)
Histones	40%–70%	Histones	Drug-induced SLE, RA
β_2 glycoprotein I	25%	Polypeptide on endothelial cells, hepatocytes, and trophoblast cells; interacts with phospholipids	High risk of thrombosis in SLE and primary antiphospholipid antibody syndrome (95%–100%); more specific than anticardiolipin antibodies
Rheumatoid factor	25%	Fc portion of IgG	Sjögren's (70%–80%), SS (20%–30%), RA (>80%)
La (SSB)	10%–20%	hYRNP	SCLE (30%–40%), SCLE-SjS overlap, primary SjS (20%)
Ku	10%	70- and 80-kDa heterodimer: DNA binding, repair protein complex, telomere maintenance, V(D)J recombination, brain	Overlap with other CTD such as DM/PM, SS
Alpha-fodrin	10%	Cytoskeleton protein in lacrimal and salivary glands	SjS: Sensitivity: 40%; Specificity: 83%

ANA, Antinuclear antibodies; *CTD*, connective tissue diseases; *DLE*, discoid lupus erythematosus; *DM/PM*, dermatomyositis/polymyositis; *dsDNA*, double stranded deoxyribonucleic acid; *IF*, immunofluorescence; *IgG*, immunoglobulin G; *LE*, lupus erythematosus; *MCTD*, mixed connective tissue disease; *RA*, rheumatoid arthritis; *RNP*, ribonucleoprotein; *rRNP*, ribosomal ribonucleoprotein; *SCLE*, subacute cutaneous lupus erythematosus; *SjS*, Sjögren's syndrome; *SLE*, systemic lupus erythematosus; *Sm*, Smith; *SS*, systemic sclerosis; *ssDNA*, single-stranded deoxyribonucleic protein.

Table 22.5 Autoantibodies associated with inflammatory dermatomyopathies

AUTOANTIBODY	PREVALENCE	MOLECULAR SPECIFICITY	CLINICAL ASSOCIATION
Myositis-Specific Autoantibodies in Polymyositis/Dermatomyositis (PM/DM)			
Anti-TIF1	20%–30%	Transcriptional intermediary factor 1 gamma (TIF1)	Malignancy-associated clinically amyopathic DM, classic DM; juvenile DM
Anti-MDA5	20% (Japanese)	Retinoic acid inducible gene: RIG-1 RNA helicase: melanoma differentiation-assoc gene 5 (MDA5)	Amyopathic dermatomyositis, rapidly progressive interstitial lung disease, vasculopathy and ulcers
Jo-1	20%–30%	Histidyl tRNA synthetase	Antisynthetase syndrome
PL-7	2%–5%	Threonyl tRNA synthetase	Antisynthetase syndrome
PL-12	2%–5%	Alanyl tRNA synthetase	Antisynthetase syndrome
OJ	<2%	Isoleucyl tRNA synthetase	Antisynthetase syndrome
EJ	2%–5%	Glycyl tRNA synthetase	Antisynthetase syndrome, possibly increased frequency of skin changes
KS	<2%	Asparaginyl	Antisynthetase syndrome
Zo	<1%	Phenylalanyl	Antisynthetase syndrome

Continued on following page

Table 22.5 Autoantibodies associated with inflammatory dermatomyopathies (*continued*)

AUTOANTIBODY	PREVALENCE	MOLECULAR SPECIFICITY	CLINICAL ASSOCIATION
Ha	<1%	Tyrosyl	Antisynthetase syndrome
NXP2	20%	Nuclear matrix protein	Adult and juvenile DM
Mi-2	5%–15%	Helicase/histone deacetylase nuclear protein complex	Classic adult and juvenile DM: myositis, Gottron's papules/sign, shawl sign, periungual telangiectasias, cuticular dystrophy (good prognosis)
SRP	4%–6%	Signal recognition particle ribonucleoprotein	Fulminant DM/PM, cardiac involvement
SAE	8%	Small ubiquitin-like modifier activating enzyme	
HMGCR	7%	HMG-CoA reductase	
Myositis-Associated Autoantibodies (Low Specificity for DM/PM)			
ANA (most common IF patterns: speckled, nucleolar)	40%		Clinically amyopathic DM (65%)
ssDNA	40%	Single-stranded DNA	SLE, SS, localized scleroderma
PM-Scl (PM-1)	8%–10%	Ribosomal RNA processing enzyme	Overlap with scleroderma
Ro (especially 52-kDa Ro)	15%	hYRNP	Overlap with SjS, SCLE, neonatal LE/CHB, SLE
U1RNP	10%	Spliceosome RNP	Overlap with connective tissue diseases
U2RNP	1%	Spliceosome RNP	Overlap with scleroderma
Ku	3%	DNA end-binding repair protein complex	Overlap with scleroderma

ANA, Antinuclear antibodies; *CHB*, congenital heart block; *EJ*, glycyl-tRNA synthetase antibody; *Ha*, hemagglutinin; *HMG-CoA*, β-Hydroxy β-methylglutaryl-CoA; *hYRNP*, hY ribonuclear protein; *IF*, immunofluorescence; *LE*, lupus erythematosus; *PM-Scl*, polymyositis/scleroderma; *RNP*, ribonucleoprotein; *SAE*, small ubiquitin-like modifier-1 activating enzyme; *SCLE*, subacute cutaneous lupus erythematosus; *SjS*, Sjögren's syndrome; *SLE*, systemic lupus erythematosus; *SRP*, signal recognition; *SS*, systemic sclerosis; *ssDNA*, single-strand deoxyribonucleic acid; *tRNA*, transfer ribonucleic acid.
From Ghirardello A, Bassi N, Palma L, et al. Autoantibodies in polymyositis and dermatomyositis. *Curr Rheumatol Rep.* 2013;15(6):335.

Table 22.6 Autoantibodies associated with systemic sclerosis and scleroderma

AUTOANTIBODY	SS, ALL SUBTYPES	SS WITH DIFFUSE CUTANEOUS SCLERODERMA	SS WITH LIMITED CUTANEOUS SCLERODERMA (CREST SYNDROME)	LOCALIZED SCLERODERMA (LINEAR SCLERODERMA; MORPHEA, LOCALIZED AND GENERALIZED)
ANA (most common IF patterns: speckled, nucleolar, centromere)	>90%			40%
Centromere (CENP-B) (better prognosis)		20%–30%	80% (+ pulmonary hypertension) (also associated with biliary cirrhosis) 10%–15%	

Table 22.6 Autoantibodies associated with systemic sclerosis and scleroderma (*continued*)

AUTOANTIBODY	SS, ALL SUBTYPES	SS WITH DIFFUSE CUTANEOUS SCLERODERMA	SS WITH LIMITED CUTANEOUS SCLERODERMA (CREST SYNDROME)	LOCALIZED SCLERODERMA (LINEAR SCLERODERMA; MORPHEA, LOCALIZED AND GENERALIZED)
Scl-70 (topo 1) (DNA topoisomerase I) (poor prognosis)		28%–70% (40%) (pulmonary fibrosis, renal crisis, internal malignancy)		
Fibrillin-1 (major component of microfibrils in the extracellular matrix)		5%	10%	30%
Histones	40%			35%
Rheumatoid factor	25%			25%
ssDNA	10%			50%
U3RNP-Fibrillarin (part of U3RNP complex)	5%	4%–10% diffuse skin, vasculopathy, ulcers, digit necrosis, pulmonary hypertension, renal		
RM-Scl (PM-Scl) (good prognosis)	4%–11%	2% (scleroderma) 25% (scleroderma + myositis)		
Ku (80- and 70-kDa DNA binding dimeric protein)		PM/SS overlap		
RNA polymerase I/III (poor prognosis)	5%–20%	20% diffuse skin and renal crisis (no pulmonary)		
U1RNP (overlap features with SLE, RA, and myositis)		5%–6% (90% in MCTD)	Puffy hands, Raynaud's, arthritis, and esophageal dysfunction	
Th/To (RNase MRP/ RNase P RNP)		2%–5%	19% (interstitial lung disease and pulmonary hypertension)	5%
hUBF (human upstream binding factor) (NOR 90)			Limited cutaneous, mild internal organ, good prognosis	

Continued on following page

Table 22.6 Autoantibodies associated with systemic sclerosis and scleroderma (*continued*)

AUTOANTIBODY	SS, ALL SUBTYPES	SS WITH DIFFUSE CUTANEOUS SCLERODERMA	SS WITH LIMITED CUTANEOUS SCLERODERMA (CREST SYNDROME)	LOCALIZED SCLERODERMA (LINEAR SCLERODERMA; MORPHEA, LOCALIZED AND GENERALIZED)
U11/U12RNP (components of spliceosome)		Raynaud's, gastrointestinal involvement, pulmonary fibrosis		
Phospholipid/ cardiolipin/β_2- glycoprotein, PDGFR, endothelial antibodies	25%–85%	Pathogenesis in sclerosis suspected		

ANA, Antinuclear antibodies; *IF*, immunofluorescence; *MCTD*, mixed connective tissue disease; *MRP*, mitochondrial RNA processing; *NOR*, nucleolus-organizing regions; *PDGFR*, platelet-derived growth factor receptor; *PM*, polymyositis; *PM-Scl*, polymyositis/scleroderma; *RNP*, ribonucleoprotein; *SLE*, systemic lupus erythematosus; *SS*, systemic sclerosis.

From Hamaguchi Y: Autoantibody profiles in systemic sclerosis: predictive value for clinical evaluation and prognosis, *J Dermatol* 37:42–53, 2010.

CHAPTER 23

URTICARIA AND ANGIOEDEMA

Marc Serota and Rohit K. Katial

1. What percentage of the population experiences acute urticaria during their lifetime?
   An estimated 15% to 25% of the population will experience at least one episode of urticaria during their lifetime (Fig. 23.1).

2. How is acute versus chronic urticaria defined?
   Classification of urticaria begins with duration and frequency of the wheals. Although arbitrary, 6 weeks of nearly daily symptoms has been chosen as the dividing point for differentiating between acute and chronic urticaria.

Ormerod AD. Urticaria: recognition, causes, and treatment. *Drugs*. 1994;48:717–730.

3. What are the characteristics of urticaria?
   An individual urticarial lesion should not last longer than 24 hours in a given location, although the patient's hives in general may be ongoing. Alternative diagnoses are suggested when there is a lack of pruritus, individual lesions last for days to weeks, angioedema without urticaria, lesions that are localized to only one area of the body or are very well defined, a review of systems suggestive of systemic disease, or a failure to respond to therapy.

4. What are the common causes of acute urticaria?
   Acute urticaria is more common in children and young adults and is most often idiopathic or caused by acute viral infections (50% to 60% in most studies). External causes should be assessed but are far less common and include drugs, foods, and insect stings.

5. What eight foods account for 90% of all food allergic reactions in the United States?
   Milk, eggs, peanuts, tree nuts, wheat, soy, fish, and shellfish.

6. Are all urticarial reactions from medications allergic (IgE–mediated) in nature?
   No. Some medication reactions may not be truly allergic but may be caused by nonspecific mast cell–releasing or anaphylactoid properties. Common drugs with this mechanism of action include opiates, vancomycin, radiocontrast media (especially, high-osmolar, ionic forms), and nonsteroidal antiinflammatory drugs.

7. What is the cause of most chronic urticaria?
   In most patients seen in referral centers, chronic urticaria remains unexplained despite extensive workup. However, the two largest subgroups of chronic urticaria patients have lesions, induced from physical stimuli (e.g., heat, pressure, vibratory, and cold) or with an autoimmune basis.

8. Is chronic urticaria primarily of allergic etiology?
   No. In a large series of patients with chronic urticaria, a personal or family history of allergy was no more common than in the general population, suggesting that there is no connection between chronic urticaria and allergy.

9. How common are the physical urticarias?
   Of 554 patients with urticaria seen in a university clinic in England, physical urticarias constituted 17.5% of the total; most of the remainder were idiopathic. The most frequent of the physical urticarias were dermographism (8.5%) (Fig. 23.2), cholinergic urticaria (5.1%), and acquired cold urticaria (2.5%).

10. Is laboratory testing helpful for chronic urticaria?
    Very rarely. In a Cleveland Clinic study, 356 cases of chronic urticaria/angioedema were assessed with 1872 lab tests. Of these, there were 319 (17%) abnormal tests, which were mostly insignificant (complete blood count with differential or basic metabolic profile). Thirty patients (8.4%) underwent additional testing. Only one patient improved as the result of a lab test (hypothyroidism improved with increased levothyroxine dose). In a systematic review of 6462 patients in 29 studies, internal disease was an underlying cause of chronic urticaria in 105 patients. Among these, the most common was urticarial vasculitis (60 cases), thyroid disease (17 cases), lupus erythematosus (7 cases), connective tissue disorders (16 cases), paraproteinemia (3 cases), polycythemia vera (4 cases), and various cancers (5 cases).

Tarbox J, Gutta R, Radojicic C, et al. Utility of routine laboratory testing in management of chronic urticaria/angioedema. *Ann Allergy Asthma Immunol*. 2011;107:239–243.
Kozel M, Bossuyt P, Mekkes J, et al. Laboratory tests and identified diagnoses in patients with physical and chronic urticaria and angioedema: a systematic review. *J Am Acad Dermatol*. 2003;48:409–416.

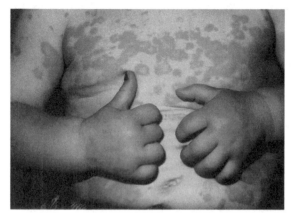

Fig. 23.1 Urticaria in a child. Note that some lesions demonstrate an annular appearance. (Courtesy James E. Fitzpatrick, MD.)

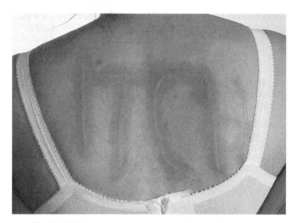

Fig. 23.2 Dermographism: whealing immediately following pressure.

11. **Is β-lactam allergy a common cause of acute urticaria?**
    Despite the perception of many patients, β-lactam allergy remains a relatively less common cause of acute urticaria. In one study, 47 children with acute urticaria while on β-lactams were evaluated for the presence of viral infection. In fact, 31 of 47 had a positive viral study while only 4 of 47 had a reaction when rechallenged with the same β-lactam.

Caubet JC, Kaiser L, Lemaître B, et al. The role of penicillin in benign skin rashes in childhood: a prospective study based on drug rechallenge. *J Allergy Clin Immunol.* 2011;127:218.

12. **What association has been described between autoantibodies and chronic urticaria?**
    Autoimmune urticaria is likely an underdiagnosed phenomenon. Up to 30% to 50% of "idiopathic" urticaria has been found to be associated with autoimmune mechanisms leading to a separate entity referred to as *autoimmune chronic urticaria*. Evidence suggests immunoglobulin G (IgG) antibodies directed against both the immunoglobulin E (IgE) receptor alpha subunit and the Fc region of IgE.

Sabroe RA, Greaves MW. Chronic idiopathic urticaria with functional autoantibodies: 12 years on. *Br J Dermatol.* 2006;154:813–819.

13. **What tests are available for autoimmune urticaria?**
    All testing methods remain controversial. The first test was the autologous serum skin test. This involves taking 0.05 mL of the patient's own serum and injecting this intradermally, typically on the volar surface of an unaffected arm

along with positive and negative controls. The sensitivity was calculated at 65% to 81% and specificity 71% to 78%. Unacceptable false-positive reactions in healthy controls with the autologous serum skin test have been shown to be as high as 56%. More recently, basophil activation and commercial assays for detecting anti-FcεRI-alpha antibodies (sometimes referred to as the chronic urticaria index) have become available, although there remains much debate regarding their clinical utility.

Sabroe RA, Grattan CE, Francis DM, et al. The autologous serum skin test: a screening test for autoantibodies in chronic idiopathic urticaria. *Br J Dermatol.* 1999;140:446–452.
Taskapan O, Kutlu A, Karabudak O. Evaluation of autologous serum skin test results in patients with chronic idiopathic urticaria, allergic/non-allergic asthma or rhinitis and healthy people, *Clin Exp Dermatol.* 2008;33:754–758.

14. What is the "triple response"? Name the components.
    The triple response (of Lewis) is responsible for producing an urticarial lesion and can classically be produced by injection of an allergen into the skin of a sensitized individual. The three components producing the reaction are as follows:
    * Vasodilatation (erythema)
    * Increased vascular permeability (wheal)
    * Axon reflex (flare)

15. What is the mechanism of the axon reflex?
    The axon reflex is produced by stimulation of cutaneous sensory nerve endings, with antidromic conduction of the impulse and release of the neurokinin substance P. Substance P is a vasodilator and it also causes the release of histamine and other mediators from cutaneous mast cells, thus augmenting the urticarial reaction.

16. List five mediators that are capable of directly causing vasodilatation and increased vascular permeability in the skin.
    * Histamine
    * Prostaglandin D_2 (PGD_2)
    * Leukotriene C_4 and D_4
    * Platelet-activating factor
    * Bradykinin

17. Name three mediators that may cause vasodilatation and increased vascular permeability indirectly through action on the mast cell.
    Substance P, the anaphylatoxins (C3a, C4a, and C5a), and histamine-releasing factors all cause release of mast cell mediators. Of these mediators, only substance P has an additional direct action on blood vessels.

18. Which cells synthesize histamine-releasing factors?
    Histamine-releasing factor may be responsible for the release of histamine and other mediators from basophils and/or mast cell. These factors have been described as products of neutrophils, platelets, alveolar macrophages, T lymphocytes, B lymphocytes, and monocytes.

19. What cytokines/chemokines may also be increased in urticarial lesions?
    There is evidence for increased production of interleukin-5; eotaxin 1, 2, 3; and regulated on activation, normal T cell expressed and secreted (RANTES), also known as chemokine ligand 5.

20. In what form of physical urticaria are subjects at risk of drowning?
    Patients with acquired cold urticaria may have massive mediator release if immersed in cold water. Such release has resulted in drowning, presumably because the patient went into shock from the massive mediator release.

21. How quickly after the application of cold does whealing develop in acquired cold urticaria?
    Whealing in cold urticaria does not develop during the exposure to the cold stimulus, but rather 2 minutes after rewarming, and a large hive appears by 10 minutes (Fig. 23.3). The delay is probably due to the decrease in cutaneous blood flow during exposure to the cold.

22. Only one form of urticaria has whealing that is sufficiently characteristic to suggest a specific diagnosis. Which one?
    The initial wheals in cholinergic urticaria are quite different from those in other forms of urticaria. They are small, punctate monomorphic (often referred to as pencil-eraser–sized, ∼0.5-cm diameter) with a prominent erythematous flare. Over time, they may become confluent, and form larger areas of whealing.

23. Where does cholinergic urticaria usually develop?
    On the upper thorax and neck, but it may spread distally to involve the entire body.

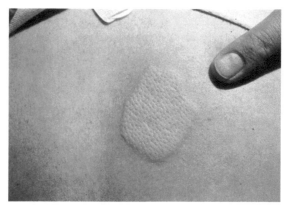

Fig. 23.3 Positive ice cube test in a patient with acquired cold urticaria. (Courtesy James E. Fitzpatrick, MD.)

24. What are the precipitating events for cholinergic urticaria? By what mechanism do they produce the whealing?

Exercise, warm baths and showers, and emotions are the classic triggers of cholinergic urticaria. There is an elevation of the core body temperature, which is perceived centrally, resulting in efferent cholinergic output to the skin and leading to mast cell degranulation.

25. How are the solar urticarias classified?

Solar urticarias (Fig. 23.4) are classified into six types according to the inciting wavelength:
- **Type I:** 280 to 320 nm
- **Type II:** 320 to 400 nm
- **Type III:** 400 to 500 nm
- **Type IV:** 320 to 500 nm
- **Type V:** 280 to 500 nm
- **Type VI:** 400 nm (protoporphyrin IX)

KEY POINTS: URTICARIA AND ANGIOEDEMA

1. Acute urticaria is usually from a secondary cause, most commonly infection, as well as food, drugs, or insect stings.
2. Chronic urticaria is most often idiopathic and not due to an allergic etiology but has an autoimmune basis in up to 50% of cases.
3. The most common physical urticaria is dermographism, but in chronic urticaria, screen for physical stimuli such as pressure, cold, and heat.
4. In angioedema without urticaria, one should screen for both hereditary and acquired angioedema by obtaining a C4 level.
5. The main medications to control urticaria are antihistamines directed toward blocking the H1 receptor, and there may be added benefit with H2 blockers.

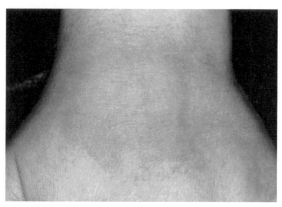

Fig. 23.4 Solar urticaria. Phototesting with ultraviolet B (290 to 320 nm) wavelength produced urticaria in this patient with a history of sun-induced anaphylaxis. (Courtesy James E. Fitzpatrick, MD.)

26. What is Darier's sign?

Darier's sign is a finding in urticaria pigmentosa. In urticaria pigmentosa, yellow-tan to red-brown macules containing increased numbers of mast cells are scattered over the body. Stroking the skin over the pigmented macules causes an urticarial wheal to form that is limited to the area of the pigmented lesion (Fig. 23.5).

27. How often does aspirin cause or exacerbate urticaria?

Aspirin is rarely a cause of urticaria in an otherwise asymptomatic patient, but many patients with chronic urticaria will have increased whealing if they take aspirin or nonsteroidal antiinflammatory drugs when their disease is active. These same patients are usually able to take aspirin with a much lower risk when their urticaria is inactive, indicating that aspirin is not the cause but a nonspecific exacerbating factor, presumably acting on a pharmacologic basis. Prospective and retrospective data suggest that aspirin administration will cause a flare in 20% to 40% of patients with active urticaria.

Moore-Robinson M, Warin RP. Effect of salicylates in urticaria. *BMJ.* 1967;4:262–264.

28. What is the prognosis of chronic urticaria?

Champion followed 554 patients with urticaria seen at a hospital clinic in England. After 6 months, 50% still had active disease. Of these patients, 40% continued to have at least intermittent symptoms 10 years later. The prognosis was somewhat worse in patients with only angioedema and even poorer if both urticaria and angioedema were present.

Champion RH, Roberts SOB, Carpenter RG, et al. Urticaria and angioedema: a review of 554 patients. *Br J Dermatol.* 1969;81:588–597.

29. Much has been discovered in recent years regarding the histopathology of chronic idiopathic urticaria. What three major types of cells may be encountered in increased numbers in these biopsies?

The characteristic histopathologic finding of nonvasculitic chronic urticaria is a subtle to modest perivascular and interstitial infiltrate. There are increased numbers of lymphocytes. Mast cells are increased some 10-fold, while there is a 4-fold increase in mononuclear cells. There is increased histamine in blisters suctioned from chronic urticaria patients. Although eosinophils are often not prominent, increased deposition of the major basic protein of the eosinophil is present in the tissue in 50% of patients, indicating eosinophil involvement in the inflammatory process, although only a fraction of these had evidence of eosinophilic accumulation.

Elias J, Boss E, Kaplan AP. Studies of the cellular infiltrate of chronic idiopathic urticaria: prominence of T lymphocytes, monocytes, and mast cells. *J Allergy Clin Immunol.* 1986;78:914–918.

Sabroe RA, Poon E, Orchard GE, et al. Cutaneous inflammatory cell infiltrate in chronic idiopathic urticaria: comparison of patients with and without anti-FcεRI or anti-IgE autoantibodies. *J Allergy Clin Immunol.* 1999;103:484–493.

Ying S, Kikuchi Y, Meng Q, et al. TH1/TH2 cytokines and inflammatory cells in skin biopsy specimens from patients with chronic idiopathic urticaria: comparison with allergen-induced late phase cutaneous reaction. *J Allergy Clin Immunol.* 2002;109:694–700.

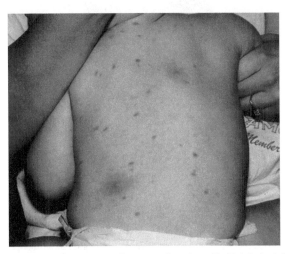

Fig. 23.5 Child with urticaria pigmentosa demonstrating multiple tan papules and a positive Darier's sign in two lesions that have been stroked. (Courtesy James E. Fitzpatrick, MD.)

30. In contrast to chronic idiopathic urticaria, what are the typical histologic features of urticarial vasculitis?

Biopsy specimens from patients with urticarial vasculitis typically reveal necrotizing vasculitis of the small venules with deposition of immunoglobulin and complement. In those with low serum complement (hypocomplementemic urticarial vasculitis), polymorphonuclear leukocytes commonly predominate, while in those with normal serum complement, a lymphocytic infiltrate is more typical.

31. Can clinical findings suggest the presence of urticarial vasculitis?

The individual lesions of vasculitis may resemble those of idiopathic urticaria; however, they may feel firmer, tend to persist for greater than 24 hours, and, on clearing, tend to leave an ecchymotic area due to leakage of red blood cells into the perivascular tissue (Fig. 23.6). Associated systemic symptoms, such as arthralgias and myalgias, are also common. The erythrocyte sedimentation rate is often increased, autoantibodies may be present, and there may be evidence of renal disease.

32. A number of clues in the patient's history may suggest that a patient with recurrent angioedema has the hereditary form. Name some.

Between 75% and 85% of patients with hereditary angioedema (HAE) give a positive family history of similar attacks. The attacks of angioedema themselves are characterized by the absence of urticaria and pruritus, both common with idiopathic angioedema. In HAE, episodes of angioedema are often triggered by trauma such as dental procedures or surgery. However, such a triggering event may not be evident. Significant upper airway obstruction is seen almost exclusively in HAE, as opposed to ordinary idiopathic angioedema. Attacks of severe abdominal pain are common in HAE, representing edema of the bowel wall. Finally, attacks of HAE typically progress for several days and respond poorly to treatment with antihistamines or epinephrine.

33. Why is C1 esterase deficiency not a part of the differential diagnosis of chronic urticaria?

Hereditary deficiency of C1 esterase inhibitor is the underlying defect in HAE. These individuals have recurring attacks of nonpruritic angioedema but do not have urticaria.

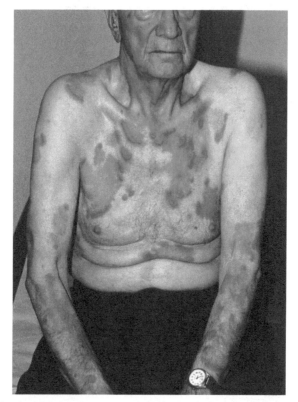

Fig. 23.6 Lesions of urticarial vasculitis demonstrating an annular appearance, with some areas showing a violaceous hue due to extravasation of red blood cells. (Courtesy JLA Collection.)

34. Name the screening tests and diagnostic pathway for HAE.
    C4 is the screening test. This should be low in HAE types I and II. C1-inhibitor level and function distinguish between HAE types I and II. A low C1q level indicates acquired forms of angioedema (autoimmune disease, B-cell malignancy).

35. Describe the different types of HAE.
    The most common type (85%) is HAE type I, which is characterized by low levels of C1-inhibitor. HAE type II (15%) is characterized by normal (or elevated) level, but abnormal qualitative function. HAE with normal C1-inhibitor (formerly known as type III) is a rare form, which is characterized by a normal C4 and C1-inhibitor level and function, despite symptomatology and inheritance pattern similar to HAE types I and II.

36. What are the clinical differences of HAE type III?
    HAE type III tends to present in early adulthood as opposed to at puberty. Facial and oral mucosal involvement tends to be more prominent. Abdominal attacks are less frequent. Females are more often and more severely affected (initially this disorder was thought to be estrogen dependent until males were also described).

37. Mutations in what genes have been associated with HAE with normal C1-inhibitor (formally known as type III)?
    The etiology of HAE with normal C1 inhibitor was previously not known, but recently, several mutations in the Factor XII, plasminogen (PLG), and angiopoieten (ANGPT1) genes have been described.

Bork K, et al. *Lancet.* 2000;356:213–217.
Binkley, Davis. *JACI.* 2000;106:546–550.
Bork K, et al. *Allergy.* 2018;73:442–450.
Bafunno V, et al. *JACI.* 2018;141:1009–1017.

38. What treatments are available for HAE?
    Traditionally, treatment with attenuated androgens, such as danazol, was used to induce synthesis of C1-inhibitor by the liver. This treatment is not as effective as newer treatments and is associated with the adverse effects of chronic androgen use. Today, the use of androgens is limited to patients who cannot afford more modern treatments due to cost. Ecallantide is a subcutaneously administered recombinant plasma kallikrein inhibitor that blocks the production of bradykinin. Allergic reactions including anaphylaxis were reported in 2% to 3% of patients, so a nurse or physician is required to give the injection. Two intravenous and one subcutaneous C1-inhibitor concentrates obtained from pooled human serum are also commercially available, with two indicated for prophylaxis and one for acute attacks. Recombinant C1-inhibitor obtained from the milk of transgenic rabbits has recently become available. Icatibant is a bradykinin B2 receptor competitive antagonist given subcutaneously. It is approved for acute attacks (not prophylaxis) and may be self-administered. Additionally, a monoclonal antibody-based kallikrein inhibitor (lanadelumab-flyo) was approved for prophylactic use in patients older than 12 years of age. Prophylactic treatment with C1-inhibitor should be initiated prior to surgical procedures. Of note, epinephrine and antihistamines are not effective for treating HAE and should not delay the use of definitive treatment.

39. A 60-year-old patient presents with a new onset of attacks of nonpruritic angioedema and a depressed C4 level. What is the first diagnosis you consider?
    Acquired C1 esterase inhibitor deficiency. This situation is usually encountered in patients with lymphoma who have a circulating low-molecular-weight immunoglobulin M (IgM), decreased C1 esterase inhibitor level, and low levels of C1 to C4 complement. The mechanism of C1 activation is by reaction with immune complexes or by binding of the C1 to anti-idiotypic antibody bound to the immunoglobulin on the surface of the tumor cells. Acquired C1 esterase deficiency has also been reported with connective tissue disorders such as systemic lupus erythematosus, with carcinoma, and with an IgG antibody directed toward C1 esterase inhibitor. In the latter circumstance, the C1 levels are usually normal.

40. Certain drugs have been identified as being particularly effective for a subset of patients with chronic urticaria or angioedema. What are these drugs, and when is a trial with them indicated?
    - Cyproheptadine has been reported to be particularly effective in controlling acquired cold urticaria.
    - Corticosteroids and nonsteroidal antiinflammatory drugs prevent the lesions of delayed pressure urticaria, whereas antihistamines are completely without benefit.
    - Hydroxychloroquine has been effective in some cases of hypocomplementemic urticarial vasculitis.
    - Omalizumab is Food and Drug Administration approved for the treatment of chronic idiopathic urticaria.

41. What three mediator antagonists have been reported to be useful in symptomatic control of urticaria?

Competitive antagonists of the H1 and H2 histamine receptor and antagonists of leukotriene D_4 receptor have been reported to be useful in treating urticaria. The latter two are usually used in conjunction with an H1 antagonist. Recent studies suggest that the nonsedating H1 antagonists are just as effective in treating urticaria as the classic, sedating antagonists.

Bensch GW, Borish L. Leukotriene receptor antagonists in the treatment of chronic idiopathic urticaria (abstract). *J Allergy Clin Immunol.* 1999;103:S154.

Monroe EW, Bernstein DI, Fox RW, et al. Relative efficacy and safety of loratadine, hydroxyzine, and placebo in chronic idiopathic urticaria. *Arzneimittelforschung.* 1992;42:1119–1121.

42. How is chronic urticaria treated?

First-line therapy includes H1-antihistamines. Second-generation H1-antihistamines are preferred to limit sedation, although first-generation H1-antihistamines may be preferable at bedtime to take advantage of their sedative effects. Some sources recommend dosages up to four times the standard dose divided twice daily to adequately control urticaria and pruritus. Second-line therapies include leukotriene receptor antagonists and short courses of oral corticosteroids. Third-line therapies include antiinflammatory medications such as dapsone, sulfasalazine, or hydroxychloroquine. In 2014, omalizumab, a monoclonal antibody that inhibits IgE binding to the high-affinity IgE receptor on mast cells, was approved in the United States for patients at least 12 years of age who failed antihistamine treatment.

Staevska M, Popov TA, Kralimarkova T, et al. The effectiveness of levocetirizine and desloratadine in up to 4 times conventional doses in difficult-to-treat urticaria. *J Allergy Clin Immunol.* 2010;125:676.

Asero R. Chronic unremitting urticaria: is the use of antihistamines above the licensed dose effective? A preliminary study of cetirizine at licensed and above-licensed doses. *Clin Exp Dermatol.* 2007;32:34.

VIRAL EXANTHEMS

Carla X. Torres-Zegarra and William L. Weston

CHAPTER 24

1. **What is the difference between an exanthem and an enanthem?**
   Any skin rash that appears abruptly and affects several areas of the body simultaneously is called an exanthem, from the Greek origin *"exanthema,"* which means *"breaking out."* If the rash occurs on mucosal surfaces, it is called an enanthem.

2. **Which viruses cause exanthems?**
   Of the hundreds of viruses that infect humans, almost all may produce an exanthem. Some viruses produce an exanthem in most infected persons. These include measles, rubella, the human herpesvirus (HHV), and parvovirus B19. A few viruses produce an exanthema in less than 1% of those infected; these include mumps, respiratory syncytial virus (RSV), and equine encephalitis.

Korman AM, Alikhan A, Kaffenberger BH. Viral exanthems: an update on laboratory testing of the adult patient. *J Am Acad Dermatol.* 2017;76(3):538–550.
Knöpfel N, Noguera-Morel L, Latour I, Torrelo A. Viral exanthems in children: a great imitator. *Clin Dermatol.* 2019;37(3):213–226.

3. **Identify the six childhood exanthems and their etiologies**
   See Table 24.1.

4. **How do viruses cause exanthems?**
   In the viral exanthems studied to date, the responsible virus is found within the skin, either in keratinocytes or endothelial cells. It is believed that the virus disseminates to skin during the viremic phase of infection, and the observed exanthem is the result of the host response to the virus.

5. **Which viruses cause morbilliform (measles-like) eruptions?**
   Measles, rubella, enteroviruses, HHV-6 and -7, Epstein-Barr virus (EBV), and cytomegalovirus (CMV) (Fig. 24.1).

6. **Which viruses cause grouped blisters on a red base?**
   Herpes simplex virus and varicella-zoster virus (Fig. 24.2A).

7. **Which viruses cause hand, foot, and mouth disease?**
   Coxsackievirus A16, ECHO 71, and other enteroviruses cause hand, foot, and mouth syndrome (Fig. 24.2B).

Gao L, Zou G, Liao Q, et al. Spectrum of enterovirus serotypes causing uncomplicated hand, foot, and mouth disease and enteroviral diagnostic yield of different clinical samples. *Clin Infect Dis.* 2018;67(11):1729–1735.
Kuntz T, Koushk-Jalali B, Tigges C, et al. Atypical variant of hand-foot-mouth disease. *Hautarzt.* 2019;70(12):964–968.

8. **What is the difference between Gianotti-Crosti syndrome and papular acrodermatitis of childhood?**
   Gianotti-Crosti syndrome and papular acrodermatitis of childhood are synonyms for a viral eruption characterized by the acute onset of a symmetrical, erythematous papular eruption that is accentuated on the face, extremities, and buttocks (Fig. 24.3). It most commonly occurs in young children between the ages of 1 and 3 years but may occur in younger children or even adolescents.

Gianotti F, Pesapane F, Gianotti R. Ferdinando Gianotti and the papular acrodermatitis of childhood: a scientist against all the odds. *JAMA Dermatol.* 2014;150(5):485.

9. **Which are the most common viruses that cause papular acrodermatitis of childhood?**
   Although originally described in association with infections with the hepatitis B virus, in the United States, it is most commonly associated with EBV infection. Less common causes include CMV, various coxsackieviruses (A16, B4, B5), adenoviruses, parvovirus B19, HHV-6, and even viral vaccinations.

Leung AKC, Sergi CM, Lam JM, Leong KF. Gianotti-Crosti syndrome (papular acrodermatitis of childhood) in the era of a viral recrudescence and vaccine opposition. *World J Pediatr.* 2019;15(6):521–527.

Table 24.1 Viral exanthems, names, and etiologies

DISEASE	NAME	ETIOLOGY
First disease	Measles (rubeola)	Measles virus
Second disease	Scarlet fever	*Streptococcus pyogenes*
Third disease	Rubella	Rubella virus
Fourth disease	Duke's disease	No longer accepted as distinct disorder
Fifth disease	Erythema infectiosum	Parvovirus B19
Sixth disease	Roseola infantum	Human herpesvirus-6 and -7

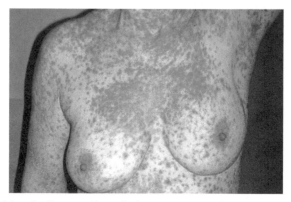

Fig. 24.1 Morbilliform viral eruption. Numerous widespread red macules and papules. (Courtesy Walter Reed Army Medical Center.)

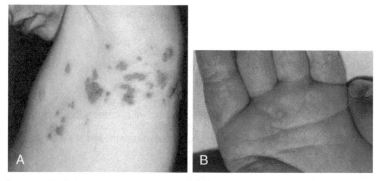

Fig. 24.2 **A,** Grouped vesicles limited to a dermatome in herpes zoster infection. **B,** Discrete palmar vesicle in epidemic hand, foot, and mouth syndrome. (Panel A courtesy James E. Fitzpatrick, MD.)

10. Which virus classically causes a lacy eruption?

Parvovirus B19, the cause of erythema infectiosum. This is the only known parvovirus to produce human infections. Patients also often demonstrate bright erythema of the cheeks that has been described as a "*slapped cheek*" appearance (Fig. 24.4A and B). The eruption is evanescent and may last from 1 to 4 hours. It becomes more prominent with sun exposure and heat. Approximately 10% of patients will have associated arthralgia or even arthritis that tends to affect the most distal joints.

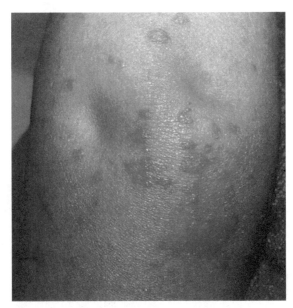

Fig. 24.3 Gianotti-Crosti syndrome. Young child with acrallylocated monomorphous edematous papules. The color can vary from skin-colored to red. (Courtesy James E. Fitzpatrick, MD.)

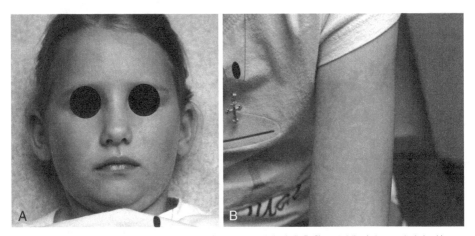

Fig. 24.4 Erythema infectiosum. **A,** Characteristic malar erythema ("slapped cheeks"). **B,** Characteristic photo-accentuated red lacy eruption on the arms. Note that it abruptly stops in the area covered by the sleeves. (Courtesy Amanda Tauscher, MD.)

11. Which populations are at risk of developing complications from parvovirus B19 infection?
    A. Pregnancy: Infection occurring during pregnancy can cause hydrops fetalis, intrauterine growth restriction, and death (risk for fetal death is between 2% and 7%).
    B. Chronic hemolytic anemia: Parvovirus B19 is the most common cause of transient aplastic crisis in patients with chronic hemolytic anemias (i.e., sickle cell disease).
    C. Immunodeficiency: Infection with parvovirus B19 can cause chronic erythroid hypoplasia with severe anemia.

Ornoy A, Ergaz Z. Parvovirus B19 infection during pregnancy and risks to the fetus. *Birth Defects Res.* 2017;109(5):311–323.

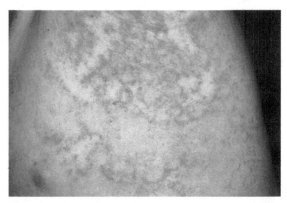

Fig. 24.5 Unilateral laterothoracic exanthem demonstrating a lacy appearance.

12. Which viruses cause scarlatina (scarlet fever–like) eruptions?

    Enteroviruses, adenoviruses, and hepatitis B and C.

13. Which virus causes purpura of the hands and feet?

    Parvovirus B19 may cause the purpuric gloves and socks syndrome. Unlike the typical rash of erythema infectiosum, patients with this presentation are viremic and contagious and should not be around those at risk.

Vázquez-Osorio I, Mallo-García S, Rodríguez-Díaz E, et al. Parvovirus B19 infection presenting concurrently as papular-purpuric gloves-and-socks syndrome and bathing-trunk eruption. *Clin Exp Dermatol.* 2017;42(1):58–60.

14. Do viral exanthems cause petechiae?

    Yes. Many viruses do, including ECHO 4, 7, and 9; EBV; measles; rubella; RSV; dengue; and parvovirus B19.

15. Can viral exanthems be on one half of the body?

    Yes. The unilateral laterothoracic exanthem, seen predominantly in children, can be unilateral at initial presentation. Some cases spread to the contralateral side but often remain accentuated on the side of initial presentation. Although it is believed to be a viral exanthem, a viral cause has not been proven (Fig. 24.5).

Leung AK, Barankin B. Unilateral laterothoracic exanthem. *J Pediatr.* 2015;167(3):775.

16. Which disorder most commonly mimics a viral morbilliform eruption?

    Drug eruptions (morbilliform drug eruptions) are often clinically indistinguishable from viral morbilliform eruptions. However, viral exanthems are more common in children, and drug eruptions tend to be more common in adults. Less commonly, urticaria, arthropod reactions, early guttate psoriasis, and early pityriasis rosea can also be morbilliform. A thorough history will aid in the diagnosis.

Stern RS. Exanthematous drug eruptions. *N Engl J Med.* 2012;366:2492–2501.

17. What are the clinical features of roseola infantum (exanthem subitum, sixth disease)?

    Roseola infantum is a disease that typically presents in infants and very young children as 2 to 5 days of high fever (103° F to 105° F) in an otherwise healthy infant, followed by defervescence and the appearance of pale, small, pink papules that are primarily located on the trunk and head (Fig. 24.6). The exanthem typically lasts from hours to 1 or 2 days. It is most commonly caused by HHV-6 and, less commonly, HHV-7. Treatment is supportive.

Stone RC, Micali GA, Schwartz RA. Roseola infantum and its causal human herpesviruses. *Int J Dermatol.* 2014;53(4):397–403.

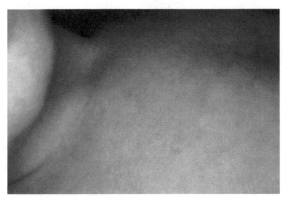

Fig. 24.6 Roseola infantum demonstrating subtle, evanescent, erythematous papular exanthem. (Courtesy Fitzsimons Army Medical Center teaching files.)

18. How does sunlight exposure affect a viral exanthem?

The erythema of viral exanthems often becomes more confluent and prominent within sun-exposed areas of skin (photodistributed).

Norval M. The effect of ultraviolet radiation on human viral infections. *Photochem Photobiol.* 2006;82(6):1495–1504.

KEY POINTS: VIRAL EXANTHEMS

1. Most viral exanthems are morbilliform (measles-like).
2. The virus is always present within the rash in either the keratinocytes or endothelial cells.
3. Any virus can produce an exanthema, including those that rarely do so.
4. Drug rashes are the most common mimics of viral exanthems.

CHAPTER 25

BULLOUS VIRAL ERUPTIONS

Carla X. Torres-Zegarra and Sylvia L. Brice

1. What do herpes simplex virus (HSV) and varicella-zoster virus (VZV) have in common?

   HSV-1, HSV-2, and VZV are all members of the human herpesvirus family. Other members of this family include cytomegalovirus, Epstein-Barr virus, human herpesvirus-6, human herpesvirus-7, and human herpesvirus-8. The human herpesviruses all contain double-stranded DNA, share certain structural features and mechanisms for infection and replication, and have the capacity to establish latent infection in the human host.

2. What happens during primary HSV infection?

   Primary infection refers to an individual's first infection with HSV, either type 1 or 2, at any site. These patients are seronegative initially but subsequently develop HSV-specific antibodies. During primary infection, HSV gains access to the host through the epithelial surface. Following active replication within the skin or mucosa, HSV infects the associated cutaneous neurons and migrates to the sensory root ganglia, where a latent infection is established. Primary HSV infection may be associated with extensive cutaneous lesions, severe pain, and systemic symptoms; however, in many cases, the primary infection is asymptomatic (or unrecognized).

3. What about recurrent HSV infection?

   Recurrent HSV infection represents reactivation of the latent virus in the sensory ganglia. "Reactivated" virus particles migrate along the nerves to the site in the skin where the primary infection occurred, with subsequent viral replication and the development of clinical lesions (Fig. 25.1A). The most common sites for recurrent herpes simplex infection are the lips (herpes labialis, "cold sores"), genitalia (herpes genitalis), and sacral area (Fig. 25.1B). Often, individuals experience a prodrome of tingling or burning in the skin prior to the development of visible lesions. Certain factors, such as fever, stress, menses, and sun exposure, may precipitate recurrent infection. The frequency of recurrent infection varies greatly between individuals. In most individuals, clinically evident recurrence becomes less frequent over time.

4. What is the difference between a primary and an initial HSV infection?

   When an individual without preexisting antibodies to either HSV-1 or HSV-2 develops an infection with HSV (either type 1 or 2), it is referred to as the primary infection. When an individual with preexisting antibodies to one type of HSV then experiences an infection with the other HSV type, it is referred to as the initial (or initial, nonprimary) infection.

5. How is HSV transmitted?

   HSV is transmitted by direct contact of the infected mucocutaneous surface(s) of one individual with the mucosa or skin of another individual. HSV does not survive long outside its normal habitat, and so transmission by contact with fomites is extremely uncommon. It is assumed that HSV-1 is generally transmitted inadvertently during childhood from infected family members, whereas infection with HSV-2 may develop later when individuals become sexually active.

6. How long is the incubation period for HSV (i.e., the time from initial infection to appearance of vesicles)?

   The time interval between exposure and development of primary disease is estimated to be 3 to 14 days. However, not all cases of primary disease are symptomatic, and so the first evidence of infection may be a recurrent episode, well after the actual exposure. This is important to note, especially in the case of genital infection, where the sudden development of "herpes" in one partner in a monogamous couple could create concerns regarding infidelity.

7. Define asymptomatic shedding.

   In individuals previously infected with HSV, virus may periodically be present at the site of infection in the absence of clinically evident lesions. This is referred to as asymptomatic shedding. During asymptomatic shedding, the presence of virus may be documented by viral culture or polymerase chain reaction (PCR). Although the viral titer is lower than during clinically active disease, transmission of the virus can nevertheless occur. In fact, contact during periods of asymptomatic shedding is thought to be responsible for many cases of disease transmission.

8. Can you be infected with HSV and not know it?

   Yes. Many individuals who give no history of HSV infection are seropositive for HSV-specific antibodies. Using viral culture or PCR, HSV can periodically be recovered from the mouth and/or anogenital region of such individuals (see "asymptomatic shedding" earlier). Based on the seroprevalence of herpes-specific antibody, 70% to 80% of the population is infected with HSV-1, and 25% to 30% with HSV-2. It is estimated that out of every four individuals with genital herpes, three do not know they are infected, and that more than half the population in the United States will become seropositive for HSV by adulthood.

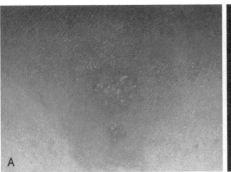 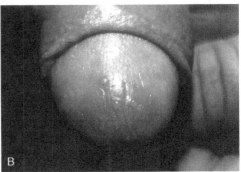

Fig. 25.1 A, Classic lesion of recurrent herpes simplex with grouped vesicles on an erythematous base. **B,** Recurrent herpes genitalis. (Courtesy Fitzsimons Army Medical Center teaching files.)

9. **How do HSV-1 and HSV-2 differ?**
   HSV types 1 and 2 are very closely related, sharing approximately 50% homology in their genetic composition. As expected, many of their viral proteins are also similar (known as type-common), although each type also produces unique proteins (type-specific). Immunohistologic techniques can be used to distinguish these type-specific proteins and differentiate HSV-1 from HSV-2 in clinical situations. Serologic testing that can accurately identify and differentiate antibodies to HSV-1 versus antibodies to HSV-2 is now also available (glycoprotein G type-specific assays). HSV-1 is usually associated with oral herpes and HSV-2 with genital herpes, although each virus can affect both sites. HSV-1 cannot be differentiated from HSV-2 based on the appearance of the skin lesions alone.

Nasrallah GK, Dargham SR, Abu-Raddad LJ. Negative epidemiological association between HSV-1 and HSV-2 infections. *Heliyon.* 2019;5 (10):e02549.

10. **How do you diagnose HSV infection?**
    The clinical history of recurrent blisters or erosions in the same site (especially in an oral or genital distribution) is highly suspicious for HSV infection. A prodrome of tingling or burning is also consistent with this diagnosis. On physical examination, the classic lesion is grouped vesicles on an erythematous base (see Fig. 25.1A), but more often, only nonspecific crusted erosions are seen. To confirm the diagnosis, laboratory assessment may be needed. The gold standard remains viral culture. However, use of many other rapid and sensitive techniques for detection of viral-specific proteins or nucleic acids is often available. For any method of detection, the age of the lesion sampled is critical. Vesicles are optimal but ulcers and erosions, if they are not dry and crusted, may also yield positive results.

11. **How is a Tzanck smear performed?**
    In a Tzanck smear, the base of the suspected herpetic lesion is gently scraped, and the skin or mucosal cells removed are placed on a glass slide. The cells are stained and then examined by light microscopy for evidence of viral-induced cytologic change, including the characteristic multinucleated giant cells (see Chapter 3, Fig. 3.5). Tzanck smears provide an efficient and inexpensive method of diagnosis, although the results are not always definitive. This technique cannot distinguish HSV-1 from HSV-2 or HSV from VZV.

12. **What are the drugs of choice for treatment of HSV?**
    There are three systemic antiviral agents routinely used for the treatment of HSV: acyclovir, valacyclovir, and famciclovir (Table 25.1). Valacyclovir is the L-valyl ester of acyclovir, with a bioavailability three to five times greater than acyclovir. Famciclovir is the diacetyl-6-deoxy analog of penciclovir. It is well absorbed and has a long intracellular half-life. Both valacyclovir and famciclovir offer the advantage of less frequent dosing compared to acyclovir. All three drugs are generally safe and highly effective because of their very specific antiviral activity. The antiviral drug is preferentially taken up by infected cells, where it must be converted to its active form by the viral enzyme thymidine kinase. The active form preferentially inhibits viral DNA synthesis, with little impact on host cell metabolism.

Whitley R, Baines J. Clinical management of herpes simplex virus infections: past, present, and future. *F1000Res.* 2018;7. pii: F1000 Faculty Rev-1726.

13. **When is chronic suppressive therapy indicated?**
    Once an episode of recurrent HSV infection (whether oral or genital) has begun, initiation of antiviral therapy often provides only mild symptomatic improvement. If antiviral therapy is initiated during the prodromal phase, the response may be somewhat better. In patients with frequently recurrent or severe disease, especially with genital herpes,

Table 25.1 Recommendations for systemic antiviral treatment of mucocutaneous herpes simplex virus (HSV) infection[*]

	DRUG	RECOMMENDED DOSAGE
Genital HSV		
Primary/first episode	Acyclovir	400 mg PO tid or 200 mg PO five times per day for 7–10 days (mild to moderate)
		5 mg/kg IV q8h for 5 days (severe)
	Valacyclovir	1 g PO bid for 7–10 days
	Famciclovir	250 mg PO tid for 10 days
Recurrent episode (start at prodrome)	Acyclovir	400 mg PO tid or 200 mg PO five times per day for 5 days
	Valacyclovir	500 mg PO bid for 3 days
		1 g daily for 5 days
	Famciclovir	1 g PO bid for 1 day
		125 mg PO bid for 5 days
Chronic suppression	Acyclovir	400 mg PO bid or 200 mg PO tid; adjust up or down according to response (six or more outbreaks per year)
	Valacyclovir	500 mg PO qd[*] (10 or more outbreaks per year)
		1 g PO qd (10 or more outbreaks per year)
	Famciclovir	250 mg PO bid (six or more outbreaks per year)
Orofacial HSV		
Primary/first episode	Acyclovir	15 mg/kg five times per day for 7 days
	Valacyclovir	1 g bid for 7 days
	Famciclovir	500 mg bid for 7 days
Recurrent (start at prodrome)	Acyclovir	400 mg PO 5 times per day for 5 days
	Valacyclovir	2 g PO bid for 1 day
	Famciclovir	1500 mg as single dose
Chronic suppression	Acyclovir	400 mg PO bid–tid
	Valacyclovir	500 mg to 1 g PO qd
Orolabial or Genital HSV in Immunosuppressed Patients		
Recurrent/suppressive	Acyclovir	400 mg PO three times per day or 5–10 mg/kg IV q8h
	Valacyclovir	500 mg to 1 g PO bid
	Famciclovir	500 mg PO bid

[*]Dose should be adjusted in the presence of renal insufficiency.
bid, Twice daily; *IV*, intravenous; *PO*, by mouth; *qd*, daily; *tid*, three times a day.

chronic suppressive therapy may be considered. After 1 year on therapy, a "drug holiday" may be given to assess the continued need for treatment, since the natural history of recurrent infection is to decrease in frequency with time.

Pittet LF, Curtis N. Does oral antiviral suppressive therapy prevent recurrent herpes labialis in children? *Arch Dis Child.* 2019;104(9):916–919. doi:10.1136/archdischild-2019-317249.

14. **Are patients with genital herpes at greater risk for becoming infected with the human immunodeficiency virus (HIV)?**
    Genital infection with HSV-2 increases the risk for HIV infection, even between active episodes. The population of immune cells that remain at the site of genital herpes lesions even after they have healed is thought to provide a favorable environment for acquisition of HIV.

McKay SL, Guo A, Pergam SA, Dooling K. Herpes zoster risk in immunocompromised adults in the United States: a systematic review [published online ahead of print November 2, 2019]. *Clin Infect Dis.* 2019;ciz1090. doi:10.1093/cid/ciz1090.

15. **What recommendations can you make to a patient with genital herpes to reduce the risk of transmission to his or her partner?**
    At the very least, avoidance of sexual contact during clinically apparent disease (i.e., until lesions are completely dry) is advised. In light of the problem with asymptomatic shedding, the safest practice is the routine use of a condom, even between active episodes. The systemic antiviral agents decrease, but do not eliminate, asymptomatic shedding. However, in the case of monogamous but discordant (one partner has genital herpes and the other does not) couples,

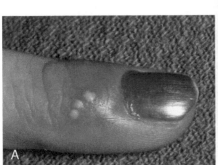
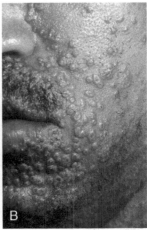

Fig. 25.2 A, Herpetic whitlow. **B,** Eczema herpeticum (Kaposi's varicelliform eruption) in a patient with atopic dermatitis. (Panel A courtesy Walter Reed Army Medical Center teaching files; panel B courtesy Scott D. Bennion, MD.)

chronic suppressive therapy taken by the infected partner may reduce the likelihood of transmitting the disease to the uninfected partner.

Garland SM, Steben M. Genital herpes. *Best Pract Res Clin Obstet Gynaecol.* 2014;28(7):1098–1110.

16. Can HSV infect the skin in areas other than around the mouth or anogenital areas?

    Yes. HSV infection may involve and recur at any location on the mucocutaneous surface. HSV infection of the hand or fingers, known as herpetic whitlow, is usually the result of autoinoculation from another site of infection (Fig. 25.2A). Herpes gladiatorum is a problem most commonly seen in athletes who participate in close contact sports such as wrestling. Typically transmitted from active herpes labialis or asymptomatic shedding in oral secretions of an infected opponent, herpes gladiatorum often affects the head, neck, or shoulders. Eczema herpeticum, also known as Kaposi's varicelliform eruption, represents a cutaneous dissemination of HSV (Fig. 25.2B). It may develop as a complication of a localized HSV infection in patients with atopic dermatitis or other underlying skin disease.

17. How does a baby get herpes? Is it a serious problem?

    In most cases, transmission of HSV to the neonate occurs by delivery through an infected birth canal. Postpartum acquisition occurs less commonly. Development of primary or initial nonprimary genital herpes by the mother at or near the time of delivery poses a significant risk for the infant. However, most cases of neonatal herpes are the result of asymptomatic shedding in women with no known history of genital herpes. Most neonatal herpes infections are the result of undiagnosed, new-onset HSV infection in the mother. Primary infection with HSV may lead to severe illness in pregnancy and may lead to intrauterine death, severe malformations, and premature birth and life-threatening infection of the newborn. The usual onset of neonatal herpes is 5 to 21 days following exposure. Approximately 80% of infected neonates have at least some characteristic skin lesions.

    In the United States, the overall incidence rate is 5–33/100,000 live births resulting in an estimated 1500 cases annually. The risk of neonatal transmission is 57% with first-episode primary infection and 25% with first-episode non-primary infection. Disease may be classified as SEM (skin, eye, mucosa), CNS, or disseminated. SEM accounts for 45% of cases; CNS with or without SEM, for 33%, and disseminated, about 20%–25%. In all, 60% will have skin lesions.

Pinninti SG, Kimberlin DW. Neonatal herpes simplex virus infections. *Semin Perinatol.* 2018;42(3):168–175.

18. How does intrapartum versus intrauterine HSV infection differ?

    Intrapartum infection accounts for 86% of neonatal HSV cases versus 4% to 5% for intrauterine transmission. Assuming an incidence of HSV infection of 1 in 5000 deliveries, intrauterine infection occurs in 1 in 100,000 deliveries. Despite this low incidence, intrauterine HSV infection is important because it can have potentially catastrophic consequences such as death or severe neurodevelopmental disability. Infants acquiring HSV in utero typically have a triad of clinical findings consisting of cutaneous manifestations (scarring, active lesions, hypo- and hyperpigmentation, aplasia cutis, and/or an erythematous macular exanthem), ophthalmologic findings (microphthalmia, retinal dysplasia, optic atrophy, and/or chorioretinitis), and neurologic involvement (microcephaly, encephalomalacia, hydranencephaly, and/or intracranial calcification).

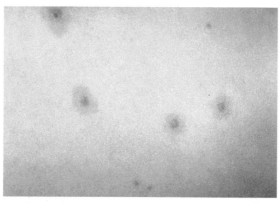

Fig. 25.3 Varicella with skin lesions at all stages of development. (Courtesy Joseph G. Morelli, MD.)

19. Which babies are at greatest risk of becoming infected with HSV?

Infants born to mothers who have a first episode of genital HSV infection near term are at much greater risk of developing neonatal herpes than are those whose mothers have recurrent genital herpes.

20. Describe the natural history of Varicella.

Varicella, or chickenpox, is the primary infection with VZV. It is characterized by the appearance of two to three successive crops of diffuse, pruritic vesicles and papules over several days. These lesions then evolve into pustules and crusted erosions, so that lesions in all stages of development are present together (Fig. 25.3). Lesions generally persist for up to 1 week.

Varicella most commonly occurs during childhood. It is highly contagious, both via respiratory secretions and contact with the cutaneous lesions. The incubation period ranges from 10 to 23 days, and the patient is considered contagious from 4 days before the onset of lesions until all lesions have crusted.

21. What is shingles?

Herpes zoster, or "shingles," is the recurrent form of infection with VZV and represents reactivation of the latent virus in the sensory ganglia. The cutaneous eruption consists of painful and/or pruritic vesicles, which tend to follow a unilateral, dermatomal distribution (Fig. 25.4). Prodromal pain may often precede the development of visible lesions. The entire course is usually 2 to 3 weeks in duration. The most common area of involvement for herpes zoster is the trunk (dermatomes innervated by the thoracic nerves), followed by the head (first branch of the trigeminal nerve). Herpes zoster is most typically seen in older and/or immunocompromised individuals.

Dayan RR, Peleg R. Herpes zoster—typical and atypical presentations. *Postgrad Med.* 2017;129(6):567–571.

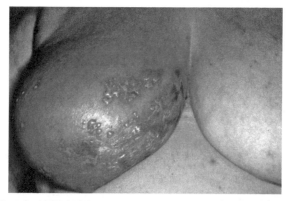

Fig. 25.4 Herpes zoster. Grouped vesicles on an erythematous base in a dermatomal distribution. (Courtesy Fitzsimons Army Medical Center teaching files.)

22. Can herpes zoster be recurrent?

Approximately 5% of patients with herpes zoster will experience a recurrence, usually in the same dermatome. However, recurrent HSV may also have a "zosteriform" distribution, indistinguishable from herpes zoster both clinically and on Tzanck smear. Although this presentation is not common, the possibility should be entertained, especially when the dermatomes involved are in the orofacial or genital distribution or the patient presents with "recurrent zoster."

23. What is disseminated zoster?

Disseminated zoster is defined as the presence of more than 20 vesicles outside the primary and adjacent dermatomes. It is uncommon in immunocompetent patients, but up to 40% of immunocompromised patients may develop this complication. In these cases, visceral involvement may also occur.

24. Is herpes zoster contagious?

Herpes zoster is the result of reactivation of latent VZV in the sensory ganglia. There is no evidence that a person can develop herpes zoster as a result of contact with patients with either varicella or herpes zoster. However, direct contact with the cutaneous lesions may result in transmission of primary varicella to a susceptible host.

25. What is postherpetic neuralgia?

Postherpetic neuralgia is the most common complication of herpes zoster. It is defined as the presence of pain after skin lesions have healed, or pain lasting more than 3 months after the onset of cutaneous lesions. The pain is often severe and debilitating. Overall, it occurs in 10% to 15% of patients, but the incidence increases dramatically with age so that over half of patients with herpes zoster who are older than 60 years develop postherpetic neuralgia. Other risk factors include prominent prodromal symptoms and moderate or severe pain at presentation. In most cases, postherpetic neuralgia resolves spontaneously within the first 12 months, but it may persist for years.

Kanamori K, Shoji K, Kinoshita N, Ishiguro A, Miyairi I. Complications of herpes zoster in children. *Pediatr Int.* 2019;61(12):1216–1220.

26. How do you diagnose VZV infection?

For varicella, the physical findings of lesions in various stages of development (papules, vesicles, pustules, and erosions), especially with a history of exposure to an individual with varicella (or zoster), is generally enough to make the diagnosis. The diagnosis of herpes zoster is also often made on the basis of physical findings. A Tzanck smear may be useful. If additional laboratory evaluation is indicated, immunohistochemical testing to detect viral-specific antigens in infected cells is recommended. A viral culture may be performed, although culturing VZV is more difficult and takes longer than culturing HSV. Use of PCR has become more commonly available. VZV serology is rarely useful for diagnosis.

27. What is the treatment for varicella?

Generally, symptomatic therapy, such as calamine lotion and oral antihistamines, is all that is required. Acyclovir is not routinely recommended for otherwise healthy children from a cost-effective standpoint. However, for varicella in an adult or immunocompromised individual, prompt initiation of systemic antiviral therapy is advised (Table 25.2). Routine childhood vaccination to prevent varicella is now recommended for children and adolescents who have not been infected. Vaccination is also recommended for susceptible adults, especially those at high risk for exposure.

28. How about herpes zoster?

Herpes zoster is a self-limited disease and in most young, otherwise healthy persons, symptomatic measures (cool compresses, antihistamines, analgesics) are sufficient. However, for persons who are over 50 years of age, have

---

Table 25.2 Recommendations for systemic antiviral treatment of varicella-zoster virus[*]

Varicella (start within 24 hours of rash onset)
Acyclovir 20 mg/kg (up to 800 mg) PO qid for 5 days (children)
Acyclovir 800 mg PO five times per day for 7 days (adult)
Acyclovir 10–12 mg/kg q8h for 7–10 days
Herpes zoster: immunocompetent patients
Acyclovir 800 mg PO five times per day for 7–10 days
Valacyclovir 1 g PO tid for 7 days
Famciclovir 500 mg PO tid for 7 days
Herpes zoster: immunosuppressed patients
Acyclovir 800 mg PO five times per day for 10 days[†]
Acyclovir 10 mg/kg/dose IV q8h for 7–10 days[†]
Valacyclovir 1 g PO tid for 10 days[†]
Famciclovir 500 mg PO tid for 10 days[†]

[*]Dose should be adjusted in the presence of renal insufficiency.
[†]Continue until there are no new lesions for 48 hours.
IV, Intravenous; *PO*, by mouth; *tid*, three times a day.

ophthalmic zoster, or are immunocompromised, systemic antiviral therapy is recommended (see Table 25.2). If started within 72 hours of the onset of skin lesions, systemic antiviral therapy reduces the discomfort and duration of the acute infection and may reduce the severity of postherpetic neuralgia.

29. Should I be concerned about the patient with herpes zoster involving the tip of the nose?
Lesions of herpes zoster involving the tip, side, or root of the nose indicate involvement of the nasociliary branch of the first division of the trigeminal nerve. This is known as Hutchinson's sign and should alert you to the possibility of herpes zoster ophthalmicus (see Fig. 25.4). Ocular disease occurs in 20% to 70% of patients with ophthalmic zoster, and antiviral therapy as well as ophthalmologic evaluation are routinely recommended. The triad of herpes zoster with cutaneous involvement of the auditory canal and auricle, ipsilateral facial palsy, and excruciating ear pain is known as the Ramsay Hunt syndrome and is the result of viral reactivation within the geniculate ganglion.

30. Who should get the herpes zoster vaccine?
Vaccination with a herpes zoster vaccine substantially reduces the incidence of noth herpes zoster and possible post-herpetic neuralgia. There are two herpes zoster vaccines available. The live attenuated vaccine (ZVL/Zostavax) has been in use since 2006 and is given as a single intramuscular injection. The Zoster Vaccine Recombinant Adjuvanted (RZV/Shingrex) received FDA approval in 2017 for immunocompetent adults 50 years and older. RZV is a non-live recombinant glycoprotein E vaccine and requires two doses given intramuscularly 2–6 moths apart. The U.S. Advisory Committee on Immunization Practices (ACIP) currently recommends the use of RZV for immunocompetent adults aged 50 years or older for the prevention of herpes zoster and related complications. The ACIP also recommends RZV for adults aged 50 years or older who previously received the live-attenuated herpes zoster vaccine (ZVL/Zostavax) and either RZV or ZVL for adults aged 60 years or older (RZV is preferred).

Gagliardi AM, Andriolo BN, Torloni MR, Soares BG. Vaccines for preventing herpes zoster in older adults. *Cochrane Database Syst Rev.* 2019;2019(11).

31. What is hand, foot, and mouth disease?
Hand, foot, and mouth disease (HFMD), or vesicular stomatitis with exanthem, is usually seen in infants or young children. Following a brief prodrome of fever, malaise, and sore throat, the characteristic enanthem develops. Red macules, vesicles, and ulcers may be seen on the buccal mucosa, tongue, palate, and pharynx (Fig. 25.5A). Lesions may also occur on the hands and feet (dorsal aspects, as well as the palms and soles) (Fig. 25.5B). HFMD is caused by one of several enteroviruses, most commonly coxsackievirus A16. It is highly contagious and spreads by direct contact via the oral-oral or oral-fecal route. Over the past 10 years, outbreaks of HFMD caused by enterovirus 71 have been reported in Asia and Australia. Although HFMD associated with coxsackievirus A16 infection is typically a mild illness, HFMD caused by enterovirus 71 has shown a higher incidence of neurologic involvement including fatal cases of encephalitis.

32. What is "eczema coxsackium"?
The presence of monomorphous erosions and vesicles in areas previously or currently affected by atopic dermatitis, similar to eczema herpeticum, caused by coxsackievirus 6 (Fig. 25.6). This virus was responsible for an HFMD outbreak in 2011–2013 that characteristically had a wide range and severe cutaneous features including widespread vesiculobullous and erosive lesions extending beyond palms and soles, eczema coxsackium, an eruption similar to Gianotti-Crosti syndrome, and a petechial or purpuric eruption.

Horsten HH, Fisker N, Bygum A. Eczema coxsackium caused by coxsackievirus A6. *Pediatr Dermatol.* 2016;33(3):e230–e231.
Mathes EF, Oza V, Frieden IJ, et al. "Eczema coxsackium" and unusual cutaneous findings in an enterovirus outbreak. *Pediatrics.* 2013;132:149–157.

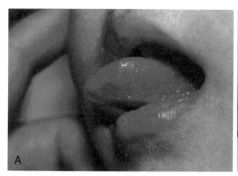
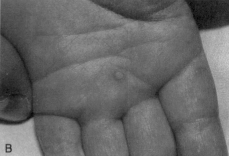

Fig. 25.5 Hand, foot, and mouth disease. **A**, Vesicular stomatitis. **B**, Typical lesions on palmar skin. The vesicular lesions are classically gray and often elliptical.

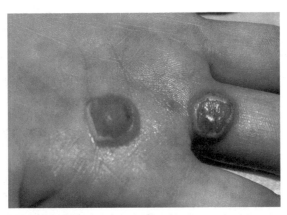

Fig. 25.6 Orf. Classic developed lesions demonstrating two vesiculobullous nodules with central ulceration developing in a man after digging in his yard that had once been a sheep farm.

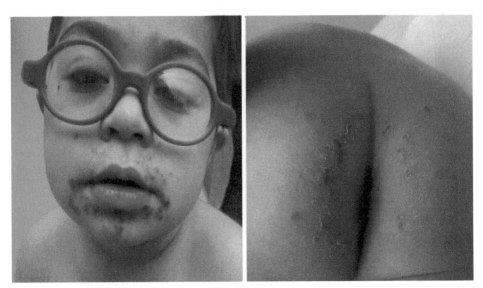

Fig. 25.7 Eczema coxsackium. Crusted eczematous papules on perioral and perianal area. Patient has a history of atopic dermatitis. (Courtesy Pediatric Dermatology Department at The Children's Hospital Colorado teaching files.)

33. What is orf?

Human orf, or ecthyma contagiosum, is caused by a parapoxvirus that is usually contracted by direct exposure to infected, or recently vaccinated, sheep or goats. Milkers' nodules are caused by a closely related virus found in cows. The lesions of both orf and milkers' nodules are identical, consisting of dome-shaped, firm bullae that develop an umbilicated crust (Fig. 25.7). One to several lesions develop, usually on the hands and forearms. They generally resolve without therapy in 4 to 6 weeks.

Caravaglio JV, Khachemoune A. Orf virus infection in humans: a review with a focus on advances in diagnosis and treatment. *J Drugs Dermatol.* 2017;16(7):684–689.

KEY POINTS: HERPES SIMPLEX VIRUS

1. HSV is transmitted by direct contact with the infected skin or mucosal surface.
2. Many cases of primary HSV are asymptomatic so that the first evidence of infection may represent a recurrence.
3. Asymptomatic shedding occurs in both orolabial and genital HSV infection.
4. For laboratory confirmation, either viral culture or an antigen detection technique is recommended.
5. Early initiation of oral antiviral therapy is the key to its success.

KEY POINTS: VARICELLA-ZOSTER VIRUS

1. Varicella (chickenpox) is the primary infection.
2. Herpes zoster (shingles) is the recurrent infection.
3. Postherpetic neuralgia is a common complication of herpes zoster, especially in older individuals.
4. Ophthalmologic evaluation and systemic antiviral therapy are recommended for patients with herpes zoster ophthalmicus.
5. The herpes zoster vaccine may substantially reduce the risk for herpes zoster and the development of postherpetic neuralgia in patients age 60 years or older.

WEBSITES

International Herpes Management Forum. www.ihmf.org.
National Institute of Allergy and Infectious Diseases. www.niaid.nih.gov.
Centers for Disease Control and Prevention. www.cdc.gov.

CHAPTER 26

WARTS AND MOLLUSCUM CONTAGIOSUM

Kristen G. Berrebi and James Fitzpatrick

You got to go all by yourself, to the middle of the woods, where you know there's a spunk-water stump, and just as it's midnight, you back up against the stump and jam your hand in and say:
Barley-corn, barley-corn, injun-meal shorts,
Spunk-water, spunk-water, swaller these warts,
and then walk away quick, 11 steps, with your eyes shut, and then turn around three times and walk home without speaking to anybody. Because if you speak the charm's busted.

Tom Sawyer to Huck Finn on Curing Warts in *The Adventures of Tom Sawyer* by Mark Twain

1. **What causes warts?**
   Warts are caused by the human papillomavirus (HPV), a nonenveloped double-stranded DNA virus. There are over 200 known HPV types, and over 100 have been totally sequenced. The virus infects basal keratinocytes, resulting in keratinocyte hyperproliferation.

2. **Do any warts come from toads?**
   No. There is no supportive scientific evidence—histologic, viral, or other—that the bumps on the skin of a toad are at all related to warts.

3. **Name the common types of warts.**
   HPV infection is highly specific for the epithelia of the skin or mucosa. Some HPV types are associated with specific clinical presentations (Table 26.1). For example, flat warts are seen primarily on the face and hands of both children and immunosuppressed patients and are often caused by HPV-3 and -10 (Fig. 26.1A). Common warts occur most often on the fingers, elbows, and knees and are frequently associated with HPV-1, -2, and -4 (Fig. 26.1B). An example of warts in an immunosuppressed patient can be seen in Fig. 26.1C.

4. **How are warts transmitted?**
   HPV is primarily transmitted via direct skin-to-skin contact with an infected individual and less frequently through fomites. Genital warts are most commonly transmitted through sexual intercourse. HPV may also be aerosolized during laser and electrocautery procedures leading to respiratory papillomatosis, which highlights the importance of wearing appropriate safety masks during these procedures. Any skin disease (i.e., atopic dermatitis) that affects the integrity of the stratum corneum may be associated with an increased risk of acquiring HPV infection. External factors may also affect barrier function. Warts can be acquired at swimming pools, where rough concrete surfaces may abrade the skin. Warts on hair-bearing skin may be spread by shaving. Periungual warts are often found in persons who have a habit of biting their cuticles.

5. **How long is the incubation period of warts?**
   Unknown. It is estimated to be several weeks to months. HPV is demonstrable by DNA hybridization and polymerase chain reaction in skin that is clinically normal, indicating the likelihood of a latent or subclinical form of HPV. In addition, it is not uncommon for a wart to recur in the same location many years following apparent resolution.

6. **Are some people more susceptible to warts than others?**
   Warts are common in healthy children and young adults; however, individuals with compromised cell-mediated immunity are more susceptible to warts than others. This includes patients with certain blood cell cancers, HIV infection, a primary immunodeficiency syndrome, or transplant patients on immunosuppressive drugs. Diseases that affect the barrier function of the skin also increase susceptibility to warts.

7. **What is epidermodysplasia verruciformis (EV)?**
   EV is a rare, inherited disorder in which cutaneous HPV infection is generalized and persistent. Most cases are autosomal recessive, but autosomal dominant and X-linked dominant forms are also reported. It is caused by mutations in either the *EVER1* or *EVER2* genes located on chromosome 17. The lesions are either flat warts or reddish-brown plaques, often developing in sun-exposed areas (Fig. 26.2A). Actinic keratosis begins to develop after the age of 30, and approximately half of EV patients will develop squamous cell carcinoma (SCC). HPV types 5 and 8 are associated with EV.

Przybyszewska J, Zlotogorski A, Ramot Y. Re-evaluation of epidermodysplasia verruciformis: reconciling more than 90 years of debate. *J Am Acad Dermatol.* 2017;76:1161–1175.

Table 26.1 Clinical Presentation of Common Types of Warts

TYPE OF WART	USUAL LOCATION	COMMON PRESENTATION	COMMON HPV TYPES
Common (verruca vulgaris)	Variable	Flesh-colored, rough, hyperkeratotic papules; single or grouped	2, 4, 29
Plantar, palmar	Soles, palms; may be painful	Thick, hyperkeratotic lesions	1, 2, 4, 10
Flat (verruca planae)	Face, hands, knees	Small, 2–5-mm, flat-topped, hyperpigmented papules; multiple	3, 10
Anogenital (condyloma acuminatum)	Genitalia, anogenital region	Moist, cauliflower-like masses, variably sized; sexually transmitted	6, 11
Epidermodysplasia verruciformis (EV)	Diffuse, most prominent on hands and feet	Diffuse verrucous hyperkeratosis with fissuring	5, 8

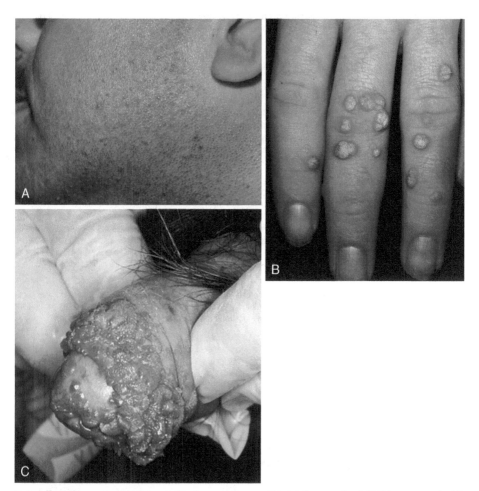

Fig. 26.1 Common types of warts. **A,** Flat warts of the face presenting as multiple 1- to 2-mm papules. **B,** Multiple common warts of the hands and feet. **C,** Condyloma acuminatum of the penis presenting as moist cauliflower-like papillomas. (Panels A and B courtesy James E. Fitzpatrick, MD; panel C courtesy Scott Norton, MD.)

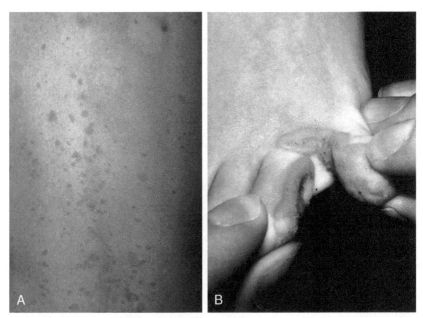

Fig. 26.2 A, Multiple reddish-brown macules of the back in a patient with epidermodysplasia verruciformis. **B,** "Kissing" warts produced by inoculation of the toe web space. (Courtesy James E. Fitzpatrick, MD.)

8. Can HPV cause cancer?

    Certain HPV types are associated with the development of malignancy. HPV-16, -18, -31, -33, or -45 are identified in most cases of cervical cancer; however, HPV-35, -39, -51, -52, -56, -58, -59, -68, -73, and -82 are also considered oncogenic. HPV does not just cause cervical cancer; some HPV types can also cause cutaneous malignancies.

Muñoz N, Bosch FX, de Sanjosé S, et al. Epidemiologic classification of human papillomavirus types associated with cervical cancer. *N Engl J Med.* 2003;348(6):518–527.

9. How does HPV cause cancer?

    High-risk HPV types are associated with E6 and E7 proteins, which inactivate the tumor suppressor proteins, p53 and Rb.

10. What is the difference between the Gardasil 9 and Cervarix HPV vaccines?

    Gardasil 9 and Cervarix are prophylactic vaccines consisting of virus-like particles derived from HPV L1 major capsid protein. Gardasil 9 is protective against seven oncogenic strains (HPV-16, -18, -31, -33, -45, -52, and -58) and HPV types 6 and 11 that are nononcogenic HPV strains that produce genital warts in both men and women. In contrast, Cervarix is a bivalent vaccine with proven protection against the oncogenic strains HPV-16 and -18 that are associated with approximately 70% of all cervical cancers. These vaccines are not protective against genotypes that cause common cutaneous warts.

11. What is verrucous carcinoma?

    Verrucous carcinoma is a locally aggressive, well-differentiated SCC that is associated with HPV-6 and -11 infection. Clinically, verrucous carcinoma can be difficult to differentiate from a large wart or condyloma acuminatum. Continued slow growth of a large wart resistant to many different treatment modalities should prompt further investigation. Three major subtypes have been described: epithelioma cuniculatum of the sole (plantar foot); *Buschke-Löwenstein tumor* (genitalia); and *proliferative verrucous hyperplasia*, also known as oral florid papillomatosis (oral mucosa) (see Chapter 62).

12. What causes the black dots within a wart?

    The small black dots, incorrectly referred to as "seeds," are actually thrombosed blood vessels.

13. Is there a best way to treat warts?

    Several treatments exist for warts; however, no single treatment method may be relied upon to eliminate warts permanently (Table 26.2). Factors influencing treatment choice include patient-specific factors (age, pain tolerance,

Table 26.2 Treatments for Warts

TREATMENT	WART TYPE	COMMENTS
Destructive Methods		
Cryotherapy	All	Dyschromia, pain, scar
Electrosurgery	Resistant	Scar, recurrence
Surgery	Resistant	Scar, recurrence
Carbon dioxide laser	Resistant	Scar, recurrence
Pulsed dye laser	Resistant	Not readily available
Caustic Acids		
Monochloroacetic, dichloroacetic, and trichloroacetic acid	Common	Irritation, blisters, scar
Cantharidin	Small, common	Irritation, blisters, hyperpigmentation, fairy ring warts
Chemotherapeutic Agents		
Podophyllotoxin*	External genital, common	Erythema, erosions, ulcers, pain
Bleomycin (intralesional)*	Common	Pain, nail loss, nail dystrophy, Raynaud's phenomenon
5-Fluorouracil (topical)*	Flat	Irritation
Immunotherapy		
Candida antigen (intralesional)	Multiple, resistant	Clearance of distant untreated warts
Imiquimod (topical)*	External genital	Erythema, burning, erosion, pruritus
Contact hypersensitivity	Resistant	Squaric acid, diphenylcyclopropenone (DPCP)
Formalin*	Plantar	Contact sensitivity
Antiviral agents	Resistant, immunosuppression	Renal toxicity
Miscellaneous		
Interferon*	Anogenital	Inject intralesional or intramuscular
Tretinoin (topical)*	Flat	Irritation
Glutaraldehyde	Plantar	Brown discoloration, allergy
Cimetidine (oral)*	Resistant	For refractory cases in children
Salicylic acid	Common, plantar	Available over the counter
Retinoids (oral)*	Immunosuppression	Relapse when drug is discontinued

*Avoid during pregnancy.

treatment anxiety), disease burden (morphology, number of lesions, distribution of lesions, associated symptoms), and cost. The physician's primary concern should be to do no harm, as warts are benign skin lesions. Resistance and recurrence are common with most treatments.

TREATMENT PEARLS

- **Flat warts:** These warts are commonly located on the face. Destructive modalities carry a higher risk of dyspigmentation. These warts respond well to treatment with topical tretinoin cream or imiquimod.
- **Multiple warts:** Destructive modalities may not be practical. Consider intralesional immunotherapy (i.e., intralesional *Candida* antigen). With immunotherapy both treated and distant untreated warts commonly resolve.
- **Filiform warts:** These warts are commonly located on the face. Using a hemostat or forceps dipped in liquid nitrogen allows one to freeze the base of the wart while minimizing damage to surrounding tissue.
- **Immunosuppressed patients:** Topical, intralesional, and intravenous cidofovir may be effective for treatment of recalcitrant warts in immunosuppressed patients.

- **Weight-bearing (plantar):** These warts are often recalcitrant to treatment. Combined salicylic acid products with pulsed dye laser are sometimes effective. Bleomycin may be used in refractory cases.
- **Children:** Many warts regress without treatment. Avoid painful modalities in younger children with multiple warts if they are not motivated to treat.

Smolinski KN, Yan AC. How and when to treat molluscum contagiosum and warts in children. *Pediatr Ann.* 2005;34:211–221.

14. What are common side effects of treatment methods?
- Scarring (liquid nitrogen, laser, acids, cantharidin).
- Blistering (liquid nitrogen, cantharidin, topical 5-fluorouracil, bleomycin) (Fig. 26.3A).
- Allergy (cantharidin, chemotherapeutic agents, tretinoin, acids, glutaraldehyde).
- Persistent hyper- or hypopigmentation (liquid nitrogen).

15. What are ring warts?
Ring warts, or satellite warts, are annular warts that may develop following any treatment that produces blisters, particularly with inadequate treatment of the peripheral edges of the lesion (Fig. 26.3B). Including a rim of surrounding skin in the treatment area may help prevent their occurrence.

16. Should all warts be eradicated?
No. Warts are benign skin growths. Two-thirds will resolve spontaneously without treatment over a 2-year period; however, there is potential for spread via autoinoculation prior to resolution. Warts may also be symptomatic or cosmetically unappealing. For these reasons, warts are often treated.

17. Should any treatments be avoided?
- Pregnancy: Chemotherapeutic agents, interferon, and retinoids should be avoided. Liquid nitrogen and laser are generally safe for use during pregnancy.
- Periungual warts: Destructive therapies (i.e., liquid nitrogen) and chemotherapeutic agents (i.e., bleomycin) may damage the nail matrix and cause permanent nail deformity.
- Bleomycin should be used with caution near the tips of digits, as Raynaud's phenomenon and sclerotic changes in the distal finger have been reported.
- IV cidofovir should be used with caution in patients with renal insufficiency.
- X-irradiation is not indicated for treatment of warts. Increased invasiveness of lesions following radiation has been reported.

18. How effective are over-the-counter (OTC) treatment options for warts?
Salicylic acid products can be effective if used consistently. OTC freezing products containing dimethyl ether and propane are less effective than in-office cryotherapy with liquid nitrogen.

Burkhart CG, Pchalek I, Adler M, et al. An in vitro study comparing temperatures of over-the-counter wart preparations with liquid nitrogen. *J Am Acad Dermatol.* 2007;57(6):1019–1020.

---

19. How can you tell if a wart is gone?
The return of normal skin lines without evidence of thrombosed vessels designates treatment success.

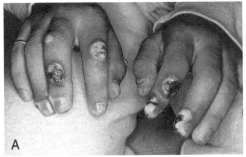 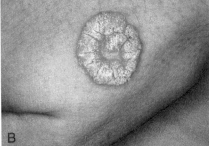

Fig. 26.3 Side effects of wart treatment. **A,** Painful blisters produced by cantharidin. (Courtesy Brenda Kokomo, MD) **B,** Fairy ring formation of warts on the wrist, at the periphery of a blister produced by previous liquid nitrogen therapy. (Courtesy James E. Fitzpatrick, MD.)

20. How can you be sure that warts will never come back?

You cannot. Given there are so many different serotypes of the HPV virus, it is possible for a patient to clear one serotype and then be infected with another.

21. Describe a few clinical scenarios involving warts that may warrant further investigation.
    - Anogenital warts in a prepubertal child generally over the age of 4 should prompt consideration of sexual abuse. However, autoinoculation must also be considered.
    - Sexual partners of patients with external genital warts (EGWs) should be evaluated for warts or other sexually transmitted diseases. Women with EGWs should be referred for cervical cancer screening using cytology +/− HPV molecular diagnostic tests per current guidelines.
    - Severe or recalcitrant warts associated with other signs of immune dysfunction should prompt consideration of an underlying primary or acquired immunodeficiency syndrome.
    - Biopsy is warranted for large, recalcitrant, and locally destructive lesions to rule out SCC.
    - Oral papillomas should be monitored frequently and biopsied early to rule out SCC.

KEY POINTS: HUMAN PAPILLOMAVIRUS INFECTION

1. There are over 200 known types of HPV, and over 100 have been totally sequenced.
2. Most HPV infections are not carcinogenic, but persistent infections with some genotypes, especially HPV-16 and HPV-18, are associated with a high risk of epithelial neoplasia.
3. Immunocompromised patients have a higher risk of HPV infection that is recalcitrant to treatment than those in immunocompetent individuals.
4. There is no single best treatment for warts.

22. Is molluscum contagiosum a type of wart?

No. Molluscum contagiosum is a viral infection of the skin produced by a poxvirus. Like warts, molluscum are more common in children and immunocompromised individuals and can be sexually acquired in adults. They may occur anywhere on the skin surface and present as firm, skin-colored umbilicated papules with a central core of keratin (Fig. 26.4A). Some lesions may demonstrate an intense host response (Fig. 26.4B). Many of the same treatments effective in treating warts are effective in treating molluscum contagiosum. In children with a normal immune system, this condition is self-limited, although resolution may take up to 2 years. In adults and immunocompromised individuals, the course may be prolonged and require treatment.

Forbat E, Al-Niaimi F, Ali FR. Molluscum contagiosum: review and update on management. *Pediatr Dermatol.* 2017;34:504–515.

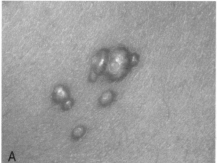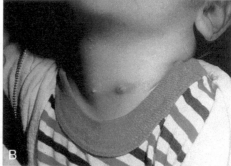

Fig. 26.4 A, Multiple papules of molluscum contagiosum demonstrating a characteristic central keratotic core. (Courtesy James E. Fitzpatrick MD) **B,** Inflammatory molluscum contagiosum in a young child demonstrating both small, waxy, umbilicated papules and an inflammatory lesion simulating a furuncle. (Courtesy Fitzsimons Army Medical Center teaching files.)

CHAPTER 27

BACTERIAL INFECTIONS

Kristen G. Berrebi and James E. Fitzpatrick

STAPHYLOCOCCAL INFECTIONS

1. Which bacterium is the most common cause of skin infections?

   Staphylococcus aureus. There are two types of *S. aureus* infections—methicillin-susceptible *S. aureus* (MSSA) infections and methicillin-resistant *S. aureus* (MRSA) infections. These two types of infections are differentiated by the classes of antibiotics to which they respond; however, clinically they look identical.

2. What kinds of skin infections does *Staphylococcus aureus* produce?

   * Impetigo (both bullous and nonbullous)—most common bacterial infection in children
   * Abscesses (occur any site)
   * Furuncles (occur only on hair-bearing sites)
   * Carbuncles (collection of furuncles)
   * Superficial folliculitis (impetigo of Bockhart)
   * Staphylococcal septicemia
   * Staphylococcal scalded skin syndrome
   * Staphylococcal cellulitis
   * Toxic shock syndrome (TSS)
   * Staphylococcal scarlet fever
   * Wound infections
   * Secondary infections of dermatitis

   The most common primary infections are impetigo and furuncles.

3. Is *Staphylococcus aureus* the only bacterium that causes impetigo?

   Older textbooks state that the most common cause of impetigo (impetigo contagiosum) is group A β-hemolytic *Streptococcus*. In recent years, most infections in the United States have been due to *S. aureus*, but the prevalence varies geographically. Although impetigo may be due to either organism, in some cases, both can be cultured. In these cases, it is thought that the streptococci are the primary infection and the staphylococci are secondary invaders after the infection has damaged the skin.

4. What does staphylococcal impetigo look like?

   Early lesions of staphylococcal impetigo appear as thin, flaccid blisters that may demonstrate cloudy contents or layering of pus (Fig. 27.1). The base of the blister may demonstrate variable erythema. Older lesions demonstrate a yellowish, "honey-colored" crust.

5. Why is staphylococcal impetigo frequently bullous?

   Bullous impetigo is caused by staphylococci that produce toxins (exfoliative toxins A and B), which cause a split in the epidermis by targeting the epidermal adhesion molecule, desmoglein 1 (Dsg-1). Phage group II staphylococci (types 55 and 71) are most commonly implicated.

   Hanawaka Y, Stanley JR. Mechanisms of blister formation by staphylococcal toxins. *J Biochem*. 2004;136:747–750.

6. How is bullous impetigo diagnosed?

   A Gram stain of the blister contents should demonstrate abundant gram-positive cocci, but the definitive test is a culture of the blister fluid. The diagnosis can also be established by doing a biopsy, which histologically demonstrates a subcorneal blister with neutrophils and cocci in the blister cavity.

7. How is bullous impetigo treated?

   There are several different classes of antibiotics that can be used to treat bullous impetigo, but typically, an oral B-lactamase resistant penicillin or first-generation cephalosporin is the first-line choice for severe infections due to MSSA. Oral clindamycin is frequently used in penicillin-allergic patients, although up to 20% or more of all staphylococci are resistant. Topical mupirocin can be used if the patient cannot take oral antibiotics or if the infection is localized to a small area. If MRSA is suspected or proven, then the first-line agent is either oral doxycycline or trimethoprim-sulfamethoxazole. For those patients who cannot take oral medication and have more complicated infections, IV cetriaxone is given for MSSA and vancomycin is administered for MRSA.

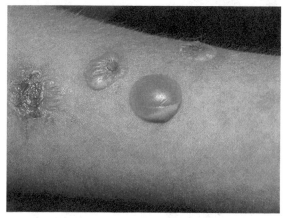

Fig. 27.1 Early lesion of bullous staphylococcal impetigo demonstrating fragile bullae with layering of the pus. A collapsed blister with lacquered appearance is also present. (Courtesy Fitzsimons Army Medical Center teaching files.)

8. What is the difference between a furuncle and a carbuncle?

A furuncle (boil) is a deep follicular abscess, and a carbuncle is a more serious subtype in which there is involvement of several adjoining follicles. A furuncle may develop into a carbuncle. Carbuncles are more likely to develop complications, such as cellulitis or septicemia.

9. How do furuncles present?

Furuncles may be solitary or multiple and present as painful, erythematous, deep-seated follicular abscesses (Fig. 27.2). Patients may demonstrate mild constitutional symptoms such as fever and regional lymphadenopathy in severe cases.

10. What is the best way to treat furuncles?

Small nonsuppurative solitary lesions are best treated with local heat until they become fluctuant and spontaneously drain. Large abscesses may require an incision, drainage, and a wick. Patients with many lesions, evidence of surrounding cellulitis, or with systemic symptoms should be treated with oral antibiotics.

The diagnosis should be confirmed with a culture and antibiotic sensitivities performed at the initial visit, since not all follicular-based abscesses are due to staphylococci.

11. Why do some patients develop recurrent staphylococcal impetigo or recurrent furunculosis?

Recurrent infections occur when *S. aureus* establishes itself as a part of the resident microbial flora. This occurs in up to 20% of individuals. The most common sites of carriage are the anterior nasal vestibule, axilla, groin, and feet.

Ibler KS, Kromann CB. Recurrent furunculosis—challenges and management: a review. *Clin Cosmet Investig Dermatol.* 2014; 18:59–64.

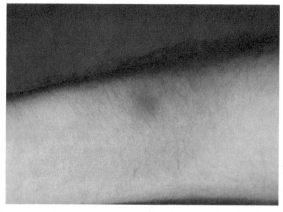

Fig. 27.2 Furuncle presenting as a very tender, erythematous follicular-based abscess.

12. **How is staphylococcal carriage eliminated?**
It is very difficult to eliminate staphylococcal carriage. Typical regimens include dilute bleach baths multiple times weekly in combination with decolonization of the nares with topical mupirocin ointment twice daily for 7–14 days. Oral treatment regimens are not preferred for decolonization, as these can induce resistance. Recolonization is common.

13. **What is staphylococcal scalded skin syndrome?**
Staphylococcal scalded skin syndrome typically occurs in infants, young children, or immunocompromised adults. Mortality is low in infants and young children (<5%) but high in adults, especially those with chronic renal failure (>50%). Like bullous impetigo, it is due to group II staphylococci that produces exfoliatoxins A and B. However, unlike bullous impetigo, a culture of the rash does not grow the pathogenic bacteria. The bacteria in staphylococcal scalded skin syndrome are located at a site distant to the rash, such as an abscess. The rash subsequently develops secondary to a buildup of exfoliatoxin systemically due to an inability of the kidneys to effectively excrete the toxins. The high level of exfoliatoxins produces diffuse, tender erythema associated with fever that rapidly progresses to flaccid bullae; the bullae wrinkle and exfoliate, leaving an oozing erythematous base (Fig. 27.3). Mortality is usually not due to the infection but is secondary to impaired temperature regulation or fluid balance.

Handler MZ, Schwartz RA. Staphylococcal scalded skin syndrome: diagnosis and management in children and adults. *J Eur Acad Dermatol Venereol.* 2014;28:1418–1423.

14. **Why *is S. aureus* frequently found in secondary infections of dermatitis and wounds?**
S. aureus has receptors that allow it to bind to fibrin that is found in abundance on wound surfaces and in dermatitic skin.

KEY POINTS: STAPHYLOCOCCAL SKIN INFECTIONS

1. *Staphylococcus aureus* is the most common cause of skin infection.
2. *Staphylococcus aureus* has replaced *Streptococcus pyogenes* as the most common cause of impetigo.
3. Bullous impetigo is always caused by *S. aureus* strains, usually phase II, type 55 and 71, that produce exfoliatoxins.
4. Approximately 20% of the population is colonized by *S. aureus*.
5. The anterior nares is the most common site of *S. aureus* colonization, but other moist sites including the axillae, groin, and toe webs can also be colonized.

STREPTOCOCCAL INFECTIONS

15. **What types of cutaneous infections are produced by β-hemolytic streptococci?**
β-Hemolytic streptococci are responsible for impetigo, blistering distal dactylitis, ecthyma, erysipelas, necrotizing fasciitis, septicemia, and TSS.

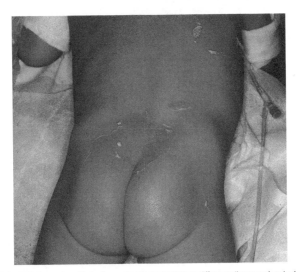

Fig. 27.3 Early staphylococcal scalded-skin syndrome demonstrating diffuse erythema and early desquamation.

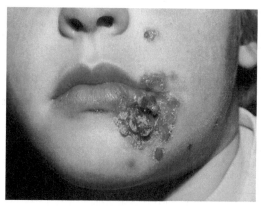

Fig. 27.4 Characteristic stuck-on, honey-colored crusts of streptococcal impetigo.

16. How does streptococcal impetigo present?

Streptococcal impetigo presents as superficial, stuck-on, honey-colored crusts overlying an erosion (Fig. 27.4). The most common location is the face, but any area may be involved. In contrast to staphylococcal impetigo, blisters are absent in the early stage. Since many patients present when lesions are old, it is often difficult to differentiate based on clinical appearance alone if streptococcus or staphylococcus is causing impetigo.

17. What is ecthyma?

Ecthyma is a severe form of streptococcal impetigo in which there is a thick crust overlying a punched-out ulceration of the epidermis (Fig. 27.5). Typically, it is surrounded by a zone of erythema. In contrast to streptococcal impetigo, which is usually found on the face and does not produce scarring, ecthyma is more commonly located on lower extremities and may heal with scarring.

18. What is blistering distal dactylitis?

Blistering distal dactylitis is an uncommon infection typically caused by *Streptococcus pyogenes* but occasionally caused by *S. aureus*. It typically presents in young children as one or more tender superficial bullae on an erythematous base on the volar fat pad of a finger (Fig. 27.6). In rare instances, toes may be affected.

19. What is erysipelas?

Erysipelas, or St. Anthony's fire, is a form of cellulitis usually caused by β-hemolytic streptococci, rarely by *S. aureus*. Patients often have a prodrome of malaise, fever, and headache. Typically, erysipelas presents on the face as an erythematous indurated plaque with a sharply demarcated border and a "cliff-drop" edge with palpation (Fig. 27.7).

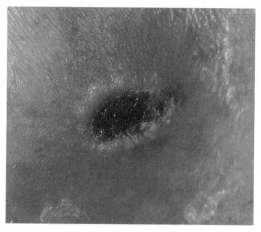

Fig. 27.5 Streptococcal ecthyma demonstrating punched-out ulceration surrounded by erythema.

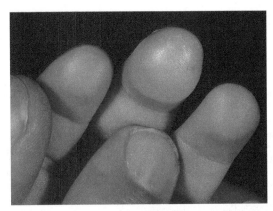

Fig. 27.6 Blistering distal dactylitis demonstrating a characteristic tender superficial blister on the volar fat pad.

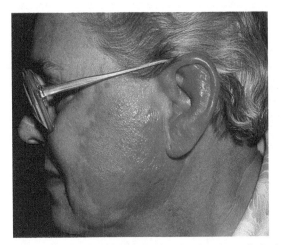

Fig. 27.7 Characteristic lesion of erysipelas demonstrating indurated, erythematous plaque with sharply demarcated border.

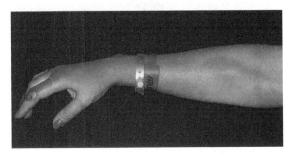

Fig. 27.8 Streptococcal cellulitis that started with an injury to the index finger. Note associated lymphangitis extending up the arm.

In severe cases, the epidermis may become bullous, pustular, or necrotic. Untreated erysipelas can be fatal due to vascular thrombosis, bacteremia, or toxin release. Streptococcal cellulitis is a more generic term that includes erysipelas but also cellulitis that lacks the characteristic cliff-drop border. Streptococcal cellulitis is most often found on extremities and is often associated with lymphangitis (Fig. 27.8). A subset of patients will develop recurrent erysipelas or streptococcal cellulitis.

20. How do you diagnose erysipelas?

The diagnosis usually is made clinically because the organism is difficult to recover in culture. Aspiration of the advancing edge following the injection of nonbacteriostatic saline produces positive cultures in about 20% of cases.

21. How is erysipelas treated?

Mild or early cases may be treated with an oral penicillin or oral erythromycin. Oral dicloxacillin is the best choice because it provides better antistaphylococcal coverage for the rare case of staphylococcal erysipelas. Severe cases or cases with central facial involvement should be hospitalized and treated with intravenous antibiotics, such as vancomycin. Erysipelas usually improves within 48 hours after institution of antibiotic therapy.

22. Describe the presentation of TSS.

TSS is an acute febrile illness that can be cause by either *S. aureus* or *Streptococcus pyogenes*. Staphylococcal TSS typically affects young, healthy adults and is classically associated with superabsorbent tampons or nasal packing. It has a mortality rate of 3%–20%, and blood cultures are often negative. Streptococcal TSS is also seen in young, healthy adults but has a higher mortality rate (30%–60%), is more frequently associated with skin and soft tissue infections, and has a higher rate of blood culture positivity (>50%). Despite being associated with more skin and soft tissue infections, having a higher rate of mortality, and having a higher rate of blood culture positivity, the rash is less impressive in streptococcal TSS than in staphylococcal TSS.

Clinically, the hallmarks of TSS are fever, hypotension, and a diffuse erythema that resembles scarlet fever. Other manifestations include pharyngeal erythema, strawberry tongue, conjunctival infection, and gastrointestinal symptoms. Desquamation of the palms and soles occurs 1 to 2 weeks following resolution of the erythema.

OTHER BACTERIAL INFECTIONS

23. What types of skin infections does *Pseudomonas aeruginosa* produce?

P. aeruginosa is one of the most feared bacterial pathogens in medicine. Cutaneous infections include:
- Ecthyma gangrenosum
- Septic vasculitis
- Pseudomonal folliculitis ("hot tub folliculitis")
- Otitis externa ("swimmer's ear")
- Toe web infection (pseudomonal pyoderma)
- *Pseudomonas* hot-foot syndrome
- Wound infections (burn wounds)
- Cellulitis
- Necrotizing fasciitis
- Green nail syndrome
- Paronychia

24. How does ecthyma gangrenosum differ from ecthyma?

- Ecthyma is caused by β-hemolytic streptococci, while ecthyma gangrenosum is most commonly caused by *P. aeruginosa*.
- Ecthyma is a localized infection that normally occurs in healthy young adults. Ecthyma gangrenosum usually follows septicemia in a neutropenic patient. Less commonly, it follows primary inoculation into the skin.
- Ecthyma responds rapidly to antibiotics, whereas ecthyma gangrenosum has a high mortality rate.
- Clinically, ecthyma gangrenosum presents as one or more red macules that become edematous and rapidly progress to hemorrhagic bullae. In the late stages, it may ulcerate (Fig. 27.9) or form an eschar surrounded by erythema.

25. Where do you usually acquire *Pseudomonas* folliculitis?

In your hot tub. *Pseudomonas* folliculitis is typically associated with hot tub use ("hot tub folliculitis"). Less commonly, it is associated with whirlpools or swimming pools. It is usually associated with *P. aeruginosa* serotype O:11, although other serotypes have also been reported. *Pseudomonas* folliculitis has also been reported as a complication of depilatories used for the removal of leg hair.

Yu Y, Chang AS, Wang L, et al. Hot tub folliculitis or hot hand-foot syndrome caused by *Pseudomonas aeruginosa*. *J Am Acad Dermatol*. 2007;57:596–600.

26. How does *Pseudomonas* folliculitis present?

Clinically, it occurs 1 to 3 days after exposure, presenting as a diffuse truncal eruption (Fig. 27.10). The primary lesion is a follicular-based erythematous papule that frequently demonstrates a follicular pustule. Less commonly, patients may also demonstrate mastitis, abscesses, lymphangitis, and fever. Another variation is seen in patients who present with painful indurated lesions of the feet and/or hand that may become pustular ("*Pseudomonas* hot hand-foot syndrome"). The disease is usually self-limited, although rare patients may continue to develop recurrent folliculitis or abscesses for up to 2 months.

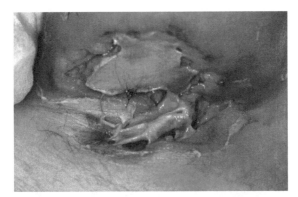

Fig. 27.9 Ecthyma gangrenosum of the axilla in a neutropenic patient demonstrating massive ulceration. (Courtesy Fitzsimons Army Medical Center teaching files.)

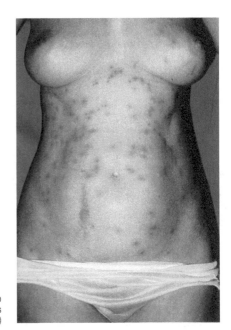

Fig. 27.10 *Pseudomonas* folliculitis. Patient with history of recent hot tub exposure and development of numerous truncal follicular-based papules and pustules. (Courtesy Fitzsimons Army Medical Center teaching files.)

27. **What is the best treatment for *Pseudomonas* folliculitis?**
    Most cases are self-limited and do not require treatment. Severe or recurrent cases can be treated with oral ciprofloxacin. Ultimately, the best treatment is prevention of infection. The most effective measures are frequent drainage of the hot tub or whirlpool to remove the buildup of desquamated skin cells that serve as the prime source of nutrients. Adequate chlorination and bromination are also necessary.

28. **How is Wood's light used in diagnosing *Pseudomonas* infections?**
    P. aeruginosa produces a pigment called pyoverdin that fluoresces yellow-green under Wood's light. The Wood's light is useful in detecting pseudomonads in burn wounds, surgical infections, ulcerated ecthyma gangrenosum, and gram-negative toe web infections.

29. **Describe the cutaneous manifestations of Lyme disease.**
    Lyme disease is a multisystem disease caused by *Borrelia burgdorferi*, a spirochete that is transmitted to humans by ticks of the genus *Ixodes*. One to 30 days after the tick bite, patients present with variable constitutional symptoms, including fever, malaise, headache, and arthralgias. Approximately of patients develop erythema chronicum migrans

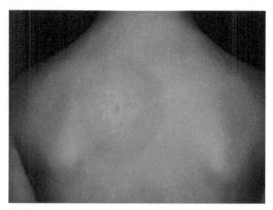

Fig. 27.11 Typical lesion of erythema chronicum migrans manifesting as central papule at the tick bite site surrounded by annular erythema.

(ECM) that begins as an erythematous papule at the bite site and progresses to an annular erythema that may reach 20 cm or more in size (Fig. 27.11). Typically, ECM presents 7–14 days after the initial tick bite. This rash spontaneously resolves regardless of treatment in 4 weeks; however, treatment for systemic Lyme disease is still required.

Gerstenblith TA, Stern TA. Lyme disease: a review of its epidemiology, evaluation, and treatment. *Psychosomatics.* 2014; 55:421–429.

30. A patient living in an endemic area for Lyme disease reports a history of a tick bite. Should that patient receive antibiotic prophylaxis?

The question of whether or not patients with tick bites in endemic areas should receive antibiotic prophylaxis is controversial. Randomized controlled trials only support the use of a 200-mg oral dose of doxycycline in a child older than 8 years of age when all of the following criteria are met: (1) The attached tick can be identified as a nymphal or adult form of *Ixodes scapularis* that has been attached for longer than 36 hours, estimated by exposure or degree of tick engorgement; (2) prophylaxis can be started within 72 hours of when tick was removed; (3) ecologic information shows that local prevalence of infection of ticks with *Borrelia burgdorferi* is greater than 20%; and (4) doxycycline is not contraindicated. For children under the age of 8 and in pregnant women, amoxicillin is the treatment of choice.

Wormser GP, Dattwyler RJ, Shapiro ED, et al. The clinical assessment, treatment, and prevention of Lyme disease, human granulocytic anaplasmosis, and babesiosis: clinical practice guidelines by the Infectious Diseases Society of America. *Clin Infect Dis.* 2006; 43:1089–1134.

KEY POINT: OTHER BACTERIAL INFECTIONS

• This chapter covers some of the most common bacterial infections in dermatology. There are many other bacterial infections affecting the skin, which are beyond the scope of this chapter.

Alikhan A, Hocker TLH. Bacterial infections. *Rev Dermatol.* 2017;288–304.

CHAPTER 28

SEXUALLY TRANSMITTED DISEASES

James E. Fitzpatrick

"Know syphilis in all of its manifestations and relations, and all other things clinical will be added unto you."
–Sir William Osler, 1897

1. What causes syphilis?
Syphilis is caused by the spirochete *Treponema pallidum*, ssp. *pallidum*, which belongs to the order Spirochaetales. *T. pallidum* ssp. *endemicum* is a subspecies that causes bejel, or endemic syphilis. Other pathogenic treponemes for humans include *T. pallidum* ssp. *pertenue*, the cause of yaws, and *T. carateum*, the cause of pinta. In recent years, there has been a surge in the number of cases of sexually transmitted disease (STDs), including syphilis, the United States. In 2011, there were 13,970 new cases of syphilis reported by the Center for Disease Control and Prevention (CDC), while in 2017, there were 30,644 new cases,

2. Describe the morphologic appearance of *T. pallidum*
T. pallidum is a delicate spiral bacterium that measures 6 to 20 μm in length and 0.10 to 0.18 μm in width (Fig. 28.1). Because of the narrow width, it is not visible by normal light microscopy and must be visualized by darkfield microscopy, by silver stains (i.e., Warthin-Starry or modified Steiner stains), or by immunoperoxidase stains. The 6 to 14 spiral coils are regularly spaced at a distance of about 1 μm. The organism reproduces by transverse fission.

3. Where did syphilis originate?
The origin of syphilis had been a point of great debate among experts, with some authorities favoring a New World origin because of an epidemic of syphilis that ravaged Europe in the last decade of the 15th century, when it was referred to as the "Great Pox." Because this epidemic coincided with the return of Columbus from America in 1493, this suggested that it was imported from the West Indies. Of interest, Columbus himself is thought to have died from syphilitic aortitis. Other authorities believe that it had always been present in the Old World. Studies on skeletal remains support that while treponemal disease was present in the Old World, epidemic syphilis was imported from the New World.

Tampa M, Sarbu I, Matei C, et al. Brief history of syphilis. *J Med Life*. 2014;7:4–10. (free online text).

4. Can I get syphilis from a toilet seat?
Probably not. Syphilis is most commonly acquired as an STD but also may be acquired congenitally or, rarely, by blood transfusions. The organism is very fragile and easily killed by heat, cold, drying, soap, and disinfectants. Since the spirochete is so fragile, the possibility that an infection could be acquired from a toilet seat is statistically very remote.

5. What are the chances of getting syphilis from having sexual intercourse with an infected individual?
The definitive study has obviously never been done, but epidemiologic studies show that the chances are about 1 in 3. It is believed that the treponemes cannot penetrate intact epidermis or mucosa and that most infections are acquired through microscopic or macroscopic breaks in the epithelium.

6. Following inoculation, how long does it take for the primary chancre to appear?
Experimental study on both rabbits and human volunteers has shown that the appearance of the primary chancre is related to the size of the inoculum. The primary chancre normally appears in 10 to 90 days, with the average time being about 3 weeks. The organism reaches the regional lymph nodes within hours.

7. Describe the typical Hunterian chancre
The classic Hunterian chancre develops at the site of inoculation as a painless ulcer with a firm, indurated border (Fig. 28.2). The size may vary from a few millimeters to several centimeters in diameter. Associated unilateral or bilateral, painless, regional, nonsuppurative lymphadenopathy develops in 50% to 85% of patients approximately 1 week after the appearance of the primary ulcer. It is important to realize that up to 50% of all chancres are atypical. Painful ulcers, multiple ulcers (Fig. 28.3), secondarily infected ulcers, and nonindurated ulcers are variations on the classic chancre.

Lee V, Kinghorn G. Syphilis: an update. *Clin Med*. 2008;8:330–333.

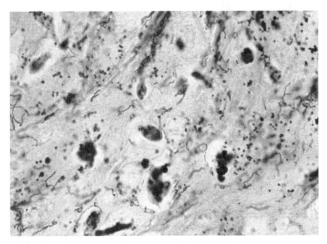

Fig. 28.1 Biopsy of secondary syphilis demonstrating numerous spirochetes in the epidermis (Warthin-Starry stain, ×1000).

8. Do syphilitic chancres occur on sites other than the genitalia?

Extragenital chancres occur in 5% of all cases of primary syphilis, although the incidence may be as high as 10%. The most common extragenital sites are the lip (Fig. 28.4A), which is associated with oral sex, and the anus, which is associated with anal intercourse. Anal intercourse may also produce rectal or colonic chancres as high as 20 cm into the bowel. Other reported sites include the tongue, tonsil, finger, thumb (Fig. 28.4B), eyelid, chin, nipple, umbilicus, axilla, and even the lower limb. A high index of suspicion is required to diagnose extragenital chancres.

Scott CM, Flint SR. Oral syphilis—reemergence of an old disease with oral manifestations. *Int J Oral Maxillofac Surg.* 2005;34:58–63.

9. What is the best way to diagnose primary syphilis?

Diagnosis cannot be based on clinical presentation alone, and, unfortunately, *T. pallidum* cannot be cultured. The most specific and rapid method of diagnosing primary syphilis is the demonstration of the spirochete utilizing darkfield examination by a trained observer. This test is not readily available to most community physicians and usually requires sending the patient to an STD clinic or medical center. The material for examination can be obtained from either the ulcer or an aspirate from an enlarged lymph node. A single negative darkfield examination does not rule out the possibility of syphilis, and it should not be regarded as negative until there are negative examinations on three consecutive days. Primary syphilis can also be diagnosed by doing a biopsy of the primary ulcer and demonstrating the organism by special stain.

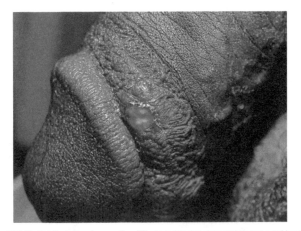

Fig. 28.2 Typical Hunterian chancre of syphilis demonstrating characteristic indurated border.

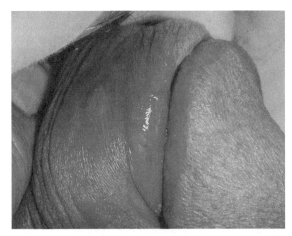

Fig. 28.3 A typical presentation of primary syphilis demonstrating two chancres. (Courtesy William James, MD.)

In lieu of these procedures, a presumptive diagnosis can be made by serologic tests (see Chapter 3). The Venereal Disease Research Laboratory (VDRL) test and rapid plasma reagin test are negative in early primary syphilis and should be repeated weekly for 1 month to be considered as negative. The diagnosis is more likely if a rising titer can be demonstrated. The fluorescent treponemal antibody–absorption test turns positive earlier and is more sensitive.

10. How is primary syphilis treated?

The current recommended treatment for primary syphilis is benzathine penicillin G, 2.4 million units in a single intramuscular dose. Patients who are allergic to penicillin (approximately 3% to 10% of the population has an immunoglobulin E–mediated allergic response to penicillin) should be skin tested to a full battery of penicillin skin test reagents, and if positive, they should ideally be desensitized before treatment. Select cases may be treated with doxycycline, tetracycline, ceftriaxone, or azithromycin; however, these choices are not preferred.

Treatment failures have been reported with all antibiotic regimens, and patients should have follow-up serologic titers at 6 and 12 months to ensure a fourfold decline in titers. Failure of nontreponemal antibody titers to fall fourfold within 6 months of treatment can be considered a probable treatment failure. Patients also need to be reported to the proper public health agency to ensure tracking of known sexual partners. Before initiating therapy for syphilis, health care providers should go to the CDC website, which was last updated in 2015, for the most current recommendations (https://www.cdc.gov/std/tg2015/syphilis.htm).

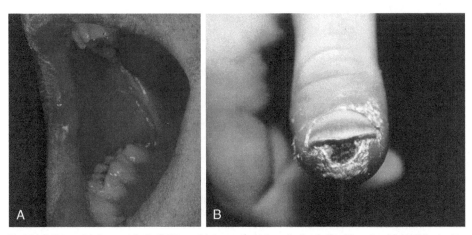

Fig. 28.4 A, Extragenital chancre of the lip. B, Extragenital chancre of syphilis on the thumb. (Panel A courtesy John L. Aeling teaching collection; Panel B courtesy Fitzsimons Army Medical Center teaching files.)

11. What is the Jarisch-Herxheimer reaction?

This acute febrile reaction, associated with shaking chills, malaise, sore throat, myalgia, headache, and localized inflammation of infected mucocutaneous sites, usually occurs 6 to 8 hours following penicillin treatment. Tetracycline, doxycycline, and ceftriaxone are less commonly associated with this reaction. It develops in 50% of patients with primary syphilis, 75% with secondary syphilis, and 30% with neurosyphilis. There is indirect evidence that this reaction is due to the release of a treponemal lipopolysaccharide that acts like a bacterial endotoxin.

12. What is the natural history of the untreated syphilitic chancre?

The untreated syphilitic chancre lasts for about 2 to 8 weeks and then disappears. The primary chancre may relapse, in which case it is referred to as chancre redux.

13. When does secondary syphilis begin?

Secondary syphilis usually begins about 6 weeks after the onset of the primary chancre. In approximately 25% of cases, the primary ulcer will still be present. In one study, 25% of patients with secondary syphilis did not recall a primary chancre.

Baughn RE, Musher DM. Secondary syphilitic lesions. *Clin Microbiol Rev*. 2005;18:205–216.

14. Do patients with secondary syphilis have any symptoms?

The most common reported symptoms include malaise (23% to 46%), headache (9% to 46%), fever (5% to 39%), pruritus (42%), and loss of appetite (25%). Less common symptoms include painful eyes, joint or bone pain, meningismus, iritis, and hoarseness. Some references incorrectly state that pruritus is uncommon in secondary syphilis.

15. List the common physical findings in secondary syphilis

- Syphiloderm (rash): 88% to 100%
- Lymphadenopathy: 85% to 89%
- Residual primary chancre: 25% to 43%
- Condylomata lata: 9% to 44%
- Hepatosplenomegaly: 23%
- Mucous patches: 7% to 12%
- Alopecia: 3% to 11% (see Chapter 20)

16. Describe the syphiloderm of secondary syphilis

The syphiloderm of secondary syphilis is most commonly a maculopapular eruption (Fig. 28.5A, B) with variable scale (70%), papular (12%), or macular (10%) lesions. Less common morphologic appearances include annular (Fig. 28.5C, D), pustular, and psoriasiform lesions. The rash typically demonstrates a widespread symmetrical distribution, although in some patients, lesions may be localized to a single anatomic region, such as the palms and soles. In a large study done in the United States, the most common sites of involvement, in descending order, were the soles, trunk, arms, genitals, palms, legs, face, neck, and scalp.

Balagula Y, Mattei PL, Wisco OJ, et al. The great imitator revisited: the spectrum of atypical cutaneous manifestations of secondary syphilis. *Int J Dermatol*. 2014;53:14341441.

17. What are condylomata lata? How do they differ from condylomata acuminata?

Condylomata lata are whitish or grayish, elevated, broad, flat papular lesions of secondary syphilis that primarily occur in moist areas, such as the penis (Fig. 28.6A), labia, inner thighs, and anal region. These papular lesions may coalesce to form verrucous plaques that are easily confused with condylomata acuminata, which are genital warts caused by human papillomavirus.

18. What are mucous patches?

Shallow, usually painless erosions of the mucous membranes (Fig. 28.6B). Some mucous patches demonstrate linear shapes and have been described as resembling "snail tracks."

19. How good are physicians at recognizing the signs and symptoms of secondary syphilis?

In a retrospective study of 34 patients with secondary syphilis who had been seen previously by community physicians, only 40% of physicians listed secondary syphilis as the primary diagnosis. Another 14% included secondary syphilis in their differential diagnosis. In sum, almost half of physicians did not consider the diagnosis.

20. What is the best way to diagnose secondary syphilis?

The diagnosis of secondary syphilis requires a health care provider with a strong index of suspicion. The cutaneous manifestations of secondary syphilis may mimic other skin diseases, including pityriasis rosea, psoriasis, erythema multiforme, pityriasis lichenoides et varioliformis acuta, and some drug reactions. It is a good rule of thumb to consider secondary syphilis in any patient having a generalized dermatitis with associated lymphadenopathy.

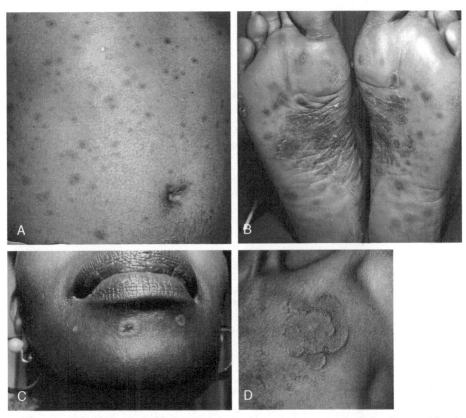

Fig. 28.5 Secondary syphilis. **A,** Hyperpigmented macules of secondary syphilis in a patient who was initially treated for chancroid. Note the strong similarity of these lesions to pityriasis rosea. **B,** Characteristic papulosquamous lesions of secondary syphilis on the soles of the feet. Macular or papulosquamous lesions on the palms are not diagnostic but are suggestive of secondary syphilis. **C,** Annular lesions of secondary syphilis on the face. **D,** Striking annular lesions of the chest in a patient with secondary syphilis. (Panel B courtesy Fitzsimons Army Medical Center teaching files; Panel D courtesy Walter Reed Army Medical Center teaching files.)

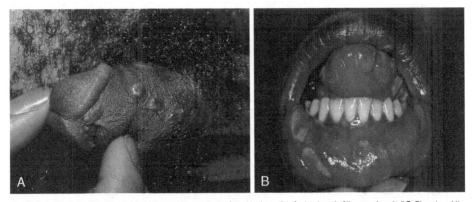

Fig. 28.6 **A,** Exophytic condylomata lata of the penis in a patient referred to the author for treatment of "venereal warts." **B,** Discrete, white, focally eroded mucous patches of secondary syphilis.

As with primary syphilis, the most specific tests are the demonstration of the spirochete either in a skin biopsy or on darkfield examination, which can be performed on either the secondary skin lesions or on aspirates from lymph nodes. In contrast to primary syphilis, serologic tests are almost invariably positive. The only exception is when there is a false-negative reaction due to a prozone phenomenon, which occurs in 1% to 2% of patients with secondary syphilis. The prozone phenomenon occurs when the titers are very high and can be eliminated by diluting the serum.

KEY POINTS: SYPHILIS

1. Syphilis is a sexually transmitted disease that can also be transmitted from the mother to the fetus.
2. Syphilis is produced by the spirochete *Treponema pallidum*, ssp. *pallidum*.
3. Secondary syphilis is protean in its clinical appearance and can be difficult to recognize, with studies showing that up to one-half of community physicians will not clinically suspect secondary syphilis.
4. The most specific and rapid method of diagnosing primary syphilis is the demonstration of the spirochete utilizing darkfield examination by a trained observer.
5. Patients with syphilis have an increased incidence of other sexually transmitted infections such as gonorrhea, human immunodeficiency virus infection, and venereal warts.

22. How should secondary syphilis be treated?
The treatment should be the same as for primary syphilis.

23. What stage follows untreated secondary syphilis?
The mucocutaneous lesions of secondary syphilis usually heal without scarring in 2 to 10 weeks, although hyperpigmentation or hypopigmentation may persist. Following the resolution of secondary syphilis, patients enter the latent stage of infection. During this stage, approximately one-fourth of patients experience relapsing secondary lesions. Most relapses occur in the first year, but these may occur for up to 5 years.

24. How is latent syphilis treated?
Latent syphilis is defined as seropositive infection without clinical evidence of disease. For the purpose of treatment, the CDC defines infections of less than 1 year as early latent syphilis and infections of greater than 1 year as late latent. The World Health Organization considers early latent syphilis to extend up to 2 years.
Like primary and secondary syphilis, early latent syphilis (also called "early nonprimary nonsecondary syphilis") is treated with 2.4 million units (mu) of benzathine penicillin G intramuscularly in a single dose. Late latent syphilis or latent syphilis of unknown duration is treated with a total of 7.2 mu of benzathine penicillin G administered as three doses of 2.4 mu intramuscularly at 1-week intervals (7.2 mu total). Penicillin-allergic patients are treated with doxycycline or tetracycline for 4 weeks; however, these therapies require close clinical and serologic follow-up.

25. When should lumbar punctures be done in patients with syphilis?
Lumbar punctures to rule out neurosyphilis are recommended for patients with late latent syphilis of more than 1-year duration or unknown duration who demonstrate neurologic symptoms, treatment failure, serum nontreponemal antibody titer equal to or greater than 1:32, other evidence of active syphilis (iritis, aortitis, gumma), nonpenicillin treatment, or positive human immunodeficiency virus (HIV) test. Syphilis frequently attacks the central nervous system, as demonstrated by the fact that 40% of patients with primary or secondary syphilis demonstrate cerebrospinal fluid pleocytosis, and 24% of patients with secondary syphilis demonstrate a reactive VDRL. In patients with syphilis/HIV coinfection, there is evidence to suggest that lumbar puncture may be indicated in all coinfected patients since the disease is more aggressive; however, this is also controversial.

Chan DJ. Syphilis and HIV co-infection: when is lumbar puncture indicated? *Curr HIV Res.* 2005;3:95–98.

26. What happens to patients with untreated latent syphilis?
Approximately one-third of patients with untreated latent syphilis develop tertiary syphilis. The other two-thirds of patients will not develop later effects of the disease.

27. Name the three major presentations of tertiary syphilis
- Late benign syphilis
- Cardiovascular disease
- Neurosyphilis (general paresis or tabes dorsalis)

28. What are the mucocutaneous features of late benign syphilis?
Late benign syphilis usually occurs 1 to 46 years after resolution of the secondary skin lesions. Although almost any organ may be involved, the most common organ is the skin (70%), followed by the mucous membranes (10%) and bones (10%). The primary lesion of late benign syphilis is the *gumma*. A gumma is a granulomatous lesion that contains treponemes only rarely; it probably represents a hypersensitivity reaction.

The skin lesions of late benign syphilis present as nodules and plaques that demonstrate a tendency for central healing and peripheral extension. The central healed areas characteristically demonstrate scarring and atrophy. The mucosal lesions may involve any mucosal surface but demonstrate a tendency to extend to and destroy the nasal cartilage, producing a "saddle nose" deformity. Involvement of the mucosa over the hard palate may produce a perforation.

Rocha N, Horta M, Sanches M, et al. Syphilitic gumma—cutaneous tertiary syphilis. *J Eur Acad Dermatol Venereol.* 2004;18:517–518.

29. What was the Tuskegee Study?

The Tuskegee Study is one of the most iniquitous prospective medical studies ever done in the United States. Untreated black men with syphilis, without their knowledge or consent, were randomized into treated and untreated groups and then followed so that the complications and mortality of untreated syphilis could be monitored. This study was part of the impetus to establish strict guidelines for biomedical research. In 1997, President Clinton formally apologized to the survivors for this U.S. Public Health Service study.

30. What are the clinical manifestations of early congenital syphilis?

In 2011, there were 360 cases of congenital syphilis reported in the United States. Early congenital syphilis has numerous mucocutaneous findings, including vesiculobullous lesions (especially the palms, sole, and anogenital area), maculopapular eruption, condylomatous lesions of the anogenital region, mucous patches, and a profuse mucosanguineous discharge from the nose due to obstruction called snuffles (Fig. 28.7). Congenital syphilis is fatal in approximately 40% of cases and untreated congenital syphilis is associated with numerous important systemic manifestations in adult life.

31. What causes chancroid?

Chancroid is a result of infection by the short gram-negative bacillus *Haemophilus ducreyi*. It is an STD that has been slowly disappearing in the United States, with 4212 cases reported in 1990 and only 6 cases in 2016; however, since the organism is difficult to culture, this infection may be underdiagnosed. The organism does not grow on routine media, and even the most commonly used media (enhanced chocolate agar with vancomycin) will miss approximately 20% of cases. Because of the difficulty in culturing this organism, the diagnosis is often made on clinical grounds and excluding primary syphilis and genital herpes infection.

32. How does chancroid present?

The infection is most common in men and frequently but not always asymptomatic in women. The primary lesion is a tender, ragged, irregularly shaped ulcer that may exhibit purulent draining (Fig. 28.8A). In general, the ulcers are less indurated than the chancre of syphilis. The ulcers frequently involve opposing cutaneous surfaces (Fig. 28.8B). More than one half of the patients will develop tender inguinal lymphadenopathy that may be either unilateral or bilateral. In some cases, the lymph node will suppurate and produce an ulcer or sinus overlying the lymph node.

Basta-Juzbašić A, Čeović R. Chancroid, lymphogranuloma venereum, granuloma inguinale, genital herpes simplex infection, and molluscum contagiosum. *Clin Dermatol.* 2014;32:290–298.

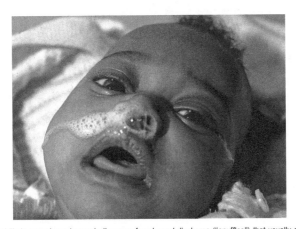

Fig. 28.7 Congenital syphilis in a newborn demonstrating a profound nasal discharge ("snuffles") that usually contains numerous viable spirochetes. (Courtesy John L. Aeling collection.)

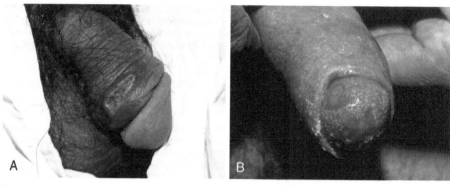

Fig. 28.8 **A,** Classic painful ulcer of chancroid demonstrating a purulent base, surrounding erythema and irregular outline. **B,** Characteristic "kissing ulcers" of chancroid in an uncircumcised man. (Courtesy Fitzsimons Army Medical Center teaching files.)

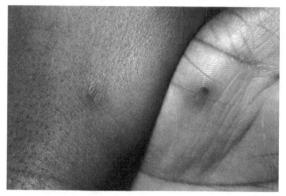

Fig. 28.9 Disseminated gonococcal infection on the hands demonstrating a typical pustule and hemorrhagic pustule. The patient also had fever, chills, and tenosynovitis of the wrists and knees. (Courtesy Fitzsimons Army Medical Center teaching files.)

33. What is the treatment of choice for chancroid?
    Treatment options include azithromycin, ceftriaxone, and erythromycin. It is important to emphasize that primary syphilis and herpes simplex infection need to be excluded.

34. A 30-year-old sexually active woman presents with a vaginal discharge, fever, chills, arthritis of the knees and wrists, with several pustules and hemorrhagic pustules of her hands and elbows. What is the most likely diagnosis?
    This is the classic presentation of disseminated gonococcal infection. Gonorrhea, which is caused by the gram-negative coccus *Neisseria gonorrhoeae*, will present as disseminated gonococcal infection in about 1% to 3% of all patients with gonorrhea. It is more common in women than men and more common in women who are menstruating. The cutaneous manifestations are typically small numbers of acral papules that vary from being pustular to hemorrhagic to being ulcerated (Fig. 28.9). Joint manifestations include tenosynovitis, migratory polyarthritis, and purulent arthritis. Less common manifestations include osteomyelitis, meningitis, and endocarditis.

Bleich AT, Sheffield JS, Wendel Jr GD, et al. Disseminated gonococcal infection in women. *Obstet Gynecol.* 2012;119:597–602.

CHAPTER 29

MYCOBACTERIAL INFECTIONS

Shannan E. McCann and Wendi E. Wohltmann

1. What is the Runyon Classification system for mycobacteria?
   The **Runyon Classification** was created in the 1950s to organize the mycobacteria based on their rate of growth, ability to form pigment, and colony characteristics.

2. What are the staining characteristics of mycobacteria?
   Mycobacteria are aerobic, non–spore-forming, nonmotile bacilli. Their most useful staining characteristic is acid fastness. Acid fastness refers to the ability to retain carbol fuchsin dye after washing with acid or alcohol as a result of a high content of cell wall mycolic acids, fatty acids, and other lipids. The acid-fast stain is also called the Ziehl-Neelsen stain.

TUBERCULOSIS

3. How many species of Mycobacterium cause infection in human beings?
   There are approximately 30 species of *Mycobacterium* that cause disease in humans. The primary culprits include *M. tuberculosis* complex, atypical mycobacteria, and *M. leprae*.

4. Name three mycobacteria in the tuberculosis complex responsible for tuberculosis.
   The three species most significant to human disease include *M. tuberculosis*, *M. bovis*, and *M. africanum*. Under certain conditions, the attenuated strain of *M. bovis*, bacillus Calmette-Guérin (BCG), may also cause disease.

5. What is tuberculosis?
   Tuberculosis (TB) is a systemic infectious disease that can affect any organ system, including the skin. Approximately 5% to 10% of infections lead to clinical disease. The lungs are the most commonly involved organ. Cutaneous TB has a broad clinical spectrum depending on the route of infection, virulence of the organism, and immune status of the host (Table 29.1). Lupus vulgaris and scrofuloderma, although rare, are the two most common forms of cutaneous TB.

6. What is the difference between a primary and secondary infection?
   Primary-inoculation TB occurs in a host not previously infected. A secondary infection occurs in a previously infected host either as a reactivation years later from a primary focus, endogenous spread to new areas, or exogenous reinfection.

Table 29.1 Classification of cutaneous tuberculosis

CLASSIFICATION	PRIMARY INFECTION (NONIMMUNE HOST)	SECONDARY INFECTION (IMMUNE HOST)
Exogenous		
Primary inoculation tuberculosis	X	
Tuberculosis verrucosa cutis		X
Endogenous		
Scrofuloderma		X
Periorificial tuberculosis		X
Hematogenous/Lymphatic		
Lupus vulgaris		X
Acute miliary tuberculosis	X	
Gummas	X	

Data from Semaan R, Traboulsi R, Kanj S. Primary Mycobacterium tuberculosis complex cutaneous infection: report of two cases and literature review. *Int J Infect Dis.* 2008; 12(5):472–477.

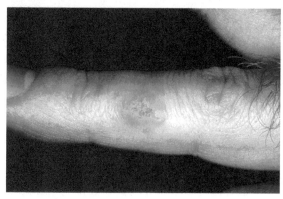

Fig. 29.1 Primary-inoculation tuberculosis presenting as an eroded papule. (Courtesy James E. Fitzpatrick, MD.)

7. **Explain the three routes of infection in cutaneous TB.**
   The first route is exogenous infection acquired from an outside source (primary-inoculation TB and TB verrucosa cutis). The second route of infection is endogenous spread. This can occur by contiguous spread (scrofuloderma) or by autoinoculation (periorificial TB) from internal organ involvement. The final route is through hematogenous or lymphatic dissemination (lupus vulgaris, miliary TB, and gummas).

8. **Who is at risk of acquiring TB?**
   One-fourth of the world's population is infected with TB. Worldwide, approximately 10 million people developed TB in 2017, with 1.3 million associated deaths. In the United States, the incidence of TB was decreasing until 1985, when it reached its nadir. Since 1985, the incidence of TB has markedly increased. In 2017, 9105 cases were reported in the United States, with over 70% of these being foreign-born persons. California, Texas, New York, and Florida account for just under 50% of the national case total. Crowded urban environments, immigration, poverty, homelessness, intravenous drug abuse, loss of TB control programs, increased use of immunosuppressive medications (e.g., tumor necrosis factor-α [TNF-α] inhibitors), and, most importantly, the HIV epidemic account for the rising incidence.

9. **Describe the histopathologic hallmark of TB.**
   The caseation granuloma (also known as tubercle) is the histopathologic hallmark of TB. This consists of giant and epithelioid cells with varying amounts of caseation necrosis. This pattern is not pathognomonic. Acid-fast bacilli (AFB) are usually easy to find in early TB lesions, but there are very few bacilli once granulomas develop.

10. **How can one acquire primary cutaneous TB?**
    Primary-inoculation TB occurs from direct inoculation of *M. tuberculosis* into the skin and includes the chancre at the site and affected regional lymph nodes. The organism cannot penetrate intact skin and requires a break in the skin, such as a minor cut or abrasion. Reports have also implicated tattooing, ear piercing, circumcision, mouth-to-mouth resuscitation, mesotherapy, blepharoplasty, acupuncture, and needle-sticks.

11. **Describe the clinical manifestation of primary-inoculation cutaneous TB.**
    Primary TB may occur in any age group but is most common in children up to 4 years of age and young adults. The face, mucous membranes (conjunctiva and oral mucosa), and lower extremity are the usual sites of infection. A tuberculous chancre develops 2 to 4 weeks after inoculation and presents as a painless, firm, red-brown papule/nodule, which slowly enlarges, eventually eroding to form a sharply demarcated ulcer (Fig. 29.1). Regional, hard, nonpainful lymphadenopathy occurs 3 to 8 weeks after infection. The purified protein derivative (PPD) may initially be negative and diagnosis is confirmed by culture.

12. **What is a tuberculid?**
    In contrast to true cutaneous TB, a tuberculid is a cutaneous or mucosal lesion that represents an immunologic hypersensitivity to mycobacterial antigens in patients with TB at a remote site (Fig. 29.2). Special stains and culture of a tuberculid lesion are negative.

13. **What cutaneous and laboratory tests are used to screen for and diagnose Mycobacterium tuberculosis?**
    Mycobacterium tuberculosis can be screened for using the tuberculin skin test or the interferon-gamma release assay (IGRA). Diagnosis is made using AFB stains, culture, polymerase chain reaction (PCR), or IGRA. Sputum samples for culture and staining are used to diagnose TB in developing countries.

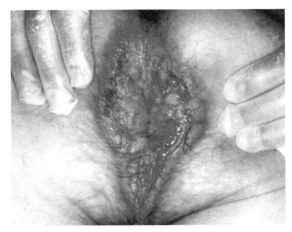

Fig. 29.2 Tuberculosis cutis orificialis. Erythematous eroded plaque of perianal area. (Courtesy James E. Fitzpatrick, MD.)

14. Is lupus vulgaris related to lupus erythematosus or lupus pernio?
    No. Lupus erythematosus is an autoimmune connective tissue disease. Lupus pernio is a cutaneous manifestation of sarcoidosis that presents as a violaceous patch on the face. Lupus vulgaris is a form of cutaneous TB. The term *lupus* is used to depict erosion as if "gnawed by a wolf." Vulgaris means common or ordinary. Both of these terms are used in a variety of unrelated diseases.

15. Describe the clinical manifestations of lupus vulgaris.
    Lupus vulgaris is a chronic progressive form of cutaneous TB that originates from another site and involves the skin or mucous membranes via contiguous, lymphatic, or hematogenous spread. In 40% of patients, there is underlying lymphadenitis, and 10% to 20% have underlying pulmonary involvement. The primary skin lesion is an asymptomatic macule or papule that is brown-red in color and has a soft gelatinous consistency (Fig. 29.3A). Squamous cell carcinoma arising in a long-standing lesion is the most serious complication (Fig. 29.3B).

16. What is diascopy?
    Diascopy is a test where a glass slide is gently pressed against the skin lesion. Lupus vulgaris lesions have a characteristic "apple jelly" color with this technique.

17. What is scrofuloderma?
    Scrofuloderma is a form of cutaneous TB that originates in tuberculous lymph nodes, bones, joints, or epididymis and spreads directly to the overlying skin. The most common locations include the lateral neck and the parotid, submandibular, and supraclavicular areas. The skin lesion presents as a firm subcutaneous nodule. As the lesion matures, there is extensive necrosis leading to a soft, doughy consistency, ulceration with bluish margins, and formation of a sinus tract. Necrotic cheesy material may drain from sinus tracts (Fig. 29.4).

18. Name the vaccination against TB. What type of vaccination is it?
    BCG is a live attenuated strain of *Mycobacterium bovis*. It has not been widely used in the United States, with the exception of a very small number of at-risk infants who cannot receive chemoprophylaxis. In third-world countries, the BCG vaccine is commonly used. This vaccination is contraindicated in immunosuppressed individuals who are at risk of disseminated *M. bovis* infection. Intravesical BCG is commonly used as treatment for bladder cancer, and cutaneous TB lesions following this therapy have been reported.

19. What drugs are used in the treatment of non-drug-resistant TB?
    First-line essential chemotherapeutic agents include isoniazid, rifampin, pyrazinamide, and ethambutol. Second-line drugs include cycloserine, ethionamide, levofloxacin, moxifloxacin, gatifloxacin, p-aminosalicylic acid, rifabutin, streptomycin, amikacin/kanamycin, and capreomycin. Isoniazid is the cornerstone of therapy, and rifampin is the second major antituberculous drug. Currently, the Centers for Disease Control and Prevention (CDC) endorses a number of 6-month and 9-month protocols. The 6-month regimens include an intensive 2-month therapy with three to four agents followed by a 4-month therapy with isoniazid plus rifampin or rifapentine.

20. What are the major side effects of antituberculous agents?
    See Table 29.2.

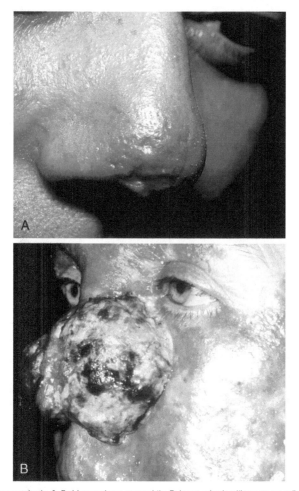

Fig. 29.3 Lupus vulgaris. **A,** Red-brown plaque on nasal tip. **B,** Lupus vulgaris with squamous cell carcinoma.

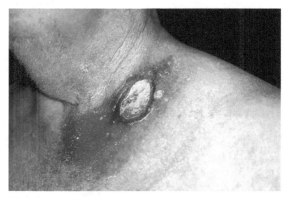

Fig. 29.4 Scrofuloderma. Erythematous to violaceous nodule with ulceration representing an extension from an underlying lymph node.

Table 29.2 First-line antituberculous agents and major side effects

DRUG	SIDE EFFECT	SPECIAL COMMENT
Isoniazid	Peripheral neuritis	From pyridoxine deficiency
	Hepatitis	Occurs with 1%–2%, increased risk with age >35
Rifampin	Hepatitis	More common when given with isoniazid
	Orange stain of secretions	May permanently stain contact lenses
Rifabutin	Neutropenia	Occurs in HIV patients
	Hepatitis	More common when given with isoniazid
	Orange stain of secretions	May permanently stain contact lenses
Rifapentine	Hepatitis	More common when given with isoniazid
	Orange stain of secretions	May permanently stain contact lenses
Pyrazinamide	Hyperuricemia	May precipitate gout
Ethambutol	Optic neuritis	Avoid in children under age 13

Data available at http://www.cdc.gov/mmwr/PDF/rr/rr5211.pdf. Accessed February 18, 2019.

21. **What factors have led to multidrug-resistant TB?**
Multidrug-resistant TB (MDRTB) is defined as combined resistance to isoniazid and rifampin and can be either primary or acquired. Primary MDRTB occurs in a person who has not previously been treated, whereas acquired MDRTB is a result of treatment failure. The main factors leading to MDRTB include patient noncompliance in drug therapy, inability or unwillingness to find adequate health care, and inappropriate treatment regimens. Homelessness, intravenous drug use, and HIV infection favor the spread of drug-resistant TB. Resistance is prevalent in Asia, South America, and Africa. In the United States, miniepidemics of drug resistance are centered in New York City, Miami, and Michigan. Spread to health care workers is a major concern.

22. **Are there any special treatment considerations for cutaneous TB?**
Treatment of cutaneous TB is the same as for systemic TB and consists of effective chemotherapeutic agents. Small lesions of lupus vulgaris or TB verrucosa cutis may be excised, but the treatment must also include standard antituberculous therapy. Surgical drainage of scrofuloderma may shorten the treatment course, and surgical intervention is necessary in any draining lesion.

23. **What is the mechanism of action of TNF-α in TB?**
TNF-α mediates host defense against infection as a key player in granuloma formation and containment of *M. tuberculosis* organisms. TNF-α inhibitors (etanercept, adalimumab, and infliximab) have been associated with reactivation of TB; therefore, patients must be screened for TB prior to TNF-α inhibitor treatment. If the PPD is positive, and the chest radiograph is negative, the patient may still receive the TNF-α inhibitor 1–2 months after starting antitubercular treatment for latent TB if immediate disease control is necessary. However, the preferred regimen is completion of 6 to 9 months of isoniazid prior to TNF-α inhibitor initiation.

KEY POINTS

1. Cutaneous tuberculosis has a broad clinical spectrum, depending on the route of infection, virulence of the organism, and immune status of the host; lupus vulgaris and scrofuloderma are the two most common forms of cutaneous tuberculosis.
2. *Mycobacterium tuberculosis* can be diagnosed using acid-fast bacilli (AFB) stains, culture, polymerase chain reaction (PCR), or interferon-gamma release assay (IGRA).
3. Atypical mycobacteria are ubiquitous and are found in soil, water, and domestic and wild animals. The presentation of these infections is quite variable, leading to frequently missed diagnoses.
4. The diagnosis of leprosy is usually made based on skin lesions, cutaneous anesthesia, enlarged superficial nerves, and by demonstrating leprosy bacilli in the skin.
5. Patients with tuberculoid leprosy have a high degree of immunity against *M. leprae* and have few skin lesions and few organisms in their skin; patients with lepromatous leprosy have low immunity against *M. leprae* and have many skin lesions and millions of organisms in their skin.

ATYPICAL MYCOBACTERIA

24. How are infections with atypical mycobacteria acquired?

Atypical mycobacteria are ubiquitous and found in soil, water, and animals. Tap water is the major reservoir for atypical mycobacteria that cause human disease. In contrast to *M. tuberculosis*, they are not transmitted from person to person. Infection has been reported with immunosuppression, Mohs micrographic surgery, cutaneous surgery, punch biopsy, acupuncture, mesotherapy, injections, cardiothoracic surgery, breast reconstruction, facial plastic surgery, laser resurfacing, liposuction, body piercing, pedicures, tattoos, and abrasions. U.S. citizens traveling to other countries for cosmetic procedures has led to a rising incidence in atypical mycobacterial infections, often with antibiotic-resistant strains.

25. How is the diagnosis of atypical mycobacteria made?

After inoculation, the incubation period ranges from 1 to 29 weeks. An eruption of painful nodules increase to 2–5 cm in size then drain purulent fluid for 7 to 14 days before forming a scar. However, infection can present with abscesses, sporotrichoid nodules, subacute or chronic nodules, superficial lymphadenitis, verrucous lesions, panniculitis, and nonhealing ulcers. The gold standard for diagnosis is skin biopsy for tissue culture followed by DNA sequencing. More rapid techniques such as nucleic acid probes, high-performance liquid chromatography, PCR-restriction length polymorphism analysis, 16S DNA sequencing, multigene sequencing, and whole genomic sequencing allow more rapid identification of isolates from specimens.

26. What is a "swimming pool granuloma"?

Mycobacterium marinum is ubiquitous in both fresh and salt water and is inoculated through minor cutaneous trauma while fishing, cleaning aquariums, or aquatic activities. Two to 3 weeks after inoculation, a small violaceous papule develops that gradually enlarges into a verrucous dark red to violaceous plaque. A sporotrichoid pattern may be seen with violaceous nodules along the afferent lymphatics (Fig. 29.5A,B). Trauma-prone sites such as the hands, feet, elbows, and knees are most commonly involved. The diagnosis is mainly clinical with supporting evidence from histologic features and culture (Fig. 29.5C), but more rapid techniques including polymerase-chain reaction are available. The lesions can heal spontaneously or invade deeper tissue but rarely disseminate. Treatment for limited cutaneous infections is monotherapy with clarithromycin, doxycycline, minocycline, or trimethoprim-sulfamethoxazole for 3 months. More significant infections require two drug combination therapy with rifampin, clarithromycin, and/or ethambutol.

27. What is a Buruli ulcer?

Buruli ulcer, caused by *Mycobacterium ulcerans*, is the third most common mycobacterial disease in immunocompetent individuals. It occurs in warm tropical climates, most notably Africa, Australia, and Mexico. Inoculation following minor trauma most commonly affects the extremities. Over 4 to 6 weeks, a painless subcutaneous swelling develops that ulcerates producing a necrotic center with undermined borders. Its unique virulence factor, mycolactone toxin, causes necrosis and local immunosuppression and can lead to extensive tissue destruction resulting in limb contractions, even amputation. Per World Health Organization (WHO) guidelines, an 8-week course of rifampin and clarithromycin is recommended.

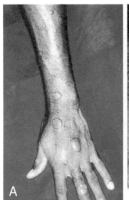
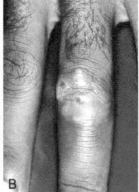
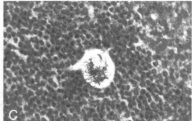

Fig. 29.5 Swimming pool granuloma caused by *M. marinum*. **A,** Erythematous nodule on the middle finger with sporotrichoid spread along the afferent lymphatics. **B,** Close-up of finger nodule. **C,** Ziehl-Neelsen staining demonstrating numerous acid-fast mycobacteria in a patient with swimming pool granuloma. (Courtesy James E. Fitzpatrick, MD.)

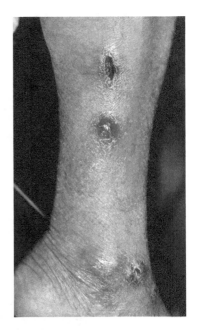

Fig. 29.6 *Mycobacterium avium-intracellulare* infection presenting as nodules and ulcerations in an HIV-infected patient. (Courtesy Margaret Muldrow, MD.)

28. Describe the clinical manifestations of Mycobacterium avium-intracellulare complex (MAC) in both non-AIDS and AIDS patients.

Mycobacterium avium complex (MAC) includes *M. avium* (most common), *M. intracellulare*, and other species. Few people who are infected develop disease but are typically susceptible with underlying lung disease or immunosuppression. HIV-negative persons most commonly present with pulmonary involvement. Disseminated disease (pulmonary, lymph node, gastrointestinal, bone) almost exclusively presents in late-stage acquired immunodeficiency syndrome patients. Cutaneous disease is rare but may occur as a manifestation of inoculation or disseminated disease. The skin lesions include ulcers, abscesses, deep nodules, or inflammatory plaques (Fig. 29.6).

29. Which atypical mycobacteria are associated with mesotherapy?

Mesotherapy is the injection of pharmaceutical and homeopathic substances into the subcutaneous fat to reduce cellulite despite a lack of evidence supporting its effectiveness. Rapidly growing mycobacteria after mesotherapy include *M. chelonae*, *M. fredericksbergense*, *M. abscessus*, and *M. fortuitum*. This procedure is popular in Europe and South America and is available in the United States.

30. Which atypical mycobacteria are associated with tattoos?

Tattoo-associated infections have been most commonly described secondary to *M. chelonae* and *M. abscessus*, with rare reports of *M. haemophilus*, *M. massiliense*, and *M. immunogenum*. Numerous reports are published of patients with pruritic papules and pustules restricted to their tattoos developing 1 to 4 weeks after the procedure. Tattoo ink and nonsterile diluent such as tap water have been implicated.

31. Which atypical mycobacteria have been associated with nail salon pedicures?

Rapidly growing furunculosis from contaminated footbath use during pedicures has been associated with *M. chelonae*, *M. abscessus*, and *M. fortuitum* (Fig. 29.7), with rare cases due to *M. bolletii* and *M. massiliense* reported.

32. How are infections with rapidly growing mycobacteria managed?

Monotherapy can induce resistance, so at least two antibiotics including trimethoprim-sulfamethoxazole, doxycycline, levofloxacin, and clarithromycin or azithromycin are recommended for a minimum of 4 months. More severe disease requires a minimum of 6 to 12 months of antibiotics. Testing for susceptibilities is advised before treatment begins in clinically significant isolates, and if treatment fails, or if there is a relapse. Surgery can be used for extensive cutaneous disease, abscesses, or medication contraindications.

33. What are some of the key features of Mycobacterium kansasii?

M. kansasii is a photochromogenic acid-fast bacillus that inhabits water sources including tap water in endemic areas worldwide, most commonly presenting as a pulmonary infection in older men with underlying chronic obstructive pulmonary disease. Dissemination to the lymph nodes, skin, soft tissue, and joints can occur in immunocompromised

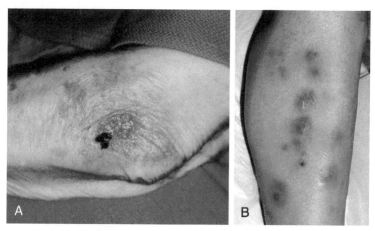

Fig. 29.7 Infections with atypical mycobacteria. **A,** Infection caused by *M. fortuitum*. Erythematous plaque with ulceration and necrosis following a puncture wound. **B,** Numerous abscesses and nodules caused by *M. chelonae* infection. (Courtesy James E. Fitzpatrick, MD.)

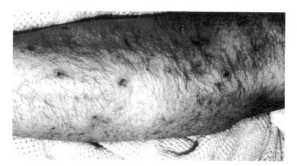

Fig. 29.8 Disseminated ulcerated lesions caused by *M. kansasii* in an HIV-infected patient.

individuals. Cutaneous involvement is heterogeneous, often appearing as an ulcer with sporotrichoid spread or cellulitis favoring HIV-infected individuals (Fig. 29.8). Treatment includes combination therapy with ethambutol, isoniazid, and rifampin.

HANSEN'S DISEASE

34. **What causes leprosy?**
    Leprosy is a chronic granulomatous infection caused by *Mycobacterium leprae*, a gram-positive acid-fast bacillus that is an obligate intracellular parasite of macrophages and the Schwann cells of nerves. It grows best around 35°C, preferring cooler areas such as the nose, ears, testes, and superficial cutaneous nerves. It cannot be grown in bacteriologic media but can be cultured in mouse foot pads.

35. **Why is leprosy called Hansen's disease?**
    Leprosy is referred to as Hansen's disease to honor Gerhard Hansen, a Norwegian physician who discovered the bacterium in 1873. *Mycobacterium leprae* was the first bacillus to be associated with human disease. Considerable social stigmata are associated with having leprosy, so it is often preferable to use the term *Hansen's disease*.

36. **How is leprosy transmitted?**
    Current evidence favors respiratory transmission via nasal and oral droplets, or rarely through breaks in the cutaneous barrier. Transmission typically requires prolonged contact with an infected individual with increasing risk associated with higher bacterial loads as in patients. Average incubation time is 4–10 years.

37. **Are children and adults equally susceptible to acquiring leprosy?**
    Children and young adults seem to be most susceptible to acquiring leprosy. Only about 5% of adults at risk, such as marriage partners, develop leprosy. As many as 60% of children who have a parent with leprosy develop the disease.

Table 29.3 Clinical features of leprosy skin lesions

CUTANEOUS LESIONS	TUBERCULOID	DIMORPHOUS	LEPROMATOUS
Number	Few	Many	Numerous
Type	Infiltrated hypopigmented plaques	Plaques, dome-shaped punched out lesions	Macules, papules, nodules, diffuse infiltration
Symmetry	Asymmetrical	Some asymmetry	Symmetrical
Sensation	Anesthetic	Variable decreased	Variable to not affected
Borders	Well defined	Less well defined	Vague
Bacilli in lesions	None detected	Many	Many

38. **Are humans the only host for *M. leprae*?**
It was once believed that humans were the only natural reservoir for *M. leprae*. However, other animals have been shown to carry the infection: the nine-banded armadillo, chimpanzee, sooty mangabey monkey, red squirrels (British Isles), and cynomolgus macaque. Up to 10% of wild armadillos in Louisiana and eastern Texas have naturally acquired leprosy.

39. **How common is leprosy?**
The WHO reported that there were 216,108 new leprosy cases registered globally in 2016, with a prevalence rate of 0.29/10,000. Leprosy is endemic in at least 53 countries, including India, where two-thirds of patients are diagnosed, as well as Brazil, Indonesia, and some countries in Africa.

40. **Are there endemic areas for leprosy in the United States?**
Southern Texas and Louisiana are considered endemic for leprosy. In 2015, 178 cases of leprosy were reported, with 72% occurring in Texas, Louisiana, Arkansas, California, Florida, Hawaii, and New York.

41. **How is leprosy recognized clinically?**
Clinical manifestations include skin lesions (Table 29.3) as well as enlarged superficial palpable nerves. Other features are nasal stuffiness, inflammatory eye changes, and loss of eyebrows or eyelashes.

42. **Is there more than one kind of leprosy?**
The four major variants of leprosy represent a spectrum of disease: indeterminate leprosy, tuberculoid leprosy, lepromatous leprosy, and borderline (dimorphous) leprosy (Fig. 29.9A–D). About 90% of the leprosy cases in the United States are the lepromatous type.

43. **Does indeterminate leprosy mean that you do not know what type it is?**
No. Indeterminate leprosy is considered the first sign of infection manifesting as a solitary, poorly demarcated, hypopigmented or erythematous, macular skin lesion. Indeterminate leprosy may clear spontaneously or progress to one of the other three types of leprosy.

44. **What are the two "polar" forms of leprosy? How do they differ?**
Tuberculoid leprosy and lepromatous leprosy are the two polar forms, and they remain stable clinically. Patients with tuberculoid leprosy have a high degree of immunity against *M. leprae*, with few skin lesions containing few organisms in their skin. Patients with lepromatous leprosy have low immunity against *M. leprae* and have generalized or diffuse cutaneous involvement harboring millions of organisms (Table 29.3).

45. **Describe dimorphous leprosy.**
Dimorphous leprosy (borderline leprosy) shows features intermediate between tuberculoid and lepromatous leprosy. It is less stable, as its clinical features and immune status may change over time. If dimorphous leprosy develops more features of lepromatous leprosy, it is referred to as dimorphous-lepromatous. If it develops features of tuberculoid leprosy, it is called dimorphous-tuberculoid.

46. **What is the unusual feature of the cell-mediated immunity in lepromatous leprosy?**
Patients with lepromatous leprosy have a specific anergy to *M. leprae*. This is in contrast to diseases such as sarcoidosis and Hodgkin's lymphoma, in which there is loss of immunity to a wide variety of antigens. The clinical spectrum of leprosy appears to depend mainly on an individual's ability to develop effective cell-mediated immunity against *M. leprae*.

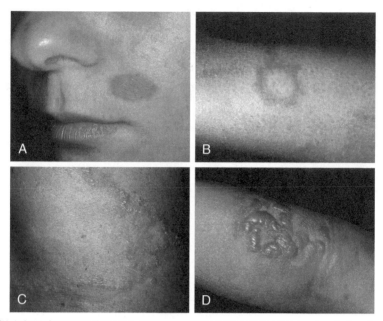

Fig. 29.9 Skin lesions in four variants of leprosy. **A,** Indeterminate leprosy. A solitary erythematous macule on the face of a young family member of a patient with lepromatous leprosy. **B,** Tuberculoid leprosy. A solitary, well-circumscribed, annular anesthetic patch. **C,** Dimorphous leprosy. A solitary anesthetic annular patch with a scaly border. **D,** Lepromatous leprosy. Coalescent brown, firm nodules.

47. How is the diagnosis of leprosy usually made?

The diagnosis of leprosy is usually made by demonstrating cutaneous anesthesia, recognizing enlarged superficial nerves, and identifying leprosy bacilli in the skin or nerves.

- In tuberculoid and dimorphous leprosy, annular cutaneous lesions lose sensation centrally. In lepromatous leprosy, the loss of light touch typically occurs first in the fingers and toes with variable anesthesia in individual skin lesions.
- Nerve enlargement in tuberculoid and dimorphous leprosy occurs within or adjacent to skin lesions. In lepromatous leprosy, large peripheral nerves can be palpated. The greater auricular nerve and the ulnar nerve at the elbow are easiest to appreciate (Fig. 29.10).
- The sensitivity using PCR in paucibacillary leprosy is 34%–80% but higher in multibacillary disease. Enzyme-linked immunosorbent assay is available for diagnosis of *M. leprae*. Per the CDC, current serological tests lack the sensitivity and specificity to be used for diagnosis.

48. What area should be biopsied to detect *M. leprae*?

The raised, active margin extending to the subcutaneous tissue of tuberculoid and dimorphous skin lesions should be biopsied. For lepromatous leprosy, the specimen should be taken from a cutaneous papule or nodule.

49. Can the same acid-fast stain used for Mycobacterium tuberculosis be used for the leprosy bacillus?

M. leprae is less acid-fast than *M. tuberculosis*, and a modified acid-fast stain known as the Fite-Faraco stain should be used to demonstrate organisms in tissue (Fig. 29.11).

50. What are Virchow cells?

Lepromatous leprosy exhibits an extensive cellular infiltrate separated from the epidermis by a narrow grenz zone of collagen. In early lesions, macrophages contain abundant live bacilli. With time or therapy, degenerated bacilli as well as lipid droplets accumulate in macrophages which are called Virchow cells. They have foamy cytoplasm and are Fite stain–positive.

51. Is the lepromin skin test helpful in making a diagnosis of leprosy?

No, but it is useful in classifying leprosy into the various subtypes. Lepromin is a crude preparation of killed *M. leprae* mycobacteria. An intradermal injection of 0.1 mL of lepromin is read at 48 hours for erythema (Fernandez reaction) or at 3 to 4 weeks for a papule or nodule (Mitsuda reaction). Patients with tuberculoid leprosy have strongly positive reactions, while lepromatous patients are usually negative.

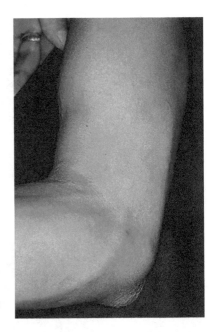

Fig. 29.10 Nerve enlargement. Palpable or visually enlarged nerves may be a sign of leprosy.

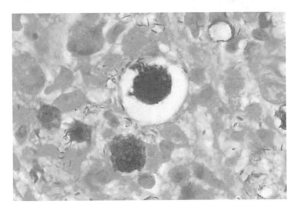

Fig. 29.11 Fite stain for *Mycobacterium leprae*. This skin biopsy shows clusters of acid-fast leprosy bacilli. The clusters are called globi. (Courtesy James E. Fitzpatrick, MD.)

52. **Is the neuropathy in lepromatous leprosy the same as that in diabetic neuropathy?**
No. Although the neuropathy is similar in the two diseases, it is a true "stocking-glove" anesthesia in diabetes mellitus. In leprosy, the cooler parts of the skin and nerves are affected, which gives the peripheral neuropathy a spotty and variable expression. For example, the dorsal aspects of the hands may be anesthetic, while the palms are partially spared resulting in patients misdiagnosed as malingerers or neurotics.

53. **Describe a patient with advanced lepromatous leprosy.**
The skin shows widespread, hyperpigmented papules and nodules with a predilection for cool parts of the body such as the earlobes, nose, fingers, and toes. There may be diffuse thickening of the dermis and loss of the lateral eyebrows (madarosis) (Fig. 29.12A,B), conjunctival erythema or corneal ulcerations, chronic rhinitis resulting in flattening of the nasal bridge producing a saddle-nose deformity (Fig. 29.13A), and a palpable postauricular nerve. Nerve involvement results in marked anesthesia of the extremities with some atrophy of the thenar and hypothenar muscles (Fig. 29.13B). Contraction of the fourth and fifth fingers may be seen. Ulcers and eschars of the hands and feet may be present secondary to minor trauma or burns (Fig. 29.13C). A plantar ulcer surrounded by hyperkeratotic skin (mal perforans ulcer) may be present over a pressure area (Fig. 29.13D).

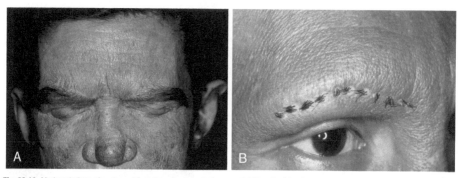

Fig. 29.12 Madarosis (loss of eyebrows) is an important sign in leprosy. **A,** This patient has heavy eyebrows due to hair transplants. He also has some destruction of the nasal cartilage and dark skin color due to the drug clofazimine. **B,** This patient has just received eyebrow transplants.

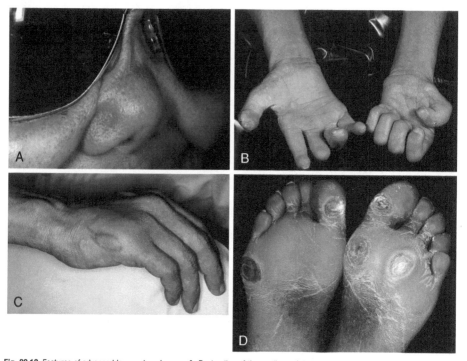

Fig. 29.13 Features of advanced lepromatous leprosy. **A,** Destruction of the cartilage of the nose producing a "saddle nose" deformity. *(Courtesy Fitzsimons Army Medical Center teaching files)* **B,** The hands often show contractures and muscle atrophy of the thenar and hypothenar eminences. **C,** Accidental burn. Because of anesthetic extremities, patients with leprosy are subject to burns and other minor trauma. **D,** Mal perforans ulcers. Patients with lepromatous leprosy develop foot ulcers surrounded by thick keratin as a result of peripheral anesthesia.

54. What are the most common complications in leprosy?
    1. Traumatic ulcers in anesthetic extremities.
    2. Reactional states that follow successful drug therapy.

55. What are the reactional states of leprosy?
    There are three types of reactions that may occur spontaneously but often follow the initiation of antibacterial therapy by months to years. Up to 30% of all leprosy patients experience one of these acute inflammatory episodes at some point in their disease course.

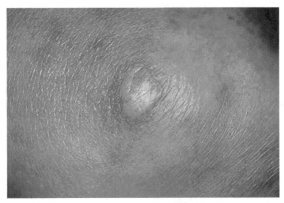

Fig. 29.14 Erythema nodosum leprosum. The reactive state in lepromatous leprosy resembles erythema nodosum but may be bullous, as seen in this patient.

Type I reaction (reversal reaction) most commonly complicates borderline leprosy due to a hypersensitivity reaction to *M. leprae* antigens presenting with the acute onset of erythema and edema of preexisting lesions. Painful neuritis with loss of sensory and motor function can occur with upgrading of the immune response. Downgrading can occur during inadequate therapy.

Type II reaction (erythema nodosum leprosum) occurs in lepromatous leprosy (Fig. 29.14) with the release of antigens from *M. leprae* during treatment. Immune complexes precipitate causing a cutaneous and systemic small vessel vasculitis. Erythematous tender nodules prone to ulceration favoring the extensor extremities and the face are associated with constitutional symptoms such as fever, arthralgias, lymphadenitis, nephritis, periostitis, and neuritis.

Type III reaction (Lucio's phenomenon) is due to an extensive necrotizing vasculitis with endothelial proliferation of *M. leprae* characterized by extensive violaceous patches and ulceration. It is typically seen in patients from Central or South America with lepromatous leprosy.

56. What drugs are used in multidrug therapy for leprosy?
The disease can be cured with multidrug therapy, and after the first dose, patients are not considered infectious. For tuberculoid leprosy, the recommended treatment is dapsone 100 mg daily and rifampin 600 mg monthly for 12 months. For lepromatous leprosy, in the United States, daily clofazimine 50 mg is added to the dapsone and rifampin regimen and the total treatment course is 24 months.

57. Do the recommendations of the WHO differ from those of the United States?
Due to economic and other factors, the WHO treatment recommendations are different from those of the United States. Paucibacillary tuberculoid leprosy is treated with dapsone 100 mg/day and rifampin 600 mg/month over 6 months. Multibacillary lepromatous leprosy is treated with rifampin 600 mg/month and clofazimine 300 mg/month, combined with dapsone 100 mg/day and clofazimine 50 mg/day for 12 months. Since 1995, WHO has provided free multidrug therapy for all leprosy patients worldwide.

58. What are the side effects of the drugs for leprosy treatment?
Dapsone is safe to use during pregnancy. Dapsone induces hemolysis of older red blood cells, causing a mild drop in hematocrit, but glucose-6-phosphatase dehydrogenase deficient patients may develop severe hemolysis. Mild methemoglobinemia is common but not a significant problem because the level usually does not exceed 12% of the total hemoglobin. Idiosyncratic reactions such as pancytopenia, peripheral neuropathies, acute psychosis, and a potentially fatal infectious mononucleosis-like condition may also develop. Rifampin, as a P450 inducer, may decrease the effect of other drugs. Hepatotoxicity and red urine are common.

59. What is the most bothersome cutaneous side effect of clofazimine?
The most bothersome side effect of clofazimine is a red to brown to purple discoloration of the skin (Fig. 29.12A). Some patients develop acquired ichthyosis.

60. How are the reactional states of leprosy treated?
For type I reactions, because of the risk of permanent nerve damage, prednisone 20 to 60 mg/day is recommended. Mild type II reactions can be controlled with aspirin or nonsteroidal anti inflammatory agents and rest. Severe type II reactions are controlled with thalidomide 100 to 200 mg/day. Thalidomide should not be given to women of childbearing age because of its severe teratogenic effects.

61. Should family members of leprosy patients be treated?

Dapsone prophylaxis of all family members is not currently recommended; however, children and spouses should be examined by experienced medical personnel at least once a year. Postexposure prophylaxis with a single dose of rifampicin to contacts of newly diagnosed patients with leprosy has demonstrated a 50%–60% reduction of the risk of developing the disease over the following 2 years.

62. Can leprosy be eliminated as a worldwide disease, as smallpox has been?

In the past 20 years, over 14 million leprosy patients have been cured, and the worldwide prevalence of leprosy has been reduced by 90%, from 10 to 12 million in 1988 to 176,176 cases in 2015. It has been eliminated from 119 of 122 countries where it was considered a public health problem in 1985 (elimination being defined as a prevalence rate of <1 case per 10,000 persons). The sequencing of the entire genome of *M. leprae* was completed in 2001.

Acknowledgment

The authors wish to acknowledge the invaluable input of Genevieve L. Egnatios, MD, Karen Warschaw, MD and Loren Golitz, MD, in coauthoring previous editions of this chapter.

BIBLIOGRAPHY

Avanzi A, Bierbauer K, Vales-Kennedy G, Guillermo C, Covino J. Nontuberculous mycobacteria infection risk in medical tourism. *JAAPA.* 2018;31(8):45–47.

Cambau E, Saunderson P, Matsuoka M, et al. Antimicrobial resistance in leprosy: results of the first prospective open survey conducted by a WHO surveillance network for the period 2009–15. *Clin Microbiol Infect.* 2018;24(12):1305–1310.

Center for Disease Control. *Leprosy.* https://www.cdc.gov/leprosy/. Accessed February 17, 2019.

Center for Disease Control. *Tuberculosis.* https://www.cdc.gov/tb/default.htm. Accessed February 17, 2019.

Espinosa OA, Ferreira SMB, Palacio FGL, et al. Accuracy of enzyme-linked immunosorbent assays (ELISAs) in detecting antibodies against Mycobacterium leprae in leprosy patients: a systematic review and meta-analysis. *Can J Infect Dis Med Microbiol.* 2018;2018:9828023.

Franco-Paredes C, Marcos LA, Hengo-Martinez AF, et al. Cutaneous mycobacterial infections. *Clin Microbiol Rev.* 2018;32(1). https://doi.org/10.1128/CMR.00069-18.

Morbidity and Mortality Weekly Report. *Treatment of tuberculosis.* http://www.cdc.gov/mmwr/PDF/rr/rr5211.pdf. Accessed February 17, 2019.

Ramos-e-Silva M, Ribeiro de Castro MC. Mycobacterial infections. In: Bolognia J, Schaffer J, Cerroni L, eds. *Dermatology.* 4th ed. Philadelphia, PA: Elsevier Saunders; 2017:1296–1318.

Resources Health, Administration Services. *National Hansen's Disease (leprosy) Program caring and curing since.* https://www.hrsa.gov/hansens-disease/index.html; 1984. Accessed 26 January 2019.

World Health Organization. *Leprosy.* https://www.who.int/lep/mdt/en/. Accessed February 17, 2019.

World Health Organization. *Treatment of Mycobacterium ulcerans disease (Buruli ulcer).* https://www.who.int/news-room/fact-sheets/detail/buruli-ulcer-(mycobacterium-ulcerans-infection). Accessed January 21, 2019.

CHAPTER 30

SUPERFICIAL FUNGAL INFECTIONS

Richard A. Keller and Deborah B. Henderson

1. What is a dermatophyte?

   A dermatophyte is a fungus that has developed the ability to live on the keratin (hair, nails, or skin scale) of animals. Dermatophytes are classed into three genera: *Microsporum*, *Trichophyton*, and *Epidermophyton*.

2. How are superficial fungal infections diagnosed?

   Superficial fungal infections can usually be suspected clinically, but definitive diagnosis requires the demonstration of fungal pathogens by microscopic examination or culture of skin, nail, or hair scrapings from the suspected lesion. During microscopic examination, hyphae are sought in the material. The material is first placed on a glass slide, and then one or two drops of 10% to 20% potassium hydroxide (KOH) are added. A fungal stain such as chlorazol black E may be added to the preparation to aid visualization of the fungal elements. The hyphae of dermatophytes will be septate and typically demonstrate branching (see Fig. 3.1). Skin scrapings can also be placed on culture media. Culturing the organism, in addition to being a diagnostic aid, permits speciation of the organism.

3. On a KOH examination, hyphal-like structures arranged in a mosaic pattern are noted. Does this indicate the presence of a dermatophyte?

   "Mosaic hyphae" are not really hyphae and do not indicate the presence of a dermatophyte. If you vary the microscope's focus, the pattern can be observed to conform to the cell walls. Mosaic hyphae actually represent thickened stratum corneum cell walls. True hyphae cross the cell walls of keratinocytes and do not conform to the contour of keratinocytes.

4. What are the three most commonly used culture media for the growth of dermatophytes?
   - **Sabouraud's dextrose agar:** A nonselective culture medium consisting of peptone, dextrose, agar, and distilled water. It allows the growth of bacteria as well as pathogenic and nonpathogenic yeast and molds.
   - **Mycosel or Mycobiotic agar:** A selective growth medium for dermatophytes. It consists of Sabouraud's agar with cycloheximide (suppresses saprophytic fungi) and chloramphenicol (suppresses bacteria). Dermatophytes and *Candida albicans* grow readily on this media, while the growth of contaminant bacteria, some yeast, and many opportunistic fungi is inhibited.
   - **Dermatophyte test media (DTM):** Sabouraud's agar with cycloheximide, gentamicin, and chlortetracycline hydrochloride. It also has a phenol red indicator. If a dermatophyte is present, the color of the media changes from yellow to red. False positives do occur.

5. Describe some of the presentations of superficial fungal infections caused by dermatophytes.

   The superficial dermatophyte infections are classified according to their location on the affected person. This location does not necessarily reveal the identity of the offending organism. The infection will cause the production of scale. The scale may or may not be associated with erythema, vesicles, or annular plaques (Table 30.1, Fig. 30.1).

6. Which dermatophyte causes the most fungal infections of skin?

   Trichophyton rubrum.

Foster KW, Ghannoum MA, Elewski BE. Epidemiologic surveillance of cutaneous fungal infections in the United States from 1999 to 2002. *J Am Acad Dermatol.* 2004;50:748–752.

Nenoff P, Krüger C, Ginter-Hanselmayer G, et al. Mycology—an update. Part 1: dermatomycoses: causative agents, epidemiology and pathogenesis. *J Dtsch Dermatol Ges.* 2014;12(3):188–209.

7. What is the most common cause of tinea capitis in the United States?

   Until the mid-1950s, *Microsporum audouinii* was the most common cause of endemic tinea capitis in the United States, but it has since been replaced by *Trichophyton tonsurans*. Several theories have been proposed to explain the almost total disappearance of *M. audouinii* from the United States, but the most plausible theory is that it was eradicated by the widespread use of griseofulvin. At the same time that *M. audouinii* disappeared, *T. tonsurans*, formerly an uncommon cause of tinea capitis, quickly spread. This species was probably introduced into the United States from Central or South America.

Foster KW, Ghannoum MA, Elewski BE. Epidemiologic surveillance of cutaneous fungal infections in the United States from 1999 to 2002. *J Am Acad Dermatol.* 2004;50:748–752.

Mirmirani P, Tucker LY. Epidemiologic trends in pediatric tinea capitis: a population-based study from Kaiser Permanente Northern California. *J Am Acad Dermatol.* 2013;69(6):916–921.

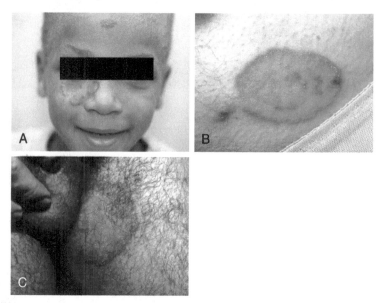

Fig. 30.1 Dermatophyte infections. **A,** Tinea faciei in a child demonstrating multiple annular scaly lesions of the face. **B,** Tinea corporis. Annular lesion with scale at the edge and clearing in the central portion of the lesion. **C,** Tinea cruris. Annular scaly lesion of the groin; note the characteristic sparing of the scrotum. (Panel A, courtesy William L. Weston, MD, collection; panels B and C courtesy Fitzsimons Army Medical Center teaching files.)

Table 30.1 Clinical presentations of dermatophyte infections

INFECTION	LOCATION
Tinea capitis	Scalp
Tinea faciei (see Fig. 30.1A)	Face
Tinea barbae	Beard
Tinea corporis (see Fig. 30.1B)	Trunk, extremities
Tinea cruris (see Fig. 30.1C)	Groin
Tinea manuum (manus)	Hands
Tinea pedis	Feet
Tinea unguium (onychomycosis)	Nails

8. Name the four clinical patterns of tinea capitis.
   1. The seborrheic pattern has a dandruff-like scaling of the scalp and should be considered in prepubertal children with suspected seborrheic dermatitis (Fig. 30.2A).
   2. In the black-dot pattern, hairs are broken off at the skin line, and black dots are seen within the areas of alopecia (Fig. 30.2B). In the United States, this pattern is primarily associated with *T. tonsurans* infections.
   3. A kerion is an inflammatory fungal infection that may mimic a bacterial folliculitis or an abscess of the scalp (Fig. 30.2C). The scalp is tender to the touch, and the patient usually has posterior cervical lymphadenopathy.
   4. Favus is a rare form of inflammatory tinea of the scalp presenting with sites of alopecia that have cup-shaped, honey-colored crusts, which are called *scutula* and are composed of fungal mats.

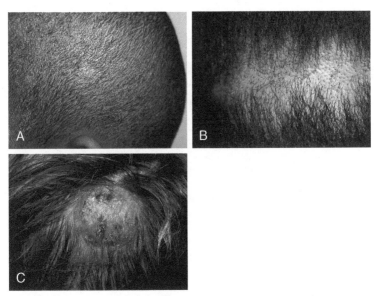

Fig. 30.2 Tinea capitis. **A,** Seborrheic pattern. **B,** Black-dot pattern. **C,** Kerion presenting as a tender boggy mass in the scalp.

Tinea capitis is one of the most commonly misdiagnosed skin infections. Any prepubertal child who presents with a scaly scalp dermatitis or carries a diagnosis of seborrheic dermatitis should be presumed to have a dermatophyte infection of the scalp until proven otherwise. Similarly, any child who presents with one or more scalp abscesses most likely has a kerion. Kerions are frequently secondarily infected with *Staphylococcus aureus*, and unsuspecting health care providers often mistakenly treat kerions as bacterial abscesses. Posterior cervical lymphadenopathy aids in identifying all forms of tinea capitis infection. Additionally, dermoscopy can often reveal "comma," "corkscrew," or dystrophic hairs within affected areas.

9. What are the types of hair invasion in tinea capitis? What dermatophytes are associated with each type?
Dermatophytes can cause three types of hair invasion:
1. **Endothrix** infections are produced by fungi that invade the inside of the hair shaft and are composed of fungal arthroconidia and hyphae (Fig. 30.3). A helpful mnemonic to remember the organisms that cause endothrix invasion is: "TVs are in houses."—T is *Trichophyton tonsurans,* V is *violaceum,* and S is *soudanense.*
2. **Ectothrix** infections are produced by fungi that primarily invade the outside of the hair shaft. Some agents of small-spore ectothrix cause a fluorescent tinea capitis. A helpful mnemonic to remember these organisms is **"Cats and Dogs Fight Grizzly."** Add *Microsporum gypseum* with the mnemonic below.
3. **Favus** infections are characterized by invasion of hair by hyphae that do not produce conidia and by the presence of linear air spaces. *T. schoenleinii* is associated with this type of invasion.

10. What is a Wood's light? What organisms are detected by this exam?
A Wood's light is an ultraviolet light source that emits in the spectrum of 325 to 400 nm. This light was used extensively for the diagnosis of tinea capitis when *Microsporum audouinii* was the major cause of this disorder. However, it is of limited usefulness today because most cases are now produced by *Trichophyton tonsurans,* which is not fluorescent. The fluorescence is caused by pteridine. The fungi responsible for fluorescent tinea capitis can be remembered by the mnemonic **"See Cats and Dogs Fight."**
- **See:** *T. schoenleinii*
- **Cats:** *M. canis*
- **And:** *M. audouinii*
- **Dogs:** *M. distortum*
- **Fight:** *T. ferrugineum*
Except for *T. schoenleinii,* all of these organisms produce a small-spore ectothrix pattern of hair invasion.

Wolf FT. Chemical nature of the fluorescent pigment produced in *Microsporum*-infected hair. *Nature.* 1957;180:860–861.

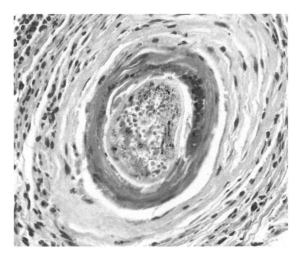

Fig. 30.3 Endothrix. Cross-section of a hair shaft filled with hyphae and arthrospores (hematoxylin and eosin [H&E]).

11. How is tinea capitis treated?

After the presence of a fungal infection is demonstrated by either culture or a positive KOH smear, treatment with an oral antifungal agent should be instituted. Most patients are placed on griseofulvin. Microsized griseofulvin at a dose of 20 to 25 mg/kg/day should be taken with meals to improve absorption. The medication is continued for at least 4 to 6 weeks, after which the site is recultured. Using antifungal shampoo may reduce shedding of the organism. Members of the patient's family also should be evaluated for infection or a carrier state, and treated if needed. A special consideration is needed in the treatment of kerions, which in addition to traditional tinea capitis antifungal treatments may also benefit for systemic glucocorticoid therapy (such as 0.5–1 mg/kg for 1 week) to diminish their significant inflammation. Patients who fail to respond to griseofulvin or are intolerant should be treated with an alternative treatment regimen:

- **Terbinafine:** 62.5 mg/day (<20 kg), 125 mg/day (20 to 40 kg), 250 mg/day (40 kg) for 2 to 6 weeks (infections by *M. canis* may require double the dose)
- **Itraconazole:** 3 to 5 mg/kg/day for 6 weeks
- **Fluconazole:** 6 mg/kg/day for 6 weeks.

Elewski BE, Hughey LC, Hunt KM, Hay RJ. Fungal disease. In: Bolognia JL, Schaffer JV, Cerroni L, et al, eds. *Dermatology.* 4th ed. Philadelphia, PA: Elsevier; 2018;1329–1363.
Chen X, Jiang X, Yang M, et al. Systemic antifungal therapy for tinea capitis in children: an abridged Cochrane review. *J Am Acad Dermatol.* 2017;76(2):368–374.

12. What is meant by a carrier state in tinea capitis?

A carrier is a person who does not have clinical signs of tinea capitis but has a positive fungal culture from the scalp. In families in whom tinea capitis is identified, the carrier rate in adults is around 30%. The presence of these carriers will reduce the cure rate for tinea capitis if they are not treated concomitantly. Treatment can include shampooing with selenium sulfide or other antifungal shampoo.

Babel D, Baughman S. Evaluation of the adult carrier state in juvenile tinea capitis caused by *Trichophyton tonsurans. J Am Acad Dermatol.* 1989;21:1209–1212.
Ilkit M, Demirhindi H. Asymptomatic dermatophyte scalp carriage: laboratory diagnosis, epidemiology and management. *Mycopathologia.* 2008;165(2):61–71.
Neil G, Hanslo D, Buccimazza S, et al. Control of the carrier state of scalp dermatophytes. *Pediatr Infect Dis J.* 1990;9:57–58.

13. Name the three types of tinea pedis. Which dermatophyte is most commonly associated with each?

The three types of tinea pedis are interdigital infection, moccasin-type infection, and vesiculobullous or inflammatory infection. Interdigital infections present as scaling, maceration, fissuring, or erythema of the webspace between the toes. This infection is usually associated with *Trichophyton rubrum* or *T. interdigitale* (recognized previously as *T. mentagrophyte var. interdigitale*). Moccasin-type tinea pedis presents as generalized scaling and hyperkeratosis of the plantar surface of the foot. This form of infection is frequently associated with nail involvement. Moccasin-type

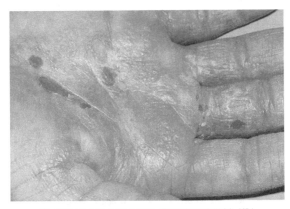

Fig. 30.4 Dermatophytid reaction. (Courtesy Mark Welch, MD.)

tinea pedis is typically caused by *T. rubrum*. The inflammatory or vesiculobullous type will cause a vesicular eruption on the arch or side of the foot and is most often caused by *T. mentagrophytes.*

14. **What nondermatophyte mold can cause mycotic infections that mimic moccasin-type tinea pedis?**
    Neoscytalidium dimidiatum (previously *Scytalidium*) has been isolated from cases of moccasin-type tinea pedis that are resistant to standard therapy. The organism will not grow on selective dermatophyte media, such as Mycosel, Mycobiotic, or DTM, but it does grow readily on Sabouraud's agar.

15. **What is a dermatophytid reaction?**
    Dermatophytid reactions are inflammatory reactions at sites distant from the site of the associated dermatophyte infection. Types of dermatophytid reactions from tinea pedis include urticaria, hand dermatitis (Fig. 30.4), or erythema nodosum. The pathogenesis of dermatophytid reactions is not fully understood, but evidence suggests that they are secondary to a strong host immunologic response against fungal antigens.

16. **Name and describe the four clinical presentations of onychomycosis.**
    1. Distal subungual onychomycosis presents as onycholysis, subungual debris, and discoloration beginning at the hyponychium that spreads proximally. The most common organism is *Trichophyton rubrum* (Fig. 30.5).
    2. Proximal subungual onychomycosis begins underneath the proximal nail fold and is typically caused by *T. rubrum*. The patient's immune status should be investigated because it is strongly associated with immunosuppressive conditions.
    3. Superficial white onychomycosis produces a white, crumbly nail surface due to invasion of the top of the nail plate. It is usually caused by *T. mentagrophytes*; however, nondermatophytes such as *Fusarium*, *Acremonium*, and *Aspergillus* have been associated with this type of infection.
    4. Candidal onychomycosis is seen in patients with chronic mucocutaneous candidiasis.

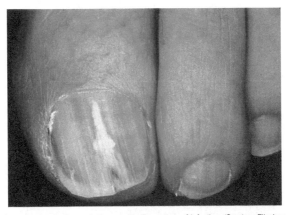

Fig. 30.5 Distal subungual onychomycosis demonstrating a spike-like pattern of infection. (Courtesy Fitzsimons Army Medical Center teaching files.)

17. Can other diseases mimic onychomycosis?

Yes. Psoriasis, Reiter's disease, lichen planus, pachyonychia congenita, Darier's disease, and Norwegian scabies are some of the diseases that can resemble onychomycosis. For this reason, the diagnosis should be established by either a KOH examination or culture before beginning prolonged and often expensive therapies to eradicate the infection.

18. How is onychomycosis treated?

Treatment of onychomycosis should be initiated only after a fungal infection of the nail is confirmed by either culture or a positive KOH smear to prevent misdiagnosis of similarly presenting nail conditions discussed earlier. Nail clippings or fragments of nail plate can also be submitted in formalin for diagnosis by hematoxylin and eosin and with fungal stains such as periodic acid–Schiff.

Traditionally, oral therapy has been shown to achieve higher complete cure rates than most topical treatments due to the low penetrance of these through the nail plate, although in 2014, two topical agents, efinaconazole and tavaborole, were approved by the Food and Drug Administration for treatment of onychomycosis. The duration of therapy is determined by which nails on the patient are being treated. For example, the first-line therapy for dermatophyte nail infections is terbinafine 250 mg/day ×6 weeks for fingernail onychomycosis and 250 mg/day ×12 weeks for toenail infections. For nondermatophyte or *Candida* infections, pulsed itraconazole has been found to be most effective at doses of 200 mg twice a day ×1 week of each month, for 2 months when treating fingernails and 3 to 4 months for toenails. It is important to note that certain populations of patients such as diabetic patients or individuals with peripheral neuropathy have a greater risk of complications from their onychomycosis, necessitating prompt treatment of their nail disease.

Del Ross JQ. The role of topical antifungal therapy for onychomycosis and the emergence of newer agents. *J Clin Aesthet Dermatol.* 2014; 7(7):10–18.

19. What are some potential risks associated with the treatment of onychomycosis?

Before initiation of therapy, patients should be screened for potential drug-drug interactions, as itraconazole may affect the half-life of commonly used medicines that are metabolized by the CYP-3A4 part of the P-450 pathway. Additionally, patients should undergo lab monitoring monthly while on these agents due to the risk of hepatotoxicity.

De Sa DC, Lamas AP, Tosti A. Oral therapy for onychomycosis: an evidence-based review. *Am J Clin Dermatol.* 2014;15(1):17–36.
Elewski B, Tavakkol A. Safety and tolerability of oral antifungal agents in the treatment of fungal nail disease: a proven reality. *Ther Clin Risk Manag.* 2005;1(4):299–306.
Gupta A., et al. Systemic antifungal agents. In: Wolverton SE, et al, ed. *Comprehensive dermatologic drug therapy.* 4th ed. Philadelphia, PA: Elsevier; 2020;99–113.

20. What is tinea versicolor?

Tinea versicolor (pityriasis versicolor) is a hypopigmented, hyperpigmented, or erythematous macular or thin papular eruption. Macules may coalesce into large patches with an adherent fine scale (Fig. 30.6). Lesions are located predominantly on the trunk but may extend to the extremities. The proper taxonomic nomenclature of the lipophilic yeast that produces this infection is debatable. Studies indicate *Malassezia globosa* is the organism most frequently associated with tinea versicolor, although older references list *M. furfur* as the most common

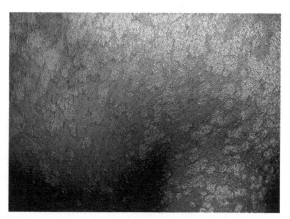

Fig. 30.6 Tinea versicolor demonstrating hypopigmented scaly patches.

organism. This eruption begins during adolescence, when the sebaceous glands become active. The eruption tends to flare when the temperatures and humidity are high. Immunosuppression, systemic corticosteroids, and sweaty or greasy skin will also cause this disease to flare.

Erchiga VC, Florencio VD. *Malassezia* species in skin diseases. *Curr Opin Infect Dis.* 2002;15:133–142.
Gupta KA, Batra R, Bluhm R, et al. Pityriasis versicolor. *Dermatol Clin.* 2003;21:413–429.
Prohic A, Ozegovic L. *Malassezia* species isolated from lesional and non-lesional skin in patients with pityriasis versicolor. *Mycoses.* 2007; 50:58–63.

21. How does *Malassezia* induce both hyperpigmentation and hypopigmentation in the skin?
    In the past, *Malassezia* has been suggested to induce hypopigmentation by production of dicarboxylic acid. These compounds do not have a direct effect on melanocytes in tissue culture. The dark lesions of tinea versicolor may be due to a variation in the inflammatory response to the infection. There is not any strong evidence that influences current thought on this question (Fig. 30.7). In hypopigmented areas melanocytes have smaller and fewer melanosomes.

Hay RJ, Ashbee HR Moore MK. Fungal infections. In: Griffiths CE, Barker J, Bleiker T, et al, eds. *Rook's textbook of dermatology.* 9th ed. Chichester, West Sussex, UK: John Wiley & Sons LTD; 2016.
Galadari I, El Komy M, Mousa A, et al. Tinea versicolor: histologic and ultrastructural investigation of pigmentary changes. *Int J Dermatol.* 1992;31:253–256.

22. How is tinea versicolor diagnosed? Why is it difficult to culture this organism?
    Tinea versicolor is diagnosed by scraping some of the scale from a lesion and looking for the characteristic "macaroni and meatballs" under the microscope. The meatballs are the yeast forms, and the macaroni are the short hyphae. This organism is a lipophilic yeast and will grow only after a source of lipid is added to the culture media. A yellow fluorescence may be seen by Wood's light examination of affected areas.

American Academy of Dermatology. https://www.aad.org/public/diseases/a-z/tinea-versicolor-treatment.

23. Does Malassezia cause any other skin disease?
    This organism can also produce a folliculitis of the trunk, arms, and neck area. *Malassezia* folliculitis presents as pruritic follicular papules and pustules that do not respond to antibiotic therapy. The yeast can be demonstrated by skin biopsies or direct examination of purulent material. The severity of seborrheic dermatitis has been reported to be associated with an increase in *Malassezia* microflora.

24. What is tinea nigra?
    A superficial dermatomycosis caused by *Hortaea (Phaeoannellomyces or Exophiala) werneckii*. This is a dematiaceous (pigment-producing) fungus. It causes an asymptomatic tan, brown, or black patch on the palms or soles. The diagnosis is made by demonstrating pigmented hyphae on a KOH examination of the lesion. Tinea nigra has been confused with acral lentiginous melanoma.

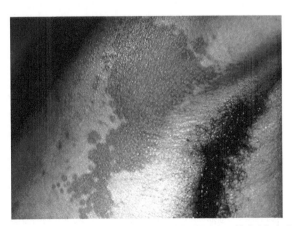

Fig. 30.7 Hyperpigmented variant of tinea versicolor. (Courtesy Walter Reed Army Medical Center teaching files.)

25. What is a Majocchi's granuloma?

Majocchi's granuloma is a follicular abscess produced when a dermatophyte infection penetrates the follicular wall into the surrounding dermis. Patients usually present with one or more tender boggy papules or plaques on the legs or, less commonly, arms. Pus may be seen draining from the hair follicle. *Trichophyton rubrum* or *T. mentagrophytes* are the species most commonly isolated from these lesions. Treatment should consist of an oral antifungal agent.

26. What is piedra?

Piedra refers to adherent deposits on the hair shaft caused by superficial fungal infections. Black piedra, which is caused by *Piedraia hortae*, presents as firm black nodules on the hair shaft. *Trichosporon ovides* is the etiologic agent that produces white piedra, which results in the formation of less adherent white concretions on scalp hair shaft. This organism has been reclassified into over six pathologic species, with the *T. inkin, T. asahii,* and *T. mucoides* being the most common causes of white piedra in pubic hair.

Hay RJ, Ashbee HR Moore MK. Fungal infections. In: Griffiths, CE, Barker J, Bleiker T, et al, eds. *Rook's textbook of dermatology.* 9th ed. Chichester, West Sussex, UK: John Wiley & Sons; 2016.

27. Name the organism most commonly isolated from cutaneous candidiasis.

Candida albicans is the most common organism isolated from lesions of candidiasis. It is normally part of the microflora of the gastrointestinal tract.

28. How do candidal infections present clinically?

The clinical presentations vary with the sites involved, duration of infection, and immune status of the host (Table 30.2). Most sites show erythema, edema, and a thin purulent discharge (Fig. 30.8).

29. What factors predispose to candidiasis?

The factors that predispose to the development of candidiasis are both endogenous and exogenous. Exogenous factors include occlusion, moisture, and warm temperature. Endogenous factors can include immunosuppression, diabetes mellitus, other endocrinopathies, antibiotics, oral contraceptives, Down syndrome, malnutrition, and pregnancy. Chronic mucocutaneous candidiasis in children and adolescents is associated with impaired response by the T helper 17 cells, which affects the response to *Candida.*

Wagner D, Sohnle P. Cutaneous defenses against dermatophytes and yeasts. *Clin Microbiol Rev.* 1995;8:317–335.
Elewski BE, Hughey LC, Hunt KM, Hay RJ. Fungal disease. In: Bolognia JL, Schaffer JV, Cerroni L, eds. *Dermatology.* 4th ed. Philadelphia, PA: Elsevier; 2018;1329–1363.

30. Which diseases are associated with adult-onset chronic mucocutaneous candidiasis?

Thymoma, myasthenia gravis, myositis, and aplastic anemia have been associated with the development of chronic mucocutaneous candidiasis after the third decade of life.

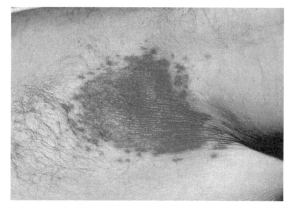

Fig. 30.8 Cutaneous candidiasis showing an erythematous plaque with characteristic satellite lesions in a body fold area. (Courtesy Larry Becker, MD.)

Table 30.2 Clinical presentations of cutaneous candidiasis

DISEASE	CLINICAL DESCRIPTION
Intertrigo	Superficial pustules, erythema, edema, creamy exudates within skin folds
Thrush	White, adherent, cottage cheese–like plaques on oral mucosa
Perlèche	Erythema, fissuring, creamy exudate at the angles of the mouth
Paronychia	Tender, erythematous, indurated proximal nail fold, with or without a purulent discharge
Erosio interdigitalis blastomycetica	Erythema, fissuring, maceration of the webspaces between the fingers

Table 30.3 Oral antifungal agents

CLASS	EXAMPLES	MECHANISMS OF ACTION
Antibiotic	Griseofulvin	Arrest of cellular division, dysfunction of spindle microtubules
Polyenes	Nystatin	Binds irreversibly with ergosterol, altering membrane permeability
Azoles	Fluconazole Itracoazole Ketoconazole	Inhibits ergosterol production by inhibiting the cytochrome P-450 lanosterol 14α-demethylase
Allylamines	Terbinafine Naftifine	Blocks ergosterol production by inhibiting squalene epoxidase

Data from Gupta A, Sauder D, Shear N. Antifungal agents: part II. J Am Acad Dermatol. 1993; 30:911–933. Gupta A., et al. Systemic antifungal agents. In: Wolverton SE, et al, ed. Comprehensive dermatologic drug therapy. 4th ed. Philadelphia, PA: Elsevier; 2020;99–113.

31. Name the different classes of oral antifungal agents and their mechanisms of action
    See Table 30.3 and Fig. 30.9.

Gupta A., et al. Systemic antifungal agents. In: Wolverton SE, et al, ed. *Comprehensive dermatologic drug therapy.* 4th ed. Philadelphia, PA: Elsevier; 2020;99–113.

32. Which hepatic cytochrome is affected by itraconazole, ketoconazole, and fluconazole?
    Cytochrome P-450 3A4. Fluconazole inhibits this enzyme at doses greater than 200 mg/day. Fluconazole is also a cytochrome 2C9 inhibitor, and it can affect the metabolism of angiotensin II inhibitors, oral hypoglycemic agents, and oral anticoagulants. Terbinafine has been associated with inhibiting cytochrome P-2D6 and caution when using with tricyclic antidepressants.

Gupta A., et al. Systemic antifungal agents. In: Wolverton SE, et al, ed. *Comprehensive dermatologic drug therapy.* 4th ed. Philadelphia, PA: Elsevier; 2020;99–113.
Venkatakrishnan K, von Moltke LL, Greenblatt DJ. Effects of the antifungal agents on oxidative drug metabolism: clinical relevance. *Clin Pharmacokinet.* 2003;38:111–180.

33. Which drugs should be used with caution when using ketoconazole, itraconazole, or fluconazole? Why?
    Warfarin, quinidine, digoxin, calcium channel blockers, busulfan, HIV protease inhibitors, cyclosporine, angiotensin II inhibitors, tacrolimus, oral hypoglycemic agents, hydantoin anticonvulsants, and alcohol. These drugs should be used with caution, because the primary effect of azole antifungal drugs on hepatic enzyme metabolism is inhibition. This results in an elevation of the serum level of any drug that requires hepatic metabolism by the cytochrome P-450 3A4 enzyme in order to be removed.

Gupta A., et al. Systemic antifungal agents. In: Wolverton SE, et al, ed. *Comprehensive dermatologic drug therapy.* 4th ed. Philadelphia, PA: Elsevier; 2020;99–113.

MECHANISM OF ACTION OF ANTIFUNGALS AGENTS

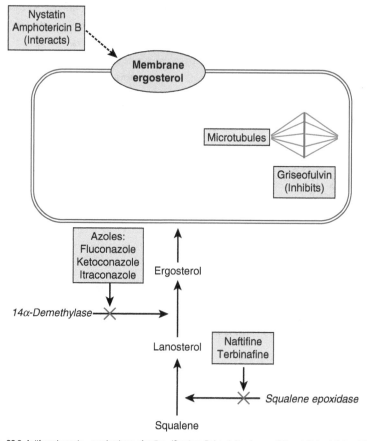

Fig. 30.9 Antifungal agents—mechanisms of action. (Courtesy Deborah Henderson, MD, and Richard Keller, MD.)

KEY POINTS: SUPERFICIAL FUNGAL INFECTIONS

1. *Trichophyton tonsurans* is the most common agent of tinea capitis in the United States and cannot be detected by Wood's light examination.
2. Asymptomatic dermatophyte carriers in households of children with tinea capitis are a source of treatment failures.
3. Check for immunosuppression in any patient with proximal subungual onychomycosis.
4. *Malassezia globosa* is the organism most commonly isolated from lesions of tinea versicolor.

34. Which drugs are contraindicated when using azole antifungal agents and why?
    Contraindicated drugs are cisapride (pulled off the U.S. market in 2000), astemizole (pulled off the U.S. market in 1999), terfenadine (pulled off the U.S. market in 1998), lovastatin, pimozide, quinidine, dofetilide, levacetylmethadol, midazolam, and triazolam. When combined with azole antifungal agents, these drugs can cause severe or life-threatening reactions. Elevated levels of cisapride, astemizole, and terfenadine are associated with cardiac arrhythmias, especially torsades de pointes. The metabolism of lovastatin is markedly reduced and can result in rhabdomyolysis. Simvastatin, atorvastatin, and cerivastatin are metabolized by the same hepatic cytochrome and also should be avoided.

Gupta A., et al. Systemic antifungal agents. In: Wolverton SE, et al, ed. *Comprehensive dermatologic drug therapy.* 4th ed. Philadelphia, PA: Elsevier; 2020;99–113.

35. Which oral antifungal agents can lower cyclosporine levels?
Griseofulvin and terbinafine.

36. Which drugs can affect antifungal drug levels?
Any drug that raises the gastric pH reduces the absorption of itraconazole and ketoconazole. Rifampin reduces the levels of oral azole and allylamines by induction of hepatic cytochromes. Isoniazid and phenytoin can induce the metabolism of azole antifungal agents. Cimetidine and oral azole antifungal agents can raise terbinafine levels.

37. Which antifungal drugs have a limited spectrum of activity in the treatment of superficial fungal infections?
Griseofulvin is not effective against tinea versicolor or cutaneous candidiasis. Oral nystatin is not absorbed from the gastrointestinal tract. Topical nystatin and amphotericin are both ineffective against dermatophyte infections. Allylamines have limited effectiveness against tinea versicolor and candidiasis.

38. Which oral antifungal is no longer a recommended treatment of tinea versicolor and other superficial fungal infections?
Ketoconazole is no longer considered a first-line therapy for superficial fungal infections due to risk of serious hepatotoxicity and QT-prolongation.

Gupta AK, Foley KA, Versteeg SG. New antifungal agents and new formulations against dermatophytes. *Mycopathologia*. 2017; 182:127–141.

KEY POINTS: SUPERFICIAL FUNGAL INFECTIONS

1. Azole antifungal agents block the cytochrome P-450 enzyme lanosterol 14α-demethylase, which depletes ergosterol from cell membranes, whereas allylamine antifungals block ergosterol production through inhibition of squalene epoxidase.
2. Systemic antifungals itraconazole, fluconazole, and ketoconazole all inhibit the cytochrome P-450 3A4 enzyme and thereby slow the metabolism of commonly used anticoagulants, hypoglycemic, and antihypertensive medicines.
3. An acidic pH increases the absorption of itraconazole and ketoconazole.

CHAPTER 31

DEEP FUNGAL INFECTIONS

Wendi E. Wohltmann

KEY POINTS: DEEP FUNGAL INFECTIONS

1. Deep fungal infections can be divided into subcutaneous (localized), systemic, and opportunistic categories.
2. Neutropenic patients are particularly at risk for systemic phaeohyphomycosis, aspergillosis, fusariosis, and mucormycosis.
3. Patients with impaired cellular immunity are particularly at risk for disseminated sporotrichosis, histoplasmosis, coccidioidomycosis, penicilliosis, *Cryptococcus*, and *Candida*.
4. The differential diagnosis of lymphocutaneous (sporotrichoid) spread includes **SLANTS: S**porotrichosis, **L**eishmaniasis, **A**typical mycobacteria, *Nocardia,* **T**ularemia, and cat **S**cratch disease.

1. What is a deep fungal infection?
   In contrast to the superficial dermatophytes, which are typically confined to dead keratinous tissue, certain mycotic infections have the capacity for deep invasion of the skin or production of skin lesions secondary to systemic infection. They are typically acquired through direct inoculation, ingestion, and/or inhalation of spores from soil or other organic matter. In this chapter, the deep fungal diseases are organized into three categories based on clinical presentation (Table 31.1).

SUBCUTANEOUS FUNGAL INFECTIONS

2. Discuss the characteristics of subcutaneous mycotic infections.
   Subcutaneous mycotic infections are caused by a heterogeneous group of fungi and are infections of implantation (inoculated directly into the skin through local trauma). The four most important infections are sporotrichosis, chromomycosis, phaeohyphomycosis, and mycetoma. Lobomycosis and rhinosporidiosis are significantly less common. As a group, these infections involve primarily the skin and subcutaneous tissues and rarely disseminate in the immunocompetent host. These organisms are ubiquitous in soil, plants, and trees.

3. What is a dimorphic fungus?
   Dimorphic fungi are capable of growing in both the mold and yeast forms. Examples of diseases caused by dimorphic fungi include sporotrichosis, histoplasmosis, blastomycosis, paracoccidioidomycosis, and penicilliosis.

4. What occupations are at increased risk of sporotrichosis?
   Sporotrichosis is caused by a dimorphic fungus, *Sporothrix schenckii*. This organism is found worldwide, except in the polar regions, and is most common in subtropical and tropical climates. It is endemic in Africa and Central and South America. In the United States, infection is most common in the Midwest. The habitat includes soil, thorny plants (especially roses), hay, sphagnum moss, and animals. Cats may carry *Sporothrix* on their paws and can cause infection by scratching their owners or animal handlers. Occupations at risk of cutaneous inoculation include farmers, gardeners (especially rose), florists, masonry workers, Christmas tree farmers, veterinarians, and animal handlers (especially cats, rodents, and armadillos).

Table 31.1 The deep fungal infections		
SUBCUTANEOUS FUNGAL INFECTIONS	**SYSTEMIC OR RESPIRATORY FUNGAL INFECTIONS**	**OPPORTUNISTIC FUNGAL INFECTIONS**
Sporotrichosis	Blastomycosis	Cryptococcosis
Phaeohyphomycosis	Histoplasmosis	Aspergillosis
Chromomycosis (chromoblastomycosis)	Coccidioidomycosis	Fusariosis
Mycetoma (Madura foot)	Paracoccidioidomycosis	Mucormycosis
Lobomycosis		Penicilliosis
Rhinosporidiosis		
Zygomycosis		

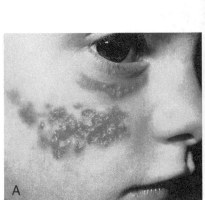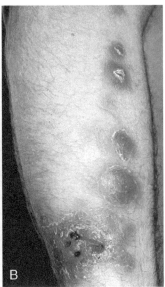

Fig. 31.1 Sporotrichosis. **A,** Linear lesions secondary to a cat scratch. **B,** Erythematous, crusted, ulcerated nodule in a lymphocutaneous pattern. (Courtesy James E. Fitzpatrick, MD.)

5. Describe the clinical manifestations of sporotrichosis.

   The classic form of sporotrichosis (lymphocutaneous) begins at the site of inoculation (most commonly, upper extremity) as a painless pink papule, pustule, or dermal nodule, which rapidly enlarges and ulcerates (Fig. 31.1A). Without treatment, the infection ascends along the lymphatics, producing secondary nodules and regional lymphadenopathy that may ulcerate (Fig. 31.1B). The fixed cutaneous variant is confined to the site of inoculation. The organisms rarely disseminate hematogenously to the joints, bone, meninges, or eye.

6. How is the diagnosis of cutaneous sporotrichosis made?

   A strong clinical suspicion is most important. Skin biopsy shows granulomatous inflammation with neutrophilic microabscesses. In the immunocompetent patient, fungal elements are only found in about 60% of cases even when special stains are utilized. When suspecting sporotrichosis, cultures (of tissue or pus) on Sabouraud's medium are both more specific and sensitive. Colonies grow rapidly in 3 to 5 days.

7. How do you treat cutaneous sporotrichosis?

   Itraconazole (100 to 200 mg/day) for 3–6 months is the treatment of choice for lymphocutaneous and fixed cutaneous sporotrichosis, with a success rate of 90% to 100%. Terbinafine (250 mg/day) is second-line treatment, and because potassium iodide (SSKI) is less costly than other agents, it is still recommended, especially in developing-world epidemics. Local hyperthermia has also been shown to be effective. Children may be safely treated with itraconazole. The treatment of choice for disseminated disease is a lipid formulation of amphotericin B (3 to 5 mg/kg per day intravenously) until the patient shows a favorable response, followed by itraconazole 200 mg twice a day for a total treatment time of at least 12 months.

8. What other organisms may present with lymphocutaneous disease?

   Several other diseases may present with a distal ulcer, proximal secondary nodules along the lymphatics, and regional lymphadenopathy. The most important include nontuberculous *Mycobacterium* (*Mycobacterium marinum*, *Mycobacterium kansasii*, *Mycobacterium fortuitum* complex), *Nocardia*, leishmaniasis, cat scratch disease, and tularemia. A patient with this clinical presentation should have tissue biopsies for routine histology and cultures to include bacteria, mycobacteria, and fungi. This pattern of disease is also called *sporotrichoid* and can be remembered using the **SLANTS mnemonic: S**porotrichosis, **L**eishmaniasis, **A**typical mycobacteria, **N**ocardia, **T**ularemia, cat **S**cratch disease.

9. What are dematiaceous fungi?

   Dematiaceous fungi are brown or black pigmented fungi. The pigment is due to melanin. They are slow growing and can be found in the soil, decaying vegetation, rotting wood, and the forest carpet. Subcutaneous-cutaneous disease is caused by traumatic inoculation into the skin. There are three broad categories of dematiaceous fungal infections, including chromoblastomycosis, phaeohyphomycosis, and eumycotic mycetoma (Madura foot).

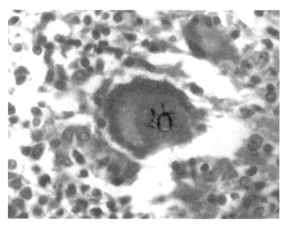

Fig. 31.2 Chromomycosis. Diagnostic golden-brown, yeastlike fungi (Medlar bodies) within a multinucleated foreign body giant cell. (Courtesy James E. Fitzpatrick, MD.)

10. How do you differentiate chromoblastomycosis from phaeohyphomycosis?

Chromoblastomycosis (also called chromomycosis) is a chronic subcutaneous infection characterized by the appearance in tissue biopsies of an intermediate, vegetative, pigmented fungal form with a yeastlike appearance that is arrested between yeast and hyphal formation. These pigmented, thick-walled fungal elements are called Medlar bodies (Fig. 31.2). Medlar bodies, also called **copper pennies** or sclerotic bodies, are diagnostic of chromoblastomycosis, differentiating it from phaeohyphomycosis. Tissue biopsies of phaeohyphomycosis are characterized by lightly pigmented filamentous hyphae.

11. Which organisms may cause chromoblastomycosis?

Five fungal species account for most infections. The most frequent organism worldwide is *Fonsecaea pedrosoi*. Other organisms include *Phialophora verrucosa*, *Fonsecaea compactum*, *Rhinocladiella aquaspersa*, and *Cladophialophora carrionii*. **Memory device: Compact** *(Fonsecaea compactum)* **dead** *(Cladophialophora carrionii)* **wet** *(Rhinocladiella aquaspersa)* **warty** *(Phialophora verrucosa)* **feet** *(Fonsecaea pedrosoi)*.

12. Which organisms cause phaeohyphomycosis?

Phaeohyphomycosis may occur in both immunocompetent and immunocompromised patients and has been attributed to over 60 genera and more than 100 species. The most important genera include *Scedosporium* (*Pseudallescheria*), *Alternaria*, *Bipolaris*, *Curvularia*, *Exophiala*, *Phialophora*, and *Wangiella*.

13. How does chromoblastomycosis present?

Chromoblastomycosis is a chronic cutaneous and subcutaneous infection that is usually present for years with minimal discomfort. The inciting injury is often not recalled. The infection is most common on the lower extremity, and 95% of cases occur in males. The typical patient is a barefoot, rural agricultural worker in the tropics. At the inoculation site, red papules develop that eventually coalesce into a plaque, which slowly enlarges and acquires a verrucous or warty surface. Lesions can evolve into a cauliflower-like mass, leading to lymphatic obstruction and elephantiasis-like edema of the lower extremity (Fig. 31.3) if left untreated. Neoplastic transformation to squamous cell carcinoma can occur.

14. How is chromoblastomycosis diagnosed and treated?

Diagnosis is made through potassium hydroxide (KOH) mounts from scrapings, biopsies of the lesions showing the organism with suppurative and granulomatous inflammation, and culture. Chromoblastomycosis is typically resistant to treatment. The treatment of choice for small lesions is surgical excision with a wide margin of normal skin. Chronic or extensive lesions should be treated with a combination of itraconazole therapy and surgical excision. Combination therapy with terbinafine, posaconazole, cryotherapy, and local heat therapy also appear to be effective. Treatment is continued for months.

15. Describe the clinical features of phaeohyphomycosis.

The spectrum of clinical infections is broad. The most typical presentation is a subcutaneous cyst or abscess at the site of trauma, and *Exophiala jeanselmei* and *E. dermatitidis* are the most common organisms. The primary lesion is a painless nodule that evolves into a fluctuant abscess. Immunocompromised patients present with multiple nodules. *Scedosporium proliferans* (42% of cases), *Bipolaris spicifera* (8%), and *Wangiella dermatitidis* (7%) are the most common causes of rare disseminated disease. The primary risk factor is decreased host immunity, especially prolonged neutropenia. The outcome is poor, despite antifungal therapy, with a 79% overall mortality rate.

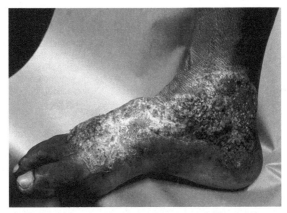

Fig. 31.3 Chromomycosis. Cauliflower-like nodules and tumors on the foot and ankle with edema. (Courtesy James E. Fitzpatrick, MD.)

16. What is Madura foot?

   Madura foot, a type of mycetoma, is a localized, destructive infection of the skin and subcutaneous tissue that eventually involves deeper structures. It may be caused by filamentous bacteria, aerobic actinomycetes (actinomycetomas), and true fungi (eumycetoma). The most common causative fungi are *Madurella mycetomatis* and *Madurella grisea*. Less frequent causes are *Acremonium kiliense*, *E. jeanselmei*, and *Scedosporium apiospermum* (also called *Pseudallescheria boydii*).

17. What are the three characteristic clinical features of Madura foot?

   The first is the formation of nodules in the skin at the site of inoculation, usually a penetrating injury. The second feature is purulent drainage and fistula formation. The third and most characteristic feature is the presence of **grains** or **granules** that are visible in the purulent drainage. Madura foot is a progressive infection leading to marked swelling and deformity in its later stages (Fig. 31.4). Additionally, the lesions have a tendency to become painful in the later stages, when bone involvement and deformity ravage the site.

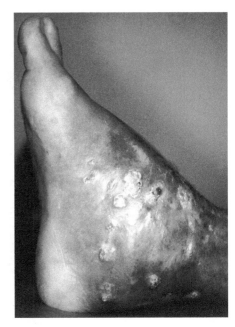

Fig. 31.4 Madura foot. Swelling and deformity of the foot and ankle with purulent drainage and fistula formation.

SYSTEMIC FUNGAL INFECTIONS

18. Discuss the pathogenesis of the systemic respiratory deep fungi

    The systemic respiratory endemic fungal infections include blastomycosis, histoplasmosis, coccidioidomycosis, paracoccidioidomycosis, and penicilliosis. These infections are all due to species that show dimorphism. These diseases are similar in pathophysiology, but each has distinct clinical characteristics. The causative organisms are found in the soil, and infection occurs with inhalation of the organism into the lung. The primary infection is pulmonary. Dissemination occurs via the lymphohematogenous route, and each fungus has a predilection for particular organ systems.

19. Where is blastomycosis endemic?

    Blastomycosis, caused by the soil saprophyte *Blastomyces dermatitidis*, is endemic in North America, especially the southeastern and south-central states bordering the Mississippi and Ohio rivers (Kentucky, Arkansas, Mississippi, Tennessee, Louisiana, Illinois, and Wisconsin), North Carolina, and the Great Lakes region (Fig. 31.5). Sporadic cases have been reported in Colorado, Texas, Kansas, and Nebraska. The typical patient is a middle-aged male with occupational or recreational exposure to the soil.

20. What are the clinical manifestations of blastomycosis?

    An important concept of blastomycosis is that it can mimic many other disease processes and has been called **"The Great Pretender."** The pulmonary manifestations range from a community-acquired pneumonia on one end of the spectrum to malignancy. Pulmonary disease is seen in 87% of patients, skin lesions in 20%, bone involvement in 15%, central nervous system (CNS) in 5% to 10%, and less commonly the genitourinary system (prostate).

21. Describe the cutaneous findings in disseminated blastomycosis

    The most characteristic cutaneous presentation is a single (or multiple) crusted, verrucous plaque on exposed skin (face, hands, arms) with color variation from gray to violet (Fig. 31.6). Microabscesses can form, and pus exudes when the crust is lifted off. As the plaque progresses, there is central clearing with graduated, elevated edges, an appearance likened to a sports stadium. Ulcerative lesions are a less common cutaneous presentation.

22. Are immunosuppressed patients at increased risk of disseminated disease with blastomycosis?

    Blastomycosis behaves as an opportunistic infection in the immunosuppressed host much less commonly than other deep fungal infections. There are, however, several reports of disseminated blastomycosis in acquired immunodeficiency syndrome patients, organ transplant recipients, diabetic patients, and patients receiving glucocorticosteroids and chemotherapy.

23. What is the treatment of blastomycosis?

    Itraconazole is the treatment of choice for mild to moderate disease. Amphotericin B is the preferred treatment of life-threatening disease, CNS involvement, and immunocompromised and pregnant patients.

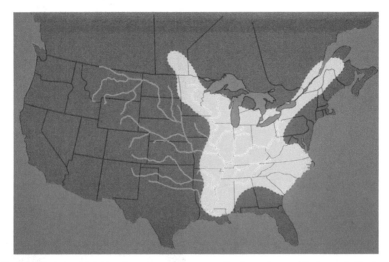

Fig. 31.5 Blastomycosis. Areas depicted in yellow represent the areas reporting the most cases of blastomycosis. (Courtesy Fitzsimons Army Medical Center teaching files.)

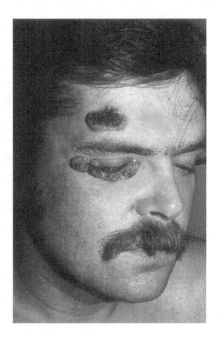

Fig. 31.6 Blastomycosis. Classic verrucous plaques located on the forehead and eyelid. (Courtesy teaching files of Fitzsimons Army Medical Center.)

24. Where is histoplasmosis endemic?

Histoplasmosis is caused by *Histoplasma capsulatum*, an environmental saprophyte. It is endemic in the Midwestern and south central United States, where 80% of the population is skin test positive. It does occur in other parts of the world, but it is not found in Europe. Soil infected with excreta from chickens, pigeons, blackbirds, starlings, and bats is inhaled, leading to a pulmonary infection. Rarely, primary cutaneous disease is contracted from traumatic inoculation.

25. What factors are necessary for production of the disease histoplasmosis?

The two most important factors are the number of organisms inhaled and immune status of the host. Only 1% of patients exposed to a small inoculum develop symptomatic disease; in contrast, 50% to 100% of persons exposed to a heavy inoculum develop symptoms.

26. Discuss the clinical manifestations of histoplasmosis.

Most patients with symptoms develop a flulike acute pulmonary illness characterized by fever, chills, headache, myalgias, chest pain, and nonproductive cough. Progressive disseminated histoplasmosis occurs in 1 of 2000 acute infections. High-risk groups for disseminated disease include patients with impaired cellular immunity such as HIV infection, lymphoma, or leukemia and also infants and the elderly. Rarely, a primary cutaneous form is seen following direct inoculation into the skin.

27. Describe the three different patterns of disseminated histoplasmosis (acute, subacute, and chronic).

The acute syndrome generally occurs in immunosuppressed patients and is characterized by fever, hepatosplenomegaly, and pancytopenia, with 18% developing **mucocutaneous ulcers**. Hilar or mediastinal lymphadenopathy and focal or patchy infiltrates are the hallmarks of the subacute form, which occurs over weeks to months. Chronic disseminated histoplasmosis is characterized by involvement of the bone marrow, gastrointestinal tract, spleen, adrenals, and CNS; 67% have **painful ulcerations on the tongue, buccal mucosa, gingiva, or larynx** (Fig. 31.7). The treatment of choice is itraconazole and, for severe diseases and immunosuppressed patients, amphotericin.

28. Are there any other cutaneous manifestations of histoplasmosis?

Erythema nodosum and, less commonly, erythema multiforme may be seen in histoplasmosis, coccidioidomycosis, and, rarely, blastomycosis. These cutaneous hypersensitivity reactions are generally associated with a good prognosis.

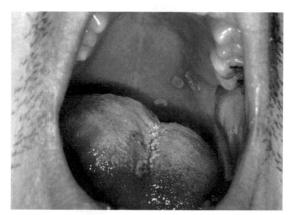

Fig. 31.7 Histoplasmosis. Oral ulcerations in an HIV-infected patient. Histoplasmosis more commonly affects the oral mucosa than the skin. (Courtesy James E. Fitzpatrick, MD.)

29. Where is coccidioidomycosis endemic?

    Coccidioidomycosis, also called San Joaquin Valley fever, is caused by *Coccidioides immitis*. It is a dimorphic fungus found in the soil of arid and semiarid regions. This organism is endemic in southern California, Arizona, New Mexico, southwestern Texas, northern Mexico, and Central and South America (Fig. 31.8).

30. What are the clinical manifestations of coccidioidomycosis?

    Primary pulmonary infection is asymptomatic in 50% of patients. In 40%, patients present with a mild flulike illness or pneumonia. Hematogenous dissemination occurs in 1% to 5% of patients. Risk factors for dissemination and fatal disease include male sex, pregnancy, immunocompromised status, and race (in order of decreasing risk by race:

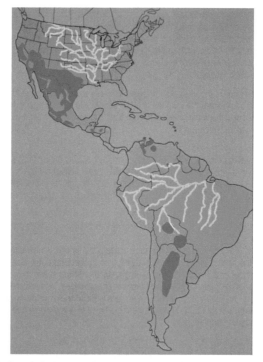

Fig. 31.8 Coccidioidomycosis. Areas depicted in red represent the regions reporting the most cases of coccidioidomycosis. (Courtesy Fitzsimons Army Medical Center teaching files.)

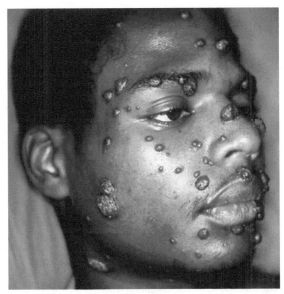

Fig. 31.9 Disseminated coccidioidomycosis. Discrete verrucous papules, plaques, and nodules. (Courtesy James E. Fitzpatrick, MD.)

Filipino, black, and white). Coccidioidomycosis is considered an AIDS-defining illness. The most common sites of extrapulmonary disease include the skin, lymph nodes, bones/joints, and CNS (meninges).

31. **What are the skin findings in coccidioidomycosis?**
Cutaneous lesions of disseminated coccidioidomycosis are protean. Warty papules, plaques, or nodules are the most characteristic (Fig. 31.9). Cellulitis, abscesses, and draining sinus tracts also may occur. Rarely, cutaneous lesions can be from primary cutaneous inoculation. Erythema nodosum is the most common reactive manifestation and indicates a robust cell-mediated immune response. Other reactive patterns include generalized morbilliform, papular, targetoid or urticarial exanthem, interstitial granulomatous dermatitis, and Sweet's syndrome.

32. **Where is paracoccidioidomycosis endemic?**
Paracoccidioidomycosis (South American blastomycosis) previously has been thought to be restricted to Latin America, especially Brazil. There have been reports of cases outside this area. The disease is confined to humid tropical and subtropical forests. *Paracoccidioides brasiliensis* is the causative dimorphic fungus.

33. **Why is paracoccidioidomycosis more common in men?**
Paracoccidioidomycosis is most common in adult men between the ages of 30 and 60 years. Skin testing indicates that the rate of infection is equal among the sexes. However, clinical disease is more common in men, with a male:female ratio of 15:1. It has been shown that this sex difference is due to the inhibitory action of estrogens on the mycelium to yeast transformation necessary for infectivity.

34. **What is the most common presenting complaint of paracoccidioidomycosis?**
Painful mucosal ulcerations involving the mouth and nose are the most common findings. Patients may also have enlarged cervical lymph nodes and verrucous, crusted, edematous facial lesions. The lung is the primary site of infection; however, respiratory complaints are the least common presenting symptom.

35. **Which organism is responsible for penicilliosis?**
Penicilliosis is caused by the dimorphic fungus *Penicillium marneffei*. It is inhaled into the lungs and causes disease in both immunocompetent and immunocompromised patients, with a predilection to the latter.

36. **Where is penicilliosis endemic?**
Penicilliosis is endemic in Southeast Asia and southern China. The increase in HIV-infected individuals in these areas has led to the emergence of this organism as a cause of infection.

37. **How does penicilliosis present clinically?**
The most common clinical presentation is subacute with weeks of intermittent fevers, headache, marked weight loss, and anemia. AIDS patients have an increased frequency of septicemia and mucocutaneous lesions. Skin lesions are a common manifestation of disseminated disease and are usually found on the upper body. Abscesses,

Table 31.2 Organisms that parasitize histiocytes mnemonic

Rare	Rhinoscleroma
Lesions	Leishmaniasis
Try	Trypanosomiasis
To	Toxoplasmosis
Grow in	Granuloma inguinale
Parasitized	Penicilliosis
Histiocytes	Histoplasmosis

subcutaneous nodules, and reactive skin diseases such as Sweet's syndrome are seen in non-HIV–infected individuals. Cutaneous lesions are more diversified in the HIV patients and include molluscum contagiosum–like papules, pustules, acneiform, and morbilliform eruptions. Delay in treatment is associated with 100% mortality in all patients. Biopsy and culture are used for diagnosis. Treatment options include itraconazole or amphotericin B in severe cases.

38. What is a parasitized histiocyte?
    It is a macrophage (histiocyte) hosting an infection. Several species of bacteria and fungi infect and proliferate and actually thrive within the cytoplasm of macrophages rather than being killed by the macrophage (Table 31.2).

OPPORTUNISTIC FUNGAL INFECTIONS

39. Define opportunistic infection
    Opportunistic infections are caused by organisms that typically produce disease in a host with lowered resistance. The four discussed in this chapter are cryptococcosis, aspergillosis, fusariosis, and mucormycosis.

40. What are the common fungal pathogens in HIV infection?
    Candida and *Cryptococcus* species are the most common fungal infections in HIV-infected patients. See Table 31.3 for other fungal pathogens and their most frequent clinical presentations.

Table 31.3 Fungal pathogens in HIV infection

ORGANISM	CLINICAL FEATURES
Candida albicans	Thrush, vaginal, and esophageal candidiasis
Cryptococcus neoformans	Pulmonary and disseminated disease, meningitis, skin, eye, prostate
Histoplasma capsulatum	Disseminated disease with fever, weight loss, and predilection for reticuloendothelial system, adrenal glands, and CNS
Coccidioides immitis	Disseminated and pulmonary disease. Predilection for skin, lymph nodes, bones/joints, and CNS
Blastomyces dermatitidis	Disseminated and pulmonary disease. Predilection for lung, skin, bone, CNS, and prostate
Aspergillus fumigatus	Disseminated and pulmonary disease
Penicillium marneffei	Disseminated disease with fever, anemia, weight loss. Mucocutaneous lesions are common
Sporotrichosis schenckii	Disseminated disease. Sites of predilection: joints/bones, eyes, and meninges

CNS, Central nervous system.

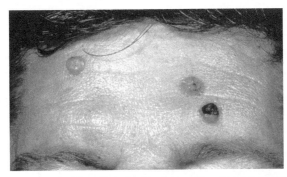

Fig. 31.10 Disseminated cryptococcosis. Multiple papules and nodules that resemble molluscum contagiosum. (Courtesy James E. Fitzpatrick, MD.)

41. Discuss the fungal infections seen in organ transplant recipients.
Organ transplant recipients are at increased risk of localized and disseminated disease from dermatophytes, yeast (candidiasis, *Malassezia*, cryptococcosis, *Trichosporon*), dimorphic organisms (histoplasmosis, coccidioidomycosis, blastomycosis), and nondermatophyte molds (aspergillosis, fusariosis, mucormycosis). Skin manifestations due to *Candida* spp., *Aspergillus* spp., dematiaceous fungi, and *Pityrosporum* typically occur shortly after transplantation. Cryptococcosis occurs 6 months or later after transplantation, and the endemic dimorphic fungi can cause disease any time following transplantation. Emerging mold pathogens in the transplant patients have included *Aspergillus fumigatus*, *Fusarium*, *Scedosporium*, and Zygomycetes (e.g., Rhizopus, Mucor, Rhizomucor).

42. What causes cryptococcosis?
Cryptococcosis is caused by *Cryptococcus neoformans*, a ubiquitous encapsulated yeast found in soil worldwide. Several strains are associated with pigeon and other avian excreta, and another strain is associated with eucalyptus trees.

43. Discuss the important epidemiologic factors of cryptococcosis.
During the pre-AIDS era (prior to 1980), cryptococcal infections were infrequent and about 50% occurred in patients with lymphoreticular malignancies. Cryptococcosis is rare in immunocompetent patients, and patients at risk are those with impaired cellular immunity (advanced HIV patients, organ transplants, lymphoreticular malignancies, patients receiving corticosteroid therapy). The incidence of cryptococcosis is inversely proportional to the CD4 lymphocyte count. The prevalence in patients infected with HIV has declined with aggressive antiretroviral therapy. The mortality rate of untreated disseminated disease is 70% to 80%.

44. How is an infection with cryptococcosis acquired?
Infection occurs primarily from inhalation of the organism leading to a primary lung infection. Immunocompetent patients generally present with a mild pulmonary infection. Disseminated disease via the hematogenous route occurs in 10% to 15% of immunosuppressed patients, with a predilection for the meninges. **It is the leading cause of fungal meningitis.** Other organs involved include the skin (10% to 20%), eye, bone, and prostate. There are a few rare reports of primary inoculation cutaneous disease, which manifests itself as a solitary papule/nodule. However, cutaneous disease is generally indicative of disseminated disease and a poor prognosis.

45. What are the cutaneous manifestations of disseminated cryptococcosis?
Cryptococcosis is a great imitator of a wide variety of cutaneous diseases. These include molluscum contagiosum–like lesions (Fig. 31.10), Kaposi sarcoma–like lesions, pyoderma gangrenosum–like lesions, herpetiform lesions, cellulitis, ulcers, subcutaneous nodules, and palpable purpura. Lesions are most commonly found on the head, neck, and genitals, but can be found anywhere. Cutaneous lesions are found in 10% to 20% of HIV-infected patients. Histologic features are characteristic with periodic acid–Schiff stain with diastase demonstrating budding yeast surrounded by a clear space representing the capsule (Fig. 31.11).

46. What patient population is at increased risk of aspergillosis?
Neutropenia and corticosteroid therapy, especially when combined, are the two most important risk factors for aspergillosis. Solid organ and bone marrow transplant recipients and leukemic patients, in particular, are at high risk. Other at-risk patients include HIV-infected individuals, patients on broad-spectrum antibiotics, and patients on immunosuppression therapy.

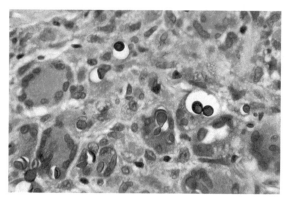

Fig. 31.11 Cryptococcosis. Periodic acid–Schiff stain with diastase demonstrating budding yeast surrounded by a clear space representing the capsule. (Courtesy Fitzsimons Army Medical Center teaching files.)

47. How common are cutaneous lesions in aspergillosis?

    Aspergillus species are ubiquitous saprophytes in the air, soil, and decaying vegetation. It is primarily a respiratory pathogen, with the lungs and sinuses as the major sites of infection. Disseminated disease occurs in 30% of aspergillosis cases, and cutaneous lesions develop in fewer than 11%. There are several documented reports of primary invasive skin infections occurring in neutropenic patients associated with intravenous catheters and adhesive tape contaminated with spores.

48. Describe the cutaneous lesions in aspergillosis

    Patients may have single or multiple lesions that begin as a well-circumscribed papule, which, over several days, enlarges into an ulcer with a necrotic base and surrounding erythematous halo (Fig. 31.12). The organism has a propensity to invade blood vessels, causing thrombosis and infarction. The skin lesions can be very destructive and extend into cartilage, bone, and fascial planes. Aspergillosis should be considered in the differential diagnosis of necrotizing lesions.

49. What opportunistic fungus is clinically and histologically similar to Aspergillus?

    Patients with prolonged neutropenia, especially leukemia patients, are susceptible to *Fusarium* infections. In this patient population, *Fusarium* species are the second most common pathogenic mold. *Fusarium* is a filamentous mold found in soil and plants. Inhalation into the lungs is the primary route of infection, although primary cutaneous infection from indwelling catheters may occur. The lung is the usual site of infection; however, 75% of patients have hematogenous spread with a predilection for the skin and sinuses. The cutaneous lesions caused by *Fusarium* are similar to aspergillosis. Histologically, the two are identical (septate hyphae with acute angle branching). The treatment of choice is amphotericin B and the mortality rate is 50% to 80%.

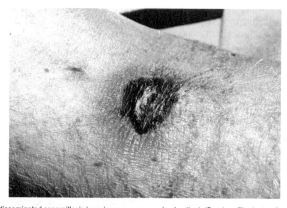

Fig. 31.12 Fatal case of disseminated aspergillosis in an immunocompromised patient. (Courtesy Fitzsimons Army Medical Center teaching files.)

50. What are the most important predisposing factors for acquiring mucormycosis?

Approximately one-third of patients have diabetes, and diabetic patients in ketoacidosis are at especially high risk. Other reported associations include malnutrition, uremia, neutropenia, hematologic malignancies, corticosteroid therapy, burns, antibiotic therapy, neonatal prematurity, iron-overload syndromes, deferoxamine therapy, and HIV-positive patients with a history of IV drug use. Neutrophils are the predominant component of host defense. Mucormycosis is caused by rapidly growing molds from several genera, including *Apophysomyces*, *Mucor*, *Rhizopus*, *Absidia*, and *Rhizomucor*. These organisms are ubiquitous in decaying vegetation, fruit, and bread.

51. Can mucormycosis be acquired from contaminated dressings?

Yes. Primary cutaneous mucormycosis can occur when the spores are directly inoculated into abraded skin. In the 1970s, there was a nationwide epidemic associated with contaminated elastic dressings. Patients presented with a cellulitis under the covered areas. Primary cutaneous mucormycosis has also been reported from gardening, intramuscular injections, intravenous lines, needle-sticks, arthropod bites, automobile accidents, and burns. Cutaneous disease accounts for approximately 10% of reported cases and can also be from hematologic spread (Fig. 31.13).

52. What is the treatment of mucormycosis?

The treatment of mucormycosis is multimodal and includes rapid diagnosis in conjunction with correction of any underlying diseases. Biopsy sample of necrotic tissue demonstrates thick, nonseptate hyphae branching at right angles. The microbiology lab should be alerted if mucormycosis is suspected, as gentle tissue handling is paramount to successful culture growth. Cultures are only positive in one-third of cases. The treatment of choice is amphotericin B, along with aggressive surgical debridement of necrotic tissue in order to minimize mortality.

53. For what fungal infections might patients on biologic therapies be at risk?

Patients on tumor necrosis factor-α antagonists most commonly are at risk for histoplasmosis, candidiasis, and aspergillosis. There may be a different degree of risk with each of the agents—infliximab creating a higher risk than etanercept or adalimumab. In endemic areas, patients are also at risk for primary or reactivation of latent coccidioidomycosis. Close monitoring of current and past residents of endemic areas is indicated.

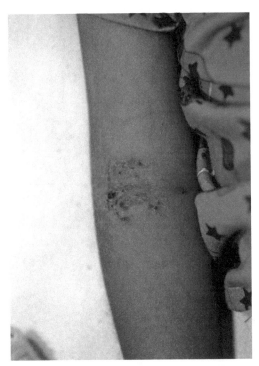

Fig. 31.13 Cutaneous mucormycosis due to Rhizopus at the site of an intravenous line. (Courtesy Joanna Burch Collection.)

BIBLIOGRAPHY

Berger AP, Ford BA, Brown-Joel Z, et al. Angioinvasive fungal infections impacting the skin: diagnosis, management, and complications (part 2). *J Am Acad Dermatol.* 2019;80(4):883–898. e2.

Elewski BE, Hughey LC, Marchiony Hunt K, et al. Fungal diseases. In: Bolognia JL, Schaffer JV, Cerroni L, eds. *Dermatology.* 4th ed. Philadelphia, PA: Elsevier; 2017:1329–1363.

Guégan S, Lanternier F, Rouzaud C, et al. Fungal skin and soft tissue infections. *Curr Opin Infect Dis.* 2016;29(2):124–130.

Shields BE, Rosenbach M, Brown-Joel Z, et al. Angioinvasive fungal infections impacting the skin: background, epidemiology, and clinical presentation (part 1). *J Am Acad Dermatol.* 2019;80(4):869–880. e5.

CHAPTER 32

PARASITIC INFESTATIONS

Brittney DeClerck

1. Where and how does one acquire cutaneous parasitic diseases?

Parasitic skin diseases may arise from systemic spread or direct penetration of the skin. Cutaneous parasitic infestations are a major source of morbidity, affecting millions worldwide. Tropical climates, crowding, poor nutrition, sanitation problems, and limited medical resources are all associated with increased variety and severity of parasitoses. Ecologically temperate climates and industrialized societies are also afflicted by significant parasitic infestations because of local vectors, distant vacations, and widespread travel to and from areas of endemic infection for business, political, humanitarian, or military purposes. Immunosuppression due to drugs or disease leads to cutaneous manifestations of parasitic diseases that may be caused by unusual organisms.

2. What is "creeping eruption?"

Properly known as cutaneous larva migrans, and popularly known as "sandworms," creeping eruption occurs when the larva of dog and cat hookworms (*Ancylostoma caninum* and *A. braziliense*, respectively) penetrate intact, exposed skin and begin migrating through the epidermis. The most common location for the eruption is the sole of the foot, although other sites such as the buttocks, back, and thighs, which may have rested on contaminated sand, are susceptible. Lacking the enzymes necessary to penetrate and survive in the deeper dermis, the larvae wander a serpiginous route at a speed up to 3 cm/day. Clinically, the primary lesion is a pruritic, erythematous, serpiginous burrow (Fig. 32.1). Although the larvae usually die in 2 to 8 weeks, survival up to 22 months has been reported. Several cases of cutaneous larva migrans–related erythema multiforme have been reported.

A variety of other animal hookworm species may also cause creeping eruption. Human hookworms may briefly cause a similar eruption, but the better-adapted parasites soon find their way into the circulation.

Richey TK, Gentry RH, Fitzpatrick JE, Morgan AM. Persistent cutaneous larva migrans due to *Ancylostoma* species. *South Med J.* 1996;89:609–611.
Vaughan TK, English JC III. Cutaneous larva migrans complicated by erythema multiforme. *Cutis.* 1998;62:33–35.

3. How do you treat creeping eruption?

An older method was to freeze the leading point of the burrow. This sometimes produced significant tissue destruction and often missed the larva, which may be up to 2 cm ahead of the visible burrow. Oral ivermectin and albendazole are treatment option. One or two sequential doses of oral ivermectin (200 mcg/kg) is the preferred treatment for uncomplicated cases given its wide availability, safety, and high cure rate (94%–100%). A classic treatment is 10% topical thiabendazole suspension applied four times a day for at least 2 days after the last sign of burrow activity. This regimen has a high cure rate and minimal toxicity, but this medication is not always readily available.

Schuster A, Lesshafft H, Reichert F, et al. Hookworm-related cutaneous larva migrans in northern Brazil: resolution of clinical pathology after a single dose of ivermectin. *Clin Infect Dis.* 2013;57(8):1155–1157.

4. What is different about larva currens?

Larva currens, or "racing larva," is caused by *Strongyloides stercoralis*, a nematode with a normal life cycle similar to the hookworm. *Strongyloides*, however, is unique in that it can complete its life cycle within the human host and bypass the obligate soil phase of the hookworms. Autoinfection may occur to a point of overwhelming infestation and host death, especially in immunocompromised patients. The serpentine eruption of larva currens appears much the same as creeping eruption but is more likely to occur on the thighs, buttocks, or perineum due to larval penetration from the nearby colon. The eruption is more fleeting and lasts no more than a few days, during which the larva's migratory speed through the dermis may be clocked at up to 10 cm/hour (Fig. 32.2). A nonspecific rash or hives may also occur because of hypersensitivity to the parasite. Ivermectin is the favored therapy for *Strongyloides* infections.

5. Are there other nematode infestations that cause skin disease?

Enterobius vermicularis (pinworms) may cause a bothersome perianal itch, but secondary complications including dermatitis, bacterial infections, and local abscesses can develop. Treatment is one dose of mebendazole or albendazole, repeated in 2 weeks. *Trichinella spiralis*, which is acquired by eating undercooked pork, may cause a diffuse rash, nail bed splinter hemorrhages, and a subtle but persistent periorbital edema (trichinosis).

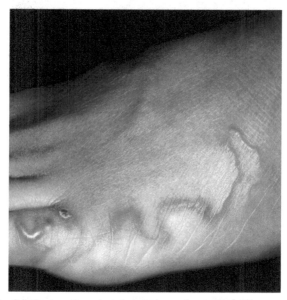

Fig. 32.1 Creeping eruption. Cutaneous larva migrans due to canine hookworm. (Courtesy Fitzsimons Army Medical Center teaching files.)

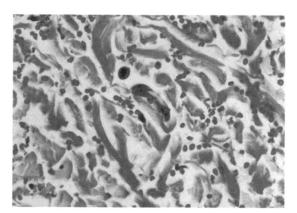

Fig. 32.2 Larva currens. Biopsy demonstrates migrating larva of Strongyloides stercoralis in the dermis. (Courtesy Fitzsimons Army Medical Center teaching files.)

6. How do filarial infections differ from other nematode infections?

All the filariae have an insect vector integral to their life cycle and live in pairs within their mammalian host. The microfilarial offspring of this couple are the primary source of morbidity. The most important filarial diseases are filariasis, loiasis, and onchocerciasis (Table 32.1).

7. Where is onchocerciasis most prevalent? How is it transmitted?

Onchocerciasis, a disease produced by the tissue nematode *Onchocerca volvulus*, affects millions of people in Africa and Central and South America. The infective larval forms are transmitted to humans through the bite of the black fly (*Simulium*) (Fig. 32.3). The common term for onchocerciasis, *river blindness*, takes its name from its feared complication and the fast-flowing rivers where the parasite and vectors are found. Elimination of onchocerciasis remains a major priority of the World Health Organization, and vaccines are under investigation.

Nguyen JC, Murphy ME, Nutman TB, et al. Cutaneous onchocerciasis in an American traveler. *Int J Dermatol.* 2005;44:125–128.

Table 32.1 Parasitic Infestations of the Skin

PARASITIC INFESTATION	VECTOR OR MODE OF TRANSMISSION
Filariasis	Mosquito
Onchocerciasis	Black fly
Creeping eruption	Soil contact and larval penetration
African trypanosomiasis	Tsetse fly
American trypanosomiasis	Kissing bug
Leishmaniasis	Sand fly
Schistosomiasis	Water contact and cercarial penetration
Dracunculiasis, sparganosis	Ingestion of larva
Echinococcosis, cysticercosis	Ingestion of cysts
Amebiasis	Direct contact or ingestion of cysts
Loiasis	Horse and deer flies
Demodex	Person-to-person contact in childhood

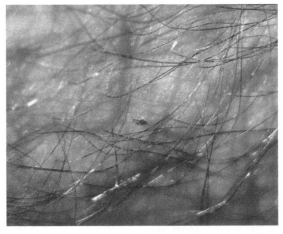

Fig. 32.3 *Simulium* species. Black fly caught in the act of biting one of the editors (JEF). Note the small size compared with the hair shafts. (Courtesy James E. Fitzpatrick, MD.)

8. Does river blindness cause cutaneous manifestations?

As the larval forms of *Onchocerca* develop into adult worms at the site of the bite, they produce subcutaneous nodules called onchocercomas, where numerous microfilariae are produced. They migrate into the skin, inducing a secondary dermatitis, skin pigmentation changes, skin thickening, frank elephantiasis, and an often disabling itching. The microfilariae also may migrate into the tissue of the eye and produce blindness due to severe uveal and corneal inflammation.

9. What are some of the problems with onchocerciasis treatment?

Diethylcarbamazine (DEC) is an effective treatment for the microfilarial stage and was used historically before 1990, but a hypersensitivity reaction to large numbers of dying parasites in the anterior chamber of the eye may cause irreversible blindness and, in some cases, death. This reaction in patients with onchocerciasis receiving DEC is considered a dangerous diagnostic sign, called the "Mazotti reaction." DEC is now contraindicated for onchocerciasis. Also a safe treatment used historically, in otherwise asymptomatic victims, was periodic "nodulectomy," which removes the adult worms and significantly lowers the morbidity of onchocerciasis. Now, however, ivermectin is the drug of choice for onchocerciasis. Ivermectin is being used for both individual treatment and as part of community onchocerciasis control. Of note, encephalopathy has been rarely reported in patients receiving ivermectin who coexistent loiasis infection.

Omura S, Crump A. Ivermectin: panacea for resource-poor communities? *Trends Parasitol.* 2014;30(9):445–455.
Turner HC, Walker M, Churcher TS, et al. Reaching the London declaration on neglected tropical diseases goals for onchocerciasis: an economic evaluation of increasing the frequency of ivermectin treatment in Africa. *Clin Infect Dis.* 2014;59(7):923–932.
Babalola OE. Ocular onchocerciasis: current management and future prospects. *Clin Ophthalmol.* 2011;5:1479–1491.

10. What is loiasis?

   Loiasis, an infection endemic in the jungles of west and central Africa, is produced by the adult form of the tissue nematode, *Loa loa*, which is transmitted through the bite of various flies including deer flies (*Chrysops* species). Usually asymptomatic, this filarial disease may cause large areas of transient edema (Calabar swelling) as the worm migrates, and it may even migrate visibly across the conjunctiva. Subcutaneous nodules may also be seen in this disease, but the worm's unique migration habits lead to the common name "eyeworm." The treatment of choice for loiasis is DEC, which should not be given if coexistent infection with onchocerciasis exists.

11. What causes elephantiasis?

   The term *elephantiasis* is applied to many dermatologic conditions that ultimately result in severe lymphatic obstruction and stasis. The affected limb may become massively enlarged, initially with pitting edema but later with a woodlike induration. The skin becomes discolored, and patches of warty growths may eventually cover the entire affected area. Lymphangitis and mechanical obstruction from lymphatic filariasis is but one way of causing elephantiasis. Offending organisms include *Wuchereria bancrofti*, *Brugia malayi*, and *B. timori*. The *Brugia* species cause elephantiasis of the extremities most commonly, while *Wuchereria* is notorious for genital disease that may eventuate in massive scrotal enlargement (Fig. 32.4).

12. Can other filarial diseases affect the skin?

   Dirofilaria tenuis, the raccoon heartworm, can cause subcutaneous nodules. *Dracunculus medinensis*, or guinea worm, wanders through the subcutaneous tissue as part of its life cycle and eventually settles down where it may cause nodules and ulceration. DEC or Ivermectin, with or without coadministration of albendazole, has been used in many of the filarial diseases described previously. The native treatment for *Dracunculus* is to snare the worm (up to 120 cm long in the female worm) through the skin and roll it up on a stick (the matchstick technique). While not proven, some medical historians postulate that the caduceus (Fig. 32.5A), the symbol for a physician, has its origins from the ancient method of extracting the *Dracuncula* worm with a stick (Fig. 32.5B).

13. What is wound myiasis?

   Wound myiasis is a disease in which various species of flies lay their eggs on or in human skin. When laid in an open wound, such as a chronic leg or decubitus ulcer, the eggs hatch into larvae (maggots) that feed on damaged skin and complete their life cycle. This is called "wound myiasis" and causes mild to severe inflammation, depending upon the fly species and wound location. In other cases, maggot nibbling of ulcer debris may actually dramatically improve the wound, and wound myiasis has been intentionally induced for this purpose.

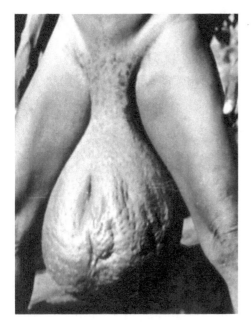

Fig. 32.4 Marked scrotal enlargement in elephantiasis. (From Zaiman H, Jong EC. Parasitic diseases of the skin and soft tissue. In: Stevens DL, ed. *Atlas of Infectious Diseases.* Vol II. New York: Churchill Livingstone; 1995.)

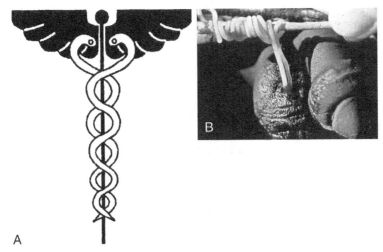

Fig. 32.5 A, Caduceus. **B,** The classic matchstick recovery technique used in extracting the adult female worm. (From Zaiman H, Jong EC. Parasitic diseases of the skin and soft tissue. In Stevens DL, ed. *Atlas of Infectious Diseases.* Vol II. New York: Churchill Livingstone; 1995.)

14. What is a warble?

More properly called *furuncular myiasis* in humans, a warble occurs when fly eggs or larvae are introduced into intact skin. Furuncular myiasis is infection of normal skin by the eggs of *Dermatobia hominis* through the bite of an infected mosquito. Once the eggs hatch, the larvae burrow into the skin, eventually producing a furuncle (boil)-like swelling.

A large larva, more than 1 cm in length in some species, grows over time. Careful examination usually reveals a "snorkel" protruding through the skin of a boil that moves when the abscess is manipulated. Surgical extirpation is the treatment of choice, although other therapies, including occlusion of the furuncle opening with petrolatum or a piece of meat, have been reported to be successful, although the mechanism for this is unclear (Fig. 32.6).

15. What is Congo floor maggot?

Unlike other forms of myiasis in which the larva feeds and pupates within the host tissue, the Congo floor maggot (*Auchmeromyia luteola*) lives in the soil or in the earthen floors of huts and crawls upon the host in the night for a blood meal. The larva, which may grow up to 18 mm long, requires 6 to 20 feedings before it pupates in the dirt. They carry no disease and may be avoided by sleeping on a raised bed.

16. What is tungiasis?

The sand flea, *Tunga penetrans*, can burrow into the foot where the female lays eggs, causing painful abscesses. Treatment is best accomplished through various possible topical agents or surgical excision. While late lesions will spontaneously ulcerate, potential complications include secondary infection and tetanus.

17. What is the difference between a chigoe and a chigger?

Chigoe is another name for *Tunga penetrans* (tungiasis). The chigger is a trombiculid mite that can cause itch with its bites.

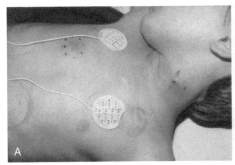
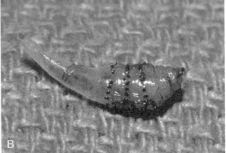

Fig. 32.6 Cutaneous myiasis. **A,** Two lesions of furuncular myiasis in a young child. The lesions were acquired in Panama. **B,** Furuncular larva after removal from patient. (Panel A courtesy Fitzsimons Army Medical Center teaching files.)

18. Do chiggers burrow into the skin to lay eggs like the sand flea?

They usually do not burrow beneath the skin, but the larval forms attach via their mouth parts (adults do not bite) and feed on tissue juices and lymph. They may feed for a few days if not removed, although the intense itching usually starts within a few hours after attachment. They prefer to feed in areas where the clothing is found in close contact with the skin, such as under socks and belts (Fig. 32.7). In some parts of Asia, they are a vector of scrub typhus and may be discouraged from attachment by wearing proper clothing, permethrin repellents, and by washing in hot, soapy water.

19. What is leishmaniasis?

Leishmaniasis, also known as Baghdad boil, kala-azar, espundia, oriental sore, and a variety of other colorful terms, is caused by *Leishmania* species, a protozoan parasite with a multicontinental distribution. Biting sand flies (*Phlebotomus* and *Lutzomyia* species) spread the disease between humans and a large variety of wild and domestic animal reservoirs. Several species and subspecies of *Leishmania* may produce infection, and the clinical manifestations and disease severity are generally species specific. Most forms cause nodules and chronic ulcerations of the skin that can spread lymphatically and can lead to widespread cutaneous disease (Fig. 32.8).

Pace D. Leishmaniasis. *J Infect.* 2014;69(suppl 1):S10–S18.

Mashayekhi-Ghoyonlo V, Kiafar B, Rohani M, Esmaeili H, Erfanian-Taghvaee MR. Correlation between socioeconomic status and clinical course in patients with cutaneous leishmaniasis. *J Cutan Med Surg.* 2015;19:40–44.

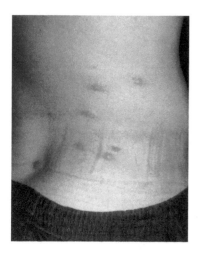

Fig. 32.7 Chigger bites. Note that they tend to accentuate under areas of pressure by clothing. (Courtesy Fitzsimons Army Medical Center teaching files.)

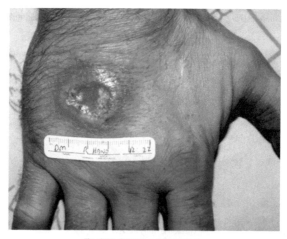

Fig. 32.8 Cutaneous leishmaniasis.

Table 32.2 Types of Leishmaniasis		
SPECIES	**DISEASE**	**DISTRIBUTION**
L. donovani group	Visceral leishmaniasis, kala-azar	India, Asia, Middle East, Africa
L. tropica group	Old World cutaneous leishmaniasis, oriental sore, newly discovered viscerotropic disease	India, Middle East
L. viannia group (*L. braziliensis* group)	New World mucocutaneous leishmaniasis, espundia	Latin America
L. mexicana group	American cutaneous leishmaniasis	Mexico, Central America, Texas, South America

20. Name the different types of leishmaniasis.
    See Table 32.2.

21. Can leishmaniasis be contracted in the United States?
    While most cases of leishmaniasis seen in the United States are acquired elsewhere, a form of cutaneous disease caused by *L. mexicana* may be acquired in central Texas and has been nicknamed "Highway 90 disease" by those familiar with its distribution. More recent cases have been reported in Oklahoma and a case reported to be locally acquired as far north as North Dakota. The standard treatment for leishmaniasis includes antimonial medications, but other medications such as ketoconazole, fluconazole, amphotericin, minocycline, and miltefosine, and physical modalities such as hyperthermia have anecdotally been shown to improve the lesions.

Davis AJ, Kedzierski L. Recent advances in antileishmanial drug development. *Curr Opin Investig Drugs.* 2005;6:163–169.
Douvoyiannis M, Khromachou T, Byers N, Hargreaves J, Murray HW. Cutaneous leishmaniasis in North Dakota. *Clin Infect Dis.* 2014;59(5): e73–e75.

22. How does cutaneous amebiasis, due to Entamoeba histolytica, present?
    Usually the result of direct extension from hepatic or colorectal disease, cutaneous amebiasis presents with serpiginous, warty ulcers of the anogenital area called *amebomas.* These ulcers may produce extensive tissue loss and predispose to severe secondary bacterial infections. Less common presentations include infection by direct inoculation of the perineum in dysenteric infants wearing diapers, and on the penis following anal intercourse with an infected person.

23. What are the skin findings in American trypanosomiasis?
    American trypanosomiasis, or Chagas disease, is caused by the parasite *Trypanosoma cruzi*, which is introduced through the conjunctiva or skin following the bite of blood-sucking reduviid bugs (kissing bugs). This insect has the unpleasant habit of defecating on the skin following its human blood meal, and the infected feces are inoculated into the conjunctiva or wound. A unilateral conjunctivitis and lid edema (Romana's sign) are usually the first clinical signs. Later, the patient may become systemically ill with various rashes and subcutaneous nodules, as well as cardiac and gastrointestinal lesions that may be fatal. Cases of native acquisition of trypanosomiasis and Chagas disease are now being reported in south Texas.

24. What are the skin findings in African trypanosomiasis?
    African trypanosomiasis, also called *sleeping sickness*, is due to *Trypanosoma gambiense* or *T. rhodesiense*. It may present with a trypanosomal chancre (primary cutaneous African trypanosomiasis) at the site of the bite, followed by nodules and dermatitis (secondary cutaneous African trypanosomiasis) (Fig. 32.9). The cardiac and neurologic complications of both forms of trypanosomiasis are the most serious clinical concerns.

McGovern TW, Williams W, Fitzpatrick JE, Cetron MS, Hepburn BC, Gentry RH. Cutaneous manifestations of African trypanosomiasis. *Arch Dermatol.* 1995;131:1178–1182.

25. Describe the cutaneous manifestations of schistosomiasis as they relate to the parasite's life cycle.
    Schistosomiasis is a trematode (fluke) infection produced by one of three species of the genus *Schistosoma.* Schistosomes have a complex life cycle that involves development in freshwater snails (intermediate host) and the release of free-swimming cercariae that penetrate the human skin. Penetration produces a transient pruritus and burning followed by blisters, bruising, and crusted papules over the next few days. As the worm reaches maturity in the portal or caval venous system, the ova are released by the adult female and passed into the feces or urine. Some ova

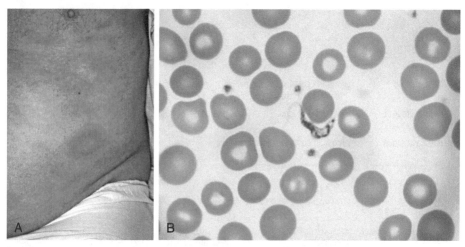

Fig. 32.9 **A,** A big game hunter returning from Africa with oval secondary lesion of African trypanosomiasis. **B,** Peripheral smear from the patient demonstrating a circulating trypanosome. (Courtesy Fitzsimons Army Medical Center teaching files.)

are deposited in the skin and may produce nodules, ulcers, and warty tumors. The anogenital region is most often involved through direct extension from the bladder or rectum, but spreading through the bloodstream and lymphatics may produce lesions at other sites.

26. Are swimmer's itch and sea bather's eruption the same thing?
No. **Swimmer's itch**, also called *clam digger's itch* and *bather's itch*, is caused by the penetration of the skin by schistosome cercariae that normally infest birds. When first exposed, the victim will have a prickly eruption within a few minutes of cercarial penetration that rapidly resolves. Repeated exposure with an allergic response leads to larger, longer-lasting, and more pruritic papules that may cause pustules, blisters, and dermatitis. As with creeping eruption, the parasite cannot complete its life cycle because it cannot penetrate the epidermis.
   Sea bather's eruption is caused by contact with larval forms of a marine jellyfish. In contrast to swimmer's itch, which presents with lesions in exposed areas, sea bather's eruption typically presents with pruritic macules and papules in areas covered by clothing. It is felt that the clothing holds the larvae close to the skin long enough to cause a small sting.

27. What is sparganosis?
Sparganosis is an infection produced by various species of the tapeworm *Spirometra*, which is seen most commonly in Asia and Southeast Asia. Sparganosis is typically acquired by drinking water containing infected copepods or the ingestion of inadequately cooked snake or frog meat. Clinically, it presents as pruritic or painful nodules that contain the encysted tapeworm. "Application sparganosis" occurs when an eye or ulcer is contaminated by a poultice made from these same animals and is characterized by similar nodules at the site of inoculation (Fig. 32.10). Sparganosis is best treated by surgical removal of the tapeworm.

Kimura S, Kashima M, Kawa Y, et al. A case of subcutaneous sparganosis: therapeutic assessment by an indirect immunofluorescence antibody titration using sections of the worm body obtained from the patient. *Br J Dermatol.* 2003;148:369–371.

28. Can other tapeworms affect the skin?
Taenia solium (pork tapeworm) may produce cysticercosis cutis, which is acquired from the oral ingestion of eggs, usually due to poor sanitary habits. Clinically, it presents as painless subcutaneous nodules containing the larval stage of the tapeworm. *Echinococcus granulosus,* a dog tapeworm, produces fluctuant, cystic tumors in the skin (hydatid disease) as well as generalized hives and itching. It is acquired from the ingestion of contaminated food or water.

29. What is *Demodex*?
These microscopic mites reside by the thousands in the hair follicles (*D. folliculorum*) and sebaceous glands (*D. brevis*) of adult humans. They resemble carrots with legs and live off sebum and squamous debris (Fig. 32.11).

30. Does *Demodex* cause skin disease?
The role of *Demodex* in facial eruptions, particularly rosacea, has been a topic of debate for decades. Many convincing reports describe a recalcitrant folliculitis, often seen in immunosuppressed patients, which responds to mite-killing

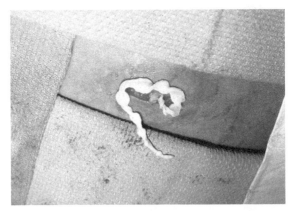

Fig. 32.10 Sparganosis. *Spirometra* species due to a poultice made from a frog. (Courtesy Fitzsimons Army Medical Center teaching files.)

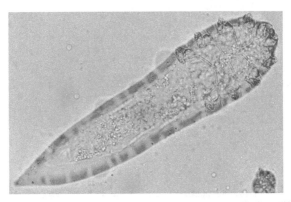

Fig. 32.11 *Demodex folliculorum* (mineral oil preparation, original magnification ×500).

topical permethrin or oral ivermectin. The contribution of *Demodex* to garden-variety rosacea is less certain, although patients with refractory rosacea pattern erythema and nodules have responded to miticidal therapy.

Forton F, Germaux MA, Brasseur T, et al. Demodicosis and rosacea: epidemiology and significance in daily dermatologic practice. *J Am Acad Dermatol.* 2005;52:74–87.

Brown M, Hernandez-Martin A, Clement A, Colmenero I, Torrelo A. Severe *Demodex folliculorum*-associated oculocutaneous rosacea in a girl successfully treated with ivermectin. *JAMA Dermatol.* 2014;150(1):61–63.

KEY POINTS: PARASITIC INFESTATIONS

1. A variety of parasitic diseases may have cutaneous manifestations.
2. Because of international travel and global conflict, what were once considered exclusively tropical diseases may show up in a North American clinic.
3. Cutaneous eruptions may be common minor nuisances, such as larval migrans and swimmer's itch, or more serious systemic infections, such as onchocerciasis and trypanosomiasis.
4. Many parasitic skin diseases are arthropod vector-borne, providing opportunities to interrupt the organisms' life cycle for both prevention and treatment.

CHAPTER 33

ARTHROPOD BITES AND STINGS

Ryan A. Stevens

1. **What are arthropods?**
   Arthropods compose the largest number and most diverse group of animals on earth. They are invertebrates that arise from eggs and share these three anatomic features: segmented bodies, hard exoskeleton, and symmetrically paired and jointed appendages.

2. **Are most arthropods harmful to humans?**
   Less than 0.5% of the 1 million named species are injurious to humans. Most are harmless, while others are even beneficial to humans.

3. **What are some examples of arthropods?**
   Arthropods may be classified as follows:
   • Arachnids (spiders, ticks, mites, scorpions)
   • Insects (e.g., bees, lice, fleas, beetles, mosquitos, butterflies, moths)
   • Millipedes, centipedes, and crustaceans

4. **Describe various ways arthropods injure humans. What insect or arachnid would cause the injury?**
   • Vesication (blisters): Blister beetle
   • Envenomation: Bees, ants, spiders
   • Allergic sensitization: Bedbugs, mosquitos, bees, and ants
   • Invasion: Human botfly; tungiasis: penetrating fleas
   • Contact urticaria: Caterpillars and setae from butterflies and moths
   • Necrosis: Brown recluse spider
   • Secondary infection: Any bite or sting, usually staphylococci
   • Vector of disease: Mosquito, tick, body louse, flies

BITES AND STINGS

5. **How do you diagnose a bite or sting?**
   The annoyance of the mosquito or the immediate pain of the bee sting rarely poses a problem of recognition. Diagnostic problems arise when the arthropod is not seen or felt but leaves a nonspecific papular rash with redness, pain, itching, or swelling. A careful history, exam, and common knowledge of local arthropod populations are necessary to make a diagnosis in this more nuanced setting.

6. **How do arthropod bites or stings typically present clinically?**
   Arthropod bites may present with itchy, red papules in a particular distribution or pattern that suggests an area of potential arthropod exposure. For example, grouped bites around an exposed ankle suggest a nonflying arthropod such as a flea, mite, chigger mite, or bedbug.

7. **Is the histopathology of an arthropod bite specific?**
   No, a biopsy of the skin lesion is nonspecific and often will show perivascular dermatitis with eosinophils.

8. **One person on a hike is "eaten alive" by mosquitos while his companions are not bothered at all. Do ectoparasites such as mosquitos, ticks, fleas, and mites bite randomly?**
   No. Most arthropods are attracted to their hosts by a number of physical and chemical stimuli such as warmth, composition of sweat, carbon dioxide, vibrations, and odor. On the other hand, lipids derived from the degenerative epidermal cells often have a repellent quality to them. Thus, to arthropods, some human hosts are far more attractive than others.

9. **Why are bite reactions to ectoparasites so much different in different people?**
   The severity of bug bite reactions depends most on the immunologic status of the patient. In general, a severely symptomatic eruption may result from only a few bites in an immunologically sensitized person, while many bites may produce no symptoms at all in a person with an acquired immunologic tolerance.

Dahl MV. Cutaneous reactions to arthropod bites and stings. *Clin Cases Dermatol.* 1991;3:11–16.

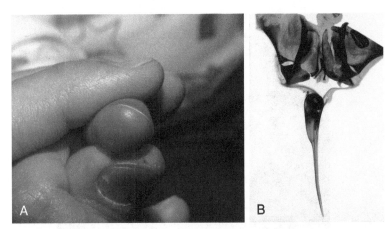

Fig. 33.1 A, Bee sting on the thumb of a young child demonstrating painful, indurated erythema. **B,** Stinger that was removed from the thumb by scraping laterally with an index card. (Courtesy Fitzsimons Army Medical teaching files.)

10. How do you treat bee stings?

The best treatment for stings is prevention. Minimize the use of perfumes and scented soaps as well as exposure to areas of wildflowers, and when confronted by agitated bees, avoid rapid movements.

When a person is stung, the venom-containing barbed stinger, if still present at the site of the sting, should be removed by gently scraping the skin horizontally with a dull knife or credit card (Fig. 33.1). Stinger removal with forceps compresses the venom gland, forcing more venom into the skin, and should be avoided. Symptomatic care with rest, elevation, and ice to the area are helpful. Antihistamines may also be useful. Early signs of systemic toxicity or allergic reactions should be noted.

11. What are the signs of serious systemic reactions to bee, wasp, or ant stings?

Anaphylaxis is the most serious systemic reaction and may occur with bronchospasm, urticaria, angioedema, and, finally, vascular collapse and even death.

12. How do you treat anaphylactic syndrome from a bee sting?

If a reaction begins, treatment includes subcutaneous injection of epinephrine, 1:1000 in aqueous solution, which can be prescribed and carried by patients at all times. This may be repeated in 15 to 20 minutes. In addition, intravenous diphenhydramine and cortisone as well as oxygen, fluids, vasopressors, and bronchodilators may also be used as needed. Since most fatalities occur within the first hour, early intervention by the allergic patient with a self-administered epinephrine injection may prevent a reaction from developing.

13. What are the unique characteristics of fire ants and their sting?

The fire ant (*Solenopsis* spp.) (Fig. 33.2), when provoked, may attack en masse, administering up to several thousand stings to a victim resulting in numerous sterile pustules (Fig. 33.3). The fire ant venom contains a hemolytic factor, solenopsin D, a piperidine alkaloid that can cause an anaphylactic reaction. Treatment of the ant stings is symptomatic.

Nguyen SA, Napoli DC. Natural history of large local and generalized cutaneous reactions to imported fire ant stings in children. *Ann Allergy Asthma Immunol.* 2005;94:387–390.

14. What species of spiders are medically important?

The female black widow (*Latrodectus mactans*) (Fig. 33.4) and the brown recluse (*Loxosceles reclusa*) (Fig. 33.5) are the most venomous spiders in the United States. The jumping spider (*Phidippus formosus*) is the most common biting spider in the United States causing a painful bite due to venom that contains hyaluronidase.

15. Does the hobo spider (Tegenaria agrestis) bite cause a necrotic reaction?

No, the latest information on this species thoroughly discredits the original reports that made claims to its importance as a dermonecrotic species. Evidence is overwhelming that this spider is not medically important.

Vetter R, Isbister G. Do hobo spider bites cause dermonecrotic injuries? *Ann Emerg Med.* 2004;44:605–607.
Gaver-Wainwright M, Zack R, Foradori M, et al. Misdiagnosis of spider bites: bacterial associates, mechanical pathogen transfer and hemolytic potential of venom from the hobo spider, *Tegeneria agrestis. J Med Entomol.* 2011;48:382–388.

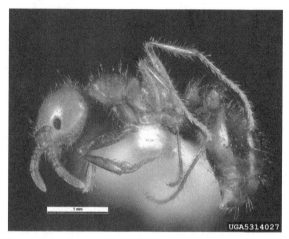

Fig. 33.2 Fire ant, *Solenopsis invicta*. (Courtesy Pest and Disease Image Library, Bugwood.org.)

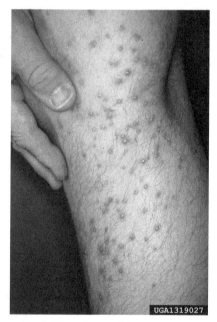

Fig. 33.3 In less than 10 seconds, an unwary scientist was stung over 250 times on one leg when he carelessly knelt on a collapsed fire ant mound. The sterile pustules developed to this stage in 3 days. (Courtesy Daniel Wojcik, Bugwood.org.)

16. How do you diagnose and treat the black widow spider bite?

The black widow (*Latrodectus mactans*) is a large black spider, often with a red hourglass figure on the ventral surface. The venom is a potent neurotoxin.

Initially, the bite is acutely painful, followed by systemic symptoms of pain and muscle cramping that can mimic an acute abdomen. Treatment of this neurotoxin with antivenin should be prompt. Calcium gluconate, muscle relaxants, and pain medications are also used.

Elston DM. What's eating you? *Latrodectus mactans* (the black widow spider). *Cutis.* 2002;69:257–258.

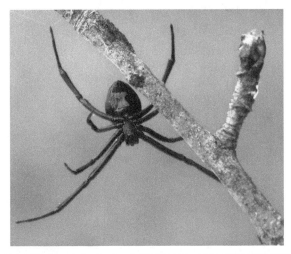

Fig. 33.4 Female black widow spider demonstrating the characteristic hour glass on the ventral surface. (Source: iStock photo 4421414. © Mark Kostich.)

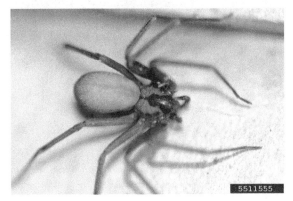

Fig. 33.5 Brown recluse spider demonstrating the characteristic violin-like marking on the dorsal thorax. (Courtesy William L. Weston Collection.)

17. How does a brown recluse spider bite present?

    Unlike the black widow, the brown recluse (*Loxosceles reclusa*) produces a dermonecrotic toxin that can cause severe necrosis of the skin (Fig. 33.6), as well as a hemolytic toxin that causes severe, even life-threatening, hemolysis. The brown recluse is a brown spider with a dark brown violin-like marking on the dorsum of the cephalothorax. The bite commonly occurs when a person is cleaning old storage rooms or woodpiles outdoors, where the spider resides. The initial bite may be painless but is followed by pain and necrosis. The bite then begins to show a central blue color (impending necrosis), a surrounding white area (a vasospasm and ischemia), and a peripheral red halo (inflammation), the "red, white, and blue" sign. If a larger area of necrosis develops after a few days, a rare but serious and life-threatening systemic reaction to the hemolytic toxin may occur.

18. How should brown recluse spider bites be treated?

    First aid measures are important and can be remembered by the mnemonic **RICE**. **R**est, **i**ce, **c**ompression, and **e**levation of the bite site decrease blood flow, temperature, and enzymatic activity of the dermonecrotic toxin. Ice should be applied immediately. General wound care, tetanus toxoid, antibiotics for secondary infection, and observation for systemic hematologic problems may be necessary until the wound heals. Dapsone and corticosteroids have been used, with variable results.

Elston DM, Miller SD, Young RJ 3rd, et al. Comparison of colchicine, dapsone, triamcinolone, and diphenhydramine therapy for the treatment of brown recluse spider envenomation: a double-blind, controlled study in a rabbit model. *Arch Dermatol.* 2005;141:595–597.
Mold JW, Thompson DM. Management of brown recluse spider bites in primary care. *J Am Board Fam Pract.* 2004;17:347–352.

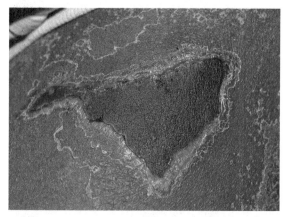

Fig. 33.6 Necrotic ulcer from the bite of a brown recluse. (Courtesy William L. Weston, MD, Collection.)

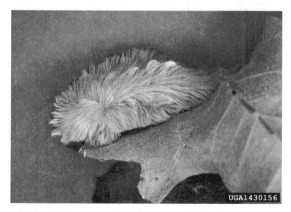

Fig. 33.7 Puss caterpillar, *Megalopyge opercularis*. (Courtesy Lacy L. Hyche, Auburn University, Bugwood.org.)

19. What is the active toxin in black widow and brown recluse spider venom?
    The black widow venom contains the neurotoxin, alpha-latrotoxin. The brown recluse venom contains the necrotoxin, sphingomyelinase D.

20. What is lepidopterism?
    Lepidopterism refers to adverse reactions to caterpillars, butterflies, and moths. Caterpillar dermatitis typically presents as painful pruritic papules and urticaria following contact with caterpillars. Contact with the puss caterpillar (*Megalopyge opercularis*) (Fig. 33.7) produces immediate pain and a characteristic tram-track pattern of hemorrhage.

Hossler EW. Caterpillars and moths: dermatologic manifestations of encounters with Lepidoptera, parts I and II. *J Am Acad Dermatol.* 2010;62:1–10, 13–28.

INFESTATIONS

21. What is scabies?
    Scabies is a contagious infestation caused by a mite that affects humans and other mammals. *Sarcoptes scabiei* var. *hominis* is the etiologic agent of human scabies. The mites burrow into the upper epidermis causing severe pruritus.

22. Is scabies self-limited?
    No, *Sarcoptes scabiei* var. *hominis* can complete its 30-day life cycle living, eating, and breeding on the human host and therefore must be treated.

23. What pertinent history is often present in patients infested with scabies?

Patients complain of severe intractable pruritus, which is almost always worse at night, with an insidious onset of red to flesh-colored pruritic papules. Secondary cases frequently occur (person-to-person transmission) in close contact or patients living in close quarters (nursing homes).

24. How does scabies present on physical exam?

The rash has a distinctive distribution involving the interdigital webs of the hands, the volar wrists, extensor elbows, axillary areas, central abdomen, genitalia, buttocks, and anterior thighs. The papular lesions affecting the shaft and glans penis, as well as the scrotum, are almost diagnostic. Scalp and facial lesions are usually absent, except in the very young.

The rash consists of pruritic papules, but a diagnostic linear burrow consisting of a very fine scale is often seen in the interdigital web area or on the volar wrists (Fig. 33.8A). Nodular lesions commonly occur on male genitalia (Fig. 33.8B).

Hicks M, Elston D. Scabies. *Dermatol Ther.* 2009;22:279–292.

25. How is the diagnosis of scabies confirmed?

The diagnosis is confirmed by scraping a small linear scaly burrow to reveal the female mite, her eggs, or fecal material under the microscope (see Chapter 3, Fig. 3.6). Less commonly, the diagnosis is established by visualizing the mite on a skin biopsy (Fig. 33.9).

26. What is Norwegian scabies?

Norwegian (crusted) scabies is a massive infestation with inordinate numbers of scabies mites due to inadequate host response. The large numbers of organisms cause a hyperplastic growth of the epithelium. Topical treatment is difficult, so oral ivermectin has been used with good success.

Tran L, Siedenberg E, Corbett S. Crusted (Norwegian) scabies. *J Emerg Med.* 2002;22:285–287.

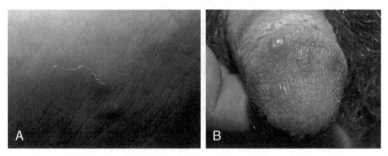

Fig. 33.8 Scabies. **A,** Characteristic linear burrow. **B,** Nodular scabies most commonly presents in male genitalia as markedly pruritic papules. The lesion is almost diagnostic. (Courtesy Fitzsimons Army Medical Center teaching files.)

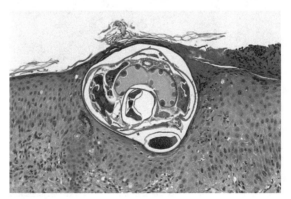

Fig. 33.9 Biopsy of scabies demonstrating mite in burrow. (Courtesy James E. Fitzpatrick, MD.)

27. What agents are used to treat scabies?

Permethrin 5% cream is the recommended first-line agent and should be applied overnight to the entire body from the neck down with a repeated application in 1 week. All members of the family should be treated to eliminate asymptomatic incubating cases. Sulfur ointment (5% to 10%) is a safe alternative in pregnant or lactating women. Topical malathion can be used for resistant cases. Oral ivermectin (200 μg/kg) is as effective as topical permethrin 5% cream when administered as two doses 1 to 2 weeks apart, although it should not be used in young children.

Manjhi PK, Sinha RI, Kumar M, et al. Comparative study of efficacy of oral ivermectin versus some topical antiscabies drugs in the treatment of scabies. *J Clin Diagn Res*. 2014;8:1–4.

28. What are the three varieties of lice that affect humans?

The head louse (*Pediculus humanus* var. *capitis*).
The body louse (*Pediculus humanus* var. *corporis*).
The pubic louse (*Phthirus pubis*).

29. Discuss head lice and how it presents clinically.

The head louse (*Pediculus humanus* var. *capitis*) is 2 to 4 mm long with three pairs of legs that are of equal length. The entire life cycle is spent in the scalp hair. The visible eggs or nits are deposited on the hair shaft, singly and close to the scalp (see Chapter 3, Fig. 3.7). Pruritus of the scalp with secondary infection is common. Associated cervical and occipital lymphadenopathy is common. Head lice are more common in school-aged children, especially young females with longer hair (Fig. 33.10).

30. Discuss body lice and how it presents clinically.

The large **body louse** (*Pediculus humanus* var. *corporis*) resembles the head louse in configuration, only being larger. It lives and reproduces in the lining of the clothes and leaves the clothing only for feeding, being rarely found on the skin. The patient presents with pruritic papules and areas of hyperpigmentation from healing. This problem occurs in the setting of poverty, overcrowding, and poor hygiene in individuals who rarely change or clean their clothes.

31. What infections are transmitted by body lice?

Epidemic typhus, trench fever, and relapsing fever can be transmitted by the body louse.

32. Discuss pubic lice and how it presents clinically.

The **pubic louse** (*Phthirus pubis*), or crabs, is smaller and broad-shouldered and has a narrow head. Eggs are found on the hair shaft. The pubic louse may also be found on short occipital scalp, body, eyebrow, eyelash, and axillary hair.

33. How should lice infestations be treated?

Head and pubic lice infestations are treated similarly. Permethrin 5% cream is applied overnight, and the treatment is repeated in 1 week (with occlusion), and the scalp is observed for viable nits. Topical malathion 0.5% and oral ivermectin can be used in resistant cases. Removal of the nits with a specially designed, fine-toothed comb ensures that the infestation is clear. All close contacts should also be treated. Body lice are eliminated by thorough cleaning of the clothes or changing them for new ones. The patient needs symptomatic relief only.

Elston DM. Drugs used in the treatment of pediculosis. *J Drugs Dermatol*. 2005;4:207–211.

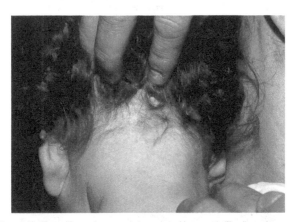

Fig. 33.10 Pediculosis. Young girl with pruritic papules on posterior scalp and lower neck. The diagnosis was established by finding nits attached to hair shafts. (Courtesy Fitzsimons Army Medical Center teaching files.)

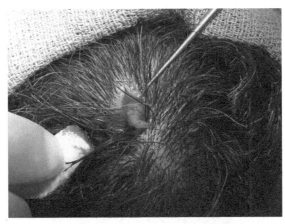

Fig. 33.11 Surgical evacuation of a human botfly larva from a furuncular nodule on the patient's scalp. (Courtesy Paige L. Neifert, MD.)

34. What is tungiasis?

Tungiasis is an infestation caused by the burrowing flea, *Tunga penetrans*. It is endemic to the Caribbean islands and Central and South America. The flea burrows into the skin, most commonly on the feet, clinically creating a black dot that evolves into a nodule with a central black punctum.

35. What dermatologic condition is caused by a human botfly?

Myiasis is an infestation of the skin by fly larvae (maggots). *Dermatobia hominis* (human botfly) is the cause of furuncular myiasis in which the larvae penetrate into the dermis causing a large tender and pruritic pyogenic furuncle. Surgical debridement of the larva is curative (Fig. 33.11).

Zoonotic Infestations

36. How do flea infestations typically present?

The adult flea is a small parasitic bloodsucker, approximately 3 mm in size (Fig. 33.12). The flea is tall and narrow. They are wingless but have powerful rear legs to reach the ankles of their prospective hosts (Fig. 33.13). Infestations typically present in affected pets.

Steen CJ, Carbonaro PA, Schwarz RA. Arthropods in dermatology. *J Am Acad Dermatol*. 2004;50:819–842.

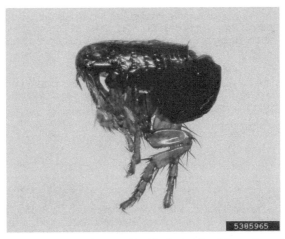

Fig. 33.12 Common cat flea, *Ctenocephalides felis*. (Courtesy Joseph Berger, Bugwood.org.)

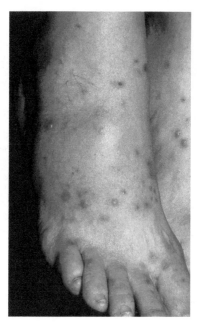

Fig. 33.13 Flea bites. Papulovesicular lesions commonly found near the exposed ankles of women. (Courtesy C. Paul Sayers, MD.)

37. How do you treat a flea infestation?

Treatment of the patient is symptomatic. The pet should be treated with insecticidal powders, shampoos, and dips. For each adult flea found on the animal, there are perhaps hundreds of adults, eggs, larvae, and pupae in the bedding material of the pet. Apply strict environmental controls such as vacuuming and washing the pet's sleeping areas.

38. Fleas serve as a vector for which disease?

Fleas serve as a vector for endemic typhus, caused by the bacteria *Rickettsia typhi*, as well as the plague, caused by *Yersinia pestis*, among others.

39. What causes "walking dandruff" in pets?

Walking dandruff presents as a dermatitis with small yellow-white scales on affected pets caused by the nonburrowing mite *Cheyletiella*.

40. What is Cheyletiella?

Cheyletiella species are free-living, nonburrowing, ectoparasitic mites of dogs, cats, and rabbits. The mite has pincer-like palpi tipped with strong claws used for grasping fur (Fig. 33.14). The eggs are attached to the hair shaft of the animal. The most common sources of the infestation are long-haired cats and new puppies, causing "walking dandruff."

41. How is Cheyletiella infestation recognized in humans?

Infested patients complain of pruritic papular eruptions, which occur most commonly in the sites that correspond to contact with an affected pet. Diagnosis is made by microscopic examination of the pet. Treatment is directed toward the pet, the pet contacts, and the environment.

Lee B. *Cheyletiella:* report of 14 cases. *Cutis.* 1992;47:11.

42. What are some other mites of medical importance?

See Table 33.1.

43. What is a bedbug?

The human bedbug, *Cimex lectularius*, is a reddish-brown, wingless insect (Fig. 33.15A). They dine at night—rapidly and painlessly—but live during the day in dark closets, behind wallpaper, or under furniture and are not usually seen. Once thought to be associated only with unclean housing, bedbugs can be found in the most pristine homes and may be passively brought in on luggage, clothing, or secondhand furniture.

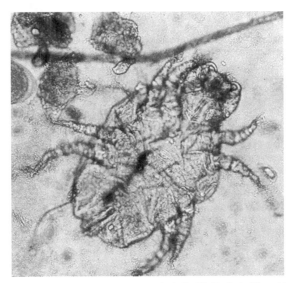

Fig. 33.14 *Cheyletiella* mite resembles scabies in size but is identified by the hooklike palpi anteriorly.

Table 33.1 Mites of medical importance

MITES	DISEASE
Acarus (grain mite)	Baker's itch
Glycyphagus (cheese mite)	Grocer's itch
Dermanyssus and *Ornithonyssus* (fowl mite)	Equine encephalitis
Liponyssoides sanguineus (house mouse mite)	Rickettsial pox
Dermatophagoides (dust mite)	Allergy
Trombicula (chigger mite)	Scrub typhus
Demodex spp.	Folliculitis, possibly rosacea

Bolognia JL, Jorizzo JL, Schaffer JV. Dermatology. Madrid, Spain: Elsevier Saunders; 2012: Chapter 85.

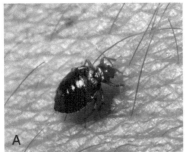
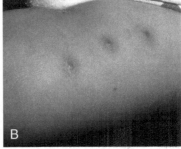

Fig. 33.15 A, Human bedbug feeding on human skin. **B,** The bedbug bite typically occurs on the trunk and extremities in a generalized asymmetrical papular eruption that may be grouped into a "breakfast, lunch, and dinner" pattern. (Courtesy C. Paul Sayers, MD.)

44. What do bedbug bites look like, and what can be done for treatment?

The pruritic bites are often multiple and grouped into a "breakfast, lunch, and dinner" pattern (Fig. 33.15B). Treatment of the patient is symptomatic, but fumigation of the home is necessary to get rid of the pest. With a good description of the bug, patients are often able to recover one to confirm the diagnosis.

Thomas I, Kihiczak GG, Schwartz RA. Bedbug bites: a review. *Int J Dermatol.* 2004;43:430–433.

Kolb A, Needham GR, Neyman KM, et al. Bedbugs. *Dermatol Ther.* 2009;22:347–352.

45. What are zoonotic dermatoses?

Zoonotic dermatoses, also called "cryptic bites," are caused by arthropods that infest animals. This can include common household pets, inhabiting pests, or nearby nesting birds or bats. These bites are chronic, recurrent, painless, and very itchy; the organisms are too small to see. Treatment is to disinfect the pet, get rid of any pests, including nearby bats and birds, then spray the area for insects and mites.

INSECT VECTORS

46. What are the kissing, or assassin, bugs?

Reduviid bugs (kissing bugs) are generally adapted to nocturnal, rapid (3 to 5 minutes), painless feedings on blood. They live in rural settings in the southern United States, Central America, and South America. The bites form pruritic edematous red papules and plaques that can lead to allergic sensitization.

Vetter R. Kissing bugs *(Triatoma)* and the skin. *Dermatol Online J.* 2001;7:6.

47. Why are kissing bugs important?

In Central and South America, reduviid bugs are infected with the etiologic agent of Chagas disease (American trypanosomiasis, *T. cruzi*), which is spread to humans from contamination of broken skin with the bug's feces. Chagas disease is a leading cause of heart disease in Central and South America.

48. What diseases are transmitted by ticks?

- **Viruses:** Colorado tick fever, tick-borne encephalitis.
- ***Rickettsia:*** Rocky Mountain spotted fever, ehrlichiosis, typhus.
- **Bacteria:** Lyme disease, relapsing fever, tularemia, babesiosis.

Dana AN. Diagnosis and treatment of tick infestation and tick-borne diseases with cutaneous manifestations. *Dermatol Ther.* 2009;22:293–326.

49. What is the most common tick-borne infectious disease in the United States?

Lyme disease. It is caused by *Borrelia burgdorferi*, a spirochete, and transmitted by the hard ticks: *Ixodes scapularis* (deer tick), in the Northeast and the upper Midwest (Minnesota and Wisconsin), and *I. pacificus* in the Pacific states.

50. How does Lyme disease present?

The classic presentation is that of a person—in spring or early summer, living in an endemic area—with a history of a tick bite associated with fever, malaise, and an annular, spreading rash called *erythema chronicum migrans.* Erythema chronicum migrans is seen in 60% to 90% of patients diagnosed with Lyme disease.

The disease may be complicated by arthritic, neurologic (facial nerve palsy), and cardiac symptoms. Treatment in the early phase consists of doxycycline for a 3-week period. Amoxicillin is the antibiotic of choice in children under 8 years old. If Lyme disease progresses to a more chronic problem, or there is evidence of neurologic symptoms, it is often necessary to use ceftriaxone in order to cross the blood–brain barrier.

51. Why do the tick bites often go unnoticed?

The nymphal form of the tick is the most common type to bite humans and is roughly the size of the dot on the letter *i* on this page, and the bite is painless.

52. How do tick bites affect humans? How are ticks removed once they are attached to the skin?

The tick bite may cause a foreign body reaction, allergic reaction to salivary proteins, reaction to a toxin (e.g., tick paralysis), or, more importantly, infectious disease carried by the tick (Fig. 33.16). Prompt removal of an attached tick with gentle steady traction by blunt forceps may prevent transmission of potential tick-borne infectious disease. The tick can be saved for identification and possible analysis for infectious disease.

Gammons M, Salam G. Tick removal. *Am Fam Physician.* 2002;15:643–645.

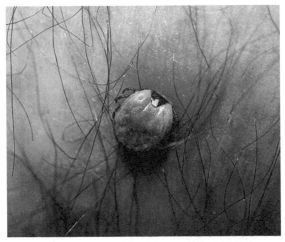

Fig. 33.16 Attached feeding tick with an allergic host response manifesting as erythema and induration. (Courtesy Fitzsimons Army Medical Center teaching files.)

53. How do you prevent tick bites?
    - Wear protective clothing, including long-sleeved shirts and pants tucked into the socks.
    - Permethrin-containing spray may be applied to the clothing, where it remains through several washings. This spray serves as a repellent as well as an insecticide.
    - Apply repellent containing N,N-diethyl-m-toluamide (DEET) on exposed areas on hands and face. The concentration of DEET in newer preparations is in the 30% to 35% range to lessen concerns about systemic absorption and toxicity.

54. Name some important arthropod-borne diseases.
    See Table 33.2.

Table 33.2 Selected diseases transmitted by arthropods

INFECTIOUS DISEASE	VECTOR
Anaplasmosis (human granulocytotropic)	Hard ticks
Arboviruses (including yellow fever, dengue, encephalitis)	Mosquitos, ticks
Babesiosis	Hard ticks
Boutonneuse fever (tick-bite fever) (*Rickettsia conorii*)	Rabbit flea
Chagas disease	Triatomid reduviid (kissing) bugs
Colorado tick fever	Hard ticks
Ehrlichiosis, monocytotropic (*Ehrlichia ewingii*)	Hard ticks
Endemic relapsing fever (*Borrelia duttoni*)	Soft ticks
Epidemic relapsing fever (*Borrelia recurrentis*)	Human body lice
Epidemic typhus (*R. prowazekii*)	Human body lice
Filariasis (*Wuchereria bancrofti, Brugia malayi*)	Mosquitos
Leishmaniasis *(Leishmania* spp.)	Phlebotomid sand flies
Loiasis (*Loa loa*)	Tabanid flies
Lyme disease (*Borrelia burgdorferi*)	Hard ticks
Malaria (*Plasmodium* spp.)	Mosquitos
Endemic murine typhus (*R. mooseri*)	Rat fleas, lice

Continued on following page

Table 33.2 Selected diseases transmitted by arthropods (*Continued*)

INFECTIOUS DISEASE	VECTOR
Onchocerciasis (*Onchocerca volvulus*)	Black flies
Plague (*Yersinia pestis*)	Rat fleas
Q fever (*Coxiella burnetii*)	Hard ticks, fleas
Rickettsial pox (*R. akari*)	Mouse mites
Rocky Mountain spotted fever (*R. rickettsii*)	Hard ticks
Scrub typhus (*R. tsutsugamushi*)	Mites (chiggers)
Trypanosomiasis, African sleeping sickness	*Glossina* (tsetse) flies
West Nile fever	Mosquitos

Adapted from Braunstein WB. Ectoparasites. In: Blaser M, Bennett JE, Dolin R, eds. Principles and Practice of Infectious Diseases. *8th ed.* Philadelphia: Elsevier; 2015:3243–3266.

55. What are the most effective insect repellents?

The most effective repellent for the prevention of bites of mosquitos, chiggers, black flies, midges, and fleas is DEET. An 8% to 10% concentration is adequate for children and a 20% to 50% concentration for adults. Other broadly effective insect repellents include icaridin (20%) and the eucalyptus-based repellent PMD (p-menthane-3,8-diol) (30%). Permethrin aerosol (Permanone) applied to clothing is the best tick repellent.

Moore SJ, Mordue Luntz AJ, Logan JG. Insect bite prevention. *Infect Dis Clin North Am.* 2012;26(3):655–673.

KEY POINTS: ARTHROPOD BITES AND STINGS

1. The brown recluse spider (*Loxosceles reclusa*) is the most common cause of dermonecrotic arachnidism.
2. Always examine the genitalia of male patients with extreme pruritus to evaluate for scabies.
3. The black widow (*Latrodectus mactans*) spider's venom is a potent neurotoxin that can cause muscle cramping simulating an acute abdomen.
4. The antibiotic of choice for Lyme disease in children under 8 years old is amoxicillin.
5. *Cheyletiella* is a nonburrowing mite which presents as "walking dandruff" on pets, and manifests as nonspecific pruritic papules and plaques on affected patients.

CHAPTER 34

CUTANEOUS MANIFESTATIONS OF INTERNAL MALIGNANCY

Ryan A. Stevens

1. **List the five criteria that establish an association between a skin disease and internal malignancy.**
   Helen Curth, while evaluating acanthosis nigricans, established the five criteria known as Curth's postulates:
   1. Concurrent onset of the cutaneous disease and internal malignancy.
   2. Parallel course of the skin disease and internal malignancy.
   3. A specific type or site of malignancy associated with the skin disease.
   4. Sound statistical evidence that the malignancy is more frequent in patients with the skin disease.
   5. A genetic link between a syndrome with skin manifestations and an internal malignancy.

2. **Describe the clinical appearance of acanthosis nigricans.**
   Acanthosis nigricans appears as velvety, hyperpigmented, papillomatous, dirty-appearing skin. It is most frequently seen on the neck, axilla, groin, and dorsal hand surfaces. It is often associated with numerous skin tags and rarely affects mucosal surfaces (Fig. 34.1).

3. **What clinical disease states are associated with acanthosis nigricans?**
   Acanthosis nigricans is a common skin finding, reported in 7.1% of children, but more common in people with darker skin pigmentation, and is frequently associated with obesity and insulin resistance. Paraneoplastic acanthosis nigricans is rare and is most commonly associated with gastrointestinal cancer, especially gastric carcinoma. When associated with malignancy, it is usually abrupt in onset, is severe, and may involve mucous membranes and palmar skin (tripe palms). Paraneoplastic acanthosis nigricans is usually accompanied by weight loss.

Stuart CA, Pate CJ, Peters EJ. Prevalence of acanthosis nigricans in an unselected population. *Am J Med.* 1989;87(3):269–272.

4. **Is the sign of Leser-Trélat (eruptive seborrheic keratoses) associated with internal malignancy?**
   The sign of Leser-Trélat is defined as the abrupt appearance of multiple seborrheic keratoses increasing in size and number caused by an associated cancer. This association remains controversial. Seborrheic keratoses are common in older patients, and so is cancer. Patients with Leser-Trélat often have coexisting paraneoplastic acanthosis nigricans and pruritus.

Schwartz R, Elston DM. The sign of Leser-Trélat. *eMedicine Online.* www.emedicine.com. Accessed April 23, 2018.

5. **What is hypertrichosis lanuginosa?**
   Hypertrichosis lanuginosa (malignant down) is an acquired excessive growth of lanugo hair, usually on the face. Glossitis is frequently an associated finding. If anorexia nervosa or drug-related causes (such as minoxidil, diazoxide, and cyclosporine) can be excluded, there is a high association with internal malignancy, such as carcinoma of the lung, breast, and colon.

6. **What is Sweet's syndrome?**
   Sweet's syndrome (acute febrile neutrophilic dermatosis) occurs mostly in women 30 to 60 years of age and consists of characteristic skin lesions, fever, malaise, and leukocytosis. Less commonly, there is involvement of the joints, eyes, lungs, kidneys, and liver. Approximately 20% of cases have an association with a hematologic malignancy, most commonly acute myelogenous leukemia.

7. **Describe the cutaneous lesions of Sweet's syndrome.**
   The clinical hallmark of Sweet's syndrome is the presence of sharply demarcated, painful, juicy, edematous plaques on the face, neck, upper trunk, and extremities (Fig. 34.2). Occasionally, papulovesicles and pustules are noted. Oral mucous membrane lesions are less common. *Pathergy* (lesions appearing in areas of trauma) can be seen.

8. **Are any laboratory abnormalities found in Sweet's syndrome?**
   Leukocytosis with neutrophilia is common and present in 60% of patients. Elevated sedimentation rates and increased C-reactive protein levels are commonly seen.

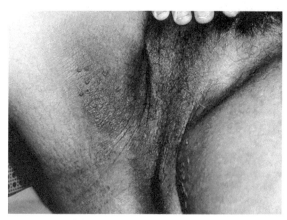

Fig. 34.1 Acanthosis nigricans with hyperpigmented velvety skin lesions and small tags on the proximal thigh and groin.

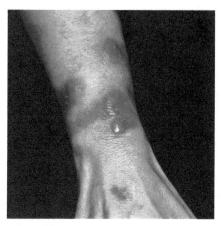

Fig. 34.2 Sweet's syndrome demonstrating painful red indurated plaques on the hand and arm. (Courtesy James E. Fitzpatrick, MD.)

9. What cancers are associated with Sweet's syndrome?

The most commonly associated malignancy is acute myelogenous leukemia, but chronic myelogenous leukemia, lymphocytic leukemia, T- and B-cell lymphomas, polycythemia, and, rarely, solid tumors also have been reported. Patients with persistent laboratory abnormalities, especially anemia, thrombocytosis, and thrombocytopenia, require close observation and thorough diagnostic evaluation.

Cohen PR. Sweet's syndrome—a comprehensive review of an acute febrile neutrophilic dermatosis. *Orphanet J Rare Dis.* 2007;2:34.

10. What other neutrophilic dermatosis can be associated with internal malignancy?

Pyoderma gangrenosum (PG) is an ulcerative skin disease with a distinctive clinical presentation. The lesions are painful, may rapidly enlarge, and are characterized by an erythematous or violaceous undermined border with a necrotic center (Fig. 34.3). The most common diseases associated with PG are inflammatory bowel disease and rheumatoid arthritis. A small subset may have monoclonal immunoglobulin A (IgA) gammopathy and other hematologic disorders. In a review of several studies, PG was associated with internal malignancy in 7.2% of patients. Leukemia is the most frequently reported malignancy, with myelocytic and myelomonocytic leukemia accounting for the majority of cases.

Callen JP, Jackson JM. Pyoderma gangrenosum: an update. *Rheum Dis Clin North Am.* 2007;33:787–802.

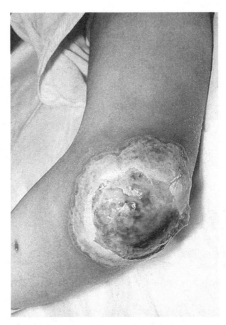

Fig. 34.3 A young woman with acute-onset pyoderma gangrenosum.

11. What is necrolytic migratory erythema?

This characteristic skin eruption is associated with an α-cell tumor of the pancreas, and most patients have elevated glucagon serum levels (glucagonoma syndrome). It presents as erythema with superficial pustules and erosions, typically involving the face, intertriginous skin, and acral extremities (Fig. 34.4). Weight loss, glossitis, stomatitis, and diabetes are frequent associations. Skin biopsy shows necrosis of the upper portion of the epidermis and is usually diagnostic.

Silva JA, Mesquita Kde C, Igreja AC, et al. Paraneoplastic cutaneous manifestations: concepts and updates. *An Bras Dermatol.* 2013;88(1):9–22.

12. What is the characteristic finding in erythema gyratum repens?

This rare skin eruption is characterized by a widespread figurate erythema composed of concentric rings with a wood grain appearance. The erythematous circinate lesions may have a fine scale and move up to 1 cm a day. Almost all patients with this unique dermatosis have an associated malignancy, most commonly carcinoma of the lung. It has also been reported with breast, bladder, cervical, and prostate cancers. The skin lesions clear within a few weeks after removal of the malignancy and usually recur if the cancer returns.

Ufkes N, Elston D. Erythema gyratum repens. *eMedicine Online.* www.emedicine.com. Accessed February 11, 2019.

13. What is Bazex syndrome (acrokeratosis paraneoplastica)?

This syndrome begins with acral violaceous psoriasiform plaques on the ears, nose, hands, and feet, likening to "blue psoriasis." Paronychia and nail dystrophy are common. Later, the eruption may generalize, and lesions on the face may appear dermatitic or lupus-like. The syndrome is more common in men and is associated with squamous cell carcinoma of the upper aerodigestive tract (Fig. 34.5).

There is another Bazex syndrome inherited as an autosomal dominant disease. This syndrome is characterized by follicular atrophoderma, early development of multiple facial basal cell carcinomas, and, in some patients, hypohidrosis.

14. What is Trousseau's sign?

Trousseau's sign consists of recurrent and migratory superficial thrombophlebitis, affecting both large and small cutaneous veins, which is associated with an internal cancer. Tender, linear, erythematous cordlike plaques are seen most commonly on the arms, legs, flanks, and abdomen. The most commonly associated cancers are pancreatic and lung carcinoma.

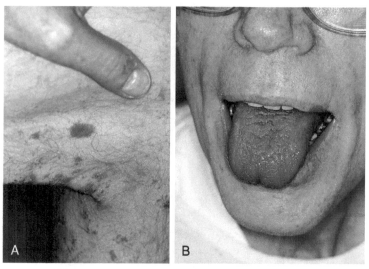

Fig. 34.4 Glucagonoma syndrome. **A,** Erosive plaques on the leg. **B,** Atrophic glossitis.

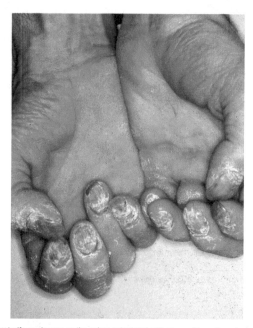

Fig. 34.5 Bazex syndrome. Psoriasiform plaques on the palms associated with paronychia and onychodystrophy. (Courtesy James E. Fitzpatrick, MD.)

15. **Is superficial migratory thrombophlebitis specific for an underlying malignancy?**
    No, superficial migratory thrombophlebitis can also be seen in Behçet's syndrome and hypercoagulable states, such as in liver disease, pregnancy, infection, oral contraceptive use, and hereditary coagulation factor deficiencies.

Varki A. Trousseau's syndrome: multiple definitions and multiple mechanisms. *Blood.* 2007;110:1723–1729.

16. **Describe the classical skin lesions of dermatomyositis.**
    The classic eruption of dermatomyositis is a reddish-purple erythema involving the face, typically the eyelids (heliotrope sign). The rash may be faint or quite inflamed and edematous (Fig. 34.6A).

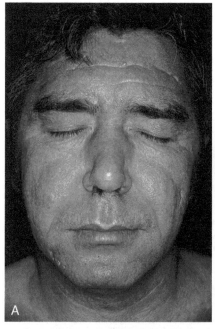
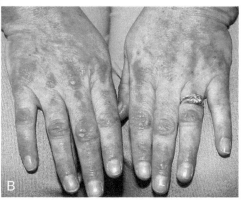

Fig. 34.6 A, Facial erythema and heliotrope sign. **B,** Classic hand lesions and Gottron's papules on the knuckles.

In addition to the facial rash, lesions on the scalp, neck, upper trunk, and extensor extremities are common. As the lesions mature, scaling and atrophy may develop. The erythema on the hands occurs over the knuckles rather than over the phalanges, as is typical of lupus erythematosus. Cuticular telangiectasias can be seen in both lupus erythematosus and dermatomyositis. Frequently, flat-topped, red-to-violaceous papules known as *Gottron's papules* develop over the knuckles of patients with dermatomyositis (Fig. 34.6B).

The skin lesions of dermatomyositis may precede clinical or laboratory evidence myositis by weeks, months, or years. A few patients may never develop muscle dysfunction. The skin lesions are notoriously resistant to topical steroid therapy.

17. **Is dermatomyositis associated with internal malignancy?**
    The true incidence of malignancy associated with dermatomyositis is difficult to define. Several large studies have reported an increased risk of malignancy with dermatomyositis. Adults should be evaluated for malignancy at diagnosis, followed by long-term surveillance. Juvenile dermatomyositis is not typically associated with an internal malignancy.

Qiang JK, Kim WB, Baibergenova A, Alhusayen R. Risk of malignancy in dermatomyositis and polymyositis. *J Cutan Med Surg.* 2017;21(2):131–136.

18. **What internal malignancy is associated with dermatomyositis?**
    The type of cancer reported to be associated with dermatomyositis parallels the incidence of cancer found in the general population, though a slight increase in ovarian carcinoma has been noted.

Callen JP, Wortman RL. Dermatomyositis. *Clin Dermatol.* 2006;24:363–373.

19. **What is Sézary's syndrome?**
    This syndrome is a subset of cutaneous T-cell lymphoma (CTCL) characterized by erythroderma, marked exfoliation, alopecia, onychodystrophy, and intolerable itching. The diagnosis is established by a skin biopsy showing CTCL, the presence of at least 15% atypical mononuclear cells in peripheral blood, and the typical clinical picture. The prognosis is generally poor.

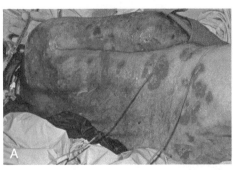
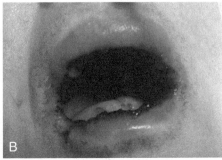

Fig. 34.7 Paraneoplastic pemphigus. **A,** Extensive superficial blisters and erosions of the trunk. **B,** Recalcitrant oral ulcers in a patient with an underlying non–Hodgkin's lymphoma.

20. What are the three components of Sézary's syndrome?

As originally described, Sézary's syndrome represents a triad of findings: (1) cutaneous erythema, (2) lymphadenopathy, and (3) 10% to 15% atypical mononuclear cells in peripheral blood.

Foss F. Mycosis fungoides and the Sézary syndrome. *Curr Opin Oncol.* 2004;5:421–428.

21. What is paraneoplastic pemphigus?

Paraneoplastic pemphigus is a superficial blistering skin disease associated with malignancy. The clinical picture may resemble pemphigus vulgaris, bullous pemphigoid, or Stevens-Johnson syndrome, with significant oral mucous membrane involvement. Recalcitrant oral erosions are often present (Fig. 34.7). The most common associated malignancies are non–Hodgkin's lymphoma and chronic lymphocytic leukemia. The disease responds poorly to immunosuppressive therapy and frequently is fatal.

22. Discuss the laboratory findings in patients with paraneoplastic pemphigus.

Skin and oral mucous membrane biopsy specimens reveal epidermal acantholysis, epidermal spongiosis, suprabasilar clefts, basal cell vacuolar changes, and dyskeratotic keratinocytes. Direct immunofluorescent examination reveals IgG and, less commonly, IgA with or without complement in the intracellular spaces and C3, IgG, or IgM at the basement membrane zone. Antibodies have been demonstrated against desmoplakins, proteins in keratinocyte attachment plaques (desmosomes), and a 230-kDa protein in the basement membrane (bullous pemphigoid antigen). Rat bladder is a useful substrate for indirect immunofluorescent examination and shows positive staining with serum from patients with paraneoplastic pemphigus but will be negative with serum from patients with classic pemphigus vulgaris.

Zhu X, Zhang B. Paraneoplastic pemphigus. *J Dermatol.* 2007;34:503–511.

23. What autoimmune blistering disorder with a tendency for scarring is associated with malignancy?

Cicatricial pemphigoid (mucous membrane pemphigoid) is a subepithelial blistering disorder with prominent involvement of mucosal surfaces, including the oral mucosa and conjunctiva, as well as the skin. Scarring of the conjunctiva can lead to symblepharon formation and, eventually, blindness. The pathogenesis is related to circulating autoantibodies to structural proteins such as bullous pemphigoid antigen 180 (BP180), integrins, and laminin 332 (laminin 5). Patients with anti-laminin 5 autoantibodies have an increased relative risk for solid organ adenocarcinomas.

Egan CA, Lazarova Z, Darling TN, Yee C, Yancey KB. Anti-epiligrin cicatricial pemphigoid: clinical findings, immunopathogenesis, and significant associations. *Medicine (Baltimore).* 2003;82:177–186.

24. Where does Paget's disease most commonly occur?

Paget's disease most commonly occurs on the female breast, although cases have been reported in men. It often begins appearing as a small eczematous patch. The borders of the lesion are sharply marginated, and the surface may be crusted, moist, erythematous, and/or scaly (Fig. 34.8). Paget's disease of the breast invariably has an underlying ductal carcinoma, although often there is no breast mass and mammograms can be normal.

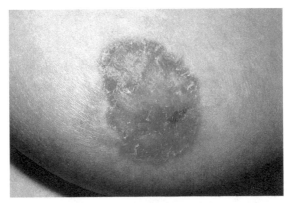

Fig. 34.8 Paget's disease. Sharply demarcated area of erythema and scale crust that had been treated as a dermatitis, showing partial destruction of the nipple. The patient had an underlying ductal breast carcinoma. (Courtesy Fitzsimons Army Medical Center teaching files.)

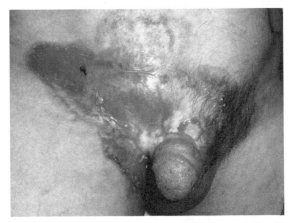

Fig. 34.9 Extramammary Paget's disease. Sharply demarcated erosive plaque with erythema and milky white "strawberries and cream" surface in inguinal region. This patient had an underlying adenocarcinoma. (Courtesy Binh Ngo, MD.)

25. Where does extramammary Paget's disease occur, and is it associated with malignancy?
    Extramammary Paget's disease occurs on the axilla, groin, or anogenital skin. The disease may present with solitary or multiple lesions resembling chronic intertrigo with a "strawberries and cream" appearance (Fig. 34.9). It is often associated with an underlying adnexal carcinoma, and about 20% of cases have carcinoma of the rectum or genitourinary tract.

Kanitakis J. Mammary and extramammary Paget's disease. *J Eur Acad Dermatol Venereol.* 2001;21(5):581–590.

26. Which disorder of abnormal extracellular protein deposition is associated with skin lesions and malignancy?
    Primary systemic amyloidosis. The cause of this disease is a plasma cell dyscrasia, including but less commonly multiple myeloma. The most common associated skin lesions are purpura or ecchymoses that are seen most frequently on thin skin areas, that is, eyelids, neck, groin, axilla, umbilicus, or oral mucosa. Other less common skin lesions include waxy papules and nodules, "pinch purpura," alopecia, nail dystrophies, scleroderma-like lesions, macroglossia, cutis verticis gyrata, bullous lesions, and dyspigmentation.

Nyirady J, Elston D. Primary systemic amyloidosis. *eMedicine Online.* www.emedicine.com. Accessed May 23, 2018.

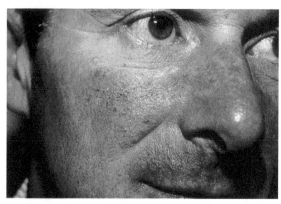

Fig. 34.10 Carcinoid syndrome. Patient with long history of flushing and development of persistent telangiectasias of the face. (Courtesy Fitzsimons Army Medical Center teaching files.)

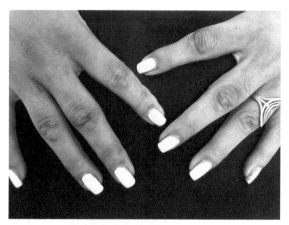

Fig. 34.11 Multicentric reticulohistiocytosis. Multiple reddish-pink papules on dorsal hands and nail folds with characteristic coral beading.

27. What is carcinoid syndrome? Does it have prognostic significance?

Carcinoid syndrome is a systemic manifestation of neuroendocrine carcinoid tumors that manifest most commonly by flushing that progresses to persistent telangiectasia (Fig. 34.10) and diarrhea. Less common findings include bronchospasm, cardiac valvular dysfunction, and pellagra-like skin changes (photodistributed dermatitis). It is estimated that 10% of patients with carcinoid tumors will develop this syndrome. Development of this syndrome has prognostic significance, as liver metastases underlie most cases, and thus, it signifies metastatic, unresectable disease.

Kleyn CE, Lai-Cheong JE, Bell HK. Cutaneous manifestations of internal malignancy: diagnosis and management. *Am J Clin Dermatol.* 2006;7(2):71–84.

28. What is multicentric reticulohistiocytosis?

Multicentric reticulohistiocytosis is a rare disease characterized by multiple skin papules and nodules in patients with severe arthritis. The papules characteristically cluster on the hands and periungual areas (coral-beading) (Fig. 34.11). Skin biopsy shows a diffuse histiocytic cellular infiltrate with large multinucleate giant cells with ground-glass cytoplasm. Associated malignancy was reported in 28% of the patients in 82 cases reported in the literature. The disease preceded the development of cancer in 73% of the patients.

Sroa N, Zirwas MJ, Bechtel M. Multicentric reticulohistiocytosis: a case report and review of the literature. *Cutis.* 2010;85(3):153–155.

29. What is erythromelalgia?

Erythromelalgia is a rare skin disease characterized by erythematous, painful, burning of the feet, ankles, and lower extremities. The disease is aggravated by heat exposure and relieved by cooling. Many patients can find relief only by soaking their legs in ice water. Erythromelalgia is most commonly idiopathic, but when associated with malignancy, it is usually hematologic, including polycythemia vera or essential thrombocythemia.

30. **Is vasculitis associated with malignancy?**

Vasculitis is rarely associated with internal malignancy. In multiple large reviews of vasculitis and cancer, vasculitis was most commonly associated with hematologic malignancy (63%–77%).

Paydas S, Zorludemir S, Sahin B. Vasculitis and leukemia. *Leuk Lymphoma.* 2000;40:105–112.
Fain O, Hamidou M, Cacoub P, et al. Vasculitides associated with malignancies: analysis of sixty patients. *Arthritis Rheum.* 2007;57(8):1473–1480.

31. **Is dry scaly skin associated with internal malignancy?**

Yes. Acquired ichthyosis may be associated with malignancy, most commonly Hodgkin's lymphoma.

Moore RL, Devere TS. Epidermal manifestations of internal malignancy. *Dermatol Clin.* 2008;26(1):17–29, vii.

32. **Can pruritus be a sign of malignancy?**

Generalized pruritus without skin lesions has been reported as a symptom of internal malignancy. Paraneoplastic pruritus is most commonly caused by lymphoproliferative malignancies such as Hodgkin's lymphoma. One-third of non-melanoma skin cancers present locally with pruritus.

Rowe B, Yosipovitch G. Malignancy-associated pruritus. *Eur J Pain.* 2016;20(1):19–23.

33. **List the autosomal dominant diseases that have prominent skin findings and internal cancer.**

See Table 34.1.

34. **Describe the cutaneous features of Gardner's syndrome.**

The cutaneous hallmark of the syndrome is epidermoid cysts, which often appear before puberty, frequently on the extremities. These cysts may be many or few. The syndrome is also characterized by osteomas (typically on facial bones), fibrous and desmoid tumors, abnormal dentition, lipomas, hypertrophy of retinal pigmented epithelium, and leiomyomas of the gastrointestinal tract. The syndrome is characterized by the early onset of colonic polyposis and has a very high incidence of colon cancer.

35. **What are the clinical findings in Cowden's syndrome (multiple hamartoma syndrome)?**

This syndrome is characterized by a triad of findings: (1) small keratotic facial papules (Fig. 34.12A), (2) cobblestoning of the oral mucosa (Fig. 34.12B), and (3) acral keratotic skin lesions. These patients also have benign tumors of neural, fibrous, vascular, and epithelial origin. Multiple small tumors of facial hair follicles (trichilemmomas) and sclerotic fibromas are pathognomonic of this syndrome. Fibrocystic disease of the breast is common, and 30% of women will develop breast cancer. Many other associated cancers have been reported, with thyroid cancer being the second most common malignancy.

36. **When do the characteristic skin lesions of Peutz-Jeghers syndrome appear?**

Brown to blue-black macules (lentigines) are present at birth or early infancy on the lips, oral mucosa, nasal mucosa, palms, soles, dorsal hand surfaces, central face, and elbows. The lentigines typically resolve with time. Polyps of the small intestine develop in 90% of patients; polyps may also occur in the stomach, colon, and rectum. There is an increased incidence of gastrointestinal malignancy, but it is not nearly as common as in patients with Gardner's syndrome. Intussusception occurs in about 50% of cases.

37. **How does multiple mucosal neuroma syndrome (multiple endocrine neoplasia, MEN2B) typically present?**

As the name implies, this syndrome is characterized by the development of multiple flesh-colored papules on the tongue, lips, and, occasionally, other mucosal surfaces early in life. These patients have a characteristic appearance with thick prominent lips and a marfanoid habitus. Ninety percent of these patients develop medullary thyroid carcinoma, and half will suffer from pheochromocytoma that is often multifocal and/or bilateral.

38. **What is Muir-Torre syndrome?**

This syndrome includes cutaneous sebaceous neoplasia and a high incidence of low-grade colon cancer. The sebaceous tumors include sebaceous adenomas, carcinomas, and sebaceomas. In addition, about one-third of patients develop keratoacanthomas. The sebaceous skin tumors may be few or many, but even one sebaceous adenoma should alert the clinician that the patient may have this syndrome.

Winship IM, Dudding T. Lessons from the skin-cutaneous features of familial cancer. *Lancet Oncol.* 2008;9:462–472.

Table 34.1 Autosomal dominant diseases with skin findings and malignancy

DISORDER	SKIN FINDINGS	CANCER	ASSOCIATIONS	AFFECTED GENE
Cowden's syndrome	Keratotic facial papules Acral keratosis Soft tissue tumors	Breast Thyroid	Mucosal papules Fibrocystic disease of the breast	PTEN
Muir-Torre syndrome	Sebaceous tumors Keratoacanthomas	Colon	Colon polyps	MSH2, MLH1
Gardner's syndrome	Epidermoid cysts	Colon	Colon polyps Osteomas Desmoids Abnormal dentition	APC
Peutz-Jeghers syndrome	Pigmented macules on mucosa, face, acral extremities	Intestinal	Intestinal polyps	STK11
Multiple mucosal neuroma syndrome	Neuromas of lips, tongue, and oral mucosa	Thyroid	Pheochromocytoma Marfanoid habitus	RET
Neurofibromatosis	Neurofibromas Café-au-lait macules	Neurofibrosarcoma (rare)	Lisch nodules Seizures Deafness	Neurofibromin
Hereditary leiomyomatosis/renal cell cancer syndrome	Multiple leiomyomas of skin and uterus	Papillary renal cell carcinoma		Decreased fumarate hydratase activity

APC, Adenomatosis polyposis coli; MLH1, micronuclear linker histone; MSH2, melanocyte stimulating hormone; PTEN, phosphate and tension homolog deleted on chromosome 10; RET, RET protooncogene (rearranged during transfection); STK11, serine threonine kinase.

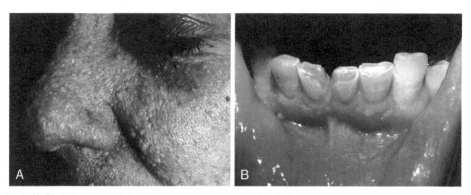

Fig. 34.12 Cowden's syndrome. **A,** Typical small keratotic papules on the face. **B,** Characteristic cobblestone papules on the mucosal surface of the lower lip.

39. Which recessively inherited diseases have skin findings and associated internal malignancy?
   See Table 34.2.

40. What is FAMMM syndrome?
   FAMMM syndrome, also known as dyplastic nevus syndrome, is the familial atypical multiple mole melanoma syndrome, and it appears to be related to germline mutations in cyclin-dependent kinase inhibitor 2A (CDKN2A). Affected patients have numerous clinically atypical nevi, increased lifetime risk for melanoma, and a family history of melanoma and/or pancreatic cancer (Fig. 34.13). Affected families benefit from screening for early detection of pancreatic cancer.

Lynch HT, Fusaro RM, Lynch JF, Brand R. Pancreatic cancer and the FAMMM syndrome. *Fam Cancer.* 2008;7:103–112.

Table 34.2 Recessively inherited diseases with skin findings and malignancy

DISORDER	INHERITANCE	CLINICAL FINDINGS	CANCER	AFFECTED GENE
Wiskott-Aldrich syndrome	X-linked recessive	Chronic dermatitis Thrombocytopenia Recurrent infections	Lymphoma, especially non–Hodgkin's	*WAS*
Bloom's syndrome	Autosomal recessive	Photosensitivity Telangiectasia of sun-exposed skin Short stature Decreased serum immunoglobulins Recurrent infections Sister chromatid exchange	Lymphomas Leukemias	*RecQ3*
Ataxia-telangiectasia (Louis-Bar syndrome)	Autosomal recessive	Progressive cerebellar ataxia Telangiectasia Recurrent sinus and pulmonary infections Decreased/absent serum immunoglobulin A Granulomas on legs	Lymphomas (increased cancer risk also seen in heterozygotes)	*ATM*
Dyskeratosis congenita	X-linked recessive Autosomal dominant	Skin atrophy and hyperpigmentation Nail dystrophy Oral precancerous leukokeratosis	Oral cancers Other malignancies	*DKC1* TERC

ATM, Ataxia telangiectasia mutated; *DKC1*, dyskerin; *RecQ3*, DNA helicase Rec Q protein-like-3; *TERC*, telomerase RNA component; *WAS*, Wiskott-Aldrich syndrome.

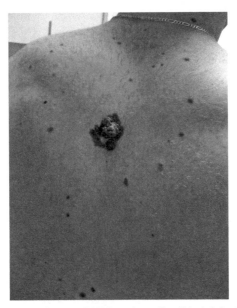

Fig. 34.13 Dysplastic nevus syndrome (FAMMM syndrome). Middle-aged man with multiple atypical nevi and a large ulcerated melanoma. (Courtesy James E. Fitzpatrick, MD.)

KEY POINTS: CUTANEOUS MANIFESTATIONS OF INTERNAL MALIGNANCY

1. Patients with biopsy-proven Sweet's syndrome should have a complete blood count to evaluate for an underlying hematologic malignancy.
2. Acanthosis nigricans is a common condition, and most cases are associated with insulin resistance. Paraneoplastic acanthosis nigricans is rare, may be of explosive onset, and is associated with tripe palms and the sign of Leser-Trélat.
3. Patients with refractory oral pemphigus vulgaris should be evaluated for paraneoplastic pemphigus.
4. Patients with dermatomyositis should have age-appropriate cancer screening, and women should be screened for ovarian carcinoma.
5. Any refractory eczematous eruption on the breast should be biopsied to exclude mammary Paget's disease.

CHAPTER 35

CUTANEOUS MANIFESTATIONS OF ENDOCRINOLOGIC DISEASE

Whitney A. High

1. How does endocrinologic disease cause skin disorders?

   Endocrinologic disease can produce cutaneous changes in several different ways:

   - Hormones interact with cell surface receptors to regulate cellular function, and many cell types in skin have such hormone receptors. This means that hormone levels can directly alter skin metabolism. For example, both skin and skin appendages express thyroid hormone receptors, and thyroid hormones can alter expression of keratins by keratinocytes.
   - Hormone excess or deficiency may affect the skin indirectly, rather than through specific hormone/hormone receptor interactions. For example, the hyperglycemia of diabetes results in impaired immune function and a predisposition to infection.
   - Other unusual skin disorders, such as necrobiosis lipoidica diabeticorum, are highly associated with endocrine disease, but the pathogenesis is poorly understood.

   Antonini D, Sibilio A, Dentice M, Missero C. An intimate relationship between thyroid hormone and skin: regulation of gene expression. *Front Endocrinol.* 2013;4:104.

2. What is necrobiosis lipoidica?

   Necrobiosis lipoidica is a granulomatous inflammatory skin condition that nearly always involves the pretibial surface. It is highly associated with diabetes, but certainly all diabetics do not get necrobiosis lipodica. Early lesions present as nondiagnostic erythematous papules or plaques that evolve yellow-brown plaques, with overlying skin atrophy and dilated blood vessels (Fig. 35.1A). Fully developed pretibial lesions are essentially diagnostic, simply because of the clinical appearance and anatomic site. Later lesions may ulcerate (Fig. 35.1B).

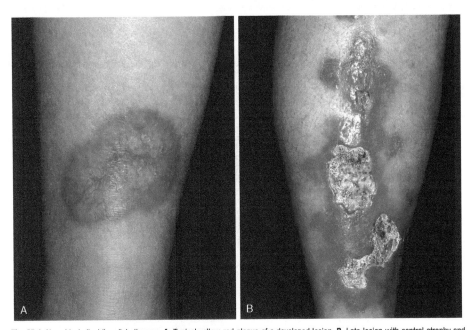

Fig. 35.1 Necrobiosis lipoidica diabeticorum. **A,** Typical yellow-red plaque of a developed lesion. **B,** Late lesion with central atrophy and extensive ulceration. (Courtesy James E. Fitzpatrick, MD.)

3. Do all patients with necrobiosis lipoidica have diabetes and how many diabetics develop the condition?

In a study of 171 patients with necrobiosis lipoidica, about 60% had diabetes. Moreover, many patients subsequently developed diabetes, had abnormal glucose tolerance tests, or had a strong family history of diabetes. Only about 10% of patients were not in a high-risk group to develop diabetes. In a more recent study with 65 patients, 22% either had or developed diabetes. Patients with necrobiosis lipoidica should be screened for diabetes. However, only about 0.3% of patients with diabetes develop necrobiosis lipoidica. The condition is most often seen in adults with type II diabetes, but it can occur in juvenile diabetes, as well. To solidify this knowledge, the following phrase if often employed: "Most cases of necrobiosis lipoidica are associated with diabetes, but no many diabetics develop necrobiosis lipoidca."

Grillo E, Rodriguez-Muñoz D, González-Garcia A, et al. Necrobiosis lipoidica. *Aust Fam Physician*. 2014;43:129–130.
Hammer E, Lilienthal E, Hofer SE, et al. Risk factors for necrobiosis lipoidica in Type 1 diabetes mellitus. *Diabet Med*. 2017;34:86–92.

5. Does glucose control affect necrobiosis lipoidica diabeticorum?

It is unclear whether tighter glycemic control (i.e., better control of diabetes) impacts the clinical course of necrobiosis lipoidica. In adults, Cohen et al. concluded that better glucose control might prevent presentation of the lesions. In children, diabetics with necrobiosis lipoidica had higher levels of hemoglobin A1c. There are several reports of resolution of necrobiosis lipoidica with pancreas transplant. At this juncture, the answer is not known with certitude.

Cohen O, Yaniv R, Karasik A, et al. Necrobiosis lipoidica and diabetic control revisited. *Med Hypotheses*. 1996;46(4):348–350.

6. What other skin findings are associated with insulin resistance?

Acanthosis nigricans is highly associated with insulin resistance, and it presents as velvety, hyperpigmented plaques, most often in intertriginous areas, such as the neck folds and axillae (Fig. 35.2). It is often described by patients as "dirty skin" that is "impossible to clean."

Insulin-like growth factors produced by the liver, in response to high levels of circulating insulin, are thought to bind epidermal growth factor receptors, or other receptors in the skin, leading to the changes of acanthosis nigricans. The condition is found in 30%–50% of patients with diabetes, and it correlates with obesity and insulin resistance. Acanthosis nigricans may predict the development of diabetes in persons at higher risk.

Videira-Silva A, Albuquerque C, Fonseca H, et al. Acanthosis nigricans as a clinical marker of insulin resistance among overweight adolescents. *Ann Pediatr Endocrinol Metab*. 2019;24:99–103.

7. Is diabetes the only condition associated with acanthosis nigricans?

No. Other endocrine diseases, such as Cushing's syndrome (with excess cortisol), acromegaly (with excess growth hormone), polycystic ovarian disease, or medications that promote hyperinsulinemia, may be associated with acanthosis nigricans. So-called "malignant" acanthosis nigricans can be a paraneoplastic condition associated

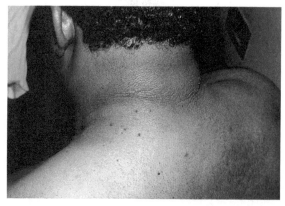

Fig. 35.2 Velvety hyperpigmentation of the neck crease in a patient with classic acanthosis nigricans. (Courtesy James E. Fitzpatrick, MD.)

with certain malignancies, most commonly gastrointestinal adenocarcinomas. In fact, oral involvement of acanthosis nigricans always suggests a paraneoplastic cause.

Higgins S, Freemark M, Prose N. Acanthosis nigricans: a practical approach to evaluation and management. *Dermaitol Online J.* 2008;14 (9):2.

8. What bacterial infections are more common in diabetic patients?

Cutaneous bacterial infections are more common and may be more severe in diabetics. Diabetic foot ulcers are a leading cause of morbidity and health care cost. Diabetic neuropathy (numbness) prevents recognition of injury, and hyperglycemia impairs white blood cell function, allowing bacterial infection. Staphylococcal folliculitis or skin abscesses are common in diabetics, but often respond well to antibiotics and surgical drainage. Diabetic patients may develop necrotizing infections of the external ear caused by *Pseudomonas aeruginosa.* There is evidence that diabetes is a risk factor for latent tuberculosis infection.

Lee MR, Huang YP, Kuo YT, et al. Diabetes mellitus and latent tuberculosis infection: a systematic review and metaanalysis. *Clin Infect Dis.* 2017;64:719–727.

9. What superficial fungal skin infections are common in diabetic patients?

Candidiasis, usually caused by *Candida albicans,* is more common in diabetics. Mucocutaneous candidiasis is characterized by white adherent exudate on erythematous skin, often with satellite pustules. Candidal vulvovaginitis is extremely common. Perianal dermatitis in men or women may be caused by *Candida.* Other forms of candidiasis include thrush (infection of oral mucosa), perlèche (angular cheilitis), intertrigo (infection of skin folds), erosio interdigitalis blastomycetica chronica (finger webspace infection), paronychia (infection of the soft tissue around the nail plate), and onychomycosis (infection of the nail). The mechanism appears to involve increased levels of glucose that serve as a substrate for *Candida* species to proliferate. Patients with recurrent cutaneous candidiasis of any form should be screened for diabetes.

Dermatophytosis is also common in diabetics, but also in the general population. A recent epidemiologic study found that among all dermatophyte infections, *Trichophyton rubrum* was the most often isolated. Tinea pedis ("athlete's foot") was most common, followed by tinea unguium (nail infection), tinea corporis ("ringworm"), tinea cruris ("jock itch"), tinea manuum (hand involvement), and tinea capitis (scalp infection), including kerion.

10. Are there more dangerous deep fungal infections associated with diabetes?

Rarely, mucormycosis will complicate diabetic ketoacidosis, and it represents a severe and progressive soft tissue infection caused by saprophytic fungi of the *Mucor, Rhizopus,* and *Absidia* families. These types of infection are poorly responsive to systemic antifungals and may be quickly and abruptly fatal.

Petrikkos G, Tsioutis C. Recent advances in the pathogenesis of mucormycoses. *Clin Ther.* 2018;40:894–902.

11. Why are diabetic patients in ketoacidosis particularly susceptible to mucormycosis?

The fungi involved in mucormycosis present in diabetic ketoacidosis because the organisms prefer a lower pH, grow rapidly with higher glucose levels, and can utilize ketones as an energy substrate.

12. What other skin disorders are often encountered in diabetic patients?

Common skin disorders in diabetics include granuloma annulare, diabetic dermopathy (atrophic, scarred, hyperpigmented papules on the anterior leg), periungual telangiectasias, yellow skin and nails, and skin tags. Less common skin disorders in diabetics include bullous diabeticorum (tense bullae of the lower extremities), vitiligo, and scleredema adultorum (stiff hands and thickened/stiff skin on the upper back).

Sanches MM, Roda Â, Pimenta R, et al. Cutaneous manifestations of diabetes mellitus and prediabetes. *Acta Med Port.* 2019;32:459–465.

13. What is pretibial myxedema?

Pretibial myxedema is characterized by brawny, indurated plaques over the pretibial areas. These plaques may be skin-colored or have a brown-red color (Fig. 35.3A). On biopsy, the skin is diffusely infiltrated by mucin (Fig. 35.3B). Pretibial myxedema is almost always caused by Graves disease, a frequent cause of hyperthyroidism, but it occurs in only 3% to 5% of patients with that disorder. Only rare cases have been reported with Hashimoto thyroiditis. Pretibial myxedema is often associated with Graves ophthalmopathy (bulging eyes or exophthalmos) and acropachy (thickened soft tissue the digits).

Fatourechi V. Pretibial myxedema: pathophysiology and treatment options. *Am J Clin Dermatol.* 2005;6:295–309.

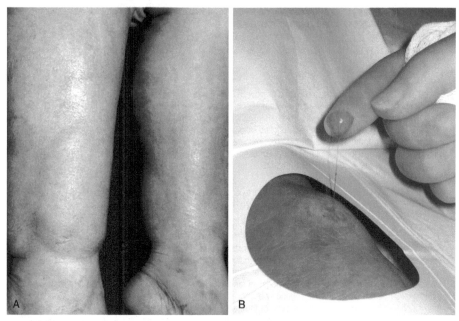

Fig. 35.3 Pretibial myxedema. **A,** Large indurated skin-colored plaques. **B,** A positive "string sign" of mucin extending from the biopsy site to the surgical glove. (Panel B courtesy Scott Freeman, MD.)

14. Does treatment of Grave disease rapidly improve pretibial myxedema?

Graves hyperthyroidism is an autoimmune disease produced by autoantibodies that bind to thyrotropin (TSH) receptors in the thyroid gland, stimulating the organ to produce and release thyroid hormone. It is thought that thyroid-stimulating hormone receptors in the connective tissue may be responsible for stimulating fibroblasts to produce large amounts of glycosaminoglycans. Localization to the pretibial area may relate to mechanical factors and dependent position. Treatment of Graves disease ameliorates the hyperthyroidism but not the underlying autoimmune condition, and hence, an immediate improvement in pretibial myxedema is not usually noted.

Daumerie C, Ludgate M, Costagliola S, et al. Evidence for thyrotropin receptor immunoreactivity in pretibial connective tissue from patients with thyroid-associated dermopathy. *Eur J Endocrinol.* 2002;146:35–38.

15. What are the skin manifestations of hypothyroidism?

Mild hypothyroidism usually makes the skin dry, scaly, cold, and pale. The dryness and scale of the skin may can lead to pruritus. Nails are often brittle. More severe and long-standing hypothyroidism can lead to yellowed and diffusely thickened skin (Fig. 35.4), loss of the outer third of the eyebrows, and thickened lips and an enlarged tongue.

16. Why do hypothyroid patients have thickened, yellow skin?

Hypothyroidism leads to reduced conversion of carotene to vitamin A in the liver. The ensuing carotenemia leads to deposition in the skin, with a resultant yellowed appearance. Increased dermal mucopolysaccharides in the skin leads to skin thickening (myxedema).

17. How does the myxedema of hypothyroidism differ from pretibial myxedema of Graves disease?

Myxedema of hypothyroidism is due to smaller accumulations of mucin over the entire surface area of skin. Pretibial myxedema is the result of marked accumulation of mucin, localized nearly exclusively to the pretibial surface.

18. Are the skin changes of hypothyroidism reversible with thyroid replacement?

Yes, the yellowed appearance of the skin and the thickened quality of the skin improve with therapy for hypothyroidism.

19. What are the skin manifestations of hyperthyroidism?

Hyperthyroidism results in warm, moist, and erythematous skin. Onycholysis (separation of the nail from the nailbed) can occur with hyperthyroidism. Pruritus may be observed. Because skin pruritus can be associated with either hypothyroidism or hyperthyroidism, patients with pruritus of unknown cause should have thyroid disease excluded.

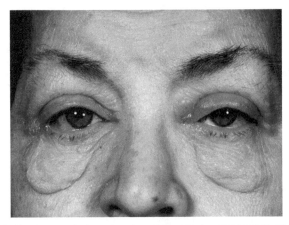

Fig. 35.4 Patient with severe generalized myxedema demonstrating intensive periocular edema and very yellow skin.

20. Which hormone gives the skin a darkened or tanned appearance?

Adrenocorticotropic hormone (ACTH) darkens the skin by stimulating melanocytes to produce melanin. In contrast to normal tanning, the darkening is often accentuated in palmar creases and upon mucous membranes (but such changes may occur without disease of the adrenocortical axis in persons of color). The most common cause of elevated ACTH levels is hypocortisolism (Addison disease) (Fig. 35.5), in which deficient adrenal production of cortisol, with low serum levels, remove feedback inhibition of the pituitary gland, with increases in ACTH production.

Slominski A, Tobin DJ, Shibahara S, et al. Melanin pigmentation in mammalian skin and its hormonal regulation. *Physiol Rev.* 2004;84:1155–1228.

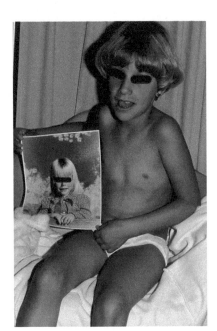

Fig. 35.5 Addison's disease. Young girl with increased unexplained darkening of her skin. Compare her skin color with the color of a photograph taken when she was younger. (Courtesy Fitzsimons Army Medical Center teaching files.)

21. **What skin disease is associated with insulin-dependent diabetes, hypothyroidism, and hypocortisolism?**

    Vitiligo; however, it is important to realize that vitiligo is not caused by a hormonal disease, but by an autoimmune disease that results in destruction of melanocytes in the skin. The condition is associated with OTHER autoimmune disease, including autoimmune endocrinopathies. Vitiligo presents as white (depigmented) macules, most often on the face and hands. Vitiligo is present in 4% of patients with insulin-dependent diabetes, 7% of patients with Graves disease, and 15% of patients with Addison disease. There is also a familial predisposition to this group of diseases.

22. **What skin findings are associated with hypercortisolism (Cushing disease)?**

    In hypercortisolism (Cushing disease), the skin is often thin and atrophic. Wound repair is inhibited. Striae can develop upon the abdomen, upper chest, and buttocks, where the skin is stretched with normal movement. The striae may be large and purple (Fig. 35.6). The skin can have a ruddy appearance, and telangiectasias may be apparent. The skin may bruise and tear easily. Other skin abnormalities may include hypertrichosis, dryness, and facial acne. Overtreatment with high-potency topical steroids for extended durations may yield similar skin changes. A broad and/or round face ("moon facies"), increased adipose accumulating on the upper back/neck ("buffalo hump"), and truncal obesity are characteristic of hypercortisolism.

23. **Are the skin changes caused by excess glucocorticoids reversible?**

    Striae and telangiectasias from hypercortisolism may fade with time but often do not disappear.

24. **Which hormones have the greatest effect on sebaceous glands and hair?**

    Androgens have the greatest effect on sebaceous glands and hair. These hormones are produced at the time of puberty, and this increased sebaceous gland activity contributes to acne. Excess androgens in women can cause acne, hirsutism (increased facial hair), and/or pattern alopecia. Hyperpigmentation of genital and/or areolar skin and clitoromegaly can result as well. Causes of hirsutism and acne in women can include adrenal or ovarian tumors, prolactin-secreting pituitary tumors, polycystic ovarian disease, and adrenal enzyme deficiencies. Familial tendencies toward acne and hirsutism can result from increased end-organ sensitivity to normal circulating levels of androgens, and may not always be related to a tumor.

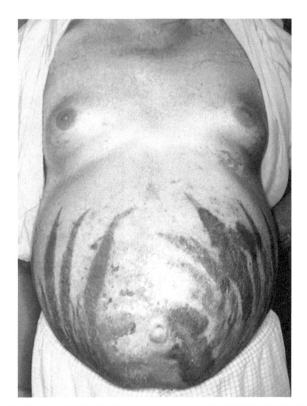

Fig. 35.6 Cushing's syndrome (excess glucocorticoids), showing truncal obesity and abdominal striae. (Courtesy James E. Fitzpatrick, MD.)

25. Are there medications and nutritional supplements that may cause acne?

Supplements and medications can have androgenic effects and may not always be reported by the patient. New-onset acne in a weightlifter may result from exogenous androgens taken as performance-enhancing drugs. New-onset acne in a young woman may be from low-estrogen oral contraceptives, as progesterone-like hormones can yield androgenic effects. New-onset acne in a later-middle-aged woman may result from small amounts of testosterone added to some perimenopausal supplements. With increased interest in transgender medicine, side effects can result from testosterone supplementation. High-dose glucocorticoid therapy can cause acne. Acne from altered hormone levels may take 4–6 weeks to appear, and resolves slowly as well.

Irwig MS. Testosterone therapy for transgender men. *Lancet Diabetes Endocrinol.* 2017;5:301–311.

26. Which hormone levels should be evaluated with acne associated with hirsutism?

Polycystic ovarian syndrome and congenital adrenal hyperplasia can result in acne that is severe or difficult to treat. Screening for these situations may include measurement of free and total testosterone, luteinizing hormone/follicle-stimulating hormone, prolactin, and dehydroepiandrosterone sulfate (DHEAS). High levels of DHEAS may indicate congenital adrenal hyperplasia, and extremely high levels can suggest an adrenal tumor.

27. How is hormonal acne treated?

Hormonal acne is ideally treated through improvement of the underlying hormonal abnormality. Low-estrogen, triphasic oral contraceptives have a net-antiandregenic effect in acne. Oral contraceptives work to decrease ovarian androgen production and free testosterone while increasing sex hormone–binding globulin (SHBG), thereby decreasing the production of sebaceous glands. Spironolactone also has an antiandregenic effect that is useful in acne and in treating pattern alopecia in women. Spironolactone inhibits testosterone and 5α-dihydrotestosterone binding and increasing SHBG, as well. It is not often used in men because of its feminizing side effects. Ultimately, all of these antiandregenic therapies are most often used in concert with more traditional acne medications.

Lortscher D, Admani S, Satur N, Eichenfield LF. Hormonal contraceptives and acne: a retrospective analysis of 2147 patients. *J Drugs Dermatol.* 2016;15:670–674.

28. What are xanthelasma?

Xanthelasma is cholesterol deposition in the skin of the eyelid that leads to distinctive yellow plaques (Fig. 35.7). Although people with xanthelasma may have normal total cholesterol and triglyceride levels, they may have more subtle lipid abnormalities that are poorly characterized in commercial assays or are associated with high cardiovascular risk and deposition of cholesterol in blood vessels. Treatment of xanthelasma is done with surgical excision, liquid nitrogen destruction, carefully performed chemical peels, various laser therapy (CO_2 laser, among others), radiofrequency ablation, or electrocautery.

Laftah Z, Al-Niaimi F. Xanthelasma—an update on treatment modalities. *J Cutan Aesthet Surg.* 2018;11:1–6.

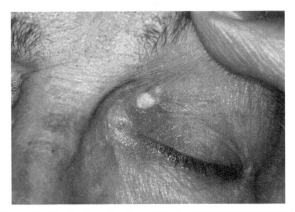

Fig. 35.7 Xanthelasma. Characteristic flat yellowish papules of the upper eyelid. (Courtesy Fitzsimons Army Medical Center teaching files.)

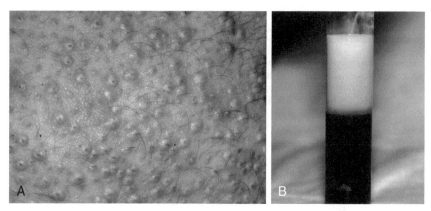

Fig. 35.8 A, Eruptive xanthomas demonstrating typical uniform yellowish papules. Many of these lesions are centered on a hair follicle. **B,** Red-top tube taken from a patient with eruptive xanthomas. The blood has separated into a triglyceride layer and blood layer. The triglycerides level was over 11,000. (Courtesy Fitzsimons Army Medical Center teaching files.)

29. What are eruptive xanthomas?

Eruptive xanthomas are multiple, small, skin-colored to yellow-brown papules that occur in crops, most often upon extensor surfaces such as the buttocks, thighs, or elbows (Fig. 35.8A). Triglycerides accumulate in histiocytes around blood vessels. These distinctive papules are a cutaneous sign of high triglyceride levels. Patients with eruptive xanathomata are at risk for pancreatitis, which can be severe or life-threatening. Eruptive xanthomata can be a sign of new onset of diabetes.

Abdelghany M, Massoud S. Eruptive xanthoma. *Cleve Clin J Med.* 2015;82:209–210.

30. How do eruptive xanthomas differ from tuberous xanthomas?

Tuberous xanthomas are larger and deeper than eruptive xanthomas. Large nodules are likened to a radish, small turnip, or other vegetable tuber, located in the deep dermis or subcutis (Fig. 35.9). Tubersous xanthomas are the result of cholesterol accumulation, in contrast to the smaller eruptive xanthomas that contain triglyceride. Caused by high serum cholesterol levels, patients with tuberous xanthomas are at risk for premature coronary artery disease. Tendinous xanthomas (similar lesions attached to large tendons, such as the Achilles tendon) may be present, as well.

31. What are the cutaneous features of acromegaly?

Acromegaly is caused by excess pituitary growth hormone, present after puberty. In the disease, thickening of bone leads to coarse facies and enlarged hands. Skin changes are caused by insulin-like growth factors that are

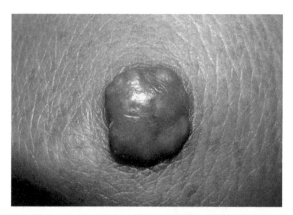

Fig. 35.9 Tuberous xanthoma manifesting as a large nodular xanthoma on the elbow. (Courtesy Fitzsimons Army Medical Center teaching files.)

produced in excess and are similar to those seen in states of insulin resistance. The skin is thickened, and acanthosis nigricans may be present. Cutis verticis gyrata (whorled furrowing of the scalp) may be seen in 30% of patients.

Degirmentepe EN, Gungor S, Kocaturk E, et al. Dermatologic manifestations of acromegaly: a case in point and a focused review. *Dermatol Online J*. 2017;23.

KEY POINTS: XANTHOMAS

1. The presence of one or more xanthomas usually indicates an abnormality of lipid metabolism or, less often, a monoclonal gammopathy.
2. Xanthomas are characterized histologically by the accumulation of lipids in tissue macrophages.
3. Eruptive xanthomas are caused by high levels of serum triglycerides.
4. Patients with eruptive xanthomas are at increased risk to develop pancreatitis.
5. Most patients with xanthelasma often have normal serum levels of triglycerides and cholesterol but often have other abnormalities of apolipoprotein metabolism.

32. How does panhypopituitarism affect the skin?

Patients with panhypopituitarism have pale skin with fine wrinkles around the eyes and mouth. Body hair and genital hair are sparse. Sweat and sebum production are diminished. Dryness and thickening of skin are not as prominent as in primary hypothyroidism, simply because there is some autonomous thyroid gland function in panhypopituitarism.

33. How do you diagnose endocrine disease based upon skin findings?

- Most skin findings in endocrinologic disease are nonspecific but relate to an effect of hormones on the skin. An example is the dry and thickened skin of hypothyroidism. However, not all dry skin is related to endocrine disease, as dry skin can result even among normal people simply from a dry environment and/or poor bathing and skin care techniques.
- Hence, nonspecific skin findings should be considered along with nonspecific findings from other organ systems to suggest an appropriate endocrine diagnosis. For example, dry, thickened skin, also with weight gain, fatigue, depression, and lethargy, would be highly suggestive of hypothyroidism.
- More specific skin findings occur in a minority of patients with endocrinologic disease, but are highly suggestive of such a diagnosis when present. For example, patients with acanthosis nigricans or necrobiosis lipoidica should be screened for diabetes. Pretibial myxedema is a feature of Graves disease. Eruptive xanthomas can occur with marked serum hypertriglyceridemia and tuberous xanthomas with high serum cholesterol.

CHAPTER 36

SKIN SIGNS OF GASTROINTESTINAL DISEASE

Whitney A. High

1. List some of the hallmark skin signs seen with diseases of the digestive tract.
   - **Cirrhosis:** Jaundice, ascites, purpura, spider angiomas
   - **Peutz-Jeghers syndrome (PJS):** Lip lentigines
   - **Inflammatory bowel disease:** Pyoderma gangrenosum (PG)
   - **Gardner syndrome:** Osteomas, epidermoid cysts

   Many diseases of the skin also involve the oral and anal mucosa. Embryologically, the foregut (forming the oral epithelium) and the hindgut (creating the anal mucosa) share a common ectodermal component in the first few weeks of fetal development. Therefore, it is entirely logical that some diseases that affect the gastrointestinal (GI) system also affect the skin.

2. What is jaundice (icterus) and when is it apparent in the skin?
   On average, 250 to 350 mg of bilirubin are generated each day, with 70% to 80% arising from senescent red blood cells and the remainder coming from heme proteins in the bone marrow and liver. Jaundice is the overaccumulation of bilirubin and various bile pigments in the skin and other organs. It may arise from obstruction in cholelithiasis, hemolysis with overproduction of bilirubin, ineffective erythropoiesis, or intrinsic liver disease. Clinically, jaundice is first apparent in ocular sclera, the skin of the face, and the sublingual tongue. The condition is best appreciated in bright daylight and may be overlooked indoors. Jaundice is not clinically apparent until serum bilirubin approximates 2.0 to 2.5 mg/dL in the adult and 5 mg/dL in the neonate. Jaundice may be the first sign of hepatic dysfunction. Conversely, yellowed skin, with normal *white* ocular sclerae, may be seen with carotenemia (excessive beta-carotene from carrots, squash, and sweet potatoes), lycopenemia (tomatoes, beets, and berries), and the drugs quinacrine and busulfan.

Frew JW, Murrell DF, Haber RM. Fifty shades of yellow: a review of the xanthodermatoses. *Int J Dermatol.* 2015;54:1109–1123.

3. What can the shade of jaundice reveal about the type of liver disease in a patient?
   Yellow discoloration of the skin is caused by bilirubin. More orange shades come from xanthorubin (intrahepatic jaundice). A deep green color is due to marked biliverdinemia and is characteristic of obstructive jaundice, such as that caused by pancreatic cancer. Patients with hepatobiliary disease, especially obstructive jaundice, often have severe pruritus. Constant scratching results in inflammation of the skin followed by postinflammatory hyperpigmentation. Postinflammatory hyperpigmentation in the presence of bile pigments imparts a bronze color to the skin. "Bronzing" is also encountered in hemochromatosis and primary Addison disease. The differential diagnosis of jaundice includes carotenemia, lycopenemia, infections with *Clonorchis sinensis* (travel to Asia) or *Fasciola hepatica* (ingesting watercress), and the sallow skin of myxedema.

4. List the top 10 skin findings suggestive of hepatic and biliary tract disease.

Jaundice	Purpura
Pigment changes	Loss of body hair
Spider angioma	Gynecomastia
Palmar erythema	Peripheral edema
Dilated abdominal wall veins	Nonpalpable gallbladder

Hepatobiliary diseases can be associated with alterations of the cutenaous vasculature, such as spider angiomas, palmar erythema, and cutaneous varices. Spider angiomas are classically associated with chronic liver disease, yet these lesions may also be seen in pregnancy, oral contraceptive use, and in normal persons, especially children. In chronic liver disease, spider angiomas may be numerous on the face, neck, upper chest, hands, and forearms. "Liver palms" refers to the mottled erythema and increased warmth of the palms (and sometimes the soles of the feet) in chronic liver disease. Palmar erythema also may be seen in pregnancy, lupus erythematosus, pulmonary disease, and hyperthyroidism.

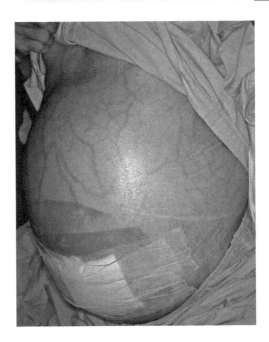

Fig. 36.1 Marked ascites with marked dilatation of the abdominal veins reflecting underlying venous portal hypertension. (Courtesy Fitzsimons Army Medical Center teaching files.)

5. **What are the most common cutaneous findings associated with portal venous hypertension?**
   Portal venous hypertension due to chronic liver disease leads to collateral circulation, with esophageal varices, as an example. In the skin, this same phenomenon may lead to dilation of abdominal wall veins (Fig. 36.1). Caput medusa refers to the dilated periumbilical veins and has been known for centuries as a marker of advanced liver disease. In men with chronic liver disease, induction of a "hyperestrogen state" (due to a decreased estrogen breakdown in the diseased liver) leads to gynecomastia; testicular atrophy; loss of axillary, truncal, and pubic hair; and a female pattern to the pubic hair. Purpura, ecchymoses, and gingival bleeding reflect impaired hepatic production of clotting factors, especially the vitamin K–dependent factors. Peripheral edema and ascites indicate hypoalbuminemia and/or portal venous hypertension.

6. **What is the most common skin symptom associated with liver disease?**
   In liver disease, pruritus is common. Primary biliary cirrhosis, diseases caused by biliary tract obstruction, and cholestatic jaundice may have severe pruritus. Moreover, constant scratching may lead to excoriations, pigment disturbances, and lichenification of the skin.

7. **What skin signs may be associated with GI bleeding?**
   See Table 36.1.

Table 36.1 Conditions associated with gastrointestinal bleeding and skin lesions

Inflammatory conditions	**Vascular malformations and tumors**
Ulcerative colitis	Hereditary hemorrhagic telangiectasia (Osler-Weber-Rendu)
Crohn's disease	Kaposi's sarcoma
Henoch-Schönlein purpura	Blue rubber bleb nevus syndrome
Polyarteritis nodosa	
Hereditary polyposis syndromes	**Miscellaneous**
Gardner's syndrome	Ehlers-Danlos syndrome
Peutz-Jeghers syndrome	Pseudoxanthoma elasticum
Multiple hamartoma syndrome (Cowden's syndrome)	

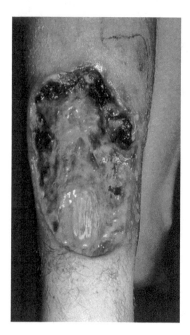

Fig. 36.2 Pyoderma gangrenosum. Large necrotic undermined ulcer of the lower leg with exposed tendon in a patient with ulcerative colitis. (Courtesy Fitzsimons Army Medical Center teaching files.)

8. What is pyoderma gangrenosum?

PG is a severe ulcerative condition that is associated with inflammatory bowel disease, autoimmune hepatitis, rheumatoid disease, and lymphoproliferative disease. The condition is more common in women, and in 70% of cases it affects the lower legs (Fig. 36.2). PG begins as a small, tender pustule that breaks down quickly to form a painful and rapidly expanding necrotic ulcer with a undermined violaceous edge. The condition manifests *pathergy*, which his development of skin lesions at sites of minor trauma. The ulcers of PG may become quite large and deep and may even become circumferential and threaten a limb. Lesions frequently heal with a thin, atrophic scar.

9. What is the cause of PG?

The cause of PG is unknown, but it is though that immune complex–mediated neutrophilic vascular reactions in the skin are involved. Impaired neutrophil phagocytosis, abnormal neutrophil trafficking, and overexpression of interleukin-8 (IL-8) or IL-16 may also play a role in pathogenesis. After the diagnosis of PG is made, the next step should be to look for an associated condition, which occurs in about 50% of cases (the remainder are considered idiopathic). Associated conditions are inflammatory bowel disease (ulcerative colitis or Crohn's disease), autoimmune hepatitis, rheumatoid arthritis, lupus erythematosus, HIV infection, and lymphoproliferative disorders. About 2% of patients with ulcerative colitis have PG, and while the diseases may present concurrently, sometimes a patient may have PG for several years before the inflammatory bowel disease becomes clinically apparent. PG is treated with high-dose oral corticosteroids with transition to steroid-sparing agents such as cyclosporine or mycophenoloate mofetil. Infliximab (tumor necrosis factor-α [TNF-α] blocker) may also be used to treat PG, as well as coexisting inflammatory bowel disease or rheumatoid arthritis. Adalimumab, another TNF-α blocker, has also been reported effective for treating some cases of PG.

Alavi A, French LE, Davis MD, et al. Pyoderma gangrenosum: an update on pathophysiology, diagnosis and treatment. *Am J Clin Dermatol.* 2017;18:355–372.

10. A patient presents with anemia, blood in the stool, and red macules on his lips/tongue. What diagnosis should be considered first?

Hereditary hemorrhagic telangiectasia (HHT), also known as Osler-Weber-Rendu syndrome, is key consideration. HHT is an autosomal dominant genetic. Two subtypes exist: HHT-1 and HHT-2, due to *ENG* (9q33-34) and *ALK-1* (2q13) transforming growth factor-β1 receptor mutations, respectively. Persons with HHT develop linear, punctate, and papular red lesions (telangiectasias) on the lips, face, mucous membranes, fingers (Fig. 36.3A,B), and toes beginning in childhood. These telangiectasias blanch with light pressure, unlike angiomas or petechiae, which are persistent.

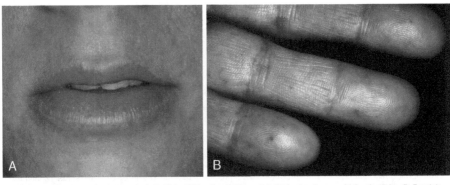

Fig. 36.3 Hereditary hemorrhagic telangiectasia (Osler-Weber-Rendu disease). **A,** Perioral and mucosal telangiectasias. **B,** Punctate telangiectasias of the fingers. (Courtesy Fitzsimons Army Medical Center teaching files.)

The entire GI tract may also be affected with similar lesions, and bleeding may be minimal (causing a chronic iron-deficiency anemia) or massive (leading to severe and sometimes fatal blood loss). The nasal mucosa may be involved, and in children, recurrent severe nosebleeds (epistaxis) may suggest the diagnosis even before other more typical findings foment. The diagnosis of HHT requires three of four criteria be met (epistaxis, telangiectasias, visceral lesions, first-degree relative with HHT). Patients continue to develop new lesions throughout life. Individuals with the HHT-1 subtype (endoglin mutation on chromosome 9) have an increased risk of arteriovenous malformations of the lungs, liver (causing cirrhosis), and brain.

Orizaga-Y-Quiroga TL, Villarreal-Martínez A, Jaramillo-Moreno G, et al. Osler-Weber-Rendu syndrome in relation to dermatology. *Actas Dermosifiliogr.* 2019;110:526–532.

11. What dermatologic conditions present with pigmented macules on the lips?
    Several conditions present with pigmented macules on the lips. The most important one concerning the GI tract is PJS. PJS presents with intestinal polyps, an increased risk of cancer, and characteristic skin findings in 95% of cases. PJS is also an autosomal dominant disorder that appears at birth or in infancy with small round to oval macules that vary from brown to blue-brown in color. These lentigines most often present on the lips and buccal mucosa (Fig. 36.4), but lesions may also involve the nose, palms, soles, fingers, hard palate, and gingiva. The lip macules are usually not present at birth but develop later.

12. What are the GI manifestations of PJS?
    Individuals with PJS have polyps in the small intestine, usually the jejunum and ileum. These polyps present around 11 to 13 years of age. When only a few polyps are present, there may be no symptoms. A large number of polyps

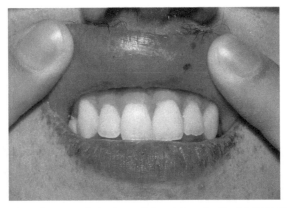

Fig. 36.4 Peutz-Jeghers syndrome. Numerous perioral and mucosal pigmented macules. (Courtesy Fitzsimons Army Medical Center teaching files.)

may lead to intussusception with abdominal pain and bleeding or obstruction. These polyps are hamartomas, which means that they are composed of benign elements normally present in the foregut. With PJS, there is a 2% to 3% risk of intestinal malignancy in patients with PJS, but a 37% chance of any type of cancer by age 65. In addition, it has been discovered that patients with this syndrome have a higher risk of developing cancer of the ovary, uterus, breast, endometrium, testicles, GI tract, lungs, and pancreas. Recent studies indicate that PJS arises from mutations in a tumor suppressor gene (19p13.5, gene *STK11/LKB1*) that normally regulates cell cycle progression. Forty percent of these mutations are spontaneous.

Sengupta S, Bose S. Peutz-Jeghers syndrome. *N Engl J Med.* 2019;380:472.

13. What is the appropriate treatment for patients with PJS?

Close ongoing surveillance and polypectomy of lesions in the small bowel are necessary. Treatment with inhibitors of cyclooxygenase-2 (COX-2 inhibitors, celecoxib) may lead to a dramatic reduction in the burden of polyps and need for surgical resection. Rapamycin (sirolimus) shows promise for PJS treatment by binding to FKBP12, and this yields an antiproliferative effects and dramatic reduction of polyp production/size.

Kopacova M, Tacheci I, Rejchrt S, et al. Peutz-Jeghers syndrome: diagnostic and therapeutic approach. *World J Gastroenterol.* 2009; 15(43):5397–5408.

14. What is pseudoxanthoma elasticum (PXE)? How does this condition cause GI bleeding?

PXE is a genetic disorder caused by mutations in the ABCC6 gene, which codes for a cellular transport protein. The condition is inherited in an autosomal recessive fashion. Cutaneous lesions associated with PXE include yellow papules on the flexural areas of the neck, axillae, and that are likened in appearance to "plucked chicken skin." The basic defect is in elastic tissue in various organs—the skin, blood vessels, eyes, and heart—and the result is calcified and dysfunctional elastic fibers. This can result in issues such as hypertension and retinal hemorrhage and vision change. Skin lesions develop in adolescence or early adulthood, and the condition is typically bilateral and symmetric. In addition to the neck, the axillae, antecubital fossae, abdomen, and thighs or other large flexor surfaces may be involved. Affected women outnumber men by 2:1.

Tsang SH, Sharma T. Inborn errors of metabolism: pseudoxanthoma elasticum. *Adv Exp Med Biol.* 2018;1085:187–189.

15. What are the internal manifestations of PXE?

Yellow papules of PXE may be seen in the mouth (Fig. 36.5), esophagus, and stomach. Involvement of the elastic tissue of the gastric arteries may result in sudden and massive gastric hemorrhage. Involvement of the eye, specifically Bruch's membrane, causes angioid streaks of the retina. Sudden hemorrhage with acute loss of vision may be a presenting sign of the disease. Involvement of larger vessels can result in claudication, hypertension, and cardiac angina, even at an early age. There is no specific treatment.

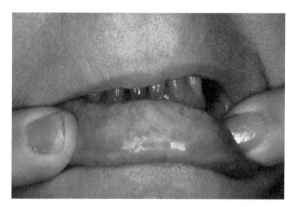

Fig. 36.5 Pseudoxanthoma elasticum. Characteristic yellow macular and papular lesions on the lip mucosa in a patient with pseudoxanthoma elasticum. (Courtesy Fitzsimons Army Medical Center teaching files.)

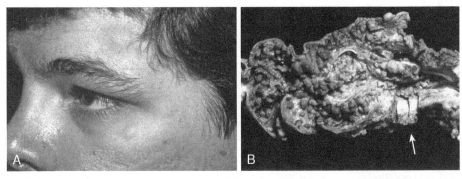

Fig. 36.6 Gardner's syndrome. **A,** Epidermoid cysts about and below the eyebrow as a cutaneous manifestation of Gardner's syndrome. **B,** Segment of colon demonstrating numerous polyps and colon adenocarcinoma at the site of the *arrow.* (Courtesy Fitzsimons Army Medical Center teaching files.)

16. **What is Gardner's syndrome?**
    Gardner syndrome is a familial adenomatous polyposis syndrome that is inherited in an autosomal dominant fashion. The condition is caused by mutations of the *APC* gene on chromosome 5c21. *APC* is a gene that yields a tumor suppressor protein with a role in cell-to-cell adhesion, signal transduction, and transcription activation. Patients with Gardner syndrome have numerous epidermoid cysts in the skin (50% to 65%), dental abnormalities including osteomas of the mandible, intra-abdominal desmoid tumors, and premalignant adenomatous polyps throughout the colon (Fig. 36.6A,B). Congenital retinal pigmentation that manifests as a dark patch on the retinal epithelium may be an early presenting sign. The incidence of Gardner syndrome in the United States is 1 in a million. The average age at onset is 22 years, and the lifetime risk of colon cancer in untreated patients is essentially 100%. Affected patients also have a predisposition to cancers of the thyroid, small intestine, brain, adrenal gland, and liver. Deforming osteomas may require excision, although the other skin manifestations of Gardner syndrome do not typically require treatment. For GI polyps, excision is preferred.

Shah KR, Boland CR, Patel M, et al. Cutaneous manifestations of gastrointestinal disease. *J Am Acad Dermatol.* 2013;68:189–245.

17. **How can cancer of the GI tract present in the skin?**
    The skin may be involved with GI tract malignancy in several ways. Metastases from a primary GI tract cancer can involve the skin. This happens most often with adenocarcinoma of the colon (see Chapter 47, Fig. 47.7). The skin and GI tract may also be both affected by a genetic disease, such as the pancreatic cancer syndrome associated with multiple atypical nevi and melanoma (chromosome 9p21, *CDKN2A*). There is also a large number of paraneoplastic dermatoses that may be associated with an underlying GI malignancy. For example, "malignant" acanthosis nigricans (AN) may be associated with gastric adenocarcinoma. Superficial migratory thrombophlebitis (SMT) (Trousseau sign) may be associated with carcinoma of the pancreas. Glucagonoma syndrome caused by pancreatic cancer may yield necrolytic migratory erythema.

18. **What is "malignant" AN?**
    AN may be caused by endocrine disorders (insulin resistance), obesity (Fig. 36.7), medications, genetic abnormalities, or underlying cancer. The sudden onset of widespread AN in an adult, particularly with unintended weight loss, should suggest an underlying malignancy. Malignant AN initially presents abruptly as a darkening and thickening of the skin, occasionally with pruritus. This morphology progresses into symmetrical hyperpigmented, velvety plaques that occur most commonly around the posterior neck, axilla, and groin. Many different cancers have been reported with "malignant" AN, but almost 60% of patients have gastric adenocarcinoma. Gastric adenocarcinoma secretes TNF-α, which stimulates the epidermal growth factor (EGF) receptor to cause proliferation of keratinocytes.

    Typically, malignant AN develops when the cancer is advanced. For paraneoplastic AN, one-third of patients have skin disease before the cancer is diagnosed, one-third have cancer and the skin disease diagnosed concurrently, and one-third present with skin disease after the internal malignancy is already known. Treatment for malignant AN is correction of the underlying pathology. In some cases, successful resection of the adenocarcinoma leads to disappearance of AN.

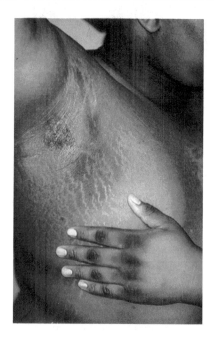

Fig. 36.7 Acanthosis nigricans. Velvety hyperpigmented lesions of the neck, axilla, and knuckles in an obese individual. (Courtesy Fitzsimons Army Medical Center teaching files.)

19. **What are tripe palms?**

"Tripe palms" is another paraneoplastic condition, related to AN, in which the palms appear velvety, with furrowing of the palmar surfaces. The condition is almost always associated with internal malignancy. When tripe palms occur in the absence of AN, squamous cell carcinoma should be suspected. The sign of Leser-Trélat (the explosive onset of a large number of seborrheic keratoses) can also be associated with AN and tripe palms. All these conditions are thought to result from the same circulating EGFs. Leser-Trélat may also be seen with tumors of the female reproductive tract and with lymphoproliferative disorders.

Thiers BH, Sahn RE, Callen JP. Cutaneous manifestations of internal malignancy. *CA Cancer J Clin*. 2009;59(2):85–86.

20. **What is SMT?**

SMT may be caused by increased blood coagulability, leading to venous thrombosis, and this can occur in the setting of pancreatic cancer. The pancreatic cancer may be asymptomatic at the time SMT develops. SMT is associated with an underlying malignancy in about 50% of cases.

SMT presents as cropped, tender, erythematous, linear cords along the course of superficial veins of the trunk and extremities. Lesions in one area may be resolving, while new lesions are developing elsewhere. It is essential that any patient presenting with SMT undergo a thorough evaluation to rule out an underlying malignancy.

21. **How do malignancies produce SMT?**

It is thought that SMT is caused by mucin-secreting abdominal adenocarcinomas because the mucin interacts with L and P selectins, which in turn yields aggregation and emboli formation. SMT is remarkably resistant to oral anticoagulant therapy such as warfarin but does respond well to low-molecular-weight heparin therapy, which is postulated to inhibit tumor growth, instead of acting though its traditional anticoagulatory mechanism. Current research indicates that dalteparin and nadroparin may elicit improved outcomes and higher survival rates. SMT is not specific for GI malignancies and has also been associated with carcinoma of the lung and breast, Hodgkin's disease, and multiple myeloma. Other associations that are not paraneoplastic include Behçet's disease and rickettsial infections.

Thayalasekaran S, Liddicoat H, Wood E. Thrombophlebitis migrans in a man with pancreatic adenocarcinoma: a case report. *Cases J*. 2009;2:6610.

KEY POINTS: JAUNDICE

1. Bilirubin has a strong affinity for tissues rich in elastic tissue, which is why it accumulates earliest in the sclera of the eye followed by the skin (especially the face), hard palate, and abdominal wall.
2. The yellow coloration in the skin is due to bilirubin, while the orange shades come from xanthorubin and the greenish hue is due to biliverdin.
3. Patients with jaundice that has an orange hue are more likely to have intrahepatic jaundice, while patients with a greenish hue are more likely to have obstructive jaundice.
4. Clinically apparent jaundice is not noticeable until the serum bilirubin exceeds 2.0 to 2.5 mg/dL in the adult.
5. Infants may have much higher levels of bilirubin in the serum (i.e., >5.0 mg/dL) before they become clinically jaundiced.

22. **How is inflammation of the fat (panniculitis) associated with pancreatic disease?**
    The pancreas is a 99% exocrine (pancreatic digestive enzyme) and a 1% endocrine (insulin, glucagon) organ. Acute pancreatitis can be caused by viral infection, drugs, alcohol, pancreatic cancer, or trauma, and this leads to a massive outpouring of digestive enzymes. Patients with pancreatitis are extremely ill with fever, vomiting, eosinophilia, and severe abdominal pain. About 2% to 3% of patients with acute pancreatitis develop tender red fluctuant nodules on the lower legs (Fig. 36.8), but lesions may also be seen on the buttocks, trunk, arms, and scalp. These nodules rupture and discharge a thick, oily liquid. The nodules are often accompanied by joint pain and swelling. Schmid's triad (panniculitis, polyarthritis, and eosinophilia) denotes a poor prognosis.
    The disease is caused by pancreatic lipase, phospholipase, trypsin, and amylase that migrate into tissue to cause the inflammation. It is felt that these pancreatic enzymes cause autodigestion of the fat in the subcutaneous tissue and periarticular fat pads. Pancreatic panniculitis may also be seen with chronic pancreatitis, pancreatic cancer (acinar type), and other pancreatic abnormalities. The histopathology is distinctive, with a lobular liquefactive necrosis and "ghost adipocytes" (granular, basophilic material in the cytoplasm secondary to calcium deposition) with neutrophils and other inflammatory cells. Administration of octreotide (inhibiting pancreatic enzyme manufacture) results in cessation of symptoms.

Zundler S, Strobel D, Manger B. Pancreatic panniculitis and polyarthritis. *Curr Rheumatol Rep.* 2017;19:62.

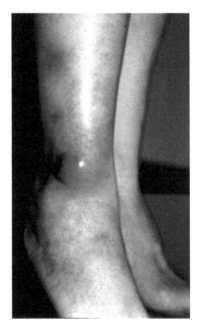

Fig. 36.8 Pancreatic panniculitis. Tender, erythematous, fluctuant nodules on the lower legs of a patient with acute pancreatitis.

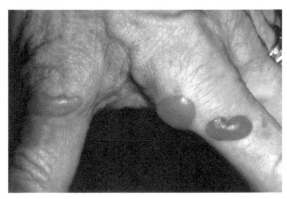

Fig. 36.9 Porphyria cutanea tarda (PCT). Vesicles and blisters, some hemorrhagic, on the digits of a patient with PCT.

23. **What chronic liver disease is associated with photosensitivity and causes blistering and scarring of the skin?**
Porphyria cutanea tarda (PCT) is a metabolic disease characterized by skin fragility, chronic blistering, and scarring of the dorsal hands, forearms, ears, and face associated with photosensitivity to sunlight (Fig. 36.9). In addition to the blistering and scarring, skin findings include thickened, coarse hairs *(hypertrichosis)* over the temples, forehead, and cheeks; occasional shiny, thickened, scleroderma-like changes *(pseudoscleroderma)* of the face, scalp, posterior neck, and torso; and hyperpigmentation or hypopigmentation.

PCT is either of autosomal dominant inheritance with incomplete penetrance or it is acquired (sporadic). It is classified into three types, I to III. Type I is sporadic with no enzyme mutation. Type II is familial with mutations in the *UROD* (uroporphyrinogen decarboxylase) gene, whereas type III is familial with no *UROD* gene mutations. The biochemical defect in chromosome 3q12 (*UROD* gene) leads to a deficiency of the hepatic and red blood cell enzyme uroporphyrinogen decarboxylase. Resultant overproduction of porphyrin precursors by the liver, which are photosensitizing compounds, leads to thickening of the dermal perivascular dermis after sunlight exposure.

There is a high incidence of liver disease and iron overload in patients with PCT. Recent studies have shown that mutations in the *HFE* gene (the hemochromatosis gene), which regulates intestinal absorption of iron, are seen with hemochromatosis and lead to an increased risk of PCT. Factors that may trigger attacks of PCT include alcohol abuse, hepatitis C infection, estrogens (especially oral contraceptives), and HIV infection.

24. **What are the best ways to establish a diagnosis of PCT?**
Bedside diagnosis may include demonstration of pink-red fluorescence of patient urine when exposed to ultraviolet light. A Wood lamp can be used for this test (see Chapter 3, Fig. 3.3). Patients also have increased total body iron stores reflected in increased serum iron and ferritin levels. Quantitative measurement of the urine porphyrins in a 24-hour urine specimen is the gold standard for making the diagnosis.

25. **How is PCT treated?**
Treatment of PCT includes elimination of alcohol and other predisposing medications, photoprotection, phlebotomy (to reduce iron stores), and ***low-dose*** antimalarial therapy (chloroquine). High-dose antimalarial therapy in this setting can be fatal. Coexisting hepatitis C should also be treated.

Stölzel U, Doss MO, Schuppan D. Clinical guide and update on porphyrias. *Gastroenterology.* 2019;157:365–381.

26. **What chronic skin disease is associated with a gluten-sensitive enteropathy?**
Dermatitis herpetiformis (DH) is an autoimmune bullous skin disease that is associated with gluten-sensitive enteropathy (celiac disease). Onset of DH usually occurs between 20 and 40 years of age. Men are affected twice as often as women. Patients with DH develop intensely itchy papules, papulovesicles, and occasionally tense blisters that are grouped (herpetiform). A symmetrical distribution over the scalp and posterior neckline, shoulders and back, elbows, knees, and the lumbosacral region is common (Fig. 36.10A). Rarely, urticarial lesions without papulovesicles may be the only manifestation of disease. Lesions on the palms are uncommon, and the mucous membranes are rarely involved. Over 90% of patients will have histologic evidence of a gluten-sensitive enteropathy, ranging from increased intraepithelial lymphocytes to complete villous atrophy of the jejunum.

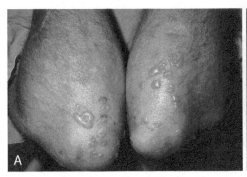
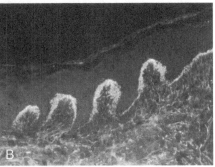

Fig. 36.10 Dermatitis herpetiformis (DH). **A,** Pruritic vesicles and bullae in a symmetrical distribution on the elbows, characteristic location for the lesions of DH. **B,** Direct immunofluorescence of lesional skin in dermatitis herpetiformis showing granular deposits of IgA in the tips of dermal papillae. (Courtesy Fitzsimons Army Medical Center teaching files.)

The disease in the skin and the intestinal tract is triggered by dietary gluten found in many grains (but not in rice, corn, or oats). There are usually no abdominal symptoms (subclinical intestinal disease), but the occasional patient may complain of bloating, cramping, and diarrhea. A gluten-free diet will result in full resolution of all skin and GI disease, but for many patients such a diet is challenge to adhere to.

Histologically, DH is characterized by the accumulation of polymorphonuclear neutrophils (PMNs) and granular deposits of immunoglobulin A (IgA) in the tips of the dermal papillae (Fig. 36.10B). These findings are considered diagnostic of DH. Direct immunofluorescence has high sensitivity in detecting the disease, and deposition of immunoreactants is retained in the skin for months after adopting a gluten-free diet.

In addition, gluten sensitivity in both DH and celiac disease is almost universally associated with human leukocyte antigens DQ2 and DQ8 located on chromosome 6. Current research indicates that epidermal transglutaminase (eTG) is the autoantigen in DH. IgA antibodies bind to eTG and are deposited in the papillary dermis of the skin, leading to recruitment of PMNs and subsequent inflammation.

Shah KR, Boland CR, Patel M, et al. Cutaneous manifestations of gastrointestinal disease. *J Am Acad Dermatol.* 2013;68:189–245.

27. How is DH treated?

Treatment of DH includes strict adherence to a gluten-free diet and/or the use of dapsone (4,4'-diaminodiphenylsulfone, also used to treat leprosy), sulfasalazine, or potent topical steroids (if oral medications are poorly tolerated or are ineffective). Dapsone is generally the most effective, and the response is so immediate that it is considered diagnostic of DH. Prior to dosing dapsone, a G6PD (glucose-6-phosphate dehydrogenase) level and complete blood count should be checked. DH is a lifelong condition, with only rare periods of brief remission. There is an increased risk of other autoimmune diseases including autoimmune thyroid disease, Sjögren's syndrome, lupus erythematosus, and insulin-dependent diabetes. There is an increased risk of lymphoma, but recent studies have indicated that this increased risk of correlates best with celiac disease where there is more villous atrophy of the GI tract.

Salmi TT. Dermatitis herpetiformis. *Clin Exp Dermatol.* 2019;44:728–731.

CHAPTER 37

CUTANEOUS MANIFESTATIONS OF RENAL DISEASE

Whitney A. High

1. **What skin changes are associated with renal disease?**
   Renal disease can manifest in the skin in three ways:
   - Skin changes that associated with renal failure
   - Systemic diseases with renal and cutaneous manifestations (e.g., Henoch-Schönlein purpura)
   - Diseases affecting the kidney where skin biopsy may be helpful in making the diagnosis, even if cutaneous findings are not prominent (e.g., primary systemic amyloidosis).

Gagnon AL, Desai T. Dermatological diseases in patients with chronic kidney disease. *J Nephropathol.* 2013;2:104–109.

2. **What cutaneous findings occur in renal failure?**
   See Table 37.1.

3. **Do cutaneous signs of chronic renal failure (CRF) resolve with hemodialysis?**
   Unfortunately, many of the cutaneous changes that are associated with CRF persist even after hemodialysis. In fact, some complaints, such as pruritus (itching), may worsen upon starting hemodialysis.

4. **What cutaneous findings are present in patients on dialysis?**
   Many skin changes described in patients with CRF are also found in patients undergoing peritoneal dialysis or hemodialysis. A large percentage of patients receiving dialysis complain of severe pruritus, although aggressive dialysis may, over time, lessen this symptom. Patients on renal dialysis may develop a bullous eruption similar to porphyria cutanea tarda (PCT) (Fig. 37.1A). Acne can occur with dialysis and with exogenous testosterone. Several perforating diseases are associated with CRF, either with or without renal dialysis, including Kyrle disease, reactive perforating collagenosis, and perforating folliculitis. Sometimes, people group these perforating diseases under one term—*acquired perforating dermatosis of CRF*. Dialysis patients may develop cutaneous complications from treatment, such as infections or contact dermatitis in the area of the peritoneal cannula or arteriovenous fistula.

Blaha T, Nigwekar S, Combs S, et al. Dermatologic manifestations in end stage renal disease. *Hemodial Int.* 2019;23:3–18.

Table 37.1 Cutaneous findings in chronic renal failure

FINDING	PERCENT AFFECTED	FINDING	PERCENT AFFECTED
Changes in pigmentation	70%	Keratotic pits of palms and soles	14%
Yellow tinge to skin	40%	Perforating disorder	4%
Hyperpigmented palmoplantar skin	30%	Finger pebbles	86%
Hyperpigmentation that is diffuse or photodistributed	22%	Calcinosis cutis	1%
Pallor	8%	Calciphylaxis	1%
Nail changes	66%	Uremic frost	3%
Half-and-half nails	39%	Porphyria and pseudoporphyria	1.2%–18%
Pale nails	23%	Cutaneous infections	70%
Splinter hemorrhages	11%	Onychomycosis	52%
Xerosis (dry skin) and/or pruritus	63%	Tinea pedis	25%

Data from Pico MR, Lugo-Somolinos A, Sanchez JL, et al. Cutaneous alterations in patients with CRF. *Int J Dermatol* 1992;31:860–863.

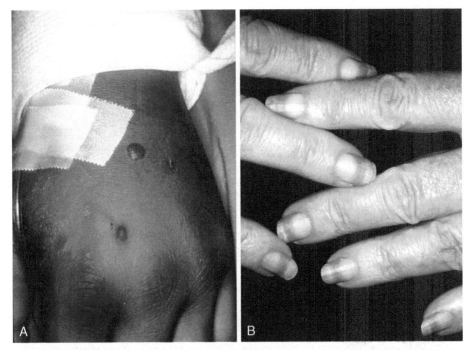

Fig. 37.1 A, Tense vesicle with pseudoporphyria on the dorsal hand of a patient undergoing renal dialysis. **B,** Half-and-half nails in a patient with chronic renal failure.

5. Describe the nail changes in CRF.
   Both "half-and-half" nails (Lindsay nails) and Muehrcke nails are associated with CRF. In "half-and-half" nails, the proximal nail is white while the distal portion retains a normal pink color (Fig. 37.1B). It is believed that edema of the nail bed leads to this appearance. Muehrcke nails are associated with hypoalbuminemia and consist of two transverse white bands, parallel, and separated by normal nailbed.

Muehrcke RC. The fingernails in chronic hypoalbuminaemia: a new physical sign. *BMJ.* 1956;9:1327–1328.

6. What is uremic frost?
   Uremic frost of the face was as a classic manifestation of CRF, but it is rarely seen in modern times. White dusty deposits were noted about the face and neck and were believed due to crystallized urea from sweat. Table 37.2 summarizes the abnormalities of skin color associated with renal failure.

Saardi KM, Schwartz RA. Uremic frost: a harbinger of impending renal failure. *Int J Dermatol.* 2016;55:17–20.

Table 37.2 Abnormalities of skin color associated with renal failure

SKIN FINDING	COLOR	DISTRIBUTION	ETIOLOGY
Uremic frost	White	Face, nostrils, neck	Deposition of crystallized urea from sweat
Pallor	Yellowish	Generalized	Anemia, urochrome deposition
Hyperpigmentation	Brown	Photodistributed or generalized	Increased β-melanocyte–stimulating hormone
Bruising	Red-purple-green-yellow-brown	Sites of trauma	Hemostatic abnormalities

7. What causes the pallor of CRF?

Pallor in CRF is due to anemia. In addition to pallor, a yellow hue to the skin may be present in CRF, believed to be due to urochrome deposition.

8. What causes the pigmentary changes of the skin seen in CR?

In CRF, increased amounts of melanin can be present in the basal layer of the epidermis and in the superficial dermis. It has been proposed that patients with such pigmentation have decreased metabolism of β-melanocyte–stimulating hormone by diseased kidneys, leading to elevated plasma levels of this hormone, in turn leading to increased melanin production by melanocytes.

9. Is pruritus a common finding in all renal failure?

While not all persons with acute renal failure develop pruritus, the symptom is common in patients with CRF. Dialysis may exacerbate this pruritus, at least early on. The precise cause of uremic pruritus is unknown. One study suggested that uremic patients have a histamine-releasing factor in sera that is depleted or diminished by ultraviolet B (UVB) light. Nitric oxide or pruritogenic cytokines may play a role in the pruritus of CRF. Another study found reduction in the total number of skin nerve terminals in uremic patients and proposed that skin innervation was altered in CRF, possibly as a consequence of this neuropathy. Secondary hyperparathyroidism, which sometimes develops in CRF, may also induce pruritus.

Swarna SS, Aziz K, Zubair T, et al. Pruritus associated with chronic kidney disease: a comprehensive literature review. *Cureus.* 2019;11: e5256.

10. How is the pruritus of renal failure treated?

First, the cause of CRF should be determined and treated. Second, patients with renal failure may still develop other unrelated skin conditions that cause pruritus, such as scabies or allergic contact dermatitis, and this must be considered. Medication reactions may cause pruritus and should be excluded. Xerosis (dry skin) causes pruritus, and frequent use of emollients, avoidance of irritants, and gentle bathing should be employed. If secondary hyperparathyroidism is thought to be involved in pruritus, surgical therapy (parathyroidectomy) may be utilized. When no specific cause for pruritus is found, treatment with UVB light may be beneficial. Other systemic treatments used with varying degrees of success include antihistamines, gabapentin/pregabalin, mast cell stabilizers (cromolyn sodium), montelukast, thalidomide, opioid agonists/antagonists, thalidomide, erythropoietin, and activated charcoal. The only definitive treatment for pruritus caused by CRF is kidney transplantation.

11. Are there skin changes associated with renal transplants?

Skin signs of CRF may resolve following successful renal transplantation (in contrast to hemodialysis). Cutaneous infections (viral, bacterial, atypical mycobacterial, and fungal) may develop, secondary to immunosuppressive therapy given following transplantation. After years of immunosuppression, benign (verrucae, premalignant keratoses, porokeratosis) and malignant cutaneous tumors (squamous cell carcinoma, malignant melanoma, Kaposi's sarcoma) may develop. Sometimes, numerous tumors may arise simultaneously or at increasingly alarming rates, often demonstrating aggressive histology and a propensity to metastasize. Lowering immunosuppressive therapy, aggressive surveillance and treatment of skin tumors, adding a systemic retinoid such as acitretin, and switching immunosuppressive transplant medications to sirolimus or everolimus (mTOR inhibitors) may help control this serious problem.

12. What is transepidermal elimination? What is its relationship to kidney disease?

Transepidermal elimination underlies a family of diseases, collectively called *perforating disorders*, in which altered components of skin are eliminated through the epidermis. Several different perforating diseases are associated with CRF, including Kyrle disease, reactive perforating collagenosis, and perforating folliculitis. Because features of more than one type of perforating disorder may be identified in patients with CRF, it has been suggested that these conditions be referred to simply as *acquired perforating dermatoses of CRF*. Perforating disorders occur up to 10% of patients on dialysis, but the condition may occur in the setting of renal failure, without dialysis. Lesions consist of keratotic papules and nodules on the trunk and extremities (Fig. 37.2). Perforating disorders are more common in blacks and diabetics. Skin biopsy establishes the diagnosis. Treatment may include antihistamines, topical keratolytics, topical or intralesional corticosteroids, topical or oral retinoids, and UVB phototherapy. The condition can spontaneously resolve over many months.

Hari Kumar KV, Prajapati J, Pavan G, et al. Acquired perforating dermatoses in patients with diabetic kidney disease on hemodialysis. *Hemodial Int.* 2010;14:73–77.
Lukács J, Schliemann S, Elsner P. Treatment of acquired reactive perforating dermatosis—a systematic review. *J Dtsch Dermatol Ges.* 2018;16:825–842.

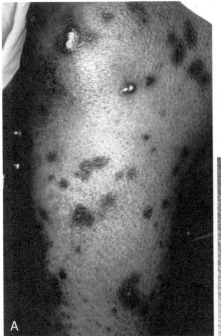
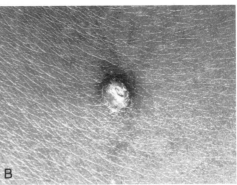

Fig. 37.2 Perforating disease of chronic renal failure. **A,** Small erythematous papules with central crusts or scales are seen on the lower legs. Central umbilication of the papules can be seen, the area of "perforation." The hyperpigmented macules are areas of prior involvement. **B,** Close-up of hyperkeratotic papule demonstrating cell area of perforation. (Courtesy James E. Fitzpatrick, MD.)

13. Describe the porphyria-like eruption of dialysis.

Patients with CRF on dialysis sometimes develop skin fragility, blisters, hyperpigmentation, and hypertrichosis that resemble cutaneous lesions of PCT. While most of these patients do not have elevated systemic porphyrins (pseudoporphyria), some do. When patients are anuric, plasma and fecal specimens must be submitted for porphyrin studies. Elevated porphyrin levels are due to decreased elimination, poor erythropoiesis, decreased activity of uroporphyrinogen decarboxylase (enzyme responsible for PCT), and failure of hemodialysis to remove porphyrins. Exacerbating factors can include hepatitis C infection, iron overload, and medications.

Quaiser S, Khan R, Khan AS. Drug induced pseudoporphyria in CKD: a case report. *Indian J Nephrol.* 2015;25:307–309.
Hamzi MA, Alayoud A, Asseraji M. Porphyria cutanea tarda in a hemodialysis patient with hepatitis virus: efficacy of treatment with multiple phlebotomies and erythropoietin. *Saudi J Kidney Dis Transpl.* 2013;24:121–123.

KEY POINTS: CUTANEOUS MANIFESTATIONS OF RENAL DISEASE

1. Uremic frost consists of white deposits on the head and neck area seen in patients with severe renal failure.
2. The pruritus of renal failure often responds to ultraviolet light B (UVB) therapy.
3. In Fabry's disease, a metabolic disorder that affects the kidney, small vascular lesions, called angiokeratomas, are often found diffusely in a bathing suit distribution.
4. Nephrogenic systemic fibrosis (NSF) is a recently described disease, consisting of papules, plaques, and thickened skin of the trunk and extremities, which is associated with impaired renal function and deposition of gadolinium in tissue from gadolinium-based contrast media used in magnetic imaging studies.

14. What is Fabry's disease?

Fabry's disease (angiokeratoma corporis diffusum, Anderson-Fabry disease) is a genetic disease caused by mutations in the GLA gene that result in a defective level of the lysosomal enzyme α-*galactosidase A*. In turn, this leads to deposition of neutral glycosphingolipids, such as trihexosyl ceramides, in cells and tissues of the body, particularly the vascular endothelium. The disease is X-linked recessive, with nearly all affected patients being male.

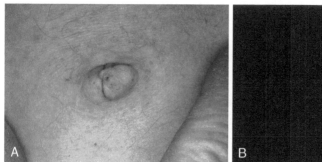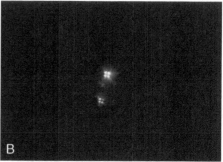

Fig. 37.3 A. Red to reddish-purple angiokeratomas in the umbilical area of a patient with Fabry's disease. **B.** Polarized urine sediment of a patient with Fabry's disease demonstrating characteristic "Maltese crosses." (Courtesy Fitzsimons Army Medical Center teaching files.)

Heterozygous females are usually asymptomatic but may have characteristic corneal opacities. A serologic test to assess enzyme function exists. Families at risk for Fabry's disease should have genetic counseling to discuss family planning options. In vitro fertilization, with a preimplantation genetic testing, is an option for mothers who are carriers. DNA from a fetus can also be assessed to determine GLA gene status. Chorionic villus sampling can be performed at 10 to 12 weeks, or amniocentesis can be performed at 13 and 20 weeks, to test for Fabry's disease.

15. Describe the skin lesions in Fabry's disease.
Diffuse angiokeratomas, seen in a "bathing suit distribution," between the waist and the knees, are seen in Fabry's disease. The lesions begin in childhood as pinpoint red to purplish macules or flat papules with slight scale, and progress in size and number (Fig. 37.3A). Lesions may be subtle on occasion. A skin biopsy may aid in diagnosis, because special stains such as Sudan black B, scarlet red, or periodic acid–Schiff may demonstrate glycolipid deposition in skin. Electron microscopy may be used to assist in diagnosis, and it demonstrates characteristic cytoplasmic glycolipid deposits in endothelial cells ("*zebra bodies*"). Polarizing microscopy of urine reveals birefringent lipid globules ("*Maltese crosses*") (Fig. 37.3B). Other findings in patients with Fabry's disease include acroparesthesias and acute attacks of severe pain, particularly in the palms and soles, often beginning in childhood. In adult life, cardiac ischemia and infarcts, transient ischemic attacks, stroke, and *progressive kidney failure* can develop. Hyperhidrosis or hypohidrosis can occur due to autonomic dysfunction. Recently, treatment with enzyme replacement therapy has become available in Europe (α-Gal A) and the United States (agalsidase β [Fabrazyme]).
NOTE: Other disorders with enzyme deficiencies may be associated with angiokeratomas such as aspartylglycosaminuria, galactosialidosis, GM1 gangliosidosis, fucosidosis, Kanzaki disease, β-mannosidosis, and sialidosis.

Giuseppe P, Daniel R, Rita BM. Cutaneous complications of Anderson-Fabry disease. *Curr Pham Des*. 2013;19:6031–6036.

16. What are five forms of vasculitis that frequently involve the kidneys and skin?
   - *Leukocytoclastic vasculitis* not otherwise specified (NOS) (immune complex–mediated postcapillary vasculitis: palpable purpura of skin, glomerulonephritis of kidneys). Etiologies may include systemic lupus erythematosus (SLE), other connective tissue diseases, infections, drugs, malignancies, etc.
   - *Henoch-Schönlein purpura* (recent streptococcal infection, palpable purpura of skin with IgA-mediated vasculitis, abdominal pain and/or hematochezia due to gastrointestinal vasculitis, arthritis, and glomerulonephritis)
   - *Polyarteritis nodosa* (small and medium vessel vasculitis with tender nodular or ulcerative cutaneous lesions, livedo racemosa, retiform purpura, efferent renal arteriole vasculitis/hypertension, neuropathy, central nervous system, cardiac, and systemic symptoms)
   - *Microscopic polyangiitis* (small vessel vasculitis of skin causing palpable purpura, glomerulonephritis of kidneys, neuropathy, systemic symptoms, perinuclear anti-neutrophil cytoplasmic antibodies [p-ANCA] positive)
   - *Granulomatosis with polyangiitis* (formerly *Wegener granulomatosis*): (small and medium vessel vasculitis, granulomatous vasculitis, granulomatous vasculitis of upper airways, lungs, glomerulonephritis of kidneys, neuropathy, cytoplasmic anti-neutrophil cytoplasmic antibodies [c-ANCA] positive)
When skin lesions that suggest vasculitis are observed (*palpable purpura*), a skin biopsy should be performed to confirm the diagnosis and determine the size of the vessel and type of inflammation (see Chapter 15). Vessels involved may vary in size from small postcapillary venules (leukocytoclastic vasculitis) to medium-sized arterioles (polyarteritis nodosa). Additional testing, to include blood pressure, renal function tests, urinalysis for proteinuria, hematuria, and red cell casts, should be performed to assess for renal involvement.

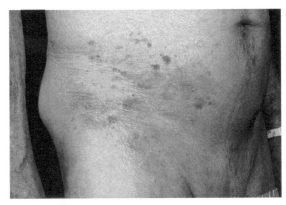

Fig. 37.4 Systemic amyloidosis. Extensive purpura in a patient with diffuse, cutaneous systemic amyloidosis. A skin biopsy demonstrated amyloid deposited in the dermis and subcutaneous tissue. (Courtesy Fitzsimons Army Medical Center teaching files.)

17. How should skin biopsy be used for the diagnosis of systemic amyloidosis?

In primary systemic amyloidosis, immunoglobulin light-chain proteins and serum amyloid P are deposited in skin, tongue, heart, spleen, joints, peripheral nerves, and carpal ligaments due to an underlying plasma cell dyscrasia or multiple myeloma. Cutaneous changes may be present, including purpura of the upper trunk, face, and eyelid, which is very characteristic of primary systemic amyloidosis (Fig. 37.4). Waxy papules, particularly on the palms and fingertips, have also been reported. Secondary systemic amyloidosis is due to chronic inflammatory diseases, such as tuberculosis and other infections, connective tissue diseases, hidradenitis suppurativa, and familial periodic fever syndromes, and is due to deposition of a distinctive non-immunoglobulin protein designated AA (amyloid A protein), of which the precursor is an acute-phase reactant produced by the liver. Cutaneous lesions due to amyloid deposits are rarely seen in this type of amyloidosis. Even when cutaneous changes are absent, a skin biopsy can assist in making a diagnosis of primary or secondary systemic amyloidosis. Biopsies of skin, abdominal fat, tongue, rectum, and minor salivary gland have been used to confirm such a diagnosis, avoiding the need for more invasive biopsies of internal organs.

Wong CK, Wang WJ. Systemic amyloidosis. A report of 19 cases. *Dermatology.* 1994;189:47–51.

18. What is NSF (nephrogenic fibrosing dermopathy)?

NSF is a systemic disorder with prominent cutaneous findings that occurs in patients with impaired renal function who received gadolinium-based contrast media for magnetic imaging studies. NSF presents as thickened or edematous skin of the extremities and trunk. In severe cases, issues with range of motion and disabling contracture of the joints occur. The fibrosis may involve extracutaneous sites, such as the sclera (yellow scleral plaques), heart, lungs, and skeletal muscle. Biopsy demonstrates increased CD34-positive and procollagen-positive fibroblasts with mucin. Using energy dispersive x-ray spectroscopy, researchers first discovered gadolinium in affected tissue, and this discovery was confirmed by other means, such as mass spectroscopy. The discovery led to a new "black-box" warning on gadolinium-based contrast media. Avoidance of these agents in persons at risk dramatically reduced disease incidence. Unfortunately, treatment of existing disease is challenging, but it has included sodium thiosulfate, imatinib mesylate, and UVA1 phototherapy.

High WA, Ayers RA, Chandler J, et al. Gadolinium is detectable within the tissue of patients with nephrogenic systemic fibrosis. *J Am Acad Dermatol.* 2007;56:21–26.

19. What is calciphylaxis?

Calciphylaxis is metastatic calcification of vasculature that occurs in patients with CRF. In the skin, it is characterized by acute, painful, ischemic necrosis. Women, diabetic patients, and obese individuals are at risk for calciphylaxis. Calciphylaxis may present initially with retiform purpura that progresses to painful, gray, bullous, or gangrenous cutaneous lesions, often leading to sepsis and death, even despite intervention. Impaired excretion of phosphate and impaired production of 1,25-dihydroxyvitamin D_3 are theorized to be initiating events. This leads to hypocalcemia and a subsequent increase in parathyroid hormone mobilization of calcium and phosphate from bone, which, in turn, leads to hyperphosphatemia and an elevated calcium-phosphorus, with resulting calcification of the small vessels in the skin and organs. Defects in matrix gla protein, a substance that inhibits vascular calcification, may also play a role. Triggers

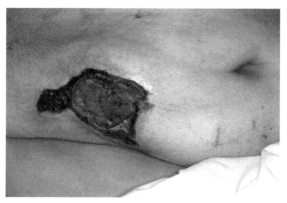

Fig. 37.5 Calciphylaxis of the lower abdomen in a patient with chronic renal failure demonstrating skin necrosis. (Courtesy Fitzsimons Army Medical Center teaching files.)

such as trauma, inflammation, infection, medication, administration of calcium, phosphate binders, and enemas with phosphate components may lead to precipitous thrombosis and calcification of vessels. A skin biopsy that includes subcutaneous fat is necessary to make the diagnosis and to exclude other conditions such as warfarin necrosis, heparin necrosis, oxalosis, or sepsis. The patient prognosis once calciphylaxis has developed is guarded, with more than 50% of patients dying within 1 year of the diagnosis. Treatment is challenging and may include parathyroidectomy, calcium/phosphorus restriction, bisphosphonates, and sodium thiosulfate.

Nigwekar SU. Calciphylaxis. *Curr Opin Nephrol Hypertens.* 2017;26:276–281.

20. What are some diseases that have both skin and renal manifestations?
See Fig. 37.5 and Table 37.3.

Table 37.3 Diseases with both skin and renal manifestations

DISEASE	PATHOGENESIS	CUTANEOUS FINDINGS	ASSOCIATED SYSTEMIC FINDINGS
Systemic sclerosis Renal crisis: abrupt onset of HTN, renal failure, HAs, fever, malaise, retinopathy, encephalopathy, pulmonary edema	Autoimmune disease involving anti–Scl-70, anticentromere, and other antinuclear antibodies resulting in progressive sclerosis of skin and internal organs	Scleroderma, morphea, sclerodactyly, telangiectatic mats, calcinosis cutis, Raynaud's syndrome	Internal organ involvement is frequent and may affect the esophagus, heart, and kidneys; lung involvement is the leading cause of death; **renal crisis** in 5%–10%
Primary systemic amyloidosis Accumulation of amyloid fibrils within vital organs leads to atrophy of normal tissue and interferes with the normal functioning of the organ	Deposits of immunoglobulin light chain (AL), or, less often, heavy chain (HL), around vessels and functional units of skin and internal organs	Pinch purpura; petechiae and ecchymosis around eyelids, neck, axilla, and anus; waxy or purpuric papules, nodules, or plaques on face, neck, scalp, and digits; hemorrhagic blisters Mucosa: macroglossia	**Renal proteinuria, renal failure,** hypoalbuminemia, edema, cardiac failure (congestive heart failure), neurologic deficits (peripheral and autonomic neuropathy), gastrointestinal (motility problems)

Table 37.3 Diseases with both skin and renal manifestations (*Continued*)

DISEASE	PATHOGENESIS	CUTANEOUS FINDINGS	ASSOCIATED SYSTEMIC FINDINGS
Secondary systemic amyloidosis Accumulation of amyloid fibrils within vital organs leads to atrophy of normal tissue and interferes with the normal functioning of the organ	Deposits of amyloid A protein (AA) (chronic inflammatory diseases and hereditary periodic fever syndromes); deposits of β_2 **microglobulin** (patients with CRF receiving **hemodialysis**)	No, or rare, cutaneous findings, but skin often biopsied for diagnosis (abdominal fat pad, minor salivary gland, rectal mucosa, buccal mucosa, tongue)	AA amyloidosis usually affects the **kidneys (proteinuria/renal failure),** liver, spleen, adrenals, and heart; synovial deposits of β_2-microglobulin: carpal tunnel syndrome, bone cysts and destructive spondyloarthropathy
Tuberous sclerosis (Bourneville disease) Epiloia (**epi**lepsy, **lo**w **i**ntelligence, **a**ngiofibroma)	TSC1 (chromosome 9q34) and TSC2 (chromosome 16p13); their protein products are hamartin and tuberin, respectively, which are integral to cell cycle and growth regulation **Polycystic kidney disease** occurs as a contiguous gene syndrome with TSC2	Skin: congenital hypopigmented macules (ash leaf macules), confetti-like hypopigmentation, facial angiofibromas, collagenomas (Shagreen patch), periungual fibromas, café-au-lait macules; mucosa: gingival fibromas and dental enamel pits	Hamartomas can be found in the eye, brain, **kidneys (angiomyolipomas),** liver, heart, lungs, and bones, sometimes progressing to malignancy; seizures, mental deficits, and neuropsychiatric disturbances are common
Nail-patella syndrome (hereditary osteo-onychodysplasia)	*LMX1B* gene: regulates collagen synthesis Dysregulation of the synthesis of collagen in the glomerular basement membrane may contribute to the nephrosis and **glomerulonephritis**	Hypoplasia of radial side of thumbnails, triangular lunula, absent or hypoplastic nails	Absent or hypoplastic patella, radial head dysplasia, iliac crest exostosis (iliac horns); **nephropathy and glomerulonephritis; renal insufficiency**
Birt-Hogg-Dube syndrome	*FLCN (BHD)* gene encodes the tumor suppressor protein folliculin	Fibrofolliculomas, trichodiscomas, and acrochordons	Lung cysts, spontaneous pneumothorax, and **renal tumors (oncocytomas and chromophobe renal cell carcinoma);** colon polyps; neural tumors
Hereditary leiomyomatosis and renal cell cancer (HLRCC) **(Reed's syndrome)**	*FH* gene: fumarate hydratase enzyme activity decreased	Multiple cutaneous leiomyomata or single leiomyoma with positive family history	Uterine leiomyomata (fibroids) and **renal tumors**

CRF, chronic renal failure; *HAs,* headaches; *HTN,* hypertension.

CUTANEOUS MANIFESTATIONS OF AIDS

George W. Turiansky and William D. James

1. How significant is the occurrence of skin disease in the setting of HIV infection?

   Dermatologic diseases are frequently encountered in HIV-infected patients. In one study of 100 serial outpatients, a 92% prevalence of skin disease was noted. Skin disease may also be the first manifestation of HIV disease and may suggest HIV infection because of increased severity of presentation, atypical clinical appearance, or increased resistance to treatment. In addition, mucocutaneous disease, such as an infection or neoplasm, may be the initial sign of a systemic process in an HIV-infected patient. Highly active antiretroviral therapy (HAART) was introduced in 1997 and has significantly decreased the occurrence and severity of many skin conditions associated with HIV infection, such as Kaposi's sarcoma (KS), eosinophilic folliculitis, oral hairy leukoplakia, and molluscum contagiosum.

2. Outline the clinical spectrum of cutaneous disease associated with HIV infection.

   See Table 38.1.

3. What are the most common dermatoses associated with HIV infection?

   Papulosquamous dermatoses are among the most commonly seen cutaneous manifestations of HIV infection, and these include seborrheic dermatitis (Fig. 38.1) and xerosis. Other common dermatologic conditions include bacterial infections, such as *Staphylococcus aureus* skin infections. Fungal infections, such as mucocutaneous candidiasis

Table 38.1 Mucocutaneous diseases seen in HIV infection*

Neoplastic diseases
Kaposi's sarcoma
Lymphoma
Squamous cell carcinoma
Basal cell carcinoma
Anogenital intraepithelial neoplasia
Invasive anogenital carcinoma

Papulosquamous diseases
Seborrheic dermatitis
Xerosis/acquired ichthyosis
Psoriasis
Reiter's syndrome

Miscellaneous diseases
Eosinophilic folliculitis
Drug eruptions
Hyperpigmentations
Photoeruptions
Pruritus
Lipodystrophy
Granuloma annulare
Aphthosis

Infectious diseases
Bacterial
Staphylococcus aureus infections
Syphilis
Bacillary angiomatosis
Botryomycosis

Table 38.1 Mucocutaneous diseases seen in HIV infection (*Continued*)

Fungal
Candida, Penicillium marneffei
Dermatophytosis
Cryptococcosis
Histoplasmosis

Viral
Human papillomavirus (HPV)
Molluscum contagiosum
Herpes simplex virus (HSV)
Varicella-zoster virus (VZV)
Cytomegalovirus (CMV)
Epstein-Barr virus

Arthropods
Scabies

*Dover JS, Johnson RA. Cutaneous manifestations of human immunodeficiency virus infection: parts 1 and 2. *Arch Dermatol.* 1991;127:1383–1391, 1549–1558.

James W, ed. AIDS: a ten-year perspective. *Dermatol Clin.* 1991;9:391–615.

Costner M, Cockerell CJ. The changing spectrum of the cutaneous manifestations of HIV disease. *Arch Dermatol.* 1998;134:1290–1292.

Kaushik SB, Cerci FB, Miracle J, et al. Chronic pruritus in HIV-positive patients in the southeastern United States: Its prevalence and effect on quality of life. *J Am Acad Dermatol.* 2014;70:659–664.

Chapter 38, Cutaneous Manifestations of AIDS, is in the public domain.

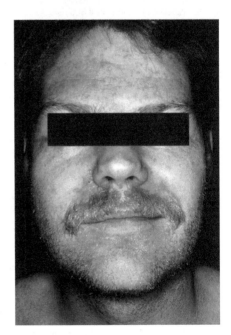

Fig. 38.1 Seborrheic dermatitis. Erythematous patches with yellow scale are present on the forehead, nose, and paranasal areas of an HIV-positive patient. (Courtesy James E. Fitzpatrick, MD.)

(oropharyngeal and vulvovaginal) and dermatophytosis (tinea pedis, tinea cruris, tinea manuum, and onychomycosis), are also commonly encountered. Frequently seen viral infections include human papillomavirus (HPV) infections (condylomata acuminata, common and plantar warts), as well as infections with herpes simplex virus, varicella-zoster virus (VZV), molluscum contagiosum, and Epstein-Barr virus (oral hairy leukoplakia). The cutaneous manifestations of HAART including lipodystrophy and the dermatologic conditions related to the immune restoration syndrome (IRS) are commonly seen.

4. Can mucocutaneous changes occur as a result of primary HIV infection?

   Yes. The earliest cutaneous sign of HIV infection is an exanthem consisting of discrete, erythematous macules and papules that usually measure 10 mm or less. They are located primarily over the trunk but also are seen on the palms and soles. These lesions may become hemorrhagic. The exanthem of acute HIV infection is not clinically or histologically specific. Mucosal changes described include oral, genital, and anal ulcers. These changes are associated with an acute febrile illness.

5. What is the most common bacterial pathogen in HIV disease? How does it manifest itself?

   Staphylococcus aureus is the most common cutaneous bacterial pathogen in HIV disease. Cutaneous infections due to *S. aureus* most commonly present as a superficial folliculitis. Less common manifestations include impetigo, ecthyma, furunculosis, cellulitis, abscesses, and botryomycosis. In addition, *S. aureus* can secondarily infect underlying primary dermatoses such as eczema, scabies, herpetic ulcers, and KS or can colonize intravenous catheter sites. Staphylococcal colonization (carriage) of the nose and flexures (perineal, toe webspaces) is known to increase in HIV disease and may account for the increased incidence of cutaneous infections. As in the general population, infections with community-acquired methicillin-resistant *S. aureus* are becoming increasingly common.

Ahuja D, Albrecht H. HIV and community-acquired MRSA. *AIDS Clin Care.* 2009;21:21–23.

6. What is known about cutaneous malignancy in HIV disease?

   KS or, more specifically, epidemic KS is the most common cutaneous malignancy in HIV disease. In the Swiss HIV Cohort Study, the risk for KS continued to be at least 20-fold higher among HAART-treated individuals compared with that of the general population. Most cases occurred in homosexual or bisexual men with HIV disease. However, KS has also been reported in HIV-negative homosexual males. Human herpesvirus-8 is associated with epidemic as well as other types of KS.

   Omland et al. reported that HIV-infected patients have an increased risk of cutaneous basal cell carcinoma (BCC) and squamous cell carcinoma (SCC) compared to a matched background cohort. The increased BCC risk was restricted to men who reported having sex with men as the route of HIV transmission. Nadir but not current CD4 count was associated with increased SCC risk.

   A study by Asgari et al. comparing HIV-infected with HIV-uninfected individuals diagnosed with at least one nonmelanoma skin cancer (NMSC), defined as BCC or SCC, and excluding genital and oral BCCs and SCCs, showed that HIV-infected individuals were at increased risk of developing subsequent primary NMSC. The risk of subsequent development of SCC but not BCC was associated with recent higher viral loads and lower CD4 counts.

Clifford GM, Polesel J, Richenbach M, et al. Cancer risk in the Swiss HIV Cohort Study: associations with immunodeficiency, smoking, and highly active antiretroviral therapy. *J Natl Cancer Inst.* 2005;97:425–432.
Schwartz RA, Micali G, Nasca MR, et al. Kaposi sarcoma: a continuing conundrum. *J Am Acad Dermatol.* 2008;59:179–206.
Omland SH, Ahlstrom MG, Gerstoft J, et al. Risk of skin cancer in patients with HIV: a Danish nationwide cohort study. *J Am Acad Dermatol.* 2018;79:689–695.
Asgari MM, Ray GT, Quesenberry Jr CP, et al. Association of multiple primary skin cancers with human immunodeficiency virus infection, CD4 count, and viral load. *JAMA Dermatol.* 2017;153:892–896.

7. What are the cutaneous clinical features of epidemic KS?

   Epidemic KS has a widespread, symmetrical distribution of rapidly progressive macules, patches, nodules, plaques, and tumors. Common areas of involvement include the trunk, extremities, face, and oral cavity. Early lesions consist of erythematous macules, patches, or papules that may have a bruise-like halo. They enlarge at different rates and tend to be oval or elongated in shape, following the lines of skin cleavage. The color varies from pink to red, purple, or brown and can easily mimic purpura, hemangiomas, nevi, sarcoidosis, pityriasis rosea, secondary syphilis, lichen planus, BCC, and melanoma. The surface may become scaly, hyperkeratotic, ulcerated, or hemorrhagic.

   Disfigurement and pain secondary to edema can occur, especially on the face, genitals, and lower extremities. *Koebnerization,* or formation of new lesions at sites of trauma, can be seen. Secondary bacterial infection can also occur. Lesions can be arranged in several known patterns, such as a follicular (clustered) pattern (Fig. 38.2), pityriasis rosea–like pattern, or dermatomal pattern.

8. How is KS treated?

   Compliance with prescribed HAART is important to improve the immune system and viral load. Therapy of localized disease may be with intralesional vinblastine, radiotherapy, liquid nitrogen cryotherapy, surgical excision, and topical alitretinoin. Treatment of more extensive disease includes α-interferon as well as single- or multiple-agent chemotherapy with vinblastine, vincristine, bleomycin, or liposomal doxorubicin.

Conant M. The International and North American Panretin Gel KS Study Groups: topical alitretinoin gel as treatment for cutaneous lesions of AIDS-related Kaposi's sarcoma: results of multicenter, double-blind, vehicle-controlled trials. Paper presented at: 6th Conference on Retroviruses and Opportunistic Infections; 1999; Chicago, IL.
Gbabe OF, Okwundu CI, Dedicoat M, et al. Treatment of severe or progressive Kaposi's sarcoma in HIV-infected adults. *Cochrane Database Syst Rev.* 2014;(8):CD003256.

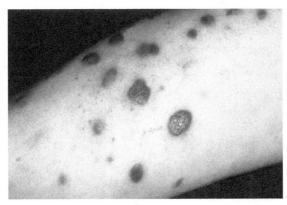

Fig. 38.2 Kaposi's sarcoma. Multiple violaceous papules and plaques. (Courtesy James E. Fitzpatrick, MD.)

9. Is the course of syphilis altered in HIV-infected individuals?
Although the course of syphilis in most HIV-infected patients is not different from that in a normal host, it may differ in several ways.
- Altered clinical manifestations of syphilis, including the usual painless chancre becoming painful secondary to bacterial infection. Lues maligna, a rare manifestation of secondary syphilis, can occur, including as the presenting sign of HIV infection, and consists of pleomorphic skin lesions with pustules, nodules, and ulcers with necrotizing vasculitis.
- Altered serologic tests for syphilis, with limited or absent antibody tests for syphilis, including repeatedly negative reagin and treponemal antibody tests. Seronegative secondary syphilis, as well as exaggerated antibody responses, has been reported. Loss of treponemal antibody positivity has also been noted.
- There may be concurrent coinfection with another sexually transmitted disease.
- There may be a decreased latency period with accelerated development of tertiary syphilis within months to years.
- There may be a lack of response to antibiotic therapy with relapses.

Gregory N, Sanchez M, Buchness MR. The spectrum of syphilis in patients with human immunodeficiency virus infection. *J Am Acad Dermatol.* 1990;22:1061–1067.
Vargas-Chandomid E, Durango NS, Ramirez-Ambriz PM. Lues maligna as primary presentation of HIV infection. *J Am Acad Dermatol.* 2018;79:AB183.

10. How does syphilis increase the risk for HIV infection?
The syphilitic chancre can itself serve as a source of HIV transmission in the HIV-infected person. An HIV-negative patient with a genital ulcer, such as in primary syphilis, can be at increased risk for acquiring HIV if exposed to an HIV-positive sexual partner.

11. What is oral hairy leukoplakia?
Oral hairy leukoplakia, which is predictive for development of AIDS, is primarily seen in HIV-infected patients but also has been described rarely in HIV-negative immunosuppressed organ transplant recipients. It is due to Epstein-Barr virus replication within clinical lesions. Oral hairy leukoplakia occurs primarily on the lateral edges of the tongue as parallel, vertically oriented, white plaques, producing a corrugated appearance (Fig. 38.3A). It can infrequently also involve the dorsal and ventral aspects of the tongue, the buccal or labial mucosa, and the soft palate. The plaque in this condition does not rub off with scraping (unlike candidal thrush) and is usually asymptomatic. Histologically, parakeratosis, acanthosis, and ballooning cells (koilocytes) are seen. In situ Epstein-Barr virus DNA hybridization of lesional scrapings or tissue sections shows positive nuclear staining within epithelial cells. Lesions may respond to acyclovir, zidovudine, podophyllin, tretinoin, or excision but do not respond to anticandidal treatment.

Resnick L, Herbst JS, Raab-Traub N. Oral hairy leukoplakia. *J Am Acad Dermatol.* 1990;22:1278–1282.

12. Name the four types of oropharyngeal candidiasis that can be seen in HIV disease.
Pseudomembranous candidiasis appears as whitish, cottage-cheese–like or creamy plaques at any site in the oropharynx. These are removable when scraped and may leave a reddish surface. *Erythematous candidiasis* appears as well-demarcated patches of erythema on the palate or dorsal tongue. Lesions of erythematous candidiasis on the

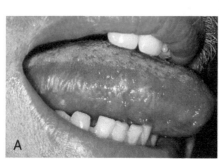
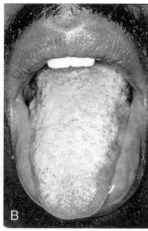

Fig. 38.3 Oral changes. **A,** Oral hairy leukoplakia. Vertically oriented white plaques with a corrugated appearance are seen on the lateral edge of the tongue. **B,** Hyperplastic candidiasis. A white coating that does not scrape off is present on the dorsal surface of the tongue in this HIV-positive patient.

tongue can look smooth and depapillated. *Hyperplastic candidiasis* appears as a white coating on the dorsum of the tongue that persists with scraping (Fig. 38.3B). *Angular cheilitis* consists of erythema, cracking, and fissuring of the mouth corners. More than one type of oropharyngeal candidiasis can coexist.

13. What is HIV-associated eosinophilic folliculitis?

HIV-associated eosinophilic folliculitis is a chronic, pruritic dermatosis of unknown etiology characterized by discrete, erythematous, follicular, urticarial papules on the head and neck, trunk, and proximal extremities (Fig. 38.4). Most cases occur in males, but the disease has been reported in females. Bacterial cultures are negative, and the eruption does not resolve with antistaphylococcal treatment. It is associated with peripheral eosinophilia, an elevated serum immunoglobulin E level, and advanced HIV infection (CD4 counts lower than 250 cells/mm^3). Eosinophilic folliculitis is not specific for HIV infection, as it has rarely been described in association with hematologic malignancies.

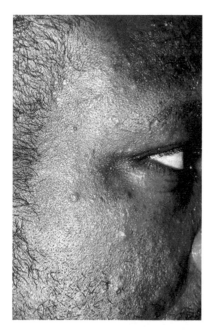

Fig. 38.4 Eosinophilic folliculitis. Multiple pruritic, firm, erythematous pink papules are present on the face of this HIV-positive patient. (Courtesy Walter Reed Army Medical Center Dermatology Clinic teaching files.)

Transverse histologic sections are superior to vertical sections in the diagnosis of this disease. Histopathologic findings include a perivascular and perifollicular mixed infiltrate with variable numbers of eosinophils and spongiosis of the follicular infundibulum or sebaceous gland with a mixed infiltrate. Treatment options include potent topical corticosteroids, antihistamines, ultraviolet B phototherapy, itraconazole, oral metronidazole, permethrin cream, and isotretinoin.

Ellis E, Scheinfeld N. Eosinophilic pustular folliculitis: a comprehensive review of treatment options. *Am J Clin Dermatol.* 2004;5:189–197.
Piantanida EW, Turiansky GW, Kenner JR, et al. HIV-associated eosinophilic folliculitis: diagnosis by transverse histologic sections. *J Am Acad Dermatol.* 1998;38:124–126.

14. **Is the incidence of drug eruptions increased in HIV disease?**
Definitely, and especially with sulfonamides and amoxicillin clavulanate. About half of HIV-infected patients with *Pneumocystis carinii* pneumonia treated with intravenous trimethoprim-sulfamethoxazole develop a widespread macular or papular erythematous eruption within weeks of initiating treatment. In HIV disease, sulfonamides are commonly used in the prophylaxis and treatment of *P. carinii* pneumonia and central nervous system toxoplasmosis. More severe drug reactions, such as hypersensitivity syndromes, Stevens-Johnson syndrome, and toxic epidermal necrolysis (TEN), have also been reported in HIV-infected patients.

Immunohistochemical evaluation of inflammatory infiltrates in TEN skin lesions in HIV-infected individuals as compared to noninfected controls revealed that the HIV-infected individuals had an eight fold increase in the ratio of CD8 + to CD4 + T cells infiltrating the dermis and a significant decrease in the number of dermal CD4 + cells. Using CD25 as a marker for regulatory T cells, investigators also found that there was a significant decrease in the ratio of CD25 + to CD4 + cells in the epidermal inflammatory infiltrates of HIV-infected individuals as compared to noninfected individuals.

Yang C, Mosam A, Mankahla A, et al. HIV infection predisposes skin to toxic epidermal necrolysis via depletion of skin-directed CD4 + T cells. *J Am Acad Dermatol.* 2014;70:1096–1102.

15. **Describe clinical features of molluscum contagiosum infection in the HIV-infected host.**
Molluscum contagiosum, a poxvirus infection, is seen in approximately 8% to 18% of patients with symptomatic HIV disease and AIDS. Although molluscum lesions often appear as dome-shaped, flesh-colored umbilicated papules, they can have an unusual appearance, involve atypical sites, and be widespread (Fig. 38.5).

In HIV disease, molluscum lesions tend to occur on the face, trunk, intertriginous areas, and buttocks as well as in the genital area. Beard area lesions are commonly seen, and these are probably spread by shaving. Lesions can be large (>1 cm, giant molluscum) or hyperkeratotic; can simulate skin cancers, common and genital warts, and keratoacanthomas; and can become confluent. Lesions can also involve the follicular epithelium with sparing of the interfollicular epithelium. Molluscum lesions can be associated with a localized chronic dermatitis surrounding a centrally located lesion (molluscum dermatitis). With progressive immune dysfunction, lesions increase in number and

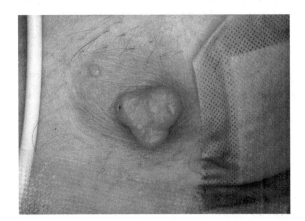

Fig. 38.5 Atypical giant molluscum contagiosum infection on the nipple in an HIV-infected patient. A more characteristic lesion of molluscum contagiosum is also present for comparison. (Courtesy Fitzsimons Army Medical Center teaching files.)

become diffuse. Disseminated cryptococcosis, histoplasmosis, and *Penicillium marneffei* infection and syphiliscan mimic facial molluscum contagiosum.

Basu S, Kumar A. Giant molluscum contagiosum—a clue to the diagnosis of human immunodeficiency virus infection. *J Epidemiology Glob Health.* 2013;3:289–291.
Brown K, Koren M, Cassler N, Turiansky GW: A unique presentation of Venus's curse—secondary syphilis mimicking molluscum contagiosum in the beard area in an AIDS patient. *Cutis,* in press.

16. How is molluscum contagiosum treated?
    Treatment options include liquid nitrogen cryotherapy, curettage, electrodesiccation, topical trichloroacetic acid, topical cantharidin, topical wart preparations including salicylic acid, topical tretinoin, topical fluorouracil and imiquimod, topical or intravenous cidofovir, and laser ablation. However, treatment of widespread lesions in advanced HIV disease is problematic, as lesions are numerous and tend to recur. Compliance with prescribed HAART is important to improve the immune system and viral load.

Buckley R, Smith K. Topical imiquimod therapy for chronic giant molluscum contagiosum in a patient with advanced human immunodeficiency virus I disease. *Arch Dermatol.* 1999; 135:1167–1169.

17. Is the prevalence of common and anogenital warts increased in HIV infection?
    The prevalence of HPV infections is increased in HIV disease, including verruca vulgaris (common warts) and condylomata acuminata (anogenital warts). Lesions can be numerous, large, confluent, and resistant to standard treatment with increasing immunodeficiency. Condylomata acuminata occur in the genital and perianal areas, where it is associated with receptive anal intercourse. In HIV disease, the incidence of HPV-associated intraepithelial neoplasia of the cervix and of the anus in homosexual men is increased. Resolution of recalcitrant hand warts temporally related to protease inhibitor–containing antiretroviral therapy has been reported.

Spach DH, Colven R. Resolution of recalcitrant hand warts in an HIV-infected patient treated with potent antiretroviral therapy. *J Am Acad Dermatol.* 1999;40:818–821.

18. What else is known about anogenital HPV infection in the setting of HIV infection?
    Patients infected with HIV infection have increased rates of anogenital HPV infection and increased severity and duration of disease. The reduced cytotoxic T-lymphocyte reactivity to the HPV oncoproteins, E6 and E7, impairs HPV clearance. HPV can cause benign, premalignant, and malignant anogenital lesions including condylomata acuminata (most commonly), Buschke-Löwenstein tumors, anal intraepithelial neoplasia, penile intraepithelial neoplasia, vulvar or vaginal intraepithelial neoplasia, and invasive anal, penile, or vulvar carcinoma. Patients are frequently infected with multiple HPV types and have a higher prevalence of high-risk HPV-16 in condylomata acuminata lesions. Patients infected with high-risk HPV are at risk for developing multiple anogenital malignancies, underscoring the importance of patient education, monitoring, and screening.
    Dysplasia-containing anogenital warts in HIV-positive men who have sex with men may clinically appear as typical anogenital warts and a high proportion may contain high-grade dysplasia or invasive carcinoma versus low-grade dysplasia only. These dysplasia-containing anogenital warts may contain low-risk HPV types only, low-risk and high-risk HPV types, or high-risk HPV types only. Anogenital warts in HIV-positive men should be evaluated histopathologically to rule out dysplasia.

Gormley RH, Kovarik CL. Human papilloma-related genital disease in the immunocompromised host. Part I. *J Am Acad Dermatol.* 2012; 66:867–880.
Gormley RH, Kovarik CL. Human papilloma-related genital disease in the immunocompromised host. Part II. *J Am Acad Dermatol.* 2012; 66:883–899.
Kreuter A, Siorokos C, Oellig F, et al. High-grade dysplasia in anogenital warts of HIV-positive men. *JAMA Dermatology.* 2016;152:1225–1230.

19. What causes bacillary angiomatosis?
    Bacillary angiomatosis is a gram-negative bacillary disease caused by *Bartonella henselae* and *B. quintana.* The disease can involve the skin, as well as the liver, spleen, lymph nodes, and bone. Cutaneous lesions consist of solitary or multiple red-to-violaceous, vascular-appearing papules and nodules that can simulate hemangiomas, pyogenic granulomas, and KS. Organisms can be demonstrated in lesional biopsies by Warthin-Starry stain. An association between bacillary angiomatosis in humans and traumatic exposure to cats having *B. henselae* blood infection has been shown. Treatment is with erythromycin or doxycycline, but clarithromycin and azithromycin have also been used.

20. How does VZV infection present in the HIV-positive patient?

Primary infection with the VZV (chickenpox) in HIV disease may be associated with complications such as pneumonia, encephalitis, hepatitis, profuse eruptions, and even death. Reactivation of latent VZV infection is increased in HIV disease. Reactivation usually manifests itself as a typical unidermatomal eruption, but with advanced immunodeficiency, multidermatomal and disseminated eruptions can occur. These eruptions may be vesiculobullous, hemorrhagic, necrotic, or poxlike and may be very painful. Chronic, painful verrucous and ecthymatous (poxlike) lesions can occur and appear as hyperkeratotic warty nodules and necrotic ulcerations, respectively.

Weinburg JM, Mysliwiec A, Turiansky GW, et al. Viral folliculitis: atypical presentations of herpes simplex, herpes zoster, and molluscum contagiosum. *Arch Dermatol.* 1997;133:983–986.

KEY POINTS: CUTANEOUS MANIFESTATIONS OF HIV INFECTION

1. *Staphylococcus aureus* is the most common cause of bacterial infection in the HIV-infected population.
2. Atypical molluscum contagiosum manifestations in the HIV-infected population include giant molluscum, disseminated lesions, confluent lesions, lesions distributed in atypical sites such as the perianal area, and lesions mimicking warts, skin cancers, and keratoacanthomas.
3. Chronic varicella-zoster infection can manifest as verrucous, hyperkeratotic nodules and as ecthymatous, poxlike ulcerations.
4. Bacillary angiomatosis is caused by *Bartonella henselae* and *B. quintana*.
5. Side effects of HAART include the lipodystrophy syndrome, new or recurrent skin disease associated with the IRS, painful periungual inflammation (paronychia), and injection site reactions (enfuvirtide).

21. Do any photosensitive dermatoses occur in HIV disease?

Various photosensitive dermatoses have been described in HIV disease, and these include porphyria cutanea tarda (PCT), lichenoid photoeruptions, and chronic actinic dermatitis. Photosensitivity may, in fact, be the presenting sign of HIV infection.

Most cases of PCT in HIV infection are acquired and many are associated with historical or serologic evidence of hepatitis B or C infection, as well as with elevated transaminase levels and history of alcohol abuse. Patients present with blisters, erosions, crusting, scarring, and increased skin fragility on the face and dorsal hands. In one study, urinary and stool porphyrin excretion patterns classic for PCT occurred in hepatitis C–positive AIDS patients without any clinical evidence of porphyria.

Lichenoid photoeruptions in HIV infection occur most often in black individuals with advanced HIV disease and may be associated with photosensitizing drug use. Patients present with pruritic, violaceous plaques that begin on the face, neck, dorsal hands, and arms. The plaques may become hyperpigmented, hypopigmented, or depigmented and may extend to non–sun-exposed sites. Histopathologic features are primarily those of lichenoid drug eruption or hypertrophic lichen planus, but some patients have findings of lichen nitidus. Patients may improve or clear with discontinuation of a photosensitizing drug, sun avoidance, and sunscreen use.

Chronic actinic dermatitis has been described in markedly immunosuppressed patients and presents as a chronic pruritic and idiopathic eczematous dermatitis in a photodistribution. Phototesting shows increased sensitivity to ultraviolet B. Histologic findings demonstrate eczematous, lymphoma-like, and psoriasiform changes.

Quansah R, Cooper CJ, Said S, et al. Hepatitis C- and HIV-induced porphyria cutanea tarda. *Am J Case Rep.* 2014;15:35–40. (free text online).

22. What is known about granuloma annulare in the setting of HIV infection?

A study of 34 consecutive HIV-positive patients with a clinical and histologic diagnosis of granuloma annulare revealed that the generalized form of granuloma annulare was a more common clinical pattern than the localized form of granuloma annulare. In this study, two patients with localized granuloma annulare had perforating lesions, both clinically and histologically. Although granuloma annulare can occur in all stages of HIV infection, it is slightly more common in patients with AIDS. Generalized granuloma annulare lesions appear as multiple, discrete, skin-colored dermal papules distributed on the trunk and extremities. Localized granuloma annulare lesions present as solitary or few discrete papules or annular plaques on one area of the body. The histologic findings of HIV-associated granuloma annulare are similar to those of non–HIV-infected individuals. There are no known cases of diabetes mellitus reported in association with HIV and granuloma annulare.

Toro JR, Chu P, Yen T-S B, et al. Granuloma annulare and human immunodeficiency virus infection. *Arch Dermatol.* 1999; 135:1341–1346.

Marzano AV, Ramoni S, Alessi E, et al. Generalized granuloma annulare and eruptive folliculitis in an HIV-positive man: resolution after antiretroviral therapy. *J Eur Acad Dermatol Venereol.* 2007;21:1114–1146.

23. **Describe some of the potential cutaneous side effects of antiretroviral therapy.**

Lipodystrophy syndrome is one of the most common cutaneous toxicities of HAART. The syndrome of lipodystrophic changes is temporally associated mainly with use of protease inhibitors, and possibly with nucleoside reverse transcriptase inhibitors. It is characterized by enlargement of the dorsocervical fat pad ("buffalo hump"), breast hypertrophy, visceral abdominal fat accumulation ("crix belly," "protease paunch") (Fig. 38.6), peripheral fat wasting with prominence of the superficial veins, and loss of fat in the buccal, temporal, and buttocks areas. Lipodystrophic changes have been associated with metabolic abnormalities including hypertriglyceridemia, hypercholesterolemia, hyperglycemia, insulin resistance, and hyperinsulinemia. Evidence of associated Cushing's syndrome or disease is lacking. Lipodystrophic changes have occasionally been reported in patients not taking protease inhibitors. Histologic findings in patients with lipoatrophy include atrophy of the subcutaneous fat, fat lobules with variably sized and often large adipocytes, prominent capillary vascular proliferation, and focal lymphocytic infiltrate and lipogranuloma formation. The exact mechanism involved in these changes is not clear. In addition, antiretroviral therapy has been temporally associated with symptomatic angiolipomatosis. Also, painful periungual inflammation (paronychia) of the fingernails and toenails has been reported with use of indinavir and lamivudine. Cutaneous side effects have been described with enfuvirtide (Fuzeon, T-20) use. This drug is a member of a class of HAART known as fusion inhibitors and is administered subcutaneously. Reported skin side effects are very common and include erythema, induration, nodules, and cysts at the injection sites (Fig. 38.7A,B). Blue or brown pigmentation of the nails and mucocutaneous hyperpigmentation has been associated with zidovudine use, while hyperpigmentation of the palms and/or soles has been associated with emtricitabine use; these changes have been most intense in darkly pigmented patients.

Introcaso CE, Hine JM, Kovarik CL. Cutaneous toxicities of antiretroviral therapy for HIV. Part I. Lipodystrophy syndrome, nucleoside reverse transcriptase inhibitors, and protease inhibitors. *J Am Acad Dermatol.* 2010;63:549–561.

Introcaso CE, Hine JM, Kovarik CL. Cutaneous toxicities of antiretroviral therapy for HIV. Part II. Nonnucleoside reverse transcriptase inhibitors, entry and fusion inhibitors, integrase inhibitors, and immune reconstitution syndrome. *J Am Acad Dermatol.* 2010; 63:563–569.

James J, Carruthers A, Carruthers J. HIV-associated facial lipoatrophy. *Dermatol Surg.* 2002;28:979–986.

Mirza RA, Turiansky GW. Enfuvirtide and cutaneous injection site reactions. *J Drugs Dermatol.* 2012;11(10):e35–e38.

Ward HA, Russo GG, Shrum J. Cutaneous manifestations of antiretroviral therapy. *J Am Acad Dermatol.* 2002;46:284–293.

24. **What is the IRS?**

IRS is also known as immune reconstitution syndrome, immune reactivation syndrome, and immune reconstitution inflammatory syndrome. It consists of the paradoxical recrudescence of quiescent disease or the appearance of new internal and cutaneous diseases that are temporally associated within weeks to months of HAART initiation. New or recurrent skin disease may consist of initial or recurrent herpes zoster, eosinophilic folliculitis, KS, molluscum contagiosum, HPV, herpes simplex virus, leishmaniasis, tumid lupus erythematosus, erythema nodosum with

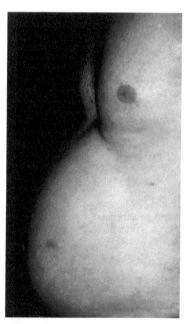

Fig. 38.6 Lipodystrophy. Visceral abdominal fat accumulation is seen in this HIV-positive patient who had been taking indinavir for 3 years. (Courtesy Walter Reed Army Medical Center Dermatology Clinic teaching files.)

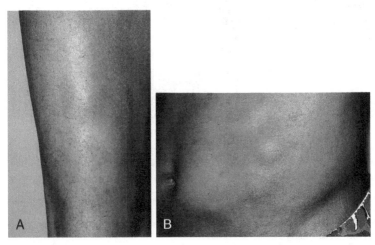

Fig. 38.7 A and **B,** Enfuvirtide injection site reactions manifesting as erythematous subcutaneous nodules. (Courtesy Walter Reed Army Medical Center Dermatology Clinic teaching files.)

pulmonary sarcoidosis with or without cutaneous sarcoidosis, extensive cytomegalovirus ulceration, reactions to prior tattoos, cutaneous mycobacterial and fungal infections, alopecia universalis and Graves' disease, leprosy complicated by type 1 reactional state, acne vulgaris, seborrheic dermatitis, and psoriasis. The IRS is attributed to the immunologic recovery produced by HAART, with restoration of pathogen-specific immunity, and is associated with decreasing viral load.

Hirsch HH, Kaufmann G, Sendi P, et al. Immune reconstitution in HIV-infected patients. *CID*. 2004;38:1159–1166.
Osei-Sekyere B, Karstaedt AS. Immune reconstitution inflammatory syndrome involving the skin. *Clin Exp Dermatol*. 2010;35:477–481.
Tripathi SV, Leslie KS, Maurer TA, et al. Psoriasis as a manifestation of HIV-related immune reconstitution inflammatory syndrome. *J Am Acad Dermatol*. 2015;72:e35–e36.

DISCLAIMER

CHAPTER 39

CUTANEOUS SIGNS OF NUTRITIONAL DISTURBANCES

Andrew T. Patterson and Wendi E. Wohltmann

KEY POINTS:

1. Pellagra is due to deficiency of niacin and/or nicotinic acid (vitamin B_3) and presents with the classic tetrad "the 4 D's": diarrhea, dermatitis, dementia, and death.
2. Patients with scurvy (vitamin C deficiency) exhibit follicular hyperkeratosis, gingival bleeding, and the development of corkscrew hairs with perifollicular hemorrhage.
3. Two important findings in vitamin A deficiency are phrynoderma ("toad skin") and Bitot's spots (gray-white corneal patches seen on ophthalmic exam).
4. Acrodermatitis enteropathica (inherited form of zinc deficiency) presents as acral, periorificial, and anogenital dermatitis; it develops 4–6 weeks after birth in bottle-fed infants and 1–2 weeks after weaning in breastfed infants.

1. When do skin abnormalities occur in association with nutritional disturbances?
   Skin manifestations occur when structural or enzymatic processes are affected by a deficiency or excess of a particular nutrient. This can be seen with dietary insufficiency or excess, malabsorption, drug interference, catabolic states, as well as metabolic, renal, hepatic, and inherited disorders. Nutrients are classified as macronutrients (protein, carbohydrate, fat), micronutrients (vitamins, minerals), and trace elements.

2. Do nutritional disturbances involve the skin exclusively?
   Absolutely not. Nutritional disorders are generalized conditions that cause adverse effects in many organ systems. Clinical history, review of systems, and physical examination are of utmost importance when determining the underlying etiology of skin findings suggestive of a nutritional disorder. As isolated nutritional disturbances are uncommon, a thorough evaluation should be undertaken when an imbalance is suspected.

3. Which skin changes are seen with protein and calorie deprivation in adults?
   In general, adults with starvation demonstrate rough, pallid, lax skin with frequent dyschromia favoring the malar and periorificial areas. Hair is thinned, and nail growth is slow with frequent fissuring. There is decreased subcutaneous fat and, with time, muscle wasting may develop.

4. What is marasmus?
   Marasmus (from the Greek meaning *wasting*) is a disorder of total calorie (energy) deficiency with resultant catabolism and utilization of muscle and fat. Infants in developing countries are at highest risk for marasmus, and affected patients often demonstrate an emaciated "monkey facies" due to loss of buccal fat that normally gives the face a rounded appearance. Other associated skin findings are nonspecific and may include dry, loose skin and thin, fragile hair.

5. What is kwashiorkor?
   Kwashiorkor (from the Ga language of Ghana, meaning "sickness of the weanling") is a result of protein deficiency with concurrent normal to excessive carbohydrate intake. Risk factors include poverty, neurologic disease, and malabsorption. There is pronounced muscle wasting with preservation of normal fat stores, failure to thrive, and marked edema that can progress to anasarca. A genetic predisposition to enterocyte loss of heparan sulfate proteoglycan (HSPG) appears to explain the clinical findings of edema, hypoalbuminemia, growth retardation, fatty liver, psychomotor disturbances, and skin changes seen in affected patients.

6. Describe the skin findings in kwashiorkor.
   Classic skin findings in kwashiorkor include mosaic skin (dry, fine areas of desquamation with cracking along skin lines) and "enamel paint" dermatosis (Fig. 39.1), which evolves into large areas of erosion and desquamation. In black children with kwashiorkor, initial circumoral pallor progresses to diffuse depigmentation, whereas affected white children often exhibit diffuse blanching erythema that rapidly progresses to dusky nonblanching purple macules and papules. Hair in affected patients is sparse, fragile, and depigmented. On trichogram analysis, the *flag sign* may be observed in the form of alternating pigmented and depigmented bands seen along the hair shafts corresponding to periods of adequate and inadequate protein consumption, respectively.

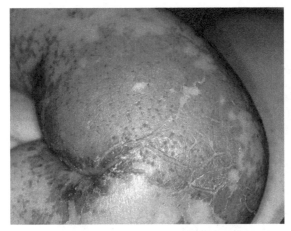

Fig. 39.1 Enamel paint dermatosis in a child with kwashiorkor. (Courtesy William Weston, MD.)

7. How can I remember the differences in skin findings associated with kwashiorkor and marasmus?
Kwashiorkor, or protein malnutrition, may be memorized by thinking of "KP," the often utilized military abbreviation for "kitchen patrol." Kwashiorkor is associated with peeling skin, akin to the often affected hands of dishwashers.

8. Do skin abnormalities occur with fat deficiency?
Essential fatty acid deficiency results from the deficiency of linoleic acid and alpha-linoleic acid, precursors of arachidonic acid that cannot be synthesized by the human body and must be obtained exogenously. It is seen primarily in the setting of malabsorption syndromes, formula-fed infants, extreme low-fat diets, and prolonged total parenteral nutrition. Skin findings may consist of a nonspecific periorificial or generalized dermatitis stemming from increased transepidermal water loss due to impaired skin barrier function. Intertriginous erosions and alopecia can also be seen. Essential fatty acid supplementation is curative.

9. Are any skin findings associated with fat excess?
Yes. Obesity researchers have documented an increased incidence of plantar hyperkeratosis (thickened soles), acanthosis nigricans, striae, and skin tags in overweight patients that may represent dermatologic manifestations of systemic insulin resistance. Excess fat deposition predisposes to intertrigo, a dermatitis occurring between skin folds, sometimes associated with secondary bacterial or candidal infection.

10. Which water-soluble vitamin abnormalities have skin findings?
Nearly all of the water-soluble vitamins demonstrate cutaneous features in deficiency states. There is considerable overlap in these skin findings, especially among the B-complex deficiencies in light of their closely related functions as coenzymes or cofactors in redox, carboxylation, or transamination reactions. Common clinical findings in riboflavin (B_2), pyridoxine (B_6), cobalamin (B_{12}), and biotin deficiencies in particular may include angular cheilitis, stomatitis, periorificial dermatitis, conjunctivitis, and glossitis.

11. What is beriberi?
Beriberi is the name applied to severe vitamin B_1 (thiamine) deficiency. Vitamin B_1 deficiency is most commonly seen in alcohol use disorder, imbalanced diets (e.g., polished rice diet), hyperemesis gravidarum, and other cases of malabsorption. Frequent mucocutaneous manifestations consist of limb edema and glossitis. Extracutaneous manifestations can include mental confusion, peripheral neuropathies, confabulation, Wernicke encephalopathy (dry type), and congestive heart failure (wet type).

12. Name the four "Ds" of pellagra.
- **D**iarrhea
- **D**ermatitis
- **D**ementia
- **D**eath

Pellagra (Italian, *pelle-*, meaning skin, and *agra-*, meaning sharp, burning, or rough) is a deficiency of niacin (vitamin B_3) that manifests classically as the "four Ds," although great variability is seen in the extent and type of gastrointestinal, neurologic, and skin manifestations. Niacin is available in animal products and enriched wheat flour and can be synthesized from tryptophan. Pellagra is most commonly seen in alcohol use disorder, prolonged isoniazid therapy, carcinoid syndrome, or Hartnup disease.

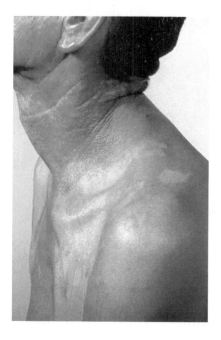

Fig. 39.2 Pellagra, showing the typical photodistributed dermatitis on the neck and chest known as "Casal's necklace." (Courtesy Richard Gentry, MD.)

13. Describe the dermatitis in pellagra.

    The dermatitis in pellagra (niacin deficiency) classically presents with a pruritic or burning erythematous eruption at sites of sun exposure. Within 2 to 3 weeks, the affected cutaneous sites become hyperpigmented, scaly, and thickened with a shellac-like appearance. "Casal's necklace" is a term used to describe the sharply demarcated distribution of the characteristic pellagra-associated eruption in a circumferential pattern involving the upper chest and neck (Fig. 39.2). Pellagra can also manifest as angular cheilitis, glossitis, stomatitis, perineal and genital erosions, and palmoplantar fissures. The skin abnormalities in pellagra respond rapidly to niacin supplementation.

14. Does scurvy still exist?

    Yes, but it is rare. Vitamin C (ascorbic acid) is present in fresh fruits and vegetables and is a necessary cofactor in collagen synthesis. Scurvy patients exhibit follicular hyperkeratosis, gingival bleeding, and the development of corkscrew hairs with perifollicular hemorrhage (Fig. 39.3). Impaired collagen synthesis results in poor wound healing. Infantile scurvy may be associated with lower extremity fractures as well as subperiosteal, gastrointestinal, and genitourinary hemorrhage.

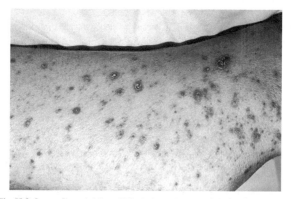

Fig. 39.3 Scurvy. Characteristic perifollicular hemorrhage and follicular hyperkeratosis.

15. Do deficiencies of the fat-soluble vitamins occur?

Yes, but less commonly because the fat-soluble vitamins (A, D, E, K) have significant storage depositories in the human body. Vitamin K deficiency is seen with malabsorption syndromes and in the newborn period prior to bacterial colonization of the intestine. Clinical features of vitamin K deficiency range from petechiae to massive hemorrhage. Vitamin D and E deficiencies are not associated with skin findings.

16. What abnormalities occur with vitamin A deficiency?

Vitamin A deficiency primarily involves the skin and eyes. Phrynoderma, meaning "toad skin," describes the characteristic cutaneous eruption of vitamin A deficiency consisting of hyperkeratotic papules with a central follicular plug involving the face, trunk, and extensor extremity surfaces. Generalized xerosis and sparse hair are also seen. Eye symptoms include night blindness and xerophthalmia. Ophthalmic exam findings may include Bitot's spots (gray-white corneal patches) and keratomalacia. Vitamin A deficiency is most commonly seen in malabsorption disorders, liver disease, and following small bowel surgery.

17. Is vitamin A excess toxic?

Yes. Hypervitaminosis A may develop following consumption of polar bear livers, chronic oversupplementation, or inappropriate use of retinoid medications. Clinically, patients develop generalized xerosis, alopecia, cheilitis, and an exfoliative dermatitis. Headache and vomiting may signify pseudotumor cerebri development. All adverse effects resolve following cessation of excess vitamin A intake.

18. What is acrodermatitis enteropathica?

Acrodermatitis enteropathica is a rare autosomal recessive disorder of intestinal and renal transport of the trace element zinc. Zinc deficiency can result in acral, periorificial, and anogenital dermatitis (Fig. 39.4). Growth failure, anemia, alopecia, depression, angular cheilitis, onychodystrophy, paronychia, and impaired wound healing are also seen. This inherited form of zinc deficiency develops 4–6 weeks after birth in bottle-fed infants and 1–2 weeks after weaning in breastfed infants.

19. How is acrodermatitis enteropathica diagnosed and treated?

Low plasma zinc levels in addition to low alkaline phosphatase (a zinc-dependent enzyme) suggest acrodermatitis enteropathica. Oral or intravenous zinc supplementation facilitates rapid improvement, with reversal of most clinical manifestations in hours to days. Affected infants can develop failure to thrive with progressive deterioration and even death if untreated.

20. Can zinc deficiency be acquired?

Yes. Acquired zinc deficiency is seen in association with diabetes mellitus, collagen vascular disease, pregnancy, Crohn's disease, nephrotic syndrome, chronic renal failure, burns, Down syndrome, alcohol use disorder, vegan diets, malabsorption syndromes, and HIV infection. Clinical findings are similar to those of the inherited form of acrodermatitis enteropathica.

21. What is carotenoderma?

Carotenoderma is a yellow to yellow-orange skin discoloration that develops when excess serum carotenoids are deposited in the stratum corneum. Most commonly affecting children, carotenoderma is most prominent on the palms, soles, and central face and is associated with ingestion of carotene found in carrots, oranges, squash, spinach, yellow corn, butter, eggs, pumpkin, yellow turnips, sweet potatoes, and dried seaweeds. The discoloration spares the conjunctivae and mucosal surfaces, which can be used to differentiate this benign condition from jaundice (Fig. 39.5). Elimination of the offending food results in normalization of skin color in weeks to months. Carotenemia can also occur in anorexia nervosa, diabetes mellitus, and hypothyroidism.

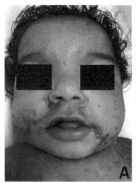 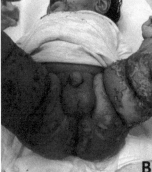 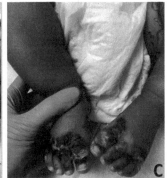

Fig. 39.4 Zinc deficiency. Clinical photographs of male infant with acrodermatitis enteropathica illustrating erosion, desquamation, and crusting in perioral (A), anogenital (B), and acral (C) regions. (Courtesy Dr. Grace Lee, MD).

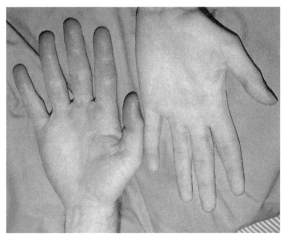

Fig. 39.5 Characteristic yellow discoloration of skin in a patient with carotenoderma contrasted with normal skin color. The patient was eating up to one bunch of carrots per day. (Courtesy James E. Fitzpatrick, MD.)

22. What skin changes are seen in eating disorders?

A number of cutaneous signs are associated with anorexia nervosa and bulimia. They include xerosis, lanugo-like hair, telogen effluvium, carotenoderma, livedo reticularis, acne, paronychia, acquired striae distensae, and Russell sign (knuckle/dorsal hand calluses from self-induced vomiting). These patients are at risk for numerous nutritional deficiencies and require psychiatric and nutritional support.

23. Has supplementation with micronutrients or homeopathic remedies been associated with any cutaneous disorders?

Yes. Ginkgo, garlic, ginger, and ginseng inhibit the activation and aggregation of platelets and may increase intraoperative bleeding, resulting in postoperative hematoma and ecchymosis. Patients should stop these supplements 1 week before surgery. Certain Chinese herbal supplements, homeopathic remedies, and illegally distilled alcohols may contain inorganic arsenic. Cutaneous features seen in chronic arsenic intoxication may include Bowen's disease (squamous cell carcinoma in situ), basal cell carcinoma, arsenical keratoses on the palms and soles, and transverse white bands across the nails due to local arsenic deposition (Mees' lines).

BIBLIOGRAPHY

Galimberti F, Mesinkovska NA. Skin findings associated with nutritional deficiencies. *Cleve Clin J Med*. 2016;83(10):731–739.
Kechichian E, Ezzedine K. Vitamin D and the skin: an update for dermatologists. *Am J Clin Dermatol*. 2018;19(2):223–235.
Ng E, Neff M. Recognising the return of nutritional deficiencies: a modern pellagra puzzle. *BMJ Case Rep*. 2018;11(1).
Noguera-Morel L, McLeish Schaefer S, Hivnor CM. Nutritional diseases. In: Bolognia JL, Schaffer JV, Cerroni L, eds. *Dermatology*. 4th ed. New York, NY: Elsevier; 2018:793–809.
Thrash B, Patel M, Shah KR, Boland CR, Menter A. Cutaneous manifestations of gastrointestinal disease: part II. *J Am Acad Dermatol*. 2013;68(2):211. e1–211.e33.

BENIGN MELANOCYTIC TUMORS

Michael R. Campoli

CHAPTER 40

1. What is a mole?

   A mole is a small burrowing mammal belonging to the family Talpidae. It is also a term commonly used to describe a melanocytic nevus.

2. What is a nevus?

   Derived from the Latin term meaning "spot" or "blemish," nevus was originally used to describe a congenital lesion or birthmark (mother's mark). In modern usage, the term describes cutaneous hamartoma, or benign proliferation of cells. However, when the term is used without a descriptive adjective, it usually refers to a melanocytic nevus. Examples of nevi used in the context of a birthmark are epidermal nevus and nevus sebaceus.

3. Are there different types of melanocytic nevi?

   Yes. Melanocytic nevi can be classified according to their histology based on (1) location of the nevus cells (e.g., junctional, compound, or intradermal nevi), (2) cytologic atypia (e.g., atypical [dysplastic] nevi), and (3) morphology and architectural arrangement of nevus cells (e.g., Spitz and spindle cell nevi). Melanocytic nevi can also be classified based on their appearance (e.g., halo nevi or blue nevi). In addition, there are congenital melanocytic and acquired nevi.

4. How do melanocytes get to the skin?

   Melanocytes arise from the cranial and truncal neural crest cells in embryonic life. The development of melanocytes from neural crest cells, as well as their ability to migrate, is dependent upon interactions between specific receptors and extracellular ligands, including endothelin 3 and the endothelin B receptors, α-melanocyte-stimulating hormone and the melanocortin-1 receptor, stem cell factor (SCF), and its receptor KIT, each of which induces the expression of microphthalmia-associated transcription factor (MITF). MITF is the most critical regulator of pigment cell development and survival. Bone morphogenic protein is a negative regulator of this process.

   Melanocytes migrate via the mesenchyme and reach their final location in the skin, uveal tract of the eye (choroid, ciliary body, and iris), leptomeninges, inner ear (cochlea), and sympathetic chain lining the colon early during embryogenesis. The melanocytes that migrate to the skin take up residence on the epidermal side of the dermal–epidermal junction and the basal layer of the hair matrix, as well as the outer root sheath of the bulge region of the hair follicle. The latter region is where melanocyte stem cells are thought to reside.

5. Explain the natural developmental history of melanocytic nevi.

   Melanocytic nevus cells are derived from melanocytes and differ from normal epidermal melanocytes in a number of ways. They are no longer dendritic, they do not distribute melanin to surrounding keratinocytes, and they are less metabolically active. The development of melanocytic nevi is multifactorial, and the molecular events underlying the development of nevi are still being investigated. Much of the available information related to the genetics of benign nevi is restricted to the analysis of genes related to melanomagenesis. Melanocytic nevi are benign clonal proliferations of cells expressing the melanocytic phenotype and are thought to be derived from precursor cells that acquire genetic mutations. These mutations activate proliferative pathways and/or suppress apoptosis, allowing for the accumulation of melanocytic cells in the skin. It is believed that at some point after proliferation, a senescence program is activated, causing termination of nevi growth. Malignant transformation of a nevus is thought to be due to the emergence of additional tumorigenic mutations, which provide an escape from oncogene-induced senescence.

   The type of nevus that is formed is thought to be dependent upon specific gene mutations as well as local environmental factors. *BRAF* gene mutations are commonly seen in acquired melanocytic nevi. Acquired melanocytic nevi are thought to begin as a proliferation of nevus cells along the dermal–epidermal junction (forming a junctional nevus; Fig. 40.1A). With continued proliferation of nevus cells, they extend from the dermal–epidermal junction into the dermis (forming a compound nevus). The junctional component of the melanocytic nevus may resolve, leaving only an intradermal component (intradermal nevus; Fig. 40.1B). However, it should be stressed that there is debate regarding the direction of nevus growth. Congenital melanocytic nevi and blue nevi frequently harbor *NRAS* and *GNAQ* mutations, respectively, while Spitz and atypical Spitz tumors usually exhibit *HRAS*, *BAP1*, and other kinase gene mutations.

   Melanocytic nevi form naturally, possibly due to ultraviolet light exposure, from the ages of 6 months to 40 years and later. They may also resolve spontaneously. However, the appearance or disappearance of any melanocytic lesion should be brought to the attention of a physician.

Cane JF, Trainor PA. Neural crest stem and progenitor cells. *Annu Rev Cell Dev Biol.* 2006;22:267–286.

Grichnik JM, Ross AL, Schneider SL, et al. How, and from which sources, do nevi really develop? *Exp Dermatol.* 2014;23:310–313.

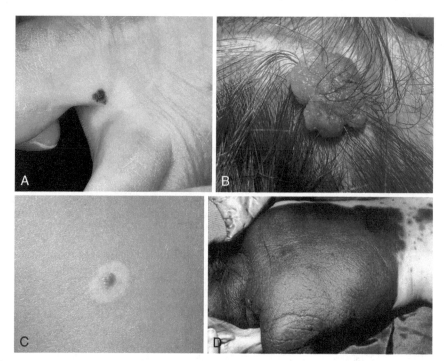

Fig. 40.1 A, Junctional nevi are typically small, flat, and dark brown in color. **B,** An intradermal nevus also may be very exophytic or papillomatous, as shown here. **C,** Typical halo nevus of the back demonstrating a central brownish-red papule. **D,** Large congenital nevus with multiple smaller congenital nevi. These lesions present a surgical challenge and a significant cosmetic problem.

Roh MR, Eliades P, Gupta S, Tsao H. Genetics of melanocytic nevi. Pigment cell. *Melanoma Res.* 2015;28:661–672.
Dimonitsas E, Liakea A, Sakellariou S, et al. An update on molecular alterations in melanocytic tumors with emphasis on Spitzoid lesions. *Ann Transl Med.* 2018;6:249.

6. What is a halo nevus?

A halo nevus, also known as a Sutton's nevus or leukoderma acquisitum centrifugum, is an acquired or congenital melanocytic nevus (CMN) with a surrounding well-circumscribed annulus of hypo- or depigmented skin (Fig. 40.1C). Halo nevi can be solitary or multiple and generally affect individuals under the age of 20 years. In general, those patients with halo nevi have an overall increased number of melanocytic nevi. Halo nevi are commonly associated with vitiligo, with 20% to 50% of vitiligo patients demonstrating halo nevi. Conversely, less than 15% to 25% of patients with halo nevi have vitiligo. Although both halo nevi and vitiligo may look similar clinically, recent studies strongly suggest that halo nevi and vitiligo have separate pathogenetic mechanisms. Nevertheless, halo nevi are strong predictors of a subset of vitiligo patients and may be an initiating factor in the pathogenesis of vitiligo. Although not completely understood, the pathogenesis of halo nevi is thought to be related to (1) an immune response against antigenically altered nevus cells or (2) a cell-mediated or humoral immune response against nonspecifically altered nevus cells. It is not completely understood whether this represents an abnormal immunologic response or whether the immune system is recognizing an atypical clone of nevomelanocytes.

Although most pigmented lesions with halos are benign, malignant melanoma can rarely be seen with an associated halo. If a pigmented lesion has an irregular border and halo or shows other atypical features, it should be biopsied.

van Geel N, Vandenhaute S, Speeckaert R, et al. Prognostic value and clinical significance of halo naevi regarding vitiligo. *Br J Dermatol.* 2011;164:743–749.
van Geel N, Mollet I, Brochez L, et al. New insights in segmental vitiligo: case report and review of theories. *Br J Dermatol.* 2014; 166:240–246.

7. What is a congenital nevus?

A CMN is a nevus that is present at birth. For the purpose of management, any melanocytic nevus that arises during the first year of life is considered "congenital." CMN are thought to arise between the 5th and 24th weeks of gestation due to morphologic error occurring in the neuroectoderm during embryogenesis, leading to unregulated growth of melanoblasts. The protooncogene *CKIT* that encodes the receptor allowing the binding of the SCF is believed to play an important role in the development of congenital nevi. CMN are permanent and grow in proportion to the child, covering the same anatomical area of skin as is affected at birth. CMN are usually characterized as small, large, or giant, although there is no universally accepted definition of these categories. Small CMN are usually defined as being up to 1.5 cm in diameter, large CMN as being between 1.5 and 20 cm in diameter, and giant CMN as being more than 20 cm in diameter. Another scheme for classifying small, large, and giant CMN considers the percentage of the body surface area the lesion covers, or the ease of surgical removal and repair of the resulting surgical defect. Still another classification scheme describes giant CMN as being as large as two of the patient's palms for lesions on the trunk and extremities, or the size of one palm for lesions on the face or neck (Fig. 40.1D). The estimated prevalence of CMN varies from 0.5% to 32%, with the majority of these lesions less than 3 to 4 cm in diameter. Large CMN are much less common and have an estimated incidence of 1 in 20,000 to 500,000 live births.

Turkmen A, Isik D, Bekercioglu M. Comparison of classification systems for congenital melanocytic nevi. *Dermatol Surg.* 2010; 36:1554–1562.
Alikhan A, Ibrahimi OA, Eisen DB. Congenital melanocytic nevi: where are we now? Part I. Clinical presentation, epidemiology, pathogenesis, histology, malignant transformation, and neurocutaneous melanosis. *J Am Acad Dermatol.* 2012;67:e1–e17.
Viana AC, Gontijo B, Bittencourt FV. Giant congenital melanocytic nevus. *An Bras Dermatol.* 2013;88:863–878.
Vourc'h-Jourdain M, Martin L, Barbarot S. Large congenital melanocytic nevi: therapeutic management and melanoma risk: a systematic review. *J Am Acad Dermatol.* 2013;68:493–498.

8. What is the histology of a CMN?

There no absolutely specific histologic findings in CMN. Studies have shown there may be differences in histology depending on the age of the patient at the time of the biopsy. Findings that support the diagnosis of a CMN include the presence of deep nevus cells, particularly within adnexal structures, vessel walls, eccrine glands, and/or perineurium.

Alikhan A, Ibrahimi OA, Eisen DB. Congenital melanocytic nevi: where are we now? Part I. Clinical presentation, epidemiology, pathogenesis, histology, malignant transformation, and neurocutaneous melanosis. *J Am Acad Dermatol.* 2012;67:e1–e17.

9. What are the genetics of CMN?

Genes that have been described as mutated in a single CMN include *NRAS, BRAF, MC1R, TP53,* and *GNAQ.* In patients with multiple CMN, postzygotic mutations in *NRAS* have been identified in 80% of CMN cases studied as well as in affected neurological and malignant tissue. In one large cohort, about one-third of CMN have been associated with a family history of CMN of any size and number in a first- or second-degree relative. In these cases, a significant increase in compound heterozygous or homozygous melanocortin-1 receptor (MC1R) variants has been identified and certain MC1R variants were associated with a more severe cutaneous phenotype of CMN. At present, the mechanism underlying MC1R variants and CMN phenotypes is not understood; however, this pattern mirrors that of sporadic adult melanoma. Whether patients with CMN with germline MC1R variants are at an increased risk of melanoma development is not yet known.

Kinsler VA, O'Hare P, Bulstrode N, et al. Melanoma in congenital melanocytic naevi. *Br J Dermatol.* 2017;176:1131–1143.

10. What is the risk of developing a malignant melanoma in a congenital nevus?

Although there is little agreement about the risk of developing melanoma within a CMN, some general guidelines can be stated. The risk appears to relate to the size of the CMN. A small or medium CMN does not appear to have any significantly greater risk for melanoma than an acquired melanocytic nevus, on the order of 1%–2%. However, this incidence varies with the severity of the congenital phenotype and size of the CMN. In this regard, while the risk for small single CMN is low, a large CMN >40 cm projected adult size, accompanied by multiple smaller CMN, is associated with a lifetime melanoma risk of has 10 to 15%. This risk of melanoma in a CMN also appears to be higher in those patients with congenital abnormalities of the CNS. It is noteworthy that in about one-third of patients with CMN who develop melanoma, the primary melanoma develops within the central nervous system. While there is evidence that melanomas tend to arise earlier in life in giant CMN, the need for removal of congenital nevi is one of the most controversial issues in pediatric dermatology. It should be stressed that surgical removal of the CMN does not decrease a patient's risk for melanoma.

Kinsler VA, Birley J, Atherton DJ. Great Ormond Street Hospital for Children Registry for Congenital Melanocytic Naevi: prospective study 1988–2007. Part 1—epidemiology, phenotype, and outcomes. *Br J Dermatol.* 2009;160:143–150.
Kinsler VA, Birley J, Atherton DJ. Great Ormond Street Hospital for Children Registry for Congenital Melanocytic Naevi: prospective study 1988–2007. Part 2—evaluation of treatments. *Br J Dermatol.* 2009;160:387–392.
Vourc'h-Jourdain M, Martin L, Barbarot S. Large congenital melanocytic nevi: therapeutic management and melanoma risk: a systematic review. *J Am Acad Dermatol.* 2013;68:493–498.
Kinsler VA, O'Hare P, Bulstrode N, et al. Melanoma in congenital melanocytic naevi. *Br J Dermatol.* 2017;176:1131–1143.

11. What is a blue nevus?

Blue nevi and related melanocytic proliferations (i.e., congenital dermal melanocytoses including Mongolian spot, nevus of Ito, and nevus of Ota) are a heterogeneous group of congenital and acquired melanocytic lesions that have in common several clinical, histologic, and immunochemical features. They have been termed dermal dendritic melanocytic proliferations because they are usually composed, at least in part, of dendritic melanocytes within the dermis. The deep dermal location of the pigment-producing cells, and therefore the pigment, causes the lesion to have its blue, black, or gray appearance due to the Tyndall effect (Fig. 40.2).

Blue nevi are usually acquired and have their onset most commonly in childhood and adolescence, but less than 25% are congenital. In general, melanocytes disappear from the dermis during embryonic migration, but some cells do remain in the scalp, sacral region, and dorsal aspect of the distal extremities. These sites correlate to the most common locations for blue nevi to occur. The three commonly identified varieties of blue nevi are the common blue nevus, cellular blue nevus, and combined blue nevus–melanocytic nevus. The vast majority of blue nevi harbor a somatic mutation in the G protein α-subunits of either *GNAQ* or *GNA11*.

12. Can blue nevi become malignant?

Yes. Malignant blue nevi can develop de novo in existing cellular blue nevi, or in a nevus of Ota (see later). Most commonly, the lesion presents as an expanding dermal nodule that may ulcerate. Malignant degeneration has an unknown incidence and prognosis, with a high rate of recurrence and metastasis, especially to lymph nodes. Malignant blue nevi are tumors of older individuals. It is more frequent in males than females. The scalp and extremities are the most common sites of occurrence. The prognosis in malignant blue nevi is poor. However, malignant blue nevi are rare, and often there is controversy regarding their histopathologic diagnosis. Moreover, the more aggressive course of malignant blue nevi may reflect the fact that most are deeply invasive tumors, since no difference in clinical outcomes has been found when compared to conventional melanoma when controlling for Breslow thickness, Clark level, and ulceration.

Zembowicz A, Mihm MC. Dermal dendritic melanocytic proliferations: an update. *Histopathology.* 2004;45:433–451.

Zembowicz A, Phadke PA. Blue nevi and variants: an update. *Arch Pathol Lab Med* 2011;135:327–336.

Sugianto JZ, Ralston JS, Metcalf JS, McFaddin CL, Smith MT. Blue nevus and "malignant blue nevus": a concise review. *Semin Diagn Pathol.* 2016;33:219–224.

13. What is a combined melanocytic nevus?

A combined melanocytic nevus is a blue nevus with an overlying melanocytic nevus. The blue nevus may be a common or cellular blue nevus. The overlying melanocytic nevus can be junctional, compound, or intradermal. This is found in 1% of all excised melanocytic nevi.

14. How does a nevus of Ota differ from a nevus of Ito?

The nevus of Ota (also called nevus fuscoceruleus ophthalmomaxillaris) is characterized clinically as a blue to gray hyperpigmentation of the skin, mucosa, and conjunctiva in the distribution of the trigeminal nerve (Fig. 40.3). Less commonly, it may also involve the meninges (meningeal melanocytoma), where it may develop a hemorrhage or, rarely, a malignant melanoma. Histologically, it is composed of heavily melanized dendritic dermal melanocytes in the upper dermis. The nevus of Ito is similar in histology to the nevus of Ota but is distributed along the neck and shoulder

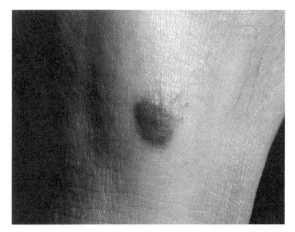

Fig. 40.2 Blue nevus on the lower leg. (Courtesy Fitzsimons Army Medical Center teaching files.)

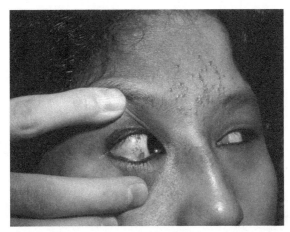

Fig. 40.3 Nevus of Ota. Unilateral macular blue-gray pigmentation of the conjunctiva, forehead, and periocular skin. The patient also has multiple syringomas of the central forehead. (Courtesy Fitzsimons Army Medical Center teaching files.)

in the distribution of the posterior supraclavicular and lateral cutaneous brachial nerves. Both lesions are considered congenital dermal melanocytoses and are more common in Asians and African-Americans. About 80% of all reported cases have been women.

15. **What is the best way to treat nevus of Ota?**
Most lesions are a cosmetic issue only, and treatment is not necessary unless it starts to affect the patient's self-esteem. In the past, scarring treatment modalities such as excision and cryotherapy were utilized. In the last 15 years, the use of Q-switched ruby, alexandrite, and Nd:YAG lasers has markedly improved the cosmetic appearance of these lesions, and they have become the treatment of choice. Although malignant changes are extremely rare, nevus of Ota patients with eye involvement should be followed closely, because a majority of associated melanomas occur in the ocular region.

16. **What is a Mongolian spot?**
A Mongolian spot is congenital dermal melanocytosis characterized as a congenital hyperpigmented spot found in the sacrococcygeal region. Most frequently found in black or Asian infants, it also occurs in infants of other races. The pigmentation often improves spontaneously in the first 3 to 5 years of life but may persist to some degree into adulthood.
    Mongolian spots usually resolve by early childhood, and hence, no treatment is generally needed; however, treatment sometimes may be required for cosmetics. The use of Q-switched ruby, alexandrite, and Nd:YAG lasers has markedly improved the cosmetic appearance of these lesions, and they have become the treatment of choice. These lesions are believed to represent the delayed disappearance of dermal melanocytes. The deep blue pigmentation is another example of the Tyndall effect. Historically, Mongolian spots have been regarded as benign, but recent data suggest that mongolian spots may be associated with inborn errors of metabolism and neurocristopathies. Neurocristopathy refers to a disorder characterized by abnormalities in neural crest migration. Examples include dermal melanocytoses, cleft lip and palate, phakomatosis pigmentovascularis, and neurofibromatosis. A close relationship between central nervous system and melanocyte population, due to their common origin from neural crest, is well known. The most common condition associated with MS is Hurler's disease, followed by GM1 gangliosidosis 1.

Snow TM. Mongolian spots in the newborn: do they mean anything? *Neonatal Netw.* 2005;24:31–33.
Gupta D, Thappa DM. Mongolian spots—a prospective study. *Pediatr Dermatol.* 2013;30:683–688.
Gupta D, Thappa DM. Mongolian spots. *Indian J Dermatol Venereol Leprol.* 2013;79:469–478.

17. **What is a Spitz nevus?**
A Spitz nevus is a benign melanocytic nevus named in honor of Dr. Sophie Spitz, who initially described this lesion as a *benign juvenile melanoma*. These most commonly occur in children but may occur at any age. Spitz nevi are most commonly acquired, but as many as 7% may be congenital. The lesion usually presents as a small, pink papule or nodule on the face or lower extremities (Fig. 40.4). Histologically, it is composed of nevus cells that are pleomorphic and cytologically atypical; these cells typically demonstrate a spindle or epithelioid appearance that share

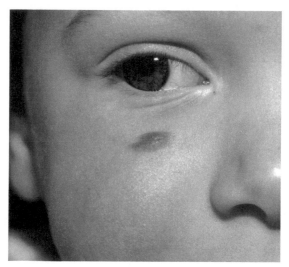

Fig. 40.4 Spitz nevus. Typical red papule on the cheek of a young child. Because of their red color, they are clinically often mistaken for vascular neoplasms. (Courtesy William L. Weston, MD Collection.)

many of the histologic characteristics found in melanoma. The histologic differentiation of Spitz nevus from malignant melanoma is one of the most difficult challenges in dermatopathology, and in some cases, the biologic behavior cannot be predicted using current criteria. It is noteworthy that *BRAF* mutations are uncommonly detected in Spitz nevi, in contrast to commonly acquired melanocytic nevi. Molecular analysis has shown three subgroups of spitzoid melanocytic tumors. The vast majority present with kinase mutations (e.g., *ALK, ROS1, NTRK1, BRAF, RET, MET*) that are rarely observed in other melanocytic tumors. The remaining two groups comprise patients with either *HRAS* or *BAP1* mutations.

Sulit DJ, Guariano RA, Krivda S. Classic and atypical Spitz nevi: review of the literature. *Cutis.* 2007;79:141–146.
Takata M, Saida T. Genetic alterations in melanocytic tumors. *J Dermatol Sci.* 2006;43:1–10.
Dimonitsas E, Liakea A, Sakellariou S, et al. An update on molecular alterations in melanocytic tumors with emphasis on Spitzoid lesions. *Ann Transl Med.* 2018;6:249.

18. What is an atypical Spitz nevus?

Atypical Spitz nevus is a poorly defined and characterized category of melanocytic tumors with histologic features of both benign Spitz nevi and malignant melanomas. The group of atypical Spitz nevi represents a mixture of Spitz nevi with atypical features and features of melanoma. At the current moment in time, it is difficult to differentiate between these two entities. The behavior of atypical spitz nevi cannot be predicted with certainty and their management is not clearly defined, with some recommending at least 1 cm surgical margins with sentinel lymph node biopsy. The utility of wide surgical margins along with the use of sentinel node lymph node biopsy has not been established for atypical spitz nevi.

Miteva M, Lazova R. Spitz nevus and atypical spitzoid neoplasm. *Semin Cutan Med Surg.* 2010;29:165-173.
Lallas A, Kyrgidis A, Ferrara G, et al. Atypical Spitz tumours and sentinel lymph node biopsy: a systematic review, *Lancet Oncol.* 2014;5(4): e178–e183.
Dimonitsas E, Liakea A, Sakellariou S, et al. An update on molecular alterations in melanocytic tumors with emphasis on Spitzoid lesions. *Ann Transl Med.* 2018;6:249.

19. Where do Becker's nevi occur?

A Becker's nevus is characterized by an area of hyperpigmentation and often hypertrichosis, most commonly on the upper back, shoulder, or chest of males (Fig. 40.5). The lesions usually become noticeable at puberty. Histologically, there are increased numbers of melanocytes, dermal melanophages, terminal hairs, and hyperpigmentation of the epidermal basal layer. Some lesions can also show increased smooth muscle and have been called smooth muscle hamartomas.

Danarti R, Konig A, Salhi A, et al. Becker's nevus syndrome revisited. *J Am Acad Dermatol.* 2004;51:965–969.

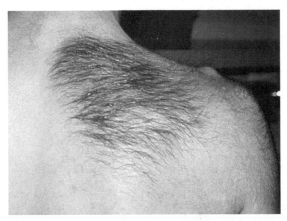

Fig. 40.5 A Becker's nevus on the upper back of a young man. This lesion has no potential for malignant degeneration.

20. What is a dysplastic (atypical) melanocytic nevus?

Dysplastic or atypical nevus is a controversial term that has eluded a precise definition. First, it should be stressed that atypical nevus is a clinical term, while dysplastic nevus is a histologic term. While atypical features may correlate with histologic dysplasia, this is not always the case. The term dysplastic or atypical nevus has been commonly used to describe an atypical-appearing melanocytic nevus believed to have increased potential for malignant transformation. Since this lesion was first described, the atypical nevus has been the subject of controversy. Argument has centered on the criteria for its histopathologic diagnosis, the incidence of melanomas developing in the lesion, and the histopathologic association of melanoma arising in an atypical nevus.

Duffy K, Grossman D. The dysplastic nevus: from historical perspective to management in the modern era: part I. Historical, histologic, and clinical aspects. *J Am Acad Dermatol.* 2012;67:1.e1–1.e16.
Duffy K, Grossman D. The dysplastic nevus: from historical perspective to management in the modern era: part II. Molecular aspects and clinical management. *J Am Acad Dermatol.* 2012;67:19.e1–19.e12.
Goldstein AM, Tucker MA. Dysplastic nevi and melanoma. *Cancer Epidemiol Biomarkers Prev.* 2013;22:528–532.

21. What is the preferred terminology for dysplastic (atypical) nevi?

The terminology used for this lesion is the subject of controversy. The lesion was first described by Clark et al. in 1978, and they used the term "B-K mole syndrome" to refer to the presence of multiple melanocytic lesions that had clinically and histologically distinct features in two families at increased risk of developing melanoma. Since then, various terms have been applied to describe this syndrome and its corresponding lesion, including the B-K mole, precancerous melanosis, atypical melanocytic hyperplasia, Clark's nevus, active junctional nevus, and melanocytic nevus with architectural disorder and cytologic atypia. "Dysplastic nevus" was first coined by Green et al. in 1980; however, some authorities have objected to this term and prefer "atypical nevus." The recognition of atypical nevi in the nonfamilial setting has also been reported and termed sporadic dysplastic (atypical) nevi. More recently, an alternative term for dysplastic (atypical) nevi was proposed by a National Institutes of Health consensus group as "nevi with architectural disorder and cytological atypia," but the designation "dysplastic nevus" continues to be used. The conference also recommended replacing atypical nevus syndrome with familial atypical melanocytic nevus syndrome. Despite their recommendations, this terminology has not been universally accepted among clinicians and pathologists.

Elder DE. Dysplastic naevi: an update. *Histopathology.* 2010;56:112–120.
Duffy K, Grossman D. The dysplastic nevus: from historical perspective to management in the modern era: part I. Historical, histologic, and clinical aspects. *J Am Acad Dermatol.* 2012;67(1):1.e1–1.e16.
Rosendahl CO, Grant-Kels JM, Que SK. Dysplastic nevus: fact and fiction. *J Am Acad Dermatol.* 2015;73:507–512.

22. What is the clinical relevance of dysplastic (atypical) melanocytic nevi?

The clinical relevance of atypical nevi relates to their association with increased melanoma risk. Several retrospective and prospective case-control studies have established that increasing numbers of atypical nevi confer an independent increasing risk of melanoma ranging from 2- to 71-fold. Patients with atypical nevi and two or more family members with melanoma seem to be at the highest risk for melanoma. Evidence that atypical nevi may be potential precursors of melanoma includes photographically documented examples of change in a preexisting nevus and the observation of histological atypia in proximity to melanomas. About 25% to 50% of melanomas have a histologically associated nevus, and the incidence rate of melanomas arising in association with atypical nevi has been estimated to be between 0.5% and 46%. The most convincing evidence for this association is the demonstration of similar or identical genetic changes in a melanoma and its associated nevus.

Despite the above findings, as well as the documented increased risk of melanoma in patients with atypical nevi, it is important to recognize that most atypical nevi are benign and do not progress to melanoma. Moreover, there is little evidence that common nevi or atypical nevi progress through sequentially higher grades of dysplasia to melanoma. Unfortunately, there is no model to examine this, because identification of any nevus results in its destruction and there are no suitable animal models. It has been estimated that the lifetime risk of any individual nevus transforming to a melanoma is 1 in 10,000. It should be stressed that many epidemiologic studies that have cited an increased risk of melanoma have evaluated dysplastic nevi primarily or exclusively using clinical criteria, which does not correlate with histologic atypia. Further, previous studies have shown that anywhere from 20% to 40% of melanomas arise from a preexisting nevus, 70% arise de novo, and in almost a 25% the historical origin cannot be assessed. The available evidence suggests that the majority of melanomas associated with nevi are found with common nevi. Although there is a clear association between nevi and increased melanoma risk, whether or not atypical nevi are at a greater risk than conventional nevi to develop melanoma is controversial. Moreover, studies of melanoma-prone families have verified that (i) members of these families without atypical nevi can develop melanoma and (ii) most melanomas in these families actually arise de novo or in clinically common nevi. Lastly, it is quite clear that a nevus precursor is not required for the majority of melanomas. It is thought that the discrepancy between melanomas arising in preexisting nevi and de novo melanomas can best be explained by the cancer stem cell theory. In this regard, the risk of melanoma associated with nevi may be due to the potential for secondary mutations within nevi, as well as to the inherent properties of the stem cell population in individuals with numerous moles.

Clark Jr WH, Reimer RR, Greene M, Ainsworth AM, Mastrangelo MJ. Origin of familial malignant melanomas from heritable melanocytic lesions. 'The B-K mole syndrome'. *Arch Dermatol.* 1978;114:732–738.

Tucker MA, Fraser MC, Goldstein AM, et al. A natural history of melanomas and dysplastic nevi: an atlas of lesions in melanoma-prone families. *Cancer.* 2002;94:3192–3209.

Chin L. The genetics of malignant melanoma: lessons from mouse and man. *Nat Rev Cancer.* 2003;3:559–570.

Duffy K, Grossman D. The dysplastic nevus: from historical perspective to management in the modern era: part I. Historical, histologic, and clinical aspects. *J Am Acad Dermatol.* 2012;67:1.e1–1.e16.

Duffy K, Grossman D. The dysplastic nevus: from historical perspective to management in the modern era: part II. Molecular aspects and clinical management. *J Am Acad Dermatol.* 2012;67:19.e1–19.e12.

Goldstein AM, Tucker MA. Dysplastic nevi and melanoma. *Cancer Epidemiol Biomarkers Prev.* 2013;22:528–532.

Rosendahl CO, Grant-Kels JM, Que SK. Dysplastic nevus: fact and fiction. *J Am Acad Dermatol.* 2015;73:507–512.

Brinckerhoff CE. Cancer stem cells (CSCs) in melanoma: there's smoke, but is there fire? *J Cell Physiol.* 2017;232:2674–2678.

Saida T. Histogenesis of cutaneous malignant melanoma: the vast majority do not develop from melanocytic nevus but arise de novo as melanoma in situ. *J Dermatol.* 2019;46(2):80–94. doi:10.1111/1346-8138.14737.

23. What objective criteria of nevi have been shown to correlate with melanoma risk?
    There are two objective criteria that have been shown to correlate with melanoma risk: (i) a high nevus count correlates with a higher risk of melanoma; and (ii) the presence of large nevi on an individual increases the relative risk of melanoma.

24. Describe the genetic mutations found in atypical melanocytic nevi.
    Like other nevi, atypical nevi arise from genetic mutations and most studies suggest that atypical nevi are clonal in origin. Although familial melanoma and atypical nevi were thought to be due to the effects of a single gene, studies have shown that the genetic causes of familial melanoma and atypical nevi are not the same. Specifically, there is little evidence for mutations in the familial melanoma genes *CDKN2A* or *CDK4* in atypical nevi. A high incidence of *BRAF* mutations has been detected in atypical nevi. It is thought that these mutations may be due to ultraviolet radiation because patients with atypical nevi may have a decreased ability to repair ultraviolet light–induced DNA damage. Compared to common nevi, atypical nevi exhibit higher proliferation index (Ki-67), alterations in the p16 and p53 tumor suppressor genes, as well as microsatellite instability at 1p, 9p, and 9p21. The phosphatase and tensin homolog (PTEN) phosphatase tumor suppressor gene is lost in a small portion of both common and atypical nevi. Mutations in various melanocytic lesions are shown in Table. 40.1.

Weatherhead SC, Haniffa M, Lawrence CM. Melanomas arising from naevi and de novo melanomas: does origin matter? *Br J Dermatol.* 2007;156:72–76.

Duffy K, Grossman D. The dysplastic nevus: from historical perspective to management in the modern era: part I. Historical, histologic, and clinical aspects. *J Am Acad Dermatol.* 2012;67:1.e1–1.e16.

Duffy K, Grossman D. The dysplastic nevus: from historical perspective to management in the modern era: part II. Molecular aspects and clinical management. *J Am Acad Dermatol.* 2012;67:19.e1–19.e12.

Rosendahl CO, Grant-Kels JM, Que SK. Dysplastic nevus: fact and fiction. *J Am Acad Dermatol.* 2015;73:507–512.

Dimonitsas E, Liakea A, Sakellariou S, et al. An update on molecular alterations in melanocytic tumors with emphasis on Spitzoid lesions. *Ann Transl Med.* 2018;6:249–266.

Table 40.1 Genetic alterations in melanocytic lesions

GENETIC ALTERATIONS	SPITZ	ATYPICAL SPITZ	CONGENITAL	ATYPICAL/ ACQUIRED	BLUE	MELANOMA
ALK	0–8%	5%				1%
BAP1		15%			17%	5% Uveal
BRAF	0–20%	0–25%	Giant 5% Small & Medium 30%	70–85%	25%	80–85%
CKIT	55%	50–56%				Acral / Mucosal
CDKN2a						5–70%
GNAQ					60–80%	Uveal
GNA11					10–20%	Uveal
HRAS	15–20%	14%				<1%
NRAS	0–5%	0–25%	Giant 95% Small & Medium 70%	6%		25%
TERT-p						20–70%

25. How common are atypical melanocytic nevi?

The exact incidence is unknown and most studies have failed to include histologic diagnosis in their methods, but it is estimated that 10% to 50% of the population have one or more atypical nevi.

26. Does clinical atypia in a nevus correlate with histologic atypia?

There is compelling evidence that atypical nevi as a histologic entity cannot reliably be correlated with any clinical entity. To this end, both common and congenital melanocytic nevi have been shown to demonstrate histologic features of dysplastic nevi.

27. Is there a difference between an atypical nevus and melanoma in situ?

Yes. The difference is determined by the histopathology. Unfortunately, consensus regarding the histologic definition of atypical nevi is lacking. When an atypical nevus has atypical melanocytic nevus cells at the dermal–epidermal interface or less commonly in the dermis, some of these cells may exhibit cytologic atypia, but this is variable and not continuous throughout the lesion. There are also often architectural abnormalities noted between melanocytic nests. In contrast, melanoma in situ has atypical melanocytes, both singly and in small nests scattered through all levels of the epidermis (pagetoid pattern). Further, a typical melanoma is often more asymmetrical; melanocytes present as solitary units in the epidermis rather than in nests, and the melanocytes demonstrate a greater degree of cytologic atypia.

28. What is the recommended treatment for an atypical nevus and melanoma in situ?

Recommended treatment for melanoma in situ is complete full-thickness excision with a minimum of a 0.5-cm margin of normal skin. However, it must be stressed that there is no evidence supporting 5-mm margins for melanoma in situ. Moreover, there is extensive evidence that the use of 5-mm margins is unsafe and will lead to positive margins, recurrence, and, in a substantial number of cases, progression to invasive melanoma. In this regard, it has been shown that 22.6% of recurrent in situ melanoma demonstrated a histologically invasive component with a mean Breslow depth of 0.94 mm. The use recommendations for 5-mm margins has been in place since the 1992 National Institutes of Health consensus panel guidelines were released, and the recommendations of 5 mm are based solely on expert opinion and not supported by data. The available scientific data argue that the guidelines should advocate for margin-controlled surgical techniques and should admonish the use of wide excision with 5-mm margins.

Controversy exists regarding the treatment of atypical nevi. Depending on the degree of cytologic atypia, full-thickness excision with margins ranging from 0.2 to 0.5 cm has been recommended. However, for any atypical nevus, the question of complete excision is controversial. The current literature suggests that re-excision of mildly to moderately dysplastic nevus is not warranted. In most cases, when a dysplastic nevus with positive biopsy margins is re-excised, the pathology shows only a scar. More importantly, long-term follow-up shows no development of melanoma at the biopsy site of dysplastic nevus incompletely or narrowly removed. This controversy regarding the treatment of atypical nevi reflects the lack of consensus about the grading of atypia in nevi, as well as the insufficient data regarding the significance of melanocytic atypia in nevi. The converse to this is that significant intraobserver and interobserver differences in the diagnosis of atypical nevi versus melanoma as well as poor interobserver agreement are often observed in the characterization of cytologic atypia. Therefore, some have argued that surgically removing severely atypical nevi prevents this inappropriate characterization of a melanoma as an atypical nevus. It should be stressed that the removal of large numbers of atypical nevi results in significant scarring and does not change a person's inherent melanoma risk. Only after thorough evaluation, and when a melanoma cannot be ruled out, should surgical removal be performed. As mentioned earlier, the vast majority of atypical nevi never become melanomas.

DeBloom JR 2nd, Zitelli JA, Brodland DG. The invasive growth potential of residual melanoma and melanoma in situ. *Dermatol Surg.* 2010; 36:1251–1257.

Campoli M, Fitzpatrick JE, High W, et al. HLA antigen expression in melanocytic lesions: is acquisition of HLA antigen expression a biomarker of atypical (dysplastic) melanocytes? *J Am Acad Dermatol.* 2012;66:911–916.

Kunishige JH, Brodland DG, Zitelli JA. Surgical margins for melanoma in situ. *J Am Acad Dermatol.* 2012;66:438–444.

Hocker TL, Alikhan A, Comfere NI, Peters MS. Favorable long-term outcomes in patients with histologically dysplastic nevi that approach a specimen border. *J Am Acad Dermatol.* 2013;68:545–551.

Abello-Poblete MV, Correa-Selm LM, Giambrone D, Victor F, Rao BK. Histologic outcomes of excised moderate and severe dysplastic nevi. *Dermatol Surg.* 2014;40:40–45.

Strazzula L, Vedak P, Hoang MP, Sober A, Tsao H, Kroshinsky D. The utility of re-excising mildly and moderately dysplastic nevi: a retrospective analysis. *J Am Acad Dermatol.* 2014;71:1071–1076.

Kunishige JH, Brodland DG, Zitelli JA. Surgical margins for melanoma in situ: when 5-mm margins are really 9 mm. *J Am Acad Dermatol.* 2015;72:745.

Stigall LE, Brodland DG, Zitelli JA. The use of Mohs micrographic surgery (MMS) for melanoma in situ (MIS) of the trunk and proximal extremities. *J Am Acad Dermatol.* 2016;75:1015–1021.

Valentín-Nogueras SM, Brodland DG, Zitelli JA, González-Sepúlveda L, Nazario CM. Mohs Micrographic Surgery Using MART-1 immunostain in the treatment of invasive melanoma and melanoma in situ. *Dermatol Surg.* 2016;42:733–744.

29. Describe the clinical appearance of dysplastic nevi.

No single feature is diagnostic of atypical nevi; instead, a collection of clinical findings is required for their diagnosis. Atypical nevi are usually larger than ordinary nevi (>6 mm) and have slightly irregular borders that fade into the surrounding normal skin (Fig. 40.6). Variation of color with an asymmetrical pattern is common. The colors vary from shades of brown to black, tan, and light red. The lesions typically have a dark center surrounded by pigment that has poor margination. Atypical nevi most frequently are located on the trunk, scalp, breast (in women), and bathing-trunk areas (in men).

30. Is there a difference between a liver spot and a freckle?

Yes. Liver spot is the term commonly used to refer to a solar or senile lentigo. A lentigo is a hyperpigmented (usually brown or black) macule that is characterized histopathologically by increased numbers of melanocytes at the dermal–epidermal junction and increased amounts of melanin in both the melanocytes and basal keratinocytes. These lesions

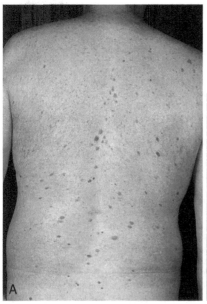
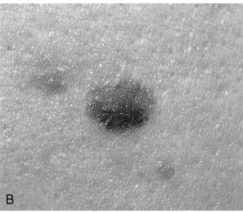

Fig. 40.6 Atypical nevi. **A,** Patient with familial atypical melanocytic nevus syndrome demonstrating numerous atypical nevi. **B,** An atypical nevus demonstrating marked variegation in color and loss of normal symmetry.

commonly arise on the dorsal aspects of the hands and face. Although solar lentigines are induced by ultraviolet radiation, they do not increase in pigmentation with exposure to the sun. Polymorphisms in the melanocortin receptor 1 gene *(MCR1)* have been associated with the development of freckles. Freckles (ephelides) are hyperpigmented macules limited to sun-exposed skin. Microscopically, they show increased amounts of melanin in basal keratinocytes, but not increased numbers of melanocytes. Freckles characteristically darken with sun exposure and lighten when the affected areas are protected from ultraviolet radiation.

31. What is a café-au-lait macule?

    Café-au-lait macules (CALMs) are uniformly light-brown (the color of coffee with cream) macules that vary in size from 2 to 20 cm and often have irregular borders. They are characterized by increased melanin in both melanocytes and keratinocytes and by giant melanosomes. CALMs grow proportionately to body growth and remain stable in size after body growth has completed. CALMs are found in 10% to 20% of the general population; however, multiple CALMs are relatively rare (0.25% to 0.5%) in the general population and should alert you to the possibility of an associated disease. Multiple CALMs are most commonly associated with neurofibromatosis (see Chapter 5), and large CALMs, with the McCune-Albright syndrome (see Chapter 18).

    Landau M, Krafchik BR. The diagnostic value of café-au-lait macules. *J Am Acad Dermatol.* 1999;40:877–890.

32. What is a nevus spilus?

    A nevus spilus is an irregularly shaped, light-brown macule with darkly pigmented macules or papules scattered randomly within the macule (Fig. 40.7). The light areas demonstrate the microscopic changes of a CALM, and areas of increased melanin with darker pigmentation show the histology of lentigines or junctional nevi. Rare cases have developed melanoma.

    Vaidya DC, Schwartz RA, Janniger CK. Nevus spilus. *Cutis.* 2007;80:465–468.

33. Can melanocytic nevi arise in locations other than the skin?

    Yes. Melanocytic nevi can occur on the retina, conjunctiva, and oral (and other) mucosal surfaces.

34. What is a labial lentigo?

    Labial lentigo (labial melanotic macule) is a hyperpigmented macule that develops on the lip. Seen most commonly in young women, there is thickening of the epidermis and increased melanin in the basal keratinocytes. These typically behave in a benign fashion.

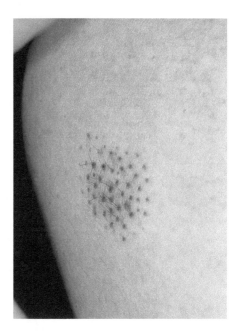

Fig. 40.7 Nevus spilus showing a large café-au-lait macule with multiple small pigmented lesions.

KEY POINTS: BENIGN MELANOCYTIC TUMORS

1. Benign melanocytic nevi may arise, grow, and regress normally. Rapid change is not normal.
2. Melanocytic nevus cells are derived from melanocytes and differ from normal epidermal melanocytes in a number of ways.
3. There appears to be a small increased risk (1% to 4%) of melanoma in patients with giant (>60 cm) CMN.
4. Patients with a large number (>100) of atypical melanocytic nevi should be followed closely for the possible development of melanoma.
5. Between 30% and 70% of melanomas arise de novo independent of a preexisting nevus.
6. Mutations in *p16*, *p52*, *PTEN*, and *BRAF* as well as microsatellite instability have been detected in atypical nevi.
7. The current literature suggests that re-excision of mildly to moderately dysplastic nevus is not warranted.
8. 5-mm surgical margins are not sufficient for melanoma in situ.
9. Multiple CALMs are most commonly associated with neurofibromatosis.
10. Ephelides and lentigines are not melanocytic nevi.

CHAPTER 41

VASCULAR AND LYMPHATIC NEOPLASMS

Nicola Natsis and Sheila Friedlander

KEY POINTS

1. Infantile hemangiomas undergo an initial rapid proliferation for several months before subsequently "leveling off" then eventually involuting, a process that may take years to complete.
2. Topical timolol gel-forming solution has been a breakthrough therapeutic option for infantile hemangiomas, performing as well as oral propranolol for smaller, thinner lesions with a lower risk of systemic adverse effects.
3. Clinicians should evaluate patients for PHACE (which stands for Posterior fossa, Hemangioma, Arterial lesions, Cardiac abnormalities, and Eye abnormalities) syndrome if they present with facial hemangiomas greater than 5 cm in size, or segmental facial hemangiomas, or if they have neurological or cardiac symptomatology.
4. While previously thought to be associated with infantile hemangioma, the consumptive coagulopathy deemed the Kasabach-Merritt phenomenon is seen almost exclusively in kaposiform hemangioendothelioma and tufted angioma.
5. Neoplasms of lymphatic tissue with or without a venous component or smooth muscle tissue may also occur, though they are rare and more common in females.

1. **Describe the natural lifecycle of an infantile hemangioma (also called hemangioma of infancy).**

   Infantile hemangiomas are present at birth or shortly thereafter. Parents may not notice precursor lesions at first, as they may be pale and flat with very subtle telangiectases prior to expanding into the classic vascular plaque that is commonly identified as an infantile hemangioma (Fig. 41.1). Infantile hemangiomas first undergo a stage of rapid proliferation, during which time the vascular lesion can become darker/deeper in color, thicker (vertical growth), and larger (longitudinal growth). This rapid growth typically occurs between 3 and 12 months of age. The rate of proliferation then slows, which is sometimes referred to as the "plateau phase." Finally, the lesions begin to involute slowly, a process that can take several years to complete. Some cases maintain a protuberant "fibrofatty residual," while others resolve with only a parchment-like scar.

2. **When should you treat an infantile hemangioma as opposed to "watchful waiting?"**

   Infantile hemangiomas should be treated if there is an imminent risk of, or existing, ulceration, skin breakdown, or if facial disfigurement is likely. This risk is increased in larger lesions with particularly rapid vertical or longitudinal growth and/or if lesions are located in areas that may be subject to increased friction or trauma such as the genitals and buttocks or medial thighs. Additionally, if the hemangioma is obstructing a critical area, for example, overlying a patient's eye, the hemangioma should be aggressively treated, since early lack of sensory input via the eye to the brain can result in permanent vision loss.[1] Facial hemangiomas near the nose and lips are also concerning, as they may lead to permanent disfigurement of these structures even after involution. Lip lesions in particular are likely to ulcerate.

3. **Describe the use of timolol for the treatment of infantile hemangioma.**

   Treatment with beta-blockers is the current gold standard of care in patients for whom treatment instead of observation is recommended. There are both topical and systemic formulations of beta-blockers for infantile hemangioma. Topical timolol—originally formulated for ophthalmologic pathologies—is now an optimal treatment option for small infantile hemangiomas. Because the medication is administered externally via liquid drops directly onto the vascular lesion, it limits the potential for absorption and systemic effects.[2] The patient's weight in kilograms is equal to the suggested maximum number of drops of topical timolol 0.5% gel-forming solution that the patient can receive in a day.[3] A common regimen is one to two drops applied directly to the lesion twice daily.

4. **Describe additional beta-blocker therapy for infantile hemangioma.**

   Propranolol is an oral option for the treatment of more problematic infantile hemangioma. The usual recommended dose is 2 to 3 mg/kg/day divided twice or three times daily.[4] Patients are usually treated on an outpatient basis with weekly incremental increase of dose starting at 1 mg/kg/day. Medically fragile or premature infants may warrant lower dosing. Inpatient treatment can be more rapidly accelerated and most patients can be increased to 2–2.5 mg/kg/day over a 36–48-hour period. An accelerated inpatient approach can also be used in patients with life or functionally threatening lesions (e.g., possible visual impairment) in whom rapid escalation to a therapeutic dose is helpful. It is important to take a blood pressure and heart rate both before and 1 to 1.5 hours after the initial administration of the

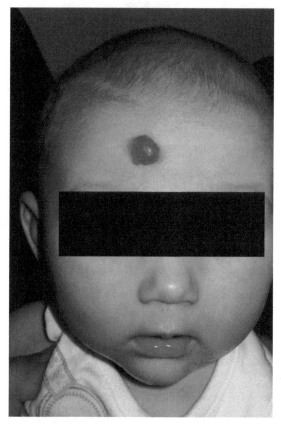

Fig. 41.1 Classic infantile hemangioma presenting of the central forehead. There is no evidence of ulceration or skin breakdown.

drug and at any time there is a dose adjustment made. Such monitoring is prudent to document any side effects such as significant bradycardia or hypotension in response to the given dose. Adjustments can be made as necessary if these side effects occur. A 2018 Cochrane review found no statistical difference between hemangioma size in patients treated with 0.5% timolol gel-forming solution at one drop twice daily compared to propranolol at 1 mg/kg/day.[5] However, another study by Léauté-Labrèze in 2008 showed a dose-response relationship to propranolol, with 3 mg/kg resulting in higher efficacy than 1 mg/kg.[6] Any infantile hemangioma that is life or function threatening should be treated with oral rather than topical therapy.

5. When is the best time to start beta-blocker therapy in patients with infantile hemangioma?
Treatment has the greatest potential for benefit if it is initiated before the rapid growth phase of the hemangioma. However, systemic therapy is not usually utilized on an outpatient basis in medically fragile infants or those less than 5 weeks of corrected gestational age. These children are usually hospitalized for initiation of systemic therapy. Smaller, thinner lesions can be initially treated with timolol but must be carefully observed over time to make sure that oral systemic therapy will not be required.

6. What is the utility of laser therapy for infantile hemangioma?
Pulsed dye laser (PDL) therapy has been used for infantile hemangioma. PDL treatment is particularly well suited for superficial hemangiomas prior to the stage of rapid proliferation. It is also an ideal treatment for the rapid resolution of ulcerated hemangiomas[7] (Fig. 41.2). PDL can also aid in the reduction of telangiectatic remnants in involuting lesions.

7. What is the most serious condition to evaluate for in patients presenting with large facial hemangiomas?
The PHACE syndrome (which stands for Posterior fossa, Hemangioma, Arterial lesions, Cardiac abnormalities, and Eye abnormalities) is a serious medical condition requiring more extensive evaluation and treatment (Fig. 41.3). PHACE syndrome is much more common in females than males, at a ratio of 9:1.[8] The diagnostic criteria for PHACE syndrome include a facial hemangioma larger than 5 cm plus one major criteria (cerebral artery anomaly, posterior fossa anomalies, aortic arch of subclavian artery anomaly, sternal defect) or two minor criteria (persistent embryonic

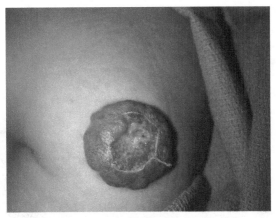

Fig. 41.2 Hemangioma with central ulceration.

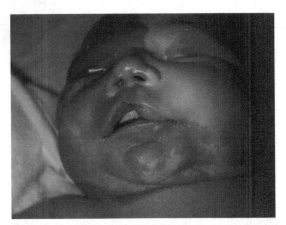

Fig. 41.3 The segmental facial hemangioma in a patient with PHACE syndrome.

arteries, midline anomalies of the brain, neuronal migration disorder, ventricular septal defect, double aortic arch, anterior segment anomalies, ectopic thyroid). In patients with large or segmental facial hemangiomas, brain and cardiovascular imaging should be performed to evaluate for possible PHACE syndrome, preferably before initiating propranolol, since this drug can induce adverse cardiac and neurologic effects. Some PHACE patients possess atretic or absent cerebral vessel anomalies that place them at risk for poor central nervous system (CNS) perfusion and ischemic stroke, particularly if treated with a beta-blocker such as propranolol. If such CNS anomalies are identified, consultation with neurology is important, as lower dosing or even withholding systemic beta-blockers may be required.

8. In a patient with more than five distinct cutaneous hemangiomas, what imaging test should you order?
   Patients with multiple cutaneous hemangiomas are at higher risk for coexisting liver hemangiomas. Thus, an ultrasound of the liver should be performed on these patients. Fig. 41.4 is representative of the multiple hemangiomas that should trigger further liver evaluation.

9. What is the second most common pediatric vascular neoplasm after infantile hemangioma?
   Pyogenic granuloma (PG, also called lobular capillary hemangioma) is the second most common pediatric vascular neoplasm (Fig. 41.5). It is characterized by a well-demarcated vascular papule or nodule, often with a friable surface and a stuck-on or pedunculated appearance. It may arise after trauma, but more commonly occurs independently of an antecedent trauma. These lesions have a propensity for bleeding, and hemostasis can then be difficult to achieve. PGs are typically removed surgically, either with shave biopsy or excision with adjuvant destruction of the vascular bed. In small, very thin lesions, some experts use pulsed-dye laser therapy or timolol.[9,10]

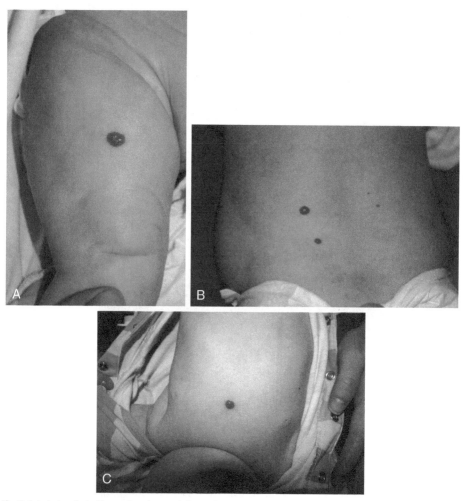

Fig. 41.4 A single patient with more than six separate hemangiomas (cutaneous hemangiomatosis) involving the back and extremities. Patient warrants a liver ultrasound.

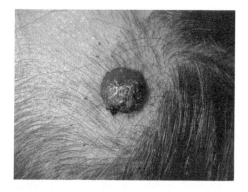

Fig. 41.5 Pyogenic granuloma of the scalp with peripheral hemorrhagic crust.

10. If an infant presents with a hemangioma at birth that is not proliferating even after months of observation, what is his or her distinct diagnosis?

    Congenital hemangioma. Congenital hemangiomas develop in utero and do not proliferate postnatally. Congenital hemangiomas may rapidly involute (RICH) (Fig. 41.6) or may never involute (NICH).

11. What lab abnormalities may be noted in a patient with certain cutaneous vascular neoplasms?

    Thrombocytopenia may be observed in patients with certain cutaneous vascular neoplasms. Platelets are sequestered into the lesion leaving a relative deficit in the circulation. This is called the Kasabach-Merritt phenomenon (KMP). This consumptive coagulopathy is not observed in hemangiomas but has been described in kaposiform hemangioendothelioma and tufted angioma.[11]

12. What are the characteristic features of kaposiform hemangioendothelioma and tufted angioma, respectively?

    Kaposiform hemangioendothelioma is a rare vascular neoplasm typically presenting at or near birth as a subcutaneous mass, often with overlying ecchymosis and telangiectases (Fig. 41.7). KMP is a common complication presenting in as many as 79% of patients with kaposiform hemangioendothelioma.[12] In patients with retroperitoneal presentations of kaposiform hemangioendothelioma, the rate of KMP is as high as 94%.[13] First-line therapy is sirolimus; surgical excision is often considered when safe. Vincristine is also used in some cases.

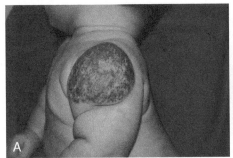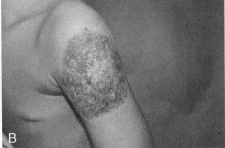

Fig. 41.6 A patient with a rapidly involuting congenital hemangioma (RICH) with images showing the progression of involution over time.

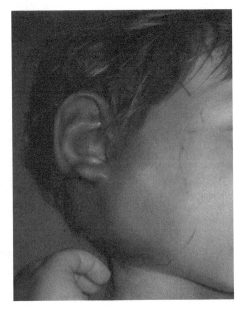

Fig. 41.7 Kaposiform hemangioendothelioma with involvement of the face, scalp, neck, and ear.

Tufted angiomas are another rare vascular neoplasm presenting at or near birth (Fig. 41.8). They most commonly arise on the extremities. They can present with overlying hair or increased sweating. Tufted angiomas may also be associated with KMP. Because of the overlap in symptoms and histology between tufted angiomas and kaposiform hemangioendothelioma, they are thought by some to be part of the same spectrum as opposed to being entirely unique entities.[13]

13. **List the benign lymphocytic neoplasms**
    a. Solitary lymphangioma: these can be cutaneous or extracutaneous. When they present on the skin, they may take on a "frog spawn," bleb network appearance (Fig. 41.9).
    b. Lymphangiomatosis: multiple lymphangiomas
    c. Lymphangiomyoma: neoplasm composed of lymphatic tissue and smooth muscle, occurring predominantly in premenopausal women.[14] It may lead to a honeycombing of smooth muscle in the lung tissue.[15]
    d. Combined venolymphatic lesions: these lesions contain both venous and lymphatic elements.

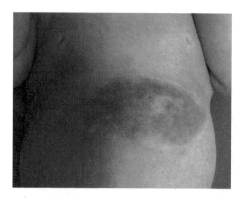

Fig. 41.8 Tufted angioma in an uncharacteristic location (abdomen as opposed to extremity).

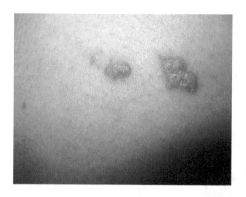

Fig. 41.9 Lymphangioma showing a globular "frog spawn" appearance.

REFERENCES

1. Bramhall RJ, Quaba A. A review of 58 patients with periorbital haemangiomas to determine appropriate cases for intervention. *J Plast Reconstr Aesthet Surg.* 2008;61(2):138–149.
2. Borok J, Gangar P, Admani S, Proudfoot J, Friedlander S. Safety and efficacy of topical timolol treatment of infantile haemangioma: a prospective trial. *Br J Dermatol.* 2018;178:e51–e52. https://doi.org/10.1111/bjd.15865.
3. Dalla Costa R, Prindaville B, Wiss K. Doing the math: a simple approach to topical timolol dosing for infantile hemangiomas. *Pediatr Dermatol.* 2018;135(2):276–277.
4. Takechi T, Kumokawa T, Kato R, Higuchi T, Kaneko T, Ieiri I. Population pharmacokinetics and pharmacodynamics of oral propranolol in pediatric patients with infantile hemangioma. *J Clin Pharmacol.* 2018;58(10):1361–1370.
5. Novoa M, Baselga E, Beltran S, et al. Interventions for infantile haemangiomas of the skin. *Cochrane Database Syst Rev.* 2018;4(4), CD006545.

6. Léauté-Labrèze C, de la Roque ED, Hubiche T, Boralevi F, Thambo JB, Taïeb A. Propranolol for severe hemangiomas of infancy. *N Engl J Med*. 2008;358(24):2649–2651. https://doi.org/10.1056/NEJMc0708819.

7. Shen L, Zhou G, Zhao J, et al. Pulsed dye laser therapy for infantile hemangiomas: a systematic review and meta-analysis. *QJM*. 2015;108(6):473–480.

8. Metry DW, Haggstrom AN, Drolet BA, et al. 2006. A prospective study of PHACE syndrome in infantile hemangiomas: demographic features, clinical findings, and complications. *Am J Med Genet*. 2010;140A:975–986.

9. Rai S, Kaur M, Bhatnagar P. Laser: a powerful tool for treatment of pyogenic granuloma. *J Cutan Aesthet Surg*. 2011;4(2):144–147.

10. Wine Lee L, Goff KL, Lam JM, et al. Treatment of pediatric pyogenic granulomas using β-adrenergic receptor antagonists. *Pediatr Dermatol*. 2014;31:203–207. https://doi.org/10.1111/pde.12217.

11. Mahajan P, Margolin J, Iacobas I. Kasabach-Merritt phenomenon: classic presentation and management options. *Clin Med Insights Blood Disord*. 2017;10 1179545X17699849.

12. Schmid I, Klenk AK, Sparber-Sauer M, et al. Kaposiform hemangioendothelioma in children: a benign vascular tumor with multiple treatment options. *World J Pediatr*. 2018;14:322–329.

13. Feito-Rodríguez M, Sánchez-Orta A, De Lucas R, et al. Congenital tufted angioma: a multicenter retrospective study of 30 cases. *Pediatr Dermatol*. 2018;35:808–816.

14. Wolff M. Lymphangiomyoma: clinicopathologic study and ultrastructural confirmation of its histogenesis. *Cancer*. 1973;31:988–1007.

15. Miller W, Cornog J, Sullivan M. Lymphangiomyomatosis. *Am J Roentgenol*. 1971;111:565–572.

CHAPTER 42

FIBROUS TUMORS OF THE SKIN

James E. Fitzpatrick and Whitney A. High

1. What are tumors of fibrous tissue?

   Tumors of fibrous tissue ("soft tissue tumors") are typically mesenchymal tumors composed of fibroblasts and variants of fibroblasts. Fibroblasts produce the structural components of the dermis, including collagen, elastin, and ground substance (dermal mucin). Some tumors are composed of myofibroblasts, which are specialized fibroblasts with contractile properties afforded by cytoplasmic actin filamets. Other specialized fibroblasts demonstrate histiocytic properties and are referred to as fibrohistiocytic. Benign soft tissue neoplasms are often divided into fibrous tumors and fibrohistiocytic tumors (Table 42.1). Malignant fibrous and fibrohistiocytic tumors are covered in Chapter 46.

2. What is an acrochordon?

   An acrochordon (skin tag, fibroma durum) is a soft, often pedunculated, flesh-colored to dark brown cutaneous papule, usually located on flexural surfaces, such as the neck, axilla, or groin (Fig. 42.1A). Acrochordons are ubiquitous. Acrochordons are most often multiple, usually 1 to 4 mm in size, but occasionally may be 3 cm or larger in diameter. Larger lesions often contain some fat and are also called fibroepithelial polyps (Fig. 42.1B).

3. What causes acrochordons?

   The precise cause is unknown. Acrochordons are associated with diabetes mellitus, obesity, pregnancy, menopause, acanthosis nigricans (see Fig. 42.1A), metabolic syndrome, and certain endocrinopathies, suggesting hormonal induction. However, the ubiquitous nature of these lesions, particularly in healthy older adults, means acrochordons may also simply be a manifestation of aging skin.

   Shah R, Jindal A, Patel N. Acrochordons as a cutaneous sign of metabolic syndrome: a case-control study. *Ann Med Health Sci Res.* 2014;4:202–205.

4. What complications are associated with acrochordons?

   The most common complications pertain to trauma, torsion, and infarction of a pedunculated lesion. When a pedunculated lesion twists on its stalk, the blood supply may be compromised with resultant tissue ischemia. Sudden pain, swelling, necrosis, and even secondary infection can result. Often, this sequence of events results in disappearance of the acrochordon.

5. Are acrochordons associated with intestinal polyposis?

   Although early studies suggested a significant association between acrochordons and colonic polyps, more recent studies, using sounder methodology, did not demonstrate an association.

6. How can acrochordons be treated?

   A simple way to treat acrochordons is scissor-snip excision (even without anesthesia). Smaller lesions can be treated by electrodessication or cryotherapy (beware of postinflammatory hypopigmentation with cryotherapy). Larger lesions (>1 cm) can be shaved off after local anesthesia.

7. What is a hypertrophic scar?

   Excessive collagen deposition at a site of wound healing leads to a hypertrophic scar. Typically, hypertrophic scars are erythematous, raised, firm, and pruritic. With time, hypertrophic scars flatten and become white. Unlike keloids, hypertrophic scars do not extend beyond the limits of the original trauma. Scars, including hypertrophic scars, are not usually considered to be neoplasms because they are reactive and eventually regress with time.

8. What is a keloid?

   A keloid is also caused by excessive collagen deposition at a wound site, but typically the deposition in a keloid is more exaggerated. Microscopically, keloids are differentiated from hypertrophic scars by the presence of large eosinophilic collagen bundles, with abundant mucin. Keloids frequently proliferate beyond the bounds of the original trauma, and this is different from hypertrophic scars. Some keloids, particularly on the sternum or upper back, may develop without identifiable preceding trauma. Keloids do not typically involute.

9. What clinical features are useful in distinguishing hypertrophic scars from keloids?

   In early lesions, it may be impossible to make this distinction, but in developed lesions, the features listed in Table 42.2 are useful.

Table 42.1 Fibrous Tumors of the Skin

BENIGN FIBROUS TUMORS	BENIGN FIBROHISTIOCYTIC TUMORS
Acquired digital fibrokeratoma	Fibrous papule
Acrochordons	Dermatofibroma
Connective tissue nevus (collagenoma, elastoma)	Giant cell tumor of tendon sheath
Dermatomyofibroma	Reticulohistiocytoma (solitary or multiple)
Desmoids (extra-abdominal and abdominal fibromatosis)	Xanthogranuloma
Fibrous hamartoma of infancy	
Infantile digital fibromatosis	
Keloid	
Knuckle pads	
Nodular fasciitis	

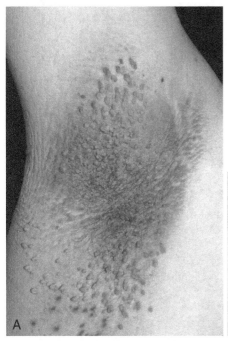
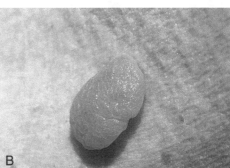

Fig. 42.1 A, Multiple, small, typical exophytic, light brown acrochordons of the axilla associated with acanthosis nigricans. **B,** Typical acrochordon demonstrating skin-colored, soft, pedunculated papule. Exophytic seborrheic keratoses and nevi may resemble acrochordons. (Panel A courtesy William L. Weston, MD collection.)

10. What factors predispose one to hypertrophic scars and keloids?

Many factors can predispose individuals to form hypertrophic scars and keloids:
- Use of certain drugs, like isotretinoin, can lead to hypertrophic scarring. For this reason, some dermatologic surgeons defer elective surgery for a year after discontinuation of isotretinoin.
- The type and degree of tissue injury also play a role in scarring. Thermal burns, with severe tissue damage, often produce hypertrophic scars or keloids.
- Anatomic site may also affect scarring. Skin that is under continuous tension or skin that is tightly stretched over bony protuberances can predispose one to hypertrophic scarring and keloid formation.
- Darker skin types are more prone to both hypertrophic scarring and keloid formation. Blacks are 2 to 19 times more likely than whites to form keloids, while Asians are 3 to 5 times more likely than whites to develop keloids. The tendency for keloids to occur in families suggests a genetic predisposition, as well.
- Certain genodermatoses such as Ehlers-Danlos syndrome, Rubinstein-Taybi syndrome, osteogenesis imperfecta, and progeria predispose one to the development of keloids.

Table 42.2 Clinical Features That Distinguish Hypertrophic Scars from Keloids

HYPERTROPHIC SCAR	KELOID
Any age group, especially children	Adolescents and young adults
All racial and ethnic groups	Blacks and Asians > Caucasians
No familial tendency	Familial tendency
Limited to sites of trauma	Sites of trauma or spontaneous
Onset within 2 months	Onset within 1 year
Any anatomic site	High-risk anatomic site
Dome-shaped lesions	Dome-shaped, exophytic, or crablike extensions
Confined to site of trauma	Extends into normal skin
Improved by corrective surgery	Often worsened by surgery
Spontaneous regression	No spontaneous regression

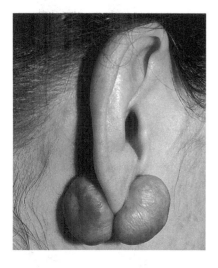

Fig. 42.2 "Dumbbell" keloids of the earlobe following ear piercing.

11. List the anatomic regions of the body that are most at risk to develop keloids.
    Presternal area, upper back, upper arms, especially over deltoids, beard area, especially over mandibular angle, and earlobes (Fig. 42.2).

12. What treatments are utilized for hypertrophic scars and keloids?
    Numerous therapies exist, although not all are particular efficacious. In general, hypertrophic scars respond to less aggressive therapy, such as potent topical steroids, intralesional steroids, chronic pressure dressings, and even silicone sheeting. Keloids often require more aggressive therapy, and even then, the response may be less than ideal. Surgical excision, injection of potent corticosteroids, and cryotherapy are often utilized treatment modalities for keloids. One study suggested that when excision is employed, it must be complete, for incomplete excision is associated with a greater chance of recurrence. Radiation is effective for keloids, but it must be used with caution and only by an experienced physician.

    Combination approaches may work best. Cryosurgery followed by corticosteroid injection is effective in some patients. Surgical excision with steroid injection at or near the time of operation is an often effective approach. One regimen calls for steroid injection to the surgical site 1 to 4 weeks postoperatively and then monthly for 6 months.

Gold DA, Sheinin R, Jacobsen G, et al. The effects of postoperative intralesional corticosteroids in the prevention of recurrent earlobe keloids: a multispecialty retrospective review. *Dermatol Surg.* 2018;44:865–869.

13. What is an acquired digital fibrokeratoma?

It is a solitary, firm, hyperkeratotic papule that often occurs around the interphalangeal joints but may occur anywhere on the hands or feet. Acquired digital fibrokeratomata often demonstrate a collarette of hyperkeratosis at the base (Fig. 42.3). Such lesions may be mistaken for warts or supernumerary digits. Histologically, lesions manifest thickened collagen bundles with an overlying attenuated epidermis and hyperkeratosis.

14. What causes acquired digital fibrokeratomas?

Some authorities believe these lesions are caused by recurrent trauma. While a history of recurrent trauma can sometimes be elicited, often patients do not recall any trauma to the site.

15. How can an acquired digital fibrokeratoma be treated?

Saucerization removal (with healing by second intention) and conservative excision are often effective. Cryotherapy is sometimes effective, but may require multiple treatments.

16. What is nodular fasciitis?

Nodular fasciitis is an uncommon, myofibroblastic tumor that many experts consider to be a pseudoneoplastic or reactive growth. Most nodular fasciitis presents in young adults as a solitary, rapidly growing, subcutaneous nodule, often on the extremities. It may follow trauma or sudden changes in activity level (i.e., military basic training, etc.). Nodules (1–3 cm in size) may be painful and may adhere to underlying fascia. Excision is curative, but untreated lesions can also spontaneously regress. Histologically, nodular fasciitis may be confused with malignant neoplasms, because the fibroblasts are large and pleomorphic, and mitotic figures are present.

17. What is a connective tissue nevus?

Connective tissue nevus is a term used for cutaneous hamartomas composed chiefly of collagen (collagenomas), elastin (elastomas), or a combination of these constituents. While the material is produced by fibroblasts, connective tissue nevi are usually no more cellular than normal dermis. Clinically, connective tissue nevi present as one or more dermal papules or plaques. Connective tissue nevi composed mostly of collagen are usually skin colored, while those composed mostly of elastin may be skin-colored or slightly yellow.

18. Why are connective tissue nevi important?

Large connective tissue nevi may be distressing to the patient for cosmetic reasons. Sometimes, multipole collagenomas may develop over a short period of time (eruptive collagenomas). Collagenomas known as shagreen patches are seen in patients with tuberous sclerosis. Multiple connective tissue nevi, called dermatofibrosis lenticularis disseminate, composed of elastic fibers and collagen, are a cutaneous marker for Buschke-Ollendorff syndrome, an autosomal dominant genetic disorder that presents also with osteopoikilosis of bones.

19. What is the gene defect in Buschke-Ollendorff syndrome?

Many but not all patients with Buschke-Ollendorff syndrome have a heterozygous, loss-of-function, germline mutation in the *LEMD3* gene on chromosome 12q14. However, absence of this mutation in affected families suggests there is some genetic heterogeneity in the disorder.

20. What is infantile digital fibromatosis?

Infantile digital fibromatosis is a rare tumor comprised of myofibroblasts. Lesions develop in infancy and early childhood, usually on fingers and toes. The lesion forms a skin-colored or red tumor located on the lateral or dorsal surface of a digit. Histologically, lesions are comprised of myofibroblasts with a characteristic eosinophilic cytoplasmic inclusion composed of actin filaments.

Heymann WR. Infantile digital fibromatosis. *J Am Acad Dermatol.* 2008;59:122–123.

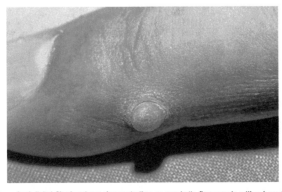

Fig. 42.3 Typical acquired digital fibrokeratoma demonstrating an exophytic firm papule with a hyperkeratotic collarette.

21. Describe the natural history of infantile digital fibromatosis.

Tumors of infantile digital fibromatosis may grow up to 2 cm but will eventually regress over a period of years (Fig. 42.4). Large lesions can produce functional impairment or joint deformities. Up to two-thirds of cases will recur after surgical excision. Because spontaneous regression is the rule, it is important that providers unfamiliar with the natural history of this tumor do not become overly aggressive and amputate a digit.

22. What is a dermatofibroma?

A dermatofibroma (DF), or fibrous histiocytoma, is the most common fibrohistiocytic tumor of the skin. DFs are usually small, firm, flat or exophytic papules located on the lower extremities of adults. Other common locations include the sides of the trunk and upper arms. While most DFs are 2 to 6 mm in diameter, some can reach sizes of 2 to 3 cm or more. DFs often demonstrate a tan or brown color, and some hypertrophy of overlying epidermis may be observed. Inexperienced examiners may mistake DFs for nevi or skin cancer.

Microscopically, most DFs are comprised of fibrohistiocytic cells that produce collagen. Some DFs have cellular areas composed of cells with round nuclei that can phagocytize lipid or hemosiderin. Multinucleated giant cells may be present. DFs that phagocytize abundant hemosiderin are sometimes referred to as hemosiderotic DFs (Fig. 42.5).

23. What is a positive "dimple" sign?

DFs usually demonstrate a "dimple sign," which is an inward dimpling of the skin when lateral pressure is applied with the thumb and forefinger. This is also called the Fitzpatrick sign, in honor of Dr. Thomas B. Fitzpatrick (Fig. 42.6).

24. Do DFs transform into skin cancer?

DFs are considered benign fibrohistiocytic tumors without malignant potential. While DFs share clinical and some general histologic similarities with dermatofibrosarcoma protuberans, a malignant tumor, the expression of immunohistochemical markers, distinguishes the two conditions. Although DFs do not become malignant, the overlying epidermis can manifest basaloid induction, and some authors believe this basaloid induction, on rare occasion, may lead to basal cell carcinoma.

Rosmaninho A, Farrajota P, Peixoto C, et al. Basal cell carcinoma overlying a dermatofibroma: a revisited controversy. *Eur J Dermatol.* 2011;21:137–138.

25. What is the best way to treat a DF?

DFs do not require any treatment. When a DF is distressing in appearance, painful, or frequently traumatized, simple excision can be utilized. The benefit of treatment should be weighed against the risk of the surgical procedure.

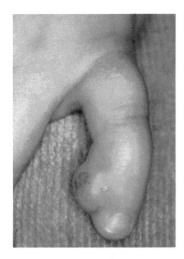

Fig. 42.4 Infantile digital fibroma. Firm skin-colored nodule with focal hemorrhage on the finger of an infant. (Courtesy Fitzsimons Army Medical Center teaching files.)

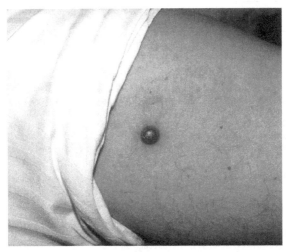

Fig. 42.5 Hemosiderotic dermatofibroma. A clinical and histologic variant of dermatofibroma with fibrohistiocytic cells demonstrating phagocytosis of hemosiderin. Because of the color, they are clinically often confused with vascular tumors, but on palpation they are typically firm. (Courtesy Fitzsimons Army Medical Center teaching files.)

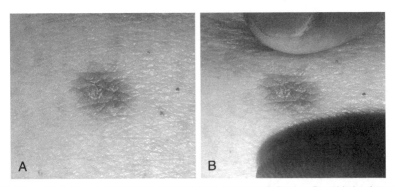

Fig. 42.6 A, Characteristic light brown dermatofibroma that is not sharply demarcated. **B,** Dimple or Fitzpatrick sign, demonstrating tendency of dermatofibromas to dimple when compressed laterally.

KEY POINTS: FIBROHISTIOCYTIC TUMORS

1. Multiple eruptive dermatofibromas are associated with an altered immune status, such as systemic lupus erythematosus and HIV/AIDS.
2. Dermatofibromas often demonstrate dimpling with lateral pressure called "dimple sign" or "Fitzpatrick sign."
3. Solitary angiofibromas on the nose and are referred to as fibrous papules of the nose and are benign but are often mistaken clinically for basal cell carcinoma.
4. Multiple angiofibromas are associated with tuberous sclerosis.
5. Buschke-Ollendorff syndrome is an autosomal dominant disorder that presents with connective tissue nevi, but also osteopoikilosis of the bones.

26. Are multiple dermatofibromas associated with any internal diseases?
    Multiple DFs have been associated with systemic lupus erythematosus, myasthenia gravis, malignancies, pregnancy, and HIV/AIDS. These associations are rare and typically involve multiple lesions erupting over a short time interval. Patients presenting with isolated DFs should not be routinely evaluated for these conditions.

Panou E, Watchorn R, Bakkour W. Multiple eruptive dermatofibromas in HIV: an immune reconstitution associated disease? *J Eur Acad Dermatol Venereol.* 2019.

Queirós C, Uva L, Soares de Almeida L, et al. Multiple eruptive dermatofibromas associated with pregnancy—a case and literature review. *Dermatol Online J.* 2019;25(5).

27. What is a "fibrous papule of the nose"?

    A fibrous papule of the nose is a common, small (usually 2 to 3 mm), asymptomatic, dome-shaped papule, usually located on nose, but also sometimes located elsewhere on the face. Lesions may be skin colored, white, red, or reddish-brown (Fig. 42.7). Microscopically, fibrous papules are composed of fusiform, stellate, or multinucleated fibroblasts with abundant slightly thick collagen bundles and dilated blood vessels. In middle-aged to older adults, these lesions may be confused with basal cell carcinoma. Fibrous papules of the nose are histologically identical to angiofibromas occurring in persons with tuberous sclerosis; hence, they represent a solitary angiofibroma.

28. How is a fibrous papule of the nose best treated?

    No treatment is required, but when desired, a shave excision, cryotherapy, and simple excision are typically effective modalities.

29. What is a "giant cell tumor of tendon sheath"?

    Giant cell tumors of the tendon sheath (GCTTS) are benign tumors that arise from the fibrous sheath that surrounds tendons, especially those of the hands/wrist, but also the feet/ankles. GCTTS usually occurs between the ages of 30 and 50 years. Although GCTTS arise from a structure deep to the skin, it is not an uncommon lesion to present initially to the dermatologist. The primary lesion is a subcutaneous nodule that seems attached to deeper structures (Fig. 42.8). X-ray examination, besides revealing a soft tissue tumor, may demonstrate erosion of cortical bone in ~10% of cases. Treatment of choice is surgical excision.

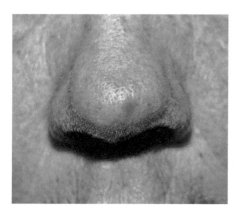

Fig. 42.7 Reddish-brown fibrous papule on the tip of the nose. (Courtesy Fitzsimons Army Medical Center teaching files.)

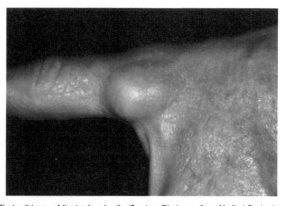

Fig. 42.8 Giant cell tumor of the tendon sheath. (Courtesy Fitzsimons Army Medical Center teaching files.)

COMMON CUTANEOUS MALIGNANCIES

CHAPTER 43

Eileen L. Axibal, Misha D. Miller, and Mariah R. Brown

1. How are skin cancers classified?

   Primary cutaneous cancers are classified on the basis of their cell of origin within the skin (Table 43.1). Skin cancers are most commonly derived from keratinocytes (e.g., squamous cell carcinoma [SCC], basal cell carcinoma [BCC]) or melanocytes (e.g., melanoma), which are normal components of the epidermis. Less commonly, they arise from other cells within the epidermis, dermis, or subcutis.

2. What are the most common nonmelanoma skin cancers (NMSCs)?

   BCC and SCC make up the majority of NMSCs. In the United States, it is estimated that 5.4 million diagnoses of NMSC occur yearly in 3.3 million patients, which makes these the most prevalent of all malignancies. Common nonmelanoma skin premalignancies include actinic keratosis and actinic cheilitis.

Rogers HW, Weinstock MA, Feldman SR, Coldiron BM. Incidence estimate of nonmelanoma skin cancer (keratinocyte carcinomas) in the U.S. population, 2012. *JAMA Dermatol.* 2015;151:1081–1086.

---

3. What is the most important cause of NMSC?

   The overwhelming majority of precancerous and cancerous skin lesions are caused by sun exposure. Several observations and epidemiologic studies support the role of ultraviolet (UV) light in the production of skin cancers:
   1. Most NMSCs develop on chronically sun exposed skin, with 80% or more occurring on the head and neck.
   2. The incidence of NMSC is lower in more polar latitudes (e.g., Minneapolis) than equatorial latitudes (e.g., Hawaii).
   3. Epidemiologic studies clearly demonstrate that NMSCs are much more common in individuals with lighter skin than in individuals with darker skin.
   4. Individuals with genetic diseases that make them sensitive to UV radiation have higher rates of skin cancer.
   5. In animal models, NMSC can be induced by solar irradiation and prevented by the use of sunscreens.
   6. The risk of skin cancer is increased with use of tanning beds. It is estimated that nearly half a million cases of NMSC and ten thousand melanoma cases can be attributed to their use.

Kim RH, Armstrong AW. Nonmelanoma skin cancer. *Dermatol Clin.* 2012;30:125–139.
Rigel D. Cutaneous ultraviolet exposure and its relationship to the development of skin cancer. *J Am Acad Dermatol.* 2008;58:S129–S132.
Wehner MR, Chren NM, Nameth D, et al. International prevalence of indoor tanning: a systematic review and meta-analysis. *JAMA Dermatol.* 2014;150:390–400.

---

4. Are there any other causes of NMSC?
   - Arsenic ingestion
   - Chronic ulcers and scars (e.g., burn wounds)
   - Environmental pollutants
   - Familial syndromes (e.g., xeroderma pigmentosum, albinism, epidermodysplasia verruciformis)
   - Local, prolonged heat exposure
   - Topical exposure to tars and oils
   - Viral infection (e.g., some strains of human papillomavirus)
   - Radiation therapy
   - Medications (voriconazole, BRAF-inhibitors, psoralen plus UVA therapy)

5. What special populations are at increased risk of NMSC?
   - **Organ transplant patients:** NMSC is the most common malignancy in solid organ transplant recipients (OTRs). OTRs are at a 65 times higher risk of SCC and 10 times higher risk of BCC than the general population. The development of skin cancer in these patients appears to be linked to the duration and degree of immunosuppression required to prevent transplant rejection. The use of calcineurin inhibitors and azathioprine has been associated with increased risk of skin cancer in this population. In addition, individuals infected with

Table 43.1 Classification of Cutaneous Malignancies

MALIGNANCY	CELL OF ORIGIN
Premalignancies/Intraepidermal Malignancies	
Actinic keratosis	Keratinocyte
Squamous cell carcinoma in situ (Bowen's disease)	Keratinocyte
Melanoma in situ	Melanocyte
Melanoma in situ, lentigo maligna variant	Melanocyte
Common Invasive Cutaneous Malignancies	
Basal cell carcinoma	Follicular keratinocyte origin (probable)
Squamous cell carcinoma	Epidermal keratinocyte
Keratoacanthoma	Follicular keratinocyte
Malignant melanoma	Melanocyte
Uncommon Cutaneous Epithelial Malignancies	
Sweat gland carcinoma (numerous variants)	Apocrine or eccrine sweat gland/duct
Follicular carcinomas (several variants)	Follicular epithelial cells
Extramammary Paget's disease	Modified keratinocytes (Toker cell)
Merkel cell carcinoma	Neuroendocrine cell (viral origin)
Cutaneous Mesenchymal Malignancies	
Atypical fibroxanthoma	Fibroblast
Dermatofibrosarcoma protuberans	CD34$^+$ dermal dendrocyte
Fibrosarcoma	Fibroblast
Angiosarcoma	Endothelial cell
Kaposi's sarcoma	Endothelial cell
Leiomyosarcoma	Smooth muscle cell
Malignant peripheral nerve sheath tumors	Schwann cells
Liposarcoma	Lipocyte

human papillomavirus (HPV) have a higher risk. The ratio of SCCs to BCCs is 4:1 in OTRs, a reversal of the normal ratio seen in the general population. SCC in particular can behave more aggressively in this population; those who develop metastatic SCC have very poor outcomes.

- **Human immunodeficiency virus (HIV) patients:** NMSC is the most common non–acquired immune deficiency syndrome (AIDS)–defining cancer seen in HIV-positive patients. HIV-positive patients appear to maintain a normal ratio of BCCs to SCCs, but are twofold to sevenfold more likely to develop NMSC than the general population.

Wheless L, Jacks S, Mooneham Potter KA, et al. Skin cancer in organ transplant recipients: more than the immune system. *J Am Acad Dermatol.* 2014;71:359–365.
Chockalingam R, Downing C, Tyring SK. Cutaneous squamous cell carcinomas in organ transplant recipients. *J Clin Med.* 2015;4 (6):1229–1239.
Zhao H, Shu G, Wang S. The risk of non-melanoma skin cancer in HIV-infected patients: new data and meta-analysis. *Int J STD AIDS.* 2016;27(7):568–575.
Honda K. HIV and skin cancer. *Dermatol Clin.* 2006;24:521–530.

6. How are NMSCs diagnosed?

A cutaneous malignancy should be considered in any patient who reports a new skin lesion, particularly in sun-exposed regions. The gold standard of diagnosis is shave, punch, or excisional biopsy, with the choice of biopsy technique depending on the size and location of the suspected malignancy. Current research is focused on developing noninvasive methods of diagnosing NMSC by using techniques such as specialized ultrasonography and microscopy. These methods, however, are currently in development and have not replaced skin biopsy with histologic examination as the gold standard for diagnosis.

Mogensen M, Jemec G. Diagnosis of nonmelanoma skin cancer/keratinocyte carcinoma: a review of the diagnostic accuracy of nonmelanoma skin cancer diagnostic tests and technologies. *Dermatol Surg.* 2007;33:1158–1174.

7. How frequently do NMSCs occur?

The exact incidence of NMSCs is unknown, both because tumor registries do not routinely track NMSC and because mortality from NMSC is low. It is estimated that 2 to 3.5 million new cases of NMSC occur each year in the United States, making them by far the most common cancers in this country. The annual cost to Medicare for the management and treatment of NMSCs is 2 billion dollars. The lifetime risk of developing NMSC in the United States is 1 in 5. Statistically, if a patient develops one NMSC, the risk of another new lesion in 5 years is 30% to 50%. Rates of NMSC increase with age and peak in the seventh and eighth decades. There is some evidence that rates of skin cancer in younger patients (<40 years old) may be increasing. Although rates of NMSC vary geographically, overall rates of NMSC have been steadily increasing in recent decades. This increase is attributed to multiple factors including increased life spans, increased sun-exposure behavior, use of tanning beds, and changes in the ozone layer affecting UV exposure.

Chen J, Fleischer A, Smith E, et al. Cost of nonmelanoma skin cancer treatment in the United States. *Dermatol Surg.* 2007;27:1035–1038.

Scotto J, Fears TR, Fraumeni Jr JF, et al. *Incidence of Nonmelanoma Skin Cancer in the United States in Collaboration with Fred Hutchinson Cancer Research Center.* Bethesda, MD: U.S. Dept. of Health and Human Services, Public Health Service, National Institutes of Health, National Cancer Institute; 1983:113, xv. NIH publication No. 83-2433.

Stern RS. Cost effectiveness of Mohs micrographic surgery. *J Invest Dermatol.* 2013;113:1129–1131.

8. How can NMSCs be prevented?

The easy answer is to avoid sun exposure. Sun protection techniques for children and adults alike include avoidance of the midday sun, liberal use of sunscreens, and wearing of protective clothing. Tans, whether received from natural sunlight or tanning booths, represent damaged skin that is more likely to develop NMSC. It is important for health care providers to promote the idea that pale skin is more attractive than tanned skin and to emphasize the risks of UV exposure.

9. What factors should you consider in treating NMSC?

The optimal treatment modality depends upon the type of malignancy (including histologic subtype, location, high-risk features such as size, recurrence, depth of invasion, and perineural invasion), patient factors (including immunosuppression and overall health of the patient), potential for recurrence and/or metastasis, and availability of various treatment methods (Table 43.2).

Neville J, Welch E, Leffell D. Management of nonmelanoma skin cancer in 2007. *Nat Clin Pract Oncol.* 2007;4:462–469.

Table 43.2 Management of Cutaneous Premalignancies and Malignancies

LESION	TREATMENT
Actinic Keratosis	Cryosurgery
	Curettage +/− electrosurgery
	Fluorouracil, topical
	Imiquimod
	Diclofenac
	Ingenol mebutate
	Chemical peel
	Dermabrasion
	Resurfacing lasers
	Photodynamic therapy
Actinic Cheilitis	Cryosurgery
	Electrosurgery
	Chemical peel
	Laser ablation
	Vermilionectomy
	Imiquimod

Continued on following page

Table 43.2 Management of Cutaneous Premalignancies and Malignancies (*Continued*)

LESION	TREATMENT
Basal Cell Carcinoma (BCC)	
Superficial	Cryosurgery
	Curettage +/− electrosurgery
	Laser ablation
	Imiquimod
	Photodynamic therapy
	Ingenol mebutate
	Excision
	Mohs surgery
Nodular	Cryosurgery
	Electrodesiccation and curettage
	Excision
	Radiation therapy
	Photodynamic therapy
	Mohs surgery
Morpheaform, aggressive BCC, or recurrent BCC	Excision
	Mohs surgery
Nonresectable BCC	Cryosurgery
	Small-molecule inhibitors of the hedgehog pathway (vismodegib, sonidegib)
	Radiation therapy
Squamous Cell Carcinoma In Situ (Bowen's Disease)	Electrodesiccation and curettage
	Fluorouracil, topical
	Imiquimod
	Cryosurgery
	Laser
	Excision
	Photodynamic therapy
	Ingenol mebutate
Squamous Cell Carcinoma (SCC)	
Low risk	Electrodesiccation and curettage
	Cryosurgery
	Excision
	Mohs surgery
High risk	Excision
	Mohs surgery
	Radiation therapy (primary or adjuvant)
	Chemotherapy, adjuvant
	Immunotherapy, Anti-PD1 (cemiplimab, pembrolizumab), primary or adjuvant
Nonresectable SCC	Radiation
	Chemotherapy
	Immunotherapy (anti-PD1)

10. **What are BCCs?**

   BCCs are the most common cutaneous malignancy and outnumber SCCs by approximately 4:1. They are low-grade malignancies of the skin and are microscopically composed of basaloid cells with characteristic peripheral palisading of the tumor cells. These basaloid tumor islands often demonstrate connections to the overlying epidermis or follicular epithelium. BCCs rarely metastasize, but can be quite locally aggressive if neglected. The origin of these common tumors has been debated, but it is believed that BCCs originate from the follicular epithelium, specifically from the stem cells of the outer root sheath. Although BCC has a very low mortality rate, the morbidity and cost from managing these tumors is high, given the large numbers of BCCs treated each year and the frequent occurrence of these tumors on cosmetically and functionally sensitive anatomic locations.

Donovan J. Review of the hair follicle origin hypothesis for basal cell carcinoma. *Dermatol Surg.* 2009;35(9):1311–1323.
Cameron MC, Lee E, Hibler BP, et al. Basal cell carcinoma: epidemiology; pathophysiology; clinical and histological subtypes; and disease associations. *J Am Acad Dermatol.* 2019;80(2):303–317.

11. **What is the molecular basis for the development of sporadic BCC?**

   The majority of sporadic BCCs are the result of UV-induced alterations in the hedgehog signaling pathway. The most common mutation in sporadic BCCs (90%) occurs in the tumor suppressor gene *PTCH*, found at locus 9q22, which encodes the PTCH1 protein. This protein is a receptor for a secreted protein ligand called sonic hedgehog (Shh), which is important in signaling processes that control cell growth and fate. Another 10% of sporadic BCCs have activating mutations in the smoothened protein (SMO), another participant in the hedgehog signaling pathway. Investigation into this pathway has led to the development of the medications vismodegib and sonidegib, which are small-molecle inhibitors, of the hedgehog pathway. They are indicated for the treatment of locally advanced and metastatic BCC, especially when surgical removal is not possible or indicated.

Epstein EH. Basal cell carcinomas: attack of the hedgehog. *Nat Rev Cancer.* 2008;8(10):743–754.
Von Hoff DD, LoRusso PM, Rudin CM, et al. Inhibition of the hedgehog pathway in advanced basal-cell carcinoma. *N Engl J Med.* 2009;361 (12):1164–1172.

12. **Describe the clinical and histologic appearance of BCCs.**

   BCCs may have more than one clinical or histologic appearance. The most common presentation is a nodular BCC, which is typically a slow-growing lesion with a smooth or pebbly surface. Nodular BCC characteristically appears translucent or pearly and often demonstrates dilated vessels (telangiectasias) (Fig. 43.1A). The tumor can gradually break down, bleed, and form ulcers (noduloulcerative BCC, Fig. 43.1B). Superficial BCCs are thin lesions that demonstrate a horizontal growth pattern. They present as erythematous, minimally indurated, slow-growing papules or plaques with variable scale (Fig. 43.1C). They can be confused with tinea corporis, nummular dermatitis, or other NMSCs such as SCC in situ (SCCIS). Morpheaform (also called desmoplastic or sclerosing) BCCs are a type of infiltrative lesion that may resemble scars or normal skin. Microscopically, they are composed of narrow cords and strands of basaloid cells that infiltrate between the collagen bundles. This variant can easily be missed, even by experienced dermatologists, and has a higher rate of recurrence after treatment than other BCC subtypes. Their true extent is often much greater than the clinical appearance suggests. BCCs can also be completely or focally pigmented and mistaken for malignant melanoma. The basosquamous variant of BCC has features of SCC and exhibits more aggressive clinical behavior. A rare variant of BCC, called a Pinkus tumor or fibroepithelioma of Pinkus, looks like a large skin tag or fibroma and is usually found in the lumbosacral region.

13. **What is basal cell nevus syndrome?**

   Basal cell nevus syndrome, also called Gorlin' syndrome, is an autosomal dominant inherited disorder characterized by a number of different germline mutations of *PTCH*—the same gene that is found to be mutated in most sporadic BCCs. It is characterized by the early onset and continued development of numerous BCCs (Fig. 43.2), in addition to other tumors and developmental abnormalities including odontogenic keratocysts of the jaw (see Chapter 62), palmar and plantar pits, skeletal abnormalities, medulloblastoma, and calcification of the falx cerebri.

Lam C, Ou JC, Billingsley EM. "PTCH"–ing it together: a basal cell nevus syndrome review. *Dermatol Surg.* 2013;39:1557–1572.

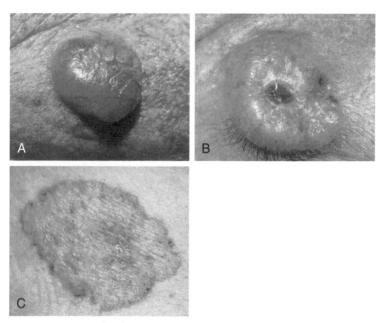

Fig. 43.1 Variants of basal cell carcinoma (BCC). **A,** Nodular BCC demonstrating characteristic dilated blood vessels. **B,** Noduloulcerative BCC above the eyebrow, demonstrating pearly appearance and central ulceration. **C,** Large superficial BCC demonstrating a plaque with focal scale and crust. (Panels A and B courtesy James E. Fitzpatrick, MD.)

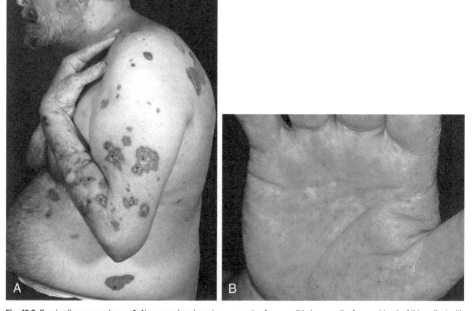

Fig. 43.2 Basal cell nevus syndrome. **A,** Numerous basal carcinomas varying from small to large on the face and trunk of this patient with several hundred basal cell carcinomas. **B,** Numerous keratotic palmar pits in a patient with basal cell nevus syndrome. (Courtesy Fitzsimons Army Medical Center teaching files.)

14. What do typical SCCs look like clinically?

SCCs may resemble BCCs, actinic keratoses, or warts, but often the initial appearance is that of an ill-defined, red lesion with a rough surface (Fig. 43.3A). SCCs are more likely to demonstrate overlying scale than are BCCs. At times, the scale may project above the skin surface, producing a cutaneous horn. Larger lesions may break down, ulcerate, and bleed. SCCs tend to be painful. Verrucous carcinomas are a variant of SCC that look like warts and are often misdiagnosed (Fig. 43.3B). Like warts, they often occur on hands and feet, but can also appear on the anogenital epithelium and oral mucosa. Verrucous carcinomas are slow growing and rarely metastasize, but they can be extremely locally aggressive.

15. What is the biologic behavior of cutaneous SCC?

Although the majority of SCCs are low risk, SCCs are more aggressive than BCCs and are more likely to metastasize. SCCs are currently estimated to metastasize at an overall rate of 2% to 6%, most commonly to the lymph nodes. Certain sites have higher rates of metastasis—SCCs arising from the vermilion lip metastasize in up to 7.6 to 14% of cases (Fig. 43.3C) and those arising from the ear metastasize in 11% of cases. SCCs arising in scars have metastatic rates of up to 30% and SCCs arising in modified epithelium (e.g., glans penis, vulva) and in immunocompromised patients are also more likely to metastasize. Disease-specific mortality rates for cutaneous SCC are thought to be 1% to 2%, with an estimated 4000 to 8000 deaths in the United States occurring each year. There are multiple staging systems available for advanced cutaneous SCC (American Joint Committee on Cancer, Brigham and Women's Hospital, International Union Against Cancer), but identifying which tumors would benefit most from aggressive therapy remains difficult. Multiple genetic mutations are associated with the development of cutaneous SCCs, in particular 90% of these tumors have UV-induced mutations in the *p53* tumor suppressor gene.

Brougham ND, Dennett ER, Cameron R, et al. The incidence of metastasis from cutaneous squamous cell carcinoma and the impact of its risk factors. *J Surg Oncol.* 2012;106:811–815.

Wang DM, Kraft S, Rohani P, et al. Association of nodal metastasis and mortality with vermilion vs cutaneous lip location in cutaneous squamous cell carcinoma of the lip. *JAMA Dermatol.* 2018;154(6):701–707.

Karia PS, Han J, Schmults CD. Cutaneous squamous cell carcinoma: estimated incidence of disease, nodal metastasis, and deaths from disease in the United States, 2012. *J Am Acad Dermatol.* 2013;68:957–966.

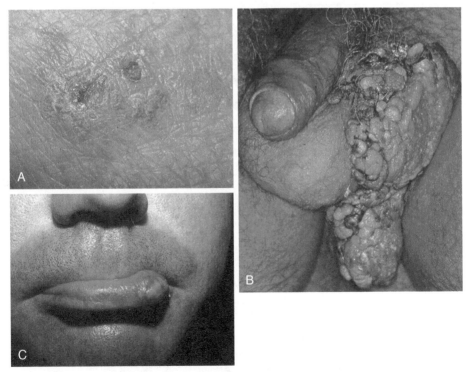

Fig. 43.3 Variants of squamous cell carcinoma (SCC). **A,** Early SCC arising in an actinic keratosis in a patient with history of chronic arsenic exposure. **B,** Large verrucous carcinoma of the genitalia. Verrucous carcinomas often reach large sizes before diagnosis because they are often treated as warts. **C,** Ulcerated squamous cell carcinoma of the lip of a 27-year-old man. This aggressive tumor was already metastatic to the cervical lymph node at the time of presentation. (Courtesy Fitzsimons Army Medical Center teaching files.)

16. What are high-risk factors for cutaneous SCC that predict a higher rate of recurrence, metastasis, and death?
    - Tumor location (ear, lip and areas of long lasting chronic ulcers or inflammation)
    - Clinical size (>2 cm)
    - Histologic depth (extension beyond the subcutaneous tissue; depth greater than 6 mm)
    - Histologic subtype (acantholytic, spindle, and desmoplastic subtypes)
    - Degree of differentiation (poorly differentiated or undifferentiated)
    - Perineural invasion of at least 0.1 mm
    - Lymphovascular invasion
    - Recurrence
    - Patient characteristics (OTRs, chronic lymphocytic leukemia, genetic syndromes)

Samarasinghe V, Madan V, Lear JT. Management of high-risk squamous cell carcinoma of the skin. *Expert Rev Anticancer Ther.* 2011;11:763–769.
Schmults CD, Karia PS, Carter JB, et al. Factors predictive of recurrence and death from cutaneous squamous cell carcinoma: a 10-year, single-institution cohort study. *JAMA Dermatol.* 2013;149:541–547.

17. What are keratoacanthomas?
    Keratoacanthomas are epidermal tumors that almost invariably appear on sun-exposed skin. They frequently appear suddenly and grow quickly as skin-colored, dome-shaped nodules that develop a central keratin-filled plug (Fig. 43.4). In the past, these lesions were considered to be a benign neoplasm, as their natural progression is to spontaneously regress without treatment. However, distinguishing a keratoacanthoma from a well-differentiated SCC based on clinical appearance or histology can be difficult. Currently, the standard of care is to treat keratoacanthomas as subtype of well-differentiated SCC, and many pathologists will describe their distinctive histology as "SCC, keratoacanthoma type." Solitary keratoacanthomas are the most common variant, but the tumor is also associated with trauma, specific genetic syndromes, and exposure to certain molecularly targeted chemotherapies. The site of origin of keratoacanthomas is uncertain, but experimental and epidemiologic studies implicate follicular epithelium.

Kwiek B, Schwartz RA. Keratoacanthoma (KA): an update and review. *J Am Acad Dermatol.* 2016;74(6):1220–1233.
Mandrell JC, Santa Cruz D. Keratoacanthoma: hyperplasia, benign neoplasm, or a type of squamous cell carcinoma? *Semin Diagn Pathol.* 2009;26:150–163.

18. What is Bowen's disease?
    Bowen's disease is an older term for SCCIS (Fig. 43.5A). Clinically, SCCIS presents as persistent, erythematous, slightly indurated plaques with variable scale. SCCIS may resemble superficial BCC, Paget's disease, or various inflammatory skin conditions. It can also appear as a pigmented plaque mimicking a melanocytic lesion. Because it is often related to HPV infection, SCCIS in the anogenital region (also called Bowenoid papulosis) may occur more prominently in young adults. Bowenoid papulosis carries a 2.6% risk of transformation to invasive SCC. SCCIS occurring on the male genitalia has also been described under the name *erythroplasia of Queyrat* (Fig. 43.5B). Microscopically, SCCIS demonstrates full-thickness cytologic atypia of the keratinocytes without invasion through the basement membrane. SCCIS is considered a precursor lesion for invasive SCC.

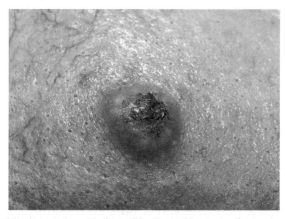

Fig. 43.4 Keratoacanthoma demonstrating a crateriform nodule with central keratin plug. (Courtesy James E. Fitzpatrick, MD.)

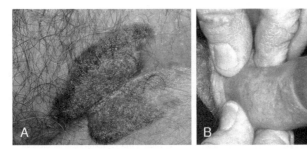

Fig. 43.5 A, Squamous cell carcinoma in situ presenting a scaly plaque on the groin. **B,** Squamous cell carcinoma of the penis (erythroplasia of Queyrat) presenting as an erythematous, minimally indurated plaque.

Prieto-Granada C, Rodriguez-Waitkus P. Cutaneous squamous cell carcinoma and related entities: epidemiology, clinical and histological features, and basic science overview. *Curr Probl Cancer.* 2015;39(4):206–215.
Dubina M, Goldenberg G. Viral-associated nonmelanoma skin cancers: a review. *Am J Dermatopathol.* 2009;31(6):561573.

19. What is an actinic keratosis?

Actinic keratoses (solar keratoses) are sun-induced precancerous lesions of the skin. They are very common in patients with light skin color and significant sun exposure. Microscopically, actinic keratoses are characterized by a proliferation of cytologically atypical keratinocytes that bud off of or replace the bottom layer of the epidermis. The atypical cells do not involve the full thickness of the epidermis. The rate of progression of untreated actinic keratoses to invasive SCCs varies widely in different studies from 0.1% to 20%, but it is most likely that the true rate of transformation is less than 5% per year for an individual actinic keratosis. About 60% of SCCs are calculated to arise in a precursor actinic keratosis, and the time for an actinic keratosis to progress to a SCC has been estimated at approximately 2 years.

Criscione VD, Weinstock MA, Naylor MF, et al. Actinic keratoses: natural history and risk of malignant transformation in the Veterans Affairs Topical Tretinoin Chemoprevention Trial. *Cancer.* 2009;115(11):2523–2530. (free online text).
Fuchs A, Marmur E. The kinetics of skin cancer: progression of actinic keratosis to squamous cell carcinoma. *Dermatol Surg.* 2007;33:1099–1101.

20. What do actinic keratoses look like?

Actinic keratoses initially appear as small, palpable bumps on normal sun-exposed skin that gradually enlarge and become red and scaly (Fig. 43.6). The overlying scale may be extensive to the point that markedly exophytic cutaneous horns are produced. Less common variants include atrophic and pigmented actinic keratoses. *Actinic cheilitis* is a term used for actinic keratoses that present on the sun-exposed vermilion lip. Many elderly patients who complain of chronic dry lower lips actually have extensive actinic cheilitis.

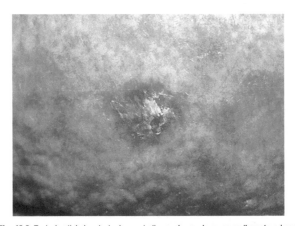

Fig. 43.6 Typical actinic keratosis demonstrating scaly papule on an erythematous base.

21. How should premalignant lesions, such as actinic keratoses and actinic cheilitis, be treated?

While a small percentage of actinic keratoses regress spontaneously, the majority will persist and a small percentage will progress to invasive SCC. Treating actinic keratoses can therefore prevent the development of SCC. Additionally, small SCCs are difficult to separate from actinic keratoses on clinical exam. The smallest SCCs are often picked up when a suspected actinic lesion does not respond to treatment or a lesion appears in a treated area.

Since these premalignancies can vary from being tiny, barely palpable lesions to involvement of an entire lip or scalp, treatment modalities depend on the size and location. Small, individual papules can be treated with cryosurgery or curettage. Patients with multiple actinic keratoses often benefit from field treatment of an entire anatomic area with destructive modalities (dermabrasion, chemical peels, laser therapy), topical therapies (imiquimod, topical 5-fluorouracil, diclofenac, ingenol mebutate, and retinoids), or photodynamic therapy. Actinic cheilitis can be treated with the same modalities as actinic keratoses. Patients with severe actinic cheilitis, especially those who have developed SCC within the lip, may benefit from complete laser ablation of the vermilion lip or surgical vermilionectomy to completely remove the affected skin.

Werner RN, Sammain A, Erdmann R, Hartmann V, Stockfleth E, Nast A. The natural history of actinic keratosis: a systematic review. *Br J Dermatol.* 2013;169(3):502–518.

CHAPTER 44

MELANOMA

Michael R. Campoli and Whitney A. High

"But what is the black spot, captain?" I asked.
"That's a summons, mate."
                    —Robert Louis Stevenson, *Treasure Island*

1. **What is melanoma?**
   Cutaneous melanoma is a malignant tumor of skin melanocytes. Other, less common sites of melanoma that are not considered "cutaneous" include melanoma of the eye, brain, oral mucosa, nasopharyngeal area, nail bed, and anal area.

2. **How common is melanoma in the United States?**
   For 2019, the American Cancer Society estimates that in the United States, about 96,500 new melanomas will be diagnosed and about 7250 people will die of melanoma. Melanoma is the most rapidly increasing form of cancer in the United States. Its incidence has increased more than 15-fold (~3% annually) over the last 40 years. For non-Hispanic white people in the United States, the yearly incidence is about 19 cases per 100,000 men and 14 cases per 100,000 women. Melanoma is now the most common cancer in young women aged 25 to 29 years. In the early 1900s, the lifetime risk of developing melanoma was about 1 in 1500, whereas it is now estimated to be about 1 in 40 for persons born in the year 2007.

American Cancer Society. *Facts & Figures 2019*. Atlanta, GA: American Cancer Society; 2019.
National Cancer Institute. *SEER Cancer stat facts: melanoma of the skin.* https://seer.cancer.gov/statfacts/html/melan.html. Accessed June 10, 2019.

3. **What is the 5-year survival rate for patients with melanoma?**
   Melanoma accounts for only about 1% of all skin cancers, but it causes the most skin cancer deaths. However, as shown in Table 44.1, the 5-year survival rate for melanoma is highly dependent upon disease stage. Men older than 65 years of age have the greatest risk of dying from melanoma. In recent years, the addition of treatments such as anti-CTLA-4 (cytotoxic T-lymphocyte-associated), anti–programmed cell death protein 1 (PD-1), and BRAF/MEK inhibitors has led to improved survival in patients with advanced melanoma. While a rising incidence of melanoma, with lesser mortality, has been attributed to improved early detection of thinner melanomas, some data indicate an increase in thicker, more advanced melanoma, suggesting other factors are at play. This controversy is unlikely to be resolved until improved prognostic markers for melanoma are discovered and utilized.

Whiteman DC, Green AC, Olsen CM. The growing burden of invasive melanoma: projections of incidence rates and numbers of new cases in six susceptible populations through 2031. *J Invest Dermatol.* 2016;136:1161–1171.
Siegel RL, Miller KD, Jemal A. Cancer statistics.*CA Cancer J Clin.* 2017;67:7–30.

4. **What causes melanoma?**
   Genetic and environmental factors impact the development of melanoma. About 10% of cutaneous melanomas are familial. Epidemiologic evidence suggests brief, intense exposure to ultraviolet A (UVA) radiation, more than ultraviolet B (UVB) radiation, contributes to development of melanoma. Sun exposure early in life, with development of more nevi, likely impacts melanoma risk. Additional potential causes of melanoma include mutations in and/or loss of tumor suppressor genes.

Armstrong BK, Cust AE. Sun exposure and skin cancer, and the puzzle of cutaneous melanoma: a perspective on Fears et al. Mathematical models of age and ultraviolet effects on the incidence of skin cancer among whites in the United States. *American Journal of Epidemiology.* 1977;105:420–427. *Cancer Epidemiol.* 2017;48:147–156.

5. **What groups have a genetic predisposition to familial melanoma?**
   A major gene locus associated with familial melanoma is *CDKN2A*, located on chromosome 9. This gene encodes p16 and p14^{ARF}, which regulate the retinoblastoma (Rb) and p53 pathways, respectively. Germline *CDKN2A* mutations are transmitted in autosomal dominant fashion and account for about 20%–50% of familial melanoma. These mutations are also found in a subset of patients with familial dysplastic mole syndrome (FDMS) who also demonstrate an

Table 44.1 2009 AJCC stage groupings and 5-year survival for primary cutaneous melanoma*

STAGE	TUMOR	NODE	METASTASES	5-YEAR SURVIVAL	10-YEAR SURVIVAL
0	Tis	N0	M0	99.5%	99%
IA	T1a	N0	M0	97%	95%
IB	T1b, 2a	N0	M0	92%	86%
IIA	T2b, 3a	N0	M0	81%	67%
IIB	T3b, 4a	N0	M0	70%	57%
IIC	T4b	N0	M0	53%	40%
IIIA	T1–4a	N1a–2a	M0	78%	68%
IIIB	T1–4b	N1a–2c	M0	59%	43%
IIIC	T1–4b	N1b–3	M0	40%	24%
IV	Any T	Any N	M1a–c	15%–20%	15%

Data from Gershenwald JE, Scolyer RA. Melanoma Staging: American Joint Committee on Cancer (AJCC) 8th Edition and Beyond. *Ann Surg Oncol.* 2018;25:2105–2110.
*Range reflects the prognostic impact of tumor burden (micrometastasis versus macrometastasis), number of nodes involved, and whether there was extracapsular extension. Patients with in-transit metastases/satellite lesions without metastatic lymph nodes are classified as N2c.

association between pancreatic cancer, and multiple nevi. Patients with FDMS present with multiple atypical nevi (>50) and a personal and/or family history of melanoma in two or more blood relatives. FDMS patients present with melanomas at a younger age (prevalence of melanoma approaches 85% by age 48) and are at a higher risk to develop a second primary melanoma.

The melanocortin receptor 1 (*MCR1*) gene has also been implicated in familial melanoma. Mutations in tumor suppressor BRCA1-associated protein 1 (BAP1) can predispose to cutaneous and ocular melanoma, other spitzoid atypical melanocytic lesions, and internal malignancies. Patients with mutations in the telomerase reverse transcriptase (*TERT*), microphthalmia-associated transcription factor (*MITF*), and phosphatase and tensin homolog (*PTEN*) genes have also been shown to have a higher incidence of cutaneous melanoma. The molecular mechanisms underlying these gene defects that are associated with cutaneous melanoma are not yet fully elucidated.

Soura E, Eliades PJ, Shannon K, Stratigos AJ, Tsao H. Hereditary melanoma: update on syndromes and management: emerging melanoma cancer complexes and genetic counseling. *J Am Acad Dermatol.* 2016;74:411–420.
Soura E, Eliades PJ, Shannon K, Stratigos AJ, Tsao H. Hereditary melanoma: update on syndromes and management: genetics of familial atypical multiple mole melanoma syndrome. *J Am Acad Dermatol.* 2016;74:395–407.

6. What are the most important risk factors for melanoma?
   Genetic and environmental factors impact melanoma risk. Genetic factors include past medical history of melanoma, family history of melanoma in a first-degree relative, fairer skin types (Fitzpatrick type I and II), larger congenital nevi, the presence of numerous atypical nevi, more than 50 benign nevi (>2 mm in size), xeroderma pigmentosum, and FDMS. Genetic variations in the *MCR1* gene, involved in pigment diversity, confer risk of melanoma. Specifically, *MC1R* variations that lead to increased production of pheomelanin (red or blond hair, freckles, and light-colored skin that tans poorly) increase the risk of melanoma. Environmental factors include intermittent high-intensity exposure to UVA and UVB radiation (especially at a young age), blistering sunburns, immunosuppression, and residence in equatorial latitudes. Ephelides (freckles), indicative of sun exposure, are associated with a two- to threefold increased risk of melanoma.

van der Leest RJ, Flohil SC, Arends LR, de Vries E, Nijsten T. Risk of subsequent cutaneous malignancy in patients with prior melanoma: a systematic review and meta-analysis. *J Eur Acad Dermatol Venereol.* 2015;29:1053–1062.
Jiang AJ, Rambhatla PV, Eide MJ. Socioeconomic and lifestyle factors and melanoma: a systematic review. *Br J Dermatol.* 2015;172:885–915.

7. List groups at higher risk for developing melanoma.
   - Persons with multiple atypical nevi
   - Persons with more than 50 benign nevi (>2 mm in size)
   - Persons with FDMS (>50 atypical nevi and a first-degree relative with melanoma)
   - Persons with *CDKN2A* mutations

- Persons with a large congenital nevus
- Persons with a past medical history of melanoma
- Persons with xeroderma pigmentosum

8. **Do all melanomas develop from atypical nevi?**

Melanoma can arise in nevi, including atypical nevi. Moreover, molecular analysis of primary melanomas that coexist with nevi suggests that melanomas arose from the nevi via intermediary lesions. Nevertheless, it is important to stress that most atypical nevi do not progress to melanoma. Around 40% to 75% of melanomas develop de novo, and of those melanomas that develop in association with a preexisting nevus, only about 50% of the nevi were histologically atypical. While there is a clear association between nevi, atypical nevi, and melanoma risk, only a portion of this risk is attributable to acquisition of genetic mutations in the nevi.

Shain AH, Bastian BC. From melanocytes to melanomas. *Nat Rev Cancer.* 2016;16:345–358.

9. **What are cancer stem cells (CSCs)?**

There is some evidence that melanoma, as well as other solid tumors, may contain a subpopulation of CSCs. CSCs are rare cells in tumors that can "self-renew" and drive tumorigenesis. CSCs are considered the source of tumor mass and are thought responsible for drug resistance and cancer recurrence. CSCs may also be responsible for metastatic disease, while less genetically capable cells grow locally. However, definitive markers for CSCs are lacking, and the inability to identify consistent markers in vivo has called into question the existence of melanoma CSCs; the issue is still one of considerable debate.

Brinckerhoff CE. Cancer stem cells (CSCs) in melanoma: there's smoke, but is there fire? *J Cell Physiol.* 2017;232:2674–2678.

10. **Is melanoma a single disease?**

No, it is likely melanoma is a common endpoint from multiple potential genetic pathways. Historically, melanoma has been divided into subsets based both upon clinical and histologic appearance and upon varied associations with skin color, sun exposure, and anatomic site. Recent molecular investigations have demonstrated that biologic subsets of disease vary in their relationship to anatomic site, sun exposure, nevus phenotype, and mutational analysis.

KEY POINTS: DIAGNOSIS OF MELANOMA

1. Melanoma is a deadly skin cancer with a rapidly increasing incidence rate.
2. When diagnosed early, and treated appropriately, melanoma can have a high cure rate.
3. Patients at higher risk for melanoma include those with FDMS, heritable *CDKN2A* mutations, multiple atypical nevi, more than 50 benign nevi, larger congenital nevi, a past medical history of melanoma, a family history of melanoma in a first-degree relative, and xeroderma pigmentosum.
4. While persons with fair skin may be at higher risk for melanoma, patients with darker skin types can also develop melanoma.
5. Melanomas do not always arise in a preexisting nevus, but melanoma can arise in a nevus.
6. Melanoma is not a single disease:
   - *B-Raf* mutations are often found in younger patients on intermittently sun-exposed skin.
   - *N-Ras* mutations are often found in older patients on chronically sun-exposed skin.
   - *c-Kit* mutations are often found in mucosal and acral melanomas.
   - *BAP1*, *GNAQ*, and *GNA11* mutations have been identified in uveal melanomas.

11. **What are the molecular pathways in melanoma?**

Although melanocytes divide rarely ($<$2 times a year), the proliferative index of melanocytes increases with genetic mutations. Although it is assumed that the mutations in melanoma originate from the mutagenic effect of UVA and UVB radiation, other indirect effects, such as free radicals produced from the biochemical interaction of UVA and melanin, may be involved in these pathologic genetic effects. Major molecular pathways implicated in melanoma include p16 (25% to 50%) and p14^{ARF} (25% to 50%), MITF (50% to 75%), B-Raf (50% to 60%), and PTEN (15% to 25%). The antiapoptotic factor Bcl-2 is often overexpressed in melanoma.

Moreover, not all melanomas are genetically similar. Melanomas that develop in younger persons, on intermittently sun-exposed skin, demonstrate a greater percentage of *B-Raf* mutations ($>$60%) than those that arise on chronically sun-exposed skin of older patients ($<$15%). In contrast, melanomas that develop on chronically sun-exposed skin in older persons demonstrate a greater percentage of *N-Ras* mutations (20% to 40%). Melanomas that develop on acral and mucosal sites demonstrate a greater percentage of *c-Kit* mutations ($>$40%) compared to non–sun-exposed (0%) and sun-exposed (30%) melanomas. Acral and mucosal melanomas also demonstrate a lower percentage of *B-Raf* mutations ($<$20% and $<$10%, respectively).

Unlike cutaneous melanoma, uveal melanoma is not characterized by mutations in *BRAF, NRAS*, or *KIT*. Despite the lack of activating mutations in *BRAF, NRAS*, and *KIT*, the mitogen-activated protein kinase (MAPK) pathway in uveal melanoma is critical to the development and progression of uveal melanoma. Activating mutations in the guanine nucleotide-binding protein Q polypeptide (GNAQ), which encodes for the alpha subunit of a heterotrimeric G protein, is found in 45% to 50% of uveal melanoma cases. More recently, mutations in *BAP1* have been linked to the development of metastatic disease in uveal melanoma.

Alexandrov LB, Nik-Zainal S, Wedge DC, et al. Signatures of mutational processes in human cancer. *Nature.* 2013;500:415–421.
Bastian BC. The molecular pathology of melanoma: an integrated taxonomy of melanocytic neoplasia. *Annu Rev Pathol.* 2014;9:239–271.
Shain AH, Yeh I, Kovalyshyn I, et al. The genetic evolution of melanoma from precursor lesions. *N Engl J Med.* 2015;373:1926–1936.
Cancer Genome Atlas Network. Genomic classification of cutaneous melanoma. *Cell.* 2015;161:1681–1696.

12. How does BRAF play a role in melanoma?

The activating BRAFv600 (Val600) mutation is typical feature of benign nevi and is also the most prevalent mutation in melanoma. The BRAF gene encodes a serine/threonine kinase involved in the mitogen-activated protein kinase (MAPK) / extracellular signal-regulated kinase (ERK) signaling pathway. Just downstream of BRAF in the MAPK signaling pathway are two other proteins—MEK1 and MEK2. Activated BRAF protein kinase phosphorylates and activates these two MEK proteins that then activate the downstream MAP kinases. This RAS/RAF/MEK/MAP kinase pathway mediates cellular responses to growth signaling and can control the survival of melanoma tumor cells. This pathway is constitutively active in BRAF-mutated melanoma, resulting in unchecked cell division and angiogenesis, evasion of cellular senescence, and loss of apoptosis (Fig. 44.1).

Catalogue of somatic mutations in cancer (COSMIC). Wellcome trust sanger institute, genome research limited. http://cancer.sanger.ac.uk/cosmic. Accessed July 15, 2015.

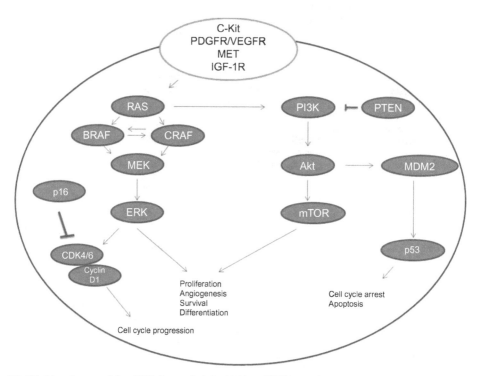

Fig. 44.1 Schematic representation of RAS/mitogen-activated protein kinase (MAPK) oncogenic signaling in melanoma. MAPK signaling can be initiated by the activation of receptor tyrosine kinases (RTKs) (e.g., c-Kit, platelet-derived growth factor receptors [PDGF-R], vascular endothelial growth factor receptors [VEGFRs], tyrosine-protein kinase Met or hepatocyte growth factor receptor [HGFR], insulin-like growth factor 1 [IGF-1] receptor, and epidermal growth factor receptor) by growth factors. Activation of RTKs stimulates the conversion of RAS from a GDP-bound state to GTP-bound (i.e., active) via the activity of guanine nucleotide exchange factors (GEF). Activated RAS can then phosphorylate RAF, leading to its activation. Once active, RAF can phosphorylate and activate MEK1 and MEK2 that then subsequently activate ERK1/2, resulting in the translocation and regulation of several transcription factors in the nucleus, such as cyclin D1, c-MYC, and microphthalmia-associated transcription factor (MITF). Besides initiation of MAPK signaling, RAS-GDP is also able to promote survival through the PI3K signaling pathway, by activating protein kinase b (AKT).

13. Is there a host immune response to melanoma?

Yes. Observations such as incomplete or complete regression of melanoma, the occurrence of vitiligo and halo nevi in patients with melanoma, and increased rates of melanoma in immunosuppressed persons indicate that the immune system plays a vital role in the course of melanoma. Tumor antigen (TA)–specific T cells play an active role in eliminating tumors and metastases. Similarly, in vitro studies employing human peripheral blood lymphocytes isolated from patients with melanoma contain TA-specific CD8$^+$ and CD4$^+$ precursor T cells, as well as natural killer cells and macrophages that kill tumor cells. CD8$^+$ T cells are thought to play a major role in controlling growth of melanoma (Fig. 44.2). These observations underpin a rationale for immunotherapy in melanoma.

Parmiani G, Castelli C, Santinami M, et al. Melanoma immunology: past, present and future. *Curr Opin Oncol.* 2007;19:121–127.
Bruttel VS, Wischhusen J. Cancer stem cell immunology: key to understanding tumorigenesis and tumor immune escape? *Front Immunol.* 2014;5:360.

14. How do melanomas evade the immune system?

Melanoma cells evade the immune system through multiple mechanisms. The Janus-kinase (JAK)/signal-transducer-and-activator-of-transcription (STAT) pathway is a major regulator of the programmed cell death protein 1 (PD-1) immune checkpoint (Fig 44.2). Upon recognition of tumor by T cells, interferons (IFNs) then released trigger JAK-STAT-mediated expression of PD-1 ligands on the surface of melanoma cells. Binding of PD-1 to PD-1 ligands (PD-1L) leads to the suppression of T-cell activity, which is undesired. This observation forms the basis for use of PD-1/PD-1L inhibition in melanoma therapy. Further immunosuppressive mechanisms of melanoma include the downregulation of class-1 major histocompatibility complex (MHC) and the secretion of inhibitory factors like tumor growth factor β.

Umansky V, Sevko A. Melanoma-induced immunosuppression and its neutralization. *Semin Cancer Biol.* 2012;22:319–326.
Garcia-Diaz A, Shin DS, Moreno BH, et al. Interferon receptor signaling pathways regulating PD-L1 and PD-L2 expression. *Cell Rep.* 2017;19:1189–1201.

15. Describe the clinical appearance of melanoma.

Cutaneous melanomas are varied in appearance. Classically, early melanoma lesions are characterized by containing different colors, such as different hues of brown, black, red, and blue. Melanoma may also appear as a brown or black discoloration of the nail or as a skin ulcer that does not heal. Melanoma can begin in a preexisting melanocytic nevus, and when this occurs, the nevus usually demonstrates a "changing" appearance, such as increased size, or asymmetry/irregularity, or it may bleed with minor trauma. A changing nevus should always be evaluated, to exclude melanoma. A "new" nevus in any patient over about 35 years of age should also be carefully evaluated. Amelanotic melanomas have no clinically visible pigment and may be pinkish-looking, reddish, purple, normal skin color or essentially clear and colorless.

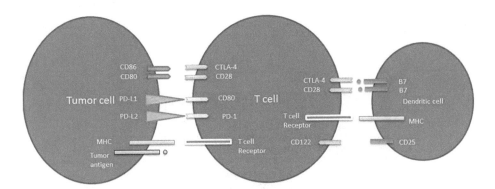

Fig. 44.2 Antigen presentation and T-cell activation via dendritic cells and tumor cells. T cells receive three signals from antigen presenting cells. Antigen presenting cells (APCs) present antigenic peptides complexed to MHC molecules to T cells through binding to their T-cell receptor (TCR) as shown. This interaction triggers intracellular signaling events (signal 1). T cells simultaneously receive additional "positive" and "negative" signals through ligand-receptor interactions within the immunological synapse. The costimulatory interaction is driven by CD80-CD28, and two inhibitory interactions driven by PD-L1/PD1 and CD80 cytotoxic T-lymphocyte-associated protein 4 (CTLA4). The integration of these signals delivers a second signal regulating the extent of T-cell activation. A third signal is also provided by cytokines released by APC. These activated T cells can recognize and destroy tumor cells by the presentation of small antigenic peptides via MHC class I on the tumor cell. Tumor cells can escape these specific T-cell immune responses in the course of somatic (genetic and phenotypic) clonal evolution. Alterations in the expression of MHC class I molecules, as well as the expression of PD-L1 and PD-L2, play a role in the molecular mechanisms underlying tumor cell immune evasion.

16. What are the ABCDEs of melanoma?

A new or changing pigmented lesion is the classic initial presentation of melanoma. A lesion that changes in size over a short period or develops pigment irregularity (black, hues of brown, red, blue, or white) should be evaluated and, quite likely, biopsied. The "ABCDEs" (Fig. 44.3) are a helpful guideline for lesions suspicious for possible melanoma.

- **A—A**symmetry. Any mole that appears unusual or shows asymmetry in shape should be evaluated.
- **B—B**order irregularity (or **B**leeding). The border of any melanocytic nevus should be relatively smooth, with a clear demarcation between the nevus and surrounding normal skin. Nevi that develop irregular or ill-defined borders should be evaluated. B is also for bleeding, and any mole that bleeds needs careful evaluation.
- **C—C**olor variegation. Most moles have relatively uniform tan or brown color. Moles that develop considerable color variegation (variable colors, particularly including grey, white and blue/black) should be carefully evaluated.
- **D—D**iameter. Most melanomas are greater than 6 mm in diameter (the diameter of a pencil eraser), but an otherwise suspicious lesion might be smaller or larger than this size.
- **E—E**volution. This emphasizes the need to evaluate any melanocytic nevus that has exhibited changing behavior over a relatively short time (weeks to months). This could include bleeding, itching, growth, or any other "evolutionary" behavior.

These "ABCDEs" are meant only to serve as general guidelines and do not take the place of a careful professional evaluation. Some physicians utilize an "ugly duckling sign," meaning a nevus with an appearance that is substantially "different" from other "signature" nevi in the same person, in the same general anatomic site, as an indication for biopsy.

Abbasi NR, Shaw HM, Rigel DS, et al. Early diagnosis of cutaneous melanoma: revisiting the ABCD criteria. *JAMA*. 2004;292:2771–2776.

17. Who should be screened for melanoma?

People with risk factors for melamoma (fair skin type, a history of atypical nevi, a strong family history of melanoma, etc.) should be screened at regular intervals, although no rigid guidelines exist. While it is thought that this will lead to identification of "thinner" melanomas, the precise benefit of regular screening on melanoma mortality is unclear. In 2016, the U.S. Preventive Services Task Force reviewed the effectiveness of skin cancer screening and concluded that "current evidence is insufficient to assess the balance of benefits and harms of visual skin examination by a clinician to screen for skin cancer in (asymptomatic) adults." The National Comprehensive Cancer Network (NCCN) recommends skin cancer screening every 6 to 12 months after a melanoma diagnosis but does not address screening guidelines for other populations. Although there is insufficient evidence to firmly conclude that skin cancer screening reduces melanoma mortality, some have argued for screening tailored to individual risk, to reduce melanoma mortality, and this is premised on improved survival for thinner (earlier) disease.

Coit DG, Thompson JA, Algazi A, et al. Melanoma, version 2.2016, NCCN Clinical Practice Guidelines in Oncology. *J Natl Compr Canc Netw*. 2016;14:450–473.

U.S. Preventive Services Task Force, Bibbins-Domingo K, Grossman DC, et al. Screening for skin cancer: US Preventive Services Task Force recommendation statement. *JAMA*. 2016;316:429–435.

Gardner LJ, Strunck JL, Wu YP, Grossman D. Current controversies in early-stage melanoma: questions on incidence, screening, and histologic regression. *J Am Acad Dermatol*. 2019;80:1–12.

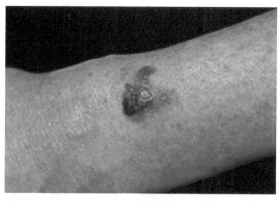

Fig. 44.3 Classic melanoma demonstrating asymmetry, irregular notched border, multiple colors, wide diameter, and a history of change and growth (evolution).

18. **What is dermoscopy?**

    Dermoscopy (dermatoscopy), also known as skin surface microscopy, or epiluminescence microscopy, is a noninvasive tool to examine melanocytic and nonmelanocytic tumors (see Chapter 3). Several dermoscopy algorithms are promulgated to aid in the assessment of melanocytic tumors but are not widely applied to lesions on the face, acral and mucosal surfaces, and nails. The sensitivity of dermoscopy in the diagnosis of melanoma ranges from 70% to 95%, compared to examination with the unaided eye, which ranges from 60% to 90%. It is critical to recognize that the success of dermoscopy depends on appropriate provider training.

    Dinnes J, Deeks JJ, Chuchu N, et al. Dermoscopy, with and without visual inspection, for diagnosing melanoma in adults. *Cochrane Database Syst Rev.* 2018;12(12):CD011902.

19. **Where on the body does melanoma most commonly arise?**

    Melanoma can arise on any part of the body. In men, primary tumors are most common on the trunk, while in women, primary tumors are most common on the lower extremity.

20. **Are there different types of melanoma?**

    Classically, melanoma was divided into the following types, but as already discussed, there is genetic evidence that these types may not be as important as was originally thought:

    - **Superficial spreading melanoma** (SSM) is the most common form of melanoma in whites (>70%). It is most often diagnosed in the fourth or fifth decade and presents as a slowly enlarging, brown (usually) or black spot with a macular and/or papular component. SSM can manifest color variegation and irregular borders (Fig. 44.4A). About 30% of SSM arises in a preexisting nevus, and 75% of these lesions demonstrate regression on exam.
    - **Nodular melanoma** is the second most common type of melanoma and represents about 15%–20% of cases. It is most often in men between the fifth and sixth decades, and it usually presents as a pigmented (usually brown or black) papule that slowly enlarges and often ulcerates (Fig. 44.4B). Nodular melanoma often presents on the head, neck, or trunk.
    - **Lentigo maligna/lentigo maligna melanoma** represents less than 15% of all cases of melanoma, but according to some evidence, it is a rapidly increasing subtype. It usually presents as an irregularly shaped, flat, pigmented lesion on actinically damaged skin on the face or other heavily sun-exposed sites. Most patients are elderly, and it is thought that a considerable length of time (years) may be spent in radial growth (**"melanoma in situ—lentigo maligna type"**) before vertical growth transpires. When invasion does occur, it is termed **lentigo maligna melanoma**.
    - **Acral lentiginous melanoma** represents 5% to 10% of all cases of melanoma. It is thought to be the commonest form of melanoma in African-Americans, Asians, and Hispanics (Fig. 44.4C). This form of melanoma usually appears as brown or black macules arising on the glabrous (non–hair-bearing) skin of an extremity (palms, soles, or nail beds). It can also occur on mucosal surfaces. The latter have an extremely poor prognosis.
    - **Amelanotic melanoma** is a non–pigment-producing variant of nodular melanoma. It is rare and comprises ~1% of all melanomas. Amelanotic melanoma can be confused with other benign skin lesions, such as pyogenic granuloma. A delayed diagnosis is not uncommon for amelanotic melanoma, and this may result in a poorer overall prognosis (Fig. 44.5).

21. **What is Clark level?**

    Clark level is a system to categorize depth of invasion for melanoma that was developed by Dr. Wallace Clark, Jr. (see below). Melanomas are classified by depth of invasion into the anatomic structures of the skin. In 2009, the American Joint Committee on Cancer (AJCC) Melanoma Staging and Classification System removed the Clark level as a regular staging parameter.

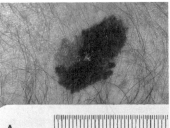

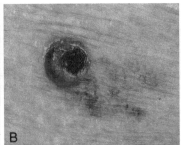
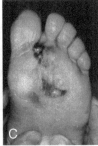

Fig. 44.4 A, Superficial spreading melanoma. The lesion shows asymmetry, notched borders, and shades of light brown. **B,** Superficial spreading malignant melanoma that has developed a nodular melanoma. **C,** Acral lentiginous melanoma on the sole of the foot demonstrating a macular and focally nodular pigmented lesion with multiple shades of black and gray with a very irregular border. (Panel A courtesy James E. Fitzpatrick, MD; panel C courtesy Fitzsimons Army Medical Center teaching files.)

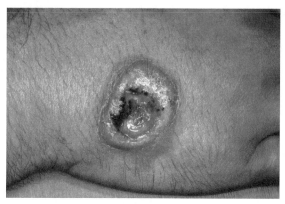

Fig. 44.5 Ulcerative amelanotic melanoma on the back of the hand. (Courtesy Fitzsimons Army Medical Center teaching files.)

- **Level I:** Tumor cells in epidermis only (melanoma in situ).
- **Level II:** Tumor cells extend from epidermis into (but do not fill) papillary dermis.
- **Level III:** Tumor cells extend from epidermis into and fill papillary dermis.
- **Level IV:** Tumor cells extend into reticular dermis.
- **Level V:** Tumor cells extend through the dermis into underlying subcutaneous fat.

22. What is Breslow depth?

Breslow depth, developed first by Dr. Alexander Breslow, is the most widely employed method for classifying the depth of invasion for primary melanoma. It is defined as the distance in millimeters as measured visually from the top of the granular layer of the epidermis, or from the base of an ulcer (in ulcerated lesions), to the deepest point of invasion by tumor cells. Breslow depth seems to be the strongest histologic predictor of survival when examining a primary lesion.

Keung EZ, Gershenwald JE. The eighth edition American Joint Committee on Cancer (AJCC) melanoma staging system: implications for melanoma treatment and care. *Expert Rev Anticancer Ther.* 2018;18:775–784.
Conic RRZ, Ko J, Damiani G, et al. Predictors of sentinel lymph node positivity in thin melanoma using the National Cancer Database. *J Am Acad Dermatol.* 2019;80:441–447.

23. What other findings should be reported in the histopathologic diagnosis of melanoma?

The AJCC recommends reporting at least the following parameters regarding the histologic diagnosis of melanoma: thickness (Breslow depth), mitoses/mm^2, presence of regression, tumor-infiltrating lymphocytes (TILs), ulceration, vascular invasion, microscopic satellites, associated nevus, and margin status. It should be noted that the AJCC classification of melanoma was updated to the eighth edition in 2017. Histopathologically, mitotic counts are not relevant for staging, and tumor depth is rounded to tenths of millimeters (due to considerations of reproducibility).

Payette MJ, Katz M III, Grant-Kels JM. Melanoma prognostic factors found in the dermatopathology report. *Clin Dermatol.* 2009;27:53–74.
Keung EZ, Gershenwald JE. The eighth edition American Joint Committee on Cancer (AJCC) melanoma staging system: implications for melanoma treatment and care. *Expert Rev Anticancer Ther.* 2018;18:775–784.

24. What immunohistochemical (IHC) markers may be utilized in the diagnosis of melanoma?

First, there is no "melanoma stain" that can be used to recognize melanoma in binary fashion. However, IHC staining can be useful in some cases to support an overall histologic impression. The most often utilized IHC stains are as follows:

- **S100:** An antibody that targets a calcium-binding protein expressed in melanocytes, Langerhans cells, and nerve cells. Although with low specificity, S100 has a high sensitivity for melanocytes.
- **HMB45:** An antibody that targets a glycoprotein of the pre-melanosome complex, HMB45 has a higher specificity for melanocytes, in general, but lesser sensitivity for some types of melanoma (desmoplastic melanoma). In common benign nevi, HMB45 often demonstrates "zonation," with more avid staining in the superior extents, and lesser staining in the deeper portions; in many (but not all) melanomas, this zonation is lost.
- **MART1/Melan-A:** MART1/Melan-A (two different clones of the antibody) targets protein antigens on the surface of melanocytes. These markers are more specific for melanocytes than is S100.

- **SOX10:** An antibody directed at nucleocytoplasmic shuttle protein of cells that originate from the neural crest (like melanocytes). It is a sensitive marker for melanocytes that yields nuclear staining, the latter of which is different from the other markers yet described.
- **P16:** An antibody directed at the tumor suppressor protein P16. Expression of P16 in melanocytic processes is generally favorable, while loss of all staining with P16 is seen in about 80% of melanoma.
- **PRAME:** **P**referentially **e**xpressed **a**ntigen in **me**lanoma is an antibody directed at an antigen predominantly expressed in human melanomas and the testis. Although studies of this antibody are new (2018 onward), expression seems to occur mostly in melanoma, and not in most benign melanocytic process, so marking in a lesion is always a point of concern.

Lezcano C, Jungbluth AA, Nehal KS, et al. PRAME expression in melanocytic tumors. *Am J Surg Pathol.* 2018;42:1456–1465.

25. Are there other factors with prognostic impact in patients with melanoma?

Prognosis is correlated strongly with Breslow depth, ulceration in the primary tumor, and the presence of nodal disease. Secondary predictors of prognosis include the number of positive lymph nodes, extranodal extension into soft tissue, age at diagnosis, sex (women > men), and anatomic site of the primary tumor. The extremities, excluding the hands and feet, have a more favorable prognosis, while lesions on the scalp, hands, feet, and mucosal surfaces have the worst.

Recently, a commercially available 31-gene expression profile (31-GEP) test has been validated in mostly (but not exclusively) industry-sponsored studies and appears to have independent prognostic value, dividing melanoma into those with lower (type I) or higher (type II) risk of metastatic disease. However, available evidence suggest that the 31-GEP test may be a helpful clinical tool in guiding use of sentinel lymph node sampling in some patients (those with pT1 and pT2 melanomas that are >65 years of age). While this test shows considerable promise in reproducibility and clinical validity, it is not yet part of the definitive NCCN guidelines for melanoma care.

Bartlett EK, Karakousis GC. Current staging and prognostic factors in melanoma. *Surg Oncol Clin N Am.* 2015;24:215–227.
Greenhaw BN, Zitelli JA, Brodland DG. Estimation of prognosis in invasive cutaneous melanoma: an independent study of the accuracy of a gene expression profile test. *Dermatol Surg.* 2018;44:1494–1500.
Gastman BR, Gerami P, Kurley SJ, et al. Identification of patients at risk for metastasis using a prognostic 31-gene expression profile in subpopulations of melanoma patients with favorable outcomes by standard criteria. *J Am Acad Dermatol.* 2019;80:149–157.

26. Are there any noninvasive technologies used to diagnosis melanoma?

Several noninvasive technologies existed, exist, or are in development to facilitate melanoma diagnosis and reduce the biopsy of benign lesions. For example, a noninvasive image analysis and pattern recognition platform known as MelaFind had received approval from the U.S. Food and Drug Administration (FDA) but was abandoned by the manufacturer. Electrical impedance spectroscopy (EIS) is a noninvasive diagnostic technique based on inherent electrical differences between benign and malignant tissues, and several EIS devices are currently being investigated in clinical trials or will soon be brought to market.

In addition to imaging technology to reduce the biopsy of benign processes, some molecular technologies are available to facilitate melanoma diagnosis. Already in existence commercially are array-based comparative genomic hybridization, fluorescence in situ hybridization, and gene expression profiling (GEP). Myriad Genetics (Salt Lake City, UT) offers a 23-gene based GEP test (myPath Melanoma) that distinguishes melanoma from benign melanocytic processes. This test has been validated on multiple occasions, but there is some concern as to its performance in truly borderline lesions, where it is most likely to be employed.

March J, Hand M, Truong A, Grossman D. Practical application of new technologies for melanoma diagnosis, part II: molecular approaches. *J Am Acad Dermatol.* 2015;72:943–958.
March J, Hand M, Grossman D. Practical application of new technologies for melanoma diagnosis, part I: noninvasive approaches. *J Am Acad Dermatol.* 2015;72:929–941.

27. How are patients with melanoma evaluated after the initial diagnosis?

In patients diagnosed with melanoma, additional evaluations should be performed to determine if there are any second primary tumors, if there is local extension of the primary tumor, or if metastatic disease is present. These should include a complete physical examination, complete skin evaluation, and lymph node exam, and it may include baseline laboratory tests, such as a complete blood count, blood chemistry studies, liver function tests, lactate dehydrogenase (LDH) level, and possibly imaging, depending on presenting signs or symptoms. There is considerable evidence to suggest that routine imaging studies and blood work have limited value in the initial evaluation of asymptomatic patients with a primary cutaneous melanoma </=4 mm in depth. The American Academy of Dermatology recommends that these tests be optional and employed based upon a thorough medical history and physical examination. Exceptions exist for asymptomatic persons with a primary tumor greater than >4 mm and/or, if necessary, for a clinical trial. Any abnormality detected with these exams needs more thorough investigation.

28. What is the most current system for staging melanoma?

The current preferred staging system for melanoma is the eighth edition of the AJCC from 2017. It is based on the TNM (tumor, lymph node, metastasis) system, and it classifies patients based chiefly on the depth of invasion in the primary tumor and whether lymph nodes or other metastases are present. Staging and survival rates for cutaneous melanoma are summarized in Fig. 44.6.

Keung EZ, Gershenwald JE. The eighth edition American Joint Committee on Cancer (AJCC) melanoma staging system: implications for melanoma treatment and care. *Expert Rev Anticancer Ther.* 2018;18:775–784.

29. How is melanoma treated?

The standard of care for treating melanoma is to:
1. Establish a histologic diagnosis of the suspected lesion.
2. Completely excise the tumor with appropriate uninvolved tissue margins.
3. Assess for the presence of detectable metastatic disease.
4. Conduct appropriate follow-up evaluations for the remainder of the patient's life.

Histologic examination remains the only gold standard for the diagnosis of melanoma. To establish a histologic diagnosis, the suspected lesion should (ideally) be excised with a thin margin of uninvolved skin (1–3 mm) to the depth of the subcuticular fat. If this is not possible, due to anatomic location or size of the lesion, a saucerization, punch, or incisional biopsy should be performed, typically on the thickest and/or most atypical portion of the lesion. Biopsy of lentigo maligna (a form of broad melanoma in situ) can be problematic, because there are often skip areas or areas of

Primary Tumor (T)

TX Primary tumor cannot be assessed (for example, curettaged or severely regressed melanoma)

T0 No evidence of primary tumor

Tis Melanoma in situ

T1 Melanomas 1.0 mm or less in thickness

T2 Melanomas 1.1 - 2.0 mm

T3 Melanomas 2.1 - 4.0 mm

T4 Melanomas more than 4.0 mm

NOTE: a and b subcategories of T are assigned based on ulceration and thickness as shown below:

CLASSIFICATION	THICKNESS mm	ULCERATION STATUS
T1	≤1.0	a: Breslow < 0.8 mm w/o ulceration b: Breslow 0.8-1.0 mm w/o ulceration or ≤ 1.0 mm w/ ulceration.
T2	1.1-2.0	a: w/o ulceration b: w/ ulceration
T3	2.1-4.0	a: w/o ulceration b: w/ ulceration
T4	>4.0	a: w/o ulceration b: w/ ulceration

Regional Lymph Nodes (N)

NX Patients in whom the regional nodes cannot be assessed (for example previously removed for another reason)

N0 No regional metastases detected

N1-3 Regional metastases based on the number of metastatic nodes, number of palpable metastatic nodes on clinical exam, and presence or absence of MSI

NOTE: N1-3 and a-c subcategories assigned as shown below:

CLASSIFICATION	# NODES	CLINICAL DETECTABLE/TVMD STATUS
N1	0-1 node	a: clinically occult, no MSI b: clinically detected, no MSI c: 0 nodes, MSI present
N2	1-3 nodes	a: 2-3 nodes clinically occult, no MSI b: 2-3 nodes clinically detected, no MSI c: 1 node clinical or occult, MSI present
N3	>1 nodes	a: >3 nodes, all clinically occult, no MSI b: >3 nodes, ≥1 clinically detected or matted, no MSI c: >1 nodes clinical or occult, MSI present

Distant Metastasis (M)

M0 No detectable evidence of distant metastases

M1a Metastases to skin, sub cutaneous, or distant lymph nodes

M1b Metastases to lung

M1c Metastases to all other visceral sites

M1d Metastases to brain

NOTE: Serum LDH is incorporated into the M category as shown below:

CLASSIFICATION	SITE	Serum LDH
M1a-d	Skin/subcutaneous/nodule (a), lung (b) other visceral (c), brain (d)	Not assessed
M1a-d(0)	Skin/subcutaneous/nodule (a), lung (b) other visceral (c), brain (d)	Normal
M1a-d(1)	Skin/subcutaneous/nodule (a), lung (b) other visceral (c), brain (d)	Elevated

ANATOMIC STAGE/PROGNOSTIC GROUPS						
Clinical Staging			Pathologic Staging			
Stage 0	Tis	N0	M0	0	Tis	N0	M0
Stage IA	T1a	N0	M0	IA	T1a	N0	M0
Stage IB	T1b	.	.		T1b	.	.
	T2a	.	.	IB	T2a	.	.
Stage IIA	T2b	N0	M0	IIA	T2b	M0	M0
	T3a	.	.		T2a	.	.
Stage IIB	T3b	.	.	IIB	T3b	.	.
	T4a	.	.		T4a	.	.
Stage IIC	T4b	.	.	IIC	T4b	.	.
Stage III	Any T	≥N1	M0	IIIA	T1-2a	N1a	M0
	.	.	.		T1-2a	N2a	.
	.	.	.	IIIB	T0	N1b-c	M0
	.	.	.		T1-2a	N1b-c	.
	.	.	.		T1-2a	N2b	.
	.	.	.		T2b-3a	N1a-2b	.
	.	.	.	IIIC	T0	N2b-c	M0
	.	.	.		T0	N3b-c	.
	.	.	.		T1a-3a	N2c-3c	.
	.	.	.		T3b-4a	Any N	.
	.	.	.		T4b	N1a-2c	.
	.	.	.	IIID	T4b	N3a-c	M0
Stage IV	Any N	Any N	M1	IV	Any T	Any N	M1

Adopted from Keung EZ, Gershenwald JE. The eighth edition American Joint Committee on Cancer (AJCC) melanoma staging system: implications for melanoma treatment and care. Expert Rev Anticancer Ther. 18:775-784, 2018.

Fig. 44.6 The eighth edition American Joint Committee on Cancer (AJCC) melanoma staging system.

regression that can lead to misdiagnosis. For lentigo maligna, it may be necessary to utilize multiple samplings or even an excisional sampling.

Once a diagnosis of melanoma is established, wide local excision of the primary tumor through the subcutis to the muscle fascia is recommended. The ideal depth of excision is unknown because there is a paucity of data regarding this aspect of surgical care. Available studies demonstrate no significant difference in the rates of local and regional recurrence between patients in whom the muscle fascia was excised and those in whom it was left intact.

Olsen G. Removal of fascia—cause of more frequent metastases of malignant melanomas of the skin to regional lymph nodes? *Cancer.* 1964;17:1159–1164.
Kenady DE, Brown BW, McBride CM. Excision of underlying fascia with a primary malignant melanoma: effect on recurrence and survival rates. *Surgery.* 1982;92:615–618.
Aloia TA, Gershenwald JE. Management of early-stage cutaneous melanoma. *Curr Probl Surg.* 2005;42:455–534.
McKenna JK, Florell SR, Goldman GD, et al. Lentigo maligna/lentigo maligna melanoma: current state of diagnosis and treatment. *Dermatol Surg.* 2006;32:493–504.
Grotz TE, Glorioso JM, Pockaj BA, Harmsen WS, Jakub JW. Preservation of the deep muscular fascia and locoregional control in melanoma. *Surgery.* 2013;153:535–541.
Hunger RE, Seyed Jafari SM, Angermeier S, Shafighi M. Excision of fascia in melanoma thicker than 2 mm: no evidence for improved clinical outcome. *Br J Dermatol.* 2014;171:1391–1396.

30. What clinical margins should be employed for melanoma?

There is ongoing controversy regarding the clinical margin of normal-appearing skin that should be excised for melanoma. Except for a handful of prospective multicenter trials, surgical margins in melanoma are based largely on consensus decision and tradition. The NIH Consensus Conference on Melanoma has recommended melanoma in situ be excised with a 0.5 cm clinical margin of normal skin; melanoma of up to 1.0 mm depth should be excised with 1 cm clinical margins; melanoma of 1 to 2 mm depth should be excised with 1 to 2 cm clinical margins; melanomas of 2 to 4 mm depth should be excised with a 2 cm clinical margin; and melanoma of 4 mm depth should be excised with 2–3 cm clinical margin. There are no randomized trials that have determined the optimal margins for excision of melanoma greater than 4 mm in thickness.

These recommendations serve only as general guidelines and surgical considerations in individual patients must be considered. In fact, there is some evidence that use of 5 mm clinical margins in melanoma is situ may be too narrow place, although the recommendation has been in place since 1992 NIH consensus panel guidelines were released, based solely on expert opinion.

Moreover, there is some evidence to suggest that tumor thickness should not influence surgical margins, at all. Use of micrographically controlled (Mohs) surgery for melanoma has been reported by multiple authors who demonstrated an equivalent or even superior result with regard to local recurrence and metastasis rates, when compared to historical controls treated with wide surgical excision. Lastly, studies suggest that definitive surgical treatment for melanoma may be delayed up to 3 weeks after biopsy of the primary lesion without affecting the 5-year survival rate.

Doepker MP, Thompson ZJ, Fisher KJ, et al. Is a wider margin (2 cm vs. 1 cm) for a 1.01–2.0 mm melanoma necessary? *Ann Surg Oncol.* 2016;23:2336–2342.
Stigall LE, Brodland DG, Zitelli JA. The use of Mohs micrographic surgery (MMS) for melanoma in situ (MIS) of the trunk and proximal extremities. *J Am Acad Dermatol.* 2016;75:1015–1021.

31. What is the most important risk factor for local recurrence of primary melanoma?

Ulceration of the primary tumor seems to be the most significant prognostic factor for increased risk of local recurrence.

32. Does a biopsy of melanoma increase the risk of spreading tumor cells or causing metastases?

Two independent studies of this question concluded that incisional biopsy of melanoma does not cause the tumor to spread locally or metastasize.

Lederman JS, Sober AJ. Does biopsy type influence survival in clinical stage I cutaneous melanoma? *J Am Acad Dermatol.* 1985;86:983–987.

33. Describe the recommended follow-up for a patient with melanoma.

Recommendations for follow-up in melanoma patients vary with the depth of the primary tumor (Table 44.2). Regardless, unlike some malignancies, melanoma can recur years after the primary tumor is removed. Patients remain at risk for recurrence and need to be followed closely for long periods of time.

Mrazek AA, Chao C. Surviving cutaneous melanoma: a clinical review of follow-up practices, surveillance, and management of recurrence. *Surg Clin North Am.* 2014;94:989–1002.
Marciano NJ, Merlin TL, Bessen T, et al. To what extent are current guidelines for cutaneous melanoma follow up based on scientific evidence? *Int J Clin Pract.* 2014;68:761–770.

Table 44.2 Recommended follow-up schedules for patients with cutaneous melanoma

STAGE	FOLLOW-UP	DURATION	THEREAFTER
0	Every 12 months	2 years	Variable
Ia	Every 6–12 months	2 years	Variable
Ib	Every 6–12 months	5 years	Variable
II	Every 3–6 months	2–3 years	Every 6–12 months for life
IIb–IV	Every 3–6 months	3 years	Every 6–12 months for life, consider imaging

34. Which tests or examinations are conducted during the routine follow-up of patients who have had melanoma?

There is no consensus regarding the routine follow-up of patients with melanoma. Close follow-up is recommended because the risk of developing a second primary melanoma is around 3% to 4.5%. Follow-up recommendations vary from one to four times per year during the first 2 years after diagnosis. During follow-up evaluations, patients should receive a physical exam directed toward detection of a local recurrence of the primary tumor, toward recognition of metastatic disease in the surrounding skin or in the draining lymphatic system, and toward detection of a second primary melanoma. As in the initial staging evaluation, any abnormality detected by physical exam, review of systems, or laboratory tests must be more fully investigated. If no abnormalities are detected by routine physical exam and review of systems, repeat laboratory tests and imaging studies are often dictated by the patient's disease stage.

Mrazek AA, Chao C. Surviving cutaneous melanoma: a clinical review of follow-up practices, surveillance, and management of recurrence. *Surg Clin North Am.* 2014;94:989–1002.
Marciano NJ, Merlin TL, Bessen T, et al. To what extent are current guidelines for cutaneous melanoma follow up based on scientific evidence? *Int J Clin Pract.* 2014;68:761–770.

35. Is local tumor recurrence an independent prognostic indicator of survival?

No. Local recurrence is defined as recurrence of a tumor within 2 cm of the excision scar of a primary melanoma. Most (<95%) recurrences occur within 5 years after excision of the primary lesion, and the risk of local recurrence depends on ulceration and the anatomic site. The risk of local recurrence is increased in ulcerated primary melanoma and in melanoma of the head, neck, hands, and feet. Local recurrence is associated with development of in-transit, regional, and distant metastatic disease, but it is not an independent prognostic factor of survival.

Bricca GM, Brodland DG, Ren D, et al. Cutaneous head and neck melanoma treated with Mohs micrographic surgery. *J Am Acad Dermatol.* 2005;52:92–100.
Thompson JF, Scolyer RA, Uren RF. Surgical management of primary cutaneous melanoma: excision margins and the role of sentinel lymph node examination. *Surg Oncol Clin N Am.* 2006;15:301–318.

36. What is sentinel lymph node biopsy?

In 1990, Morton introduced intraoperative lymphatic mapping and selective lymph node dissection or SLN biopsy (SLNB) for melanoma patients. He showed that the status of the SLN reflects the status of the entire lymph node basin, because when the sentinel node was uninvolved, the other lymph nodes in that basin were also uninvolved. Over time, the status of the SLN was confirmed as an important prognostic factor for patients with primary melanoma.

SLNB often guides further therapeutic interventions including adjuvant chemotherapy, radiation therapy, or entrance into clinical trials. However, the theoretical value of SLNB is premised on the assumption that melanoma cells migrate in an orderly fashion toward the draining lymph node. This assumption is not always correct. To this end, there is evidence that lymph node status is an indicator, but not governor, of distant metastases and survival.

37. What is the survival benefit of performing SLNB in patients with melanoma?

To date, there is no irrefutable evidence that SLNB improves melanoma survival. The final results of the Multicenter Selective Lymphadenectomy Trials (MSLT) demonstrated that for cutaneous melanoma, wide local excision and SLNB followed by immediate completion lymph node dissection (CLND) for patients with positive sentinel nodes did not provide overall or melanoma specific survival advantage over wide excision and observation. MSLT-II demonstrated that immediate CLND did not increase overall or melanoma-specific survival compared to close clinical observation and delayed CLND even among patients with melanoma and positive sentinel nodes. In sum, these results indicate that, at present, SLNB should be regarded as a staging procedure, with prognostic, but not therapeutic, value.

There remains some controversy regarding SLNB. Proponents of SLNB argue that it may identify patients who may be candidates for adjuvant therapy (see below). However, to date, there are no adjuvant drugs that prolong survival for the subgroup of patients with only microscopic disease. Most of approved therapies are for unresectable melanoma. Those agents approved for stage III have not shown improved survival for the subgroup of microscopic disease. Furthermore, the sensitivity, specificity, positive predictive value, and negative predictive value of SLN status are limited and there is no definitive evidence that SLN status provides additional prognostic information beyond that predicted by Breslow depth and ulceration alone; the latter are readily available from a pathology report and do not require a separate surgical procedure. Recent evidence has shown that after the fifth year of follow-up, SLN status is no longer an independent predictor of relapse or mortality. Patients with a Breslow depth in excess of 2 mm should be considered at higher risk for 10-year relapse, regardless of the results of SLNB.

Despite the controversies surrounding SLN, the AJCC recommends that all patients with primary melanoma greater than 1 mm in depth have an SLN biopsy prior to entry into melanoma clinical trials.

Amersi F, Morton DL. The role of sentinel lymph node biopsy in the management of melanoma. *Adv Surg.* 2007;41:241–256.

McGregor JM, Sasieni P. Sentinel node biopsy in cutaneous melanoma: time for consensus to better inform patient choice. *Br J Dermatol.* 2015;172:552–554.

Sladden M, Zagarella S, Popescu CM, Bigby M. No survival benefit for patients with melanoma undergoing sentinel lymph node biopsy: critical appraisal of the Multicenter Selective Lymphadenectomy Trial-I final report. *Br J Dermatol.* 2015;172:566–571.

Stiegel E, Xiong D, Ya J, Funchain P, et al. Prognostic value of sentinel lymph node biopsy according to Breslow thickness for cutaneous melanoma. *J Am Acad Dermatol.* 2018;78:942–948.

38. What is linear melanonychia?

Linear melanonychia is a pigmented streak of the nail (Fig. 44.7). Among many potential causes, subungual melanoma is the most serious. Longitudinal melanonychia is often seen in persons of darker skin type, particularly where it may involve more than one nail. If a pigmented nail band involves only one nail, occurs in a middle-aged or elderly white patient, shows progressive widening or darkening (meaning is it wider toward the base of the nail, rather than the tip), or if there is extension of pigment onto the surrounding nail fold, a biopsy may be warranted.

39. What is Hutchinson sign?

Hutchinson sign is pigmentation at the base of linear melanonychia involving the proximal nail fold and periungual skin (Fig. 44.8). This sign is concerning for nail unit melanoma.

Baran R, Kechijian P. Hutchinson's sign: a reappraisal. *J Am Acad Dermatol.* 2001;44:87–90.

40. What forms of chemotherapy are used in the treatment of metastatic melanoma?

Chemotherapy in metastatic melanomas yielded disappointing results, with 5-year survival rates for treated patients ranging from 3% to 14%. Dacarbazine has shown some efficacy as single-agent therapy. Response rates average around 10% to 20%, with durations averaging 6 months and a complete response rate of about 5%.

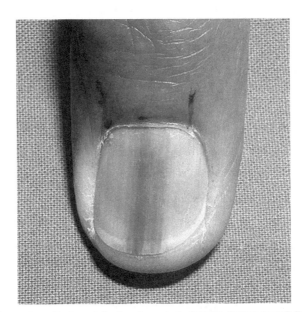

Fig. 44.7 Linear melanonychia demonstrating linear brown streak of pigment. (Courtesy James E. Fitzpatrick, MD.)

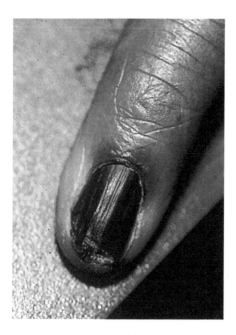

Fig. 44.8 Acral lentiginous melanoma in situ arising from the nail bed of a black woman. Note the presence of pigment in the periungual tissue (positive Hutchinson's sign). (Courtesy James E. Fitzpatrick, MD.)

Newer agents such as temozolomide are of similar efficacy to dacarbazine but offer the advantages of oral administration and penetration of the blood–brain barrier. Cisplatin has been shown to be somewhat effective as single-agent therapy, but it has significant toxicities. Other studies have shown that the nitrosoureas (carmustine, lomustine, and semustine) have an overall response rate ranging from 13% to 18%. Similarly, tubular toxins such as vinblastine, vincristine, and Taxol (paclitaxel) have led to response rates of between 12% and 15%. The combination of carboplatin and paclitaxel is currently under investigation. The approval of immunotherapies as well as inhibitors of the BRAF pathway for the treatment of melanoma has provided multiple new therapeutic options for patients. The combination of chemotherapy and immunotherapy, known as biochemotherapy, has shown high clinical responses, but it has not been shown to improve overall survival.

Flaherty LE, Othus M, Atkins MB, et al. Southwest Oncology Group S0008: a phase III trial of high-dose interferon Alfa-2b versus cisplatin, vinblastine, and dacarbazine DTIC, plus interleukin-2 and interferon in patients with high-risk melanoma—an intergroup study of cancer and leukemia Group B, Children's Oncology Group, Eastern Cooperative Oncology Group, and Southwest Oncology Group. *J Clin Oncol.* 2014;32:3771–3778.
Wilson MA, Schuchter LM. Chemotherapy for Melanoma. *Cancer Treat Res.* 2016;167:209–229.

41. Is radiation therapy effective for the eradication of melanoma?
   No. Radiation therapy is used for palliative care of cerebral metastases and for local control of unresectable disease.

Testori A, Rutkowski P, Marsden J, et al. Surgery and radiotherapy in the treatment of cutaneous melanoma. *Ann Oncol.* 2009;20(suppl 6): vi22–vi29.
Mahadevan A, Patel VL, Dagoglu N. Radiation therapy in the management of malignant melanoma. *Oncology (Williston Park).* 2015;29:743–751.

KEY POINTS: TREATMENT OF MELANOMA

1. Immunologic events appear to play a role in the clinical course of the melanoma.
2. Thickness and ulceration are key prognostic factors of the primary tumor.
3. Early dissection in SLN-positive patients does not improve survival.
4. At present there is no certain curative treatment for advanced-stage melanoma.
5. Significant progress has been made in the use of immunotherapy and inhibitors of the BRAF pathway in the treatment of patients with advanced-stage melanoma.

42. How effective is immunotherapy in melanoma?

The lack of effective treatment for advanced-stage melanoma using radiation and chemotherapy has highlighted the need to develop alternative therapeutic strategies. Among them, immunotherapy has made significant progress over the past 10 years because immunologic events appear to play a role in the clinical course of melanoma.

Ipilimumab, which targets CTLA-4, was approved by the U.S. FDA in 2011 for the treatment of unresectable or metastatic melanoma. A survival benefit was demonstrated for patients treated with ipilimumab in two randomized trials. Data suggest that a proportion of patients treated with ipilimumab can achieve survival of at least 5 years.

The success of ipilimumab led to the development of immune-checkpoint mediator-directed PD-1. These agents include nivolumab and pembrolizumab, which target PD-1 and were approved in 2014 and 2015, respectively, by the FDA for the treatment of metastatic melanoma. Several clinical trials are ongoing, using nivolumab and pembrolizumab in monotherapy or in combination with ipilimumab, chemotherapy, radiotherapy, other immunotherapies, and targeted therapies.

Recently, T-cell–based immunotherapy has been emphasized because T cells are believed to play a major role in the control of tumor growth. In general, these vaccines have been relatively successful in animals; however, these results have not translated into human trials.

Additional means of cellular immunotherapy is the adoptive transfer of immune effector cells into patients. The ex vivo expansion of lymphokine-activated killer cells or TIL, with or without interleukin-2 (IL-2), has achieved some remarkable response rates in cancer patients.

The use of biologic response modifiers, such as interferon (IFN), and other cytokines has demonstrated modest success. IFN-α, as a single-agent treatment, has yielded response rates of 15%–20% and complete response rates in up to 5% of patients. However, use of IFN-α remains controversial because its use has been associated only with an increase in disease-free interval but not overall survival.

Biochemotherapy with the chemotherapeutic drugs dacarbazine and cisplatin, and immunotherapeutic agents such as IFN-α and IL-2, yielded higher response rates, reported in the 40% to 50% range. However, most cases were limited to metastases of soft tissues, lymph nodes, and subcutaneous tissue or the lung. Few responses were observed in patients with visceral metastases.

Oncolytic viruses represent a newer approach where native or attenuated viruses are used to selectively kill melanoma cells. Talimogene laherparepvec (TVEC, Imlygic) is the first oncolytic virus that showed a therapeutic benefit in a clinical study and it was approved in 2015 for advanced stage melanoma. A number of similar oncolytic viruses are in development.

Philips GK, Atkins M. Therapeutic uses of anti-PD-1 antibodies. *Int Immunol.* 2015;27:39–46.

Franklin C, Livingstone E, Roesch A, Schilling B, Schadendorf D. Immunotherapy in melanoma: recent advances and future directions. *Eur J Surg Oncol.* 2017;43:604–611.

Ascierto PA, Flaherty K, Goff S. Emerging strategies in systemic therapy for the treatment of melanoma. *Am Soc Clin Oncol Educ Book.* 2018;23:751–758.

Domingues B, Lopes JM, Soares P, Pópulo H. Melanoma treatment in review. *Immunotargets Ther.* 2018;7:35–49.

43. Does gene therapy offer promise in the treatment of melanoma?

Several different therapeutic strategies are being explored that are termed "gene therapy":

1. Genetic modification of TILs to make them more effective at killing tumor cells.
2. Genetic modification of the tumor cells to increase the production of immunostimulatory cytokines that attract and stimulate cells involved in the immune response.
3. Genetic modification of tumor nodules to increase production of human leukocyte antigens so that the system recognizes and rejects these tumor nodules in a manner similar to that of mismatched transplanted organs.

These approaches have generated promising results in laboratory and/or limited and early clinical trials, but all are still in the early investigational phases and are not ready for wide use.

Pavlick AC, Adams S, Fink MA, et al. Novel therapeutic agents under investigation for malignant melanoma. *Expert Opin Investig Drugs.* 2003;12:1545–1558.

Heo JR, Kim NH, Cho J, Choi KC. Current treatments for advanced melanoma and introduction of a promising novel gene therapy for melanoma (Review). *Oncol Rep.* 2016;36:1779–1786.

44. How about local perfusion therapy?

The treatment of localized cutaneous and lymphatic metastases by isolated hyperthermic limb perfusion, using a combination of chemotherapeutic and immunotherapeutic agents, has generated renewed interest after a successful European trial.

In this type of treatment, the circulation of a limb is isolated, the blood is withdrawn and slowly heated, and it is then returned to the limb along with high doses of melphalan (chemotherapy) with or without tumor necrosis factor or gamma-interferon (cytokines).

Because the circulation of the limb is isolated from the systemic circulation, much higher doses of the therapeutic agents can be administered, beyond what is systemically tolerated.

Kroon BB, Noorda EM, Vrouenraets BC, et al. Isolated limb perfusion for melanoma. *Surg Oncol Clin N Am.* 2008;17:785–794.
Grünhagen DJ, Verhoef C. Isolated limb perfusion for stage III melanoma: does it still have a role in the present era of effective systemic therapy? *Oncology (Williston Park).* 2016;30:1045–1052.

45. What are other newer targeted therapies for melanoma?

Improved understanding of the molecular mechanisms of melanoma development has increased our therapeutic options. As noted earlier, the major molecular pathways that have been implicated in melanoma include p16 and p14^{ARF}, B-Raf, N-Ras, MITF, PTEN, and Bcl2.

In the RAS-RAF-MEK-ERK (MAP kinase) signaling pathway, a major driver is BRAF, which can initiate a cascade of events, including phosphorylation and activation of MEK. *BRAF* mutations are found in more than 50% of all melanomas. Along with ipilimumab and PD-1 inhibitors, biologic agents that target BRAF and MEK have emerged as key therapies for advanced melanoma.

Vemurafenib, an inhibitor of mutant *BRAF*, was approved by the FDA in 2011 for the treatment of melanomas that harbor the *BRAF* V600E mutation. In 2012, the BRAF inhibitor dabrafenib and the MEK inhibitor trametinib were also approved by the FDA, based on results showing improved median progression-free survival. Encorafenib, another BRAF-mutant inhibitor, has also been employed in melanoma therapy.

While BRAF inhibitors led to remarkable response rates with better overall survival rates in melanoma clinical trials, the clinical benefit of these therapies has been limited, due to the development of tumor resistance. In this regard, targeting other effectors downstream of BRAF has proven a valid strategy to overcome resistance. MEK is a downstream target of BRAF and, in contrast to the BRAF inhibitors, MEK inhibitors showed activity in NRAS-mutant melanomas. Trametinib, a pharmacological MEK1/2 inhibitor with antitumoral activity, was approved by the FDA in 2013 as a monotherapy for unresectable or metastatic malignant and for melanomas with BRAF mutations. In 2015, the combination of cobimetinib, an oral selective MEK inhibitor, and vemurafenib was approved for treatment of unresectable melanomas with *BRAF* mutations. Several clinical trials are ongoing with the combination of these medications with radiotherapy, immunotherapies, and other targeted therapies.

Newer small molecular inhibitors are under investigation for melanoma therapy, including inhibitors targeting cyclin dependent kinase (CDK4/6), tyrosine-protein kinase KIT (c-KIT), mammalian target of rapamycin (mTOR), and the epidermal growth factor receptor (ErbB) family of tyrosine kinase receptors.

McDermott D, Lebbé C, Hodi FS, et al. Durable benefit and the potential for long-term survival with immunotherapy in advanced melanoma. *Cancer Treat Rev.* 2014;40:1056–1064.
Domingues B, Lopes JM, Soares P, Pópulo H. Melanoma treatment in review. *Immunotargets Ther.* 2018;7:35–49.
Richtig E. ASCO Congress 2018: melanoma treatment. *Memo.* 2018;11:261–265.
Schadendorf D, van Akkooi ACJ, Berking C, et al. Melanoma. *Lancet.* 2018;392:971–984.

CHAPTER 45

LEUKEMIC AND LYMPHOMATOUS INFILTRATES OF THE SKIN

Theresa R. Pacheco

1. Define lymphoma.

    A lymphoma is a malignancy of the immune system that is characterized by an abnormal proliferation of lymphocytes. Lymphoma can arise in either B cells or T cells or natural killer lymphocytes. Lymphomas can be divided into two categories: Hodgkin's and non–Hodgkin's lymphomas (NHLs). NHLs are a heterogeneous group of malignancies. Within NHLs, there can be aggressive (fast-growing) or indolent (slow-growing) types. Indolent NHLs include follicular lymphoma and cutaneous T-cell lymphoma (CTCL), as well as other types.

MYCOSIS FUNGOIDES

2. Is there a T-cell lymphoma that begins in the skin?

    Yes. CTCL is a primarily indolent, heterogeneous group of NHLs localized to the skin.

3. What is the most common subtype of CTCL?

    Mycosis fungoides (MF) (60%) is the most common subtype of CTCL. Histologically, it has a polymorphous cellular infiltrate composed primarily of atypical mononuclear cells and a variable background infiltrate of polymorphonuclear leukocytes, eosinophils, and lymphocytes. The atypical mononuclear cells are moderately large and have a folded (cerebriform) nucleus. These cells are typically seen within the epidermis either singly or in small clusters (Pautrier's microabscesses) or may preferentially be seen in the basal cell layer. MF cells are primarily CD4-positive helper T cells.

4. How common is CTCL?

    Although CTCL only comprises a fraction of all NHL diagnoses (~3%), the annual incidence of CTCL in the United States has increased dramatically across all age groups and races. CTCL occurs more frequently in men than women, and the incidence of MF rises with age. There are approximately 16,000 to 20,000 patients with MF in the United States, with about 1500 to 3000 new cases diagnosed each year. Higher incidence may be due to changes in classification schemes, improved detection, infectious agents, or environmental exposures.

Criscione VD, Weinstock MA. Incidence of cutaneous T-cell lymphoma in the United States, 1973–2002. *Arch Dermatol.* 2007;143:854–859.

5. How does mycosis fungoides begin?

    Typically, MF begins with persistent scaly patches (Fig. 45.1) that respond poorly to topical therapy with emollients and medium potency topical steroids. In the early stages, skin biopsy is frequently not diagnostic. The average time from onset of skin lesions to diagnosis is 7 years. In time, the patches thicken and become plaques (Fig. 45.2). Eventually, skin tumors develop (Fig. 45.3) and the lymph nodes can become involved. Peripheral blood involvement can be assessment by ratings defined by Sézary counts (SCs) and more sophisticated clonal and immunohistochemical analysis. Visceral disease is a late occurrence. Median survival for persons with patch- and plaque-stage disease is 12 years; for tumor-stage disease, it is 5 years; and for nodal or visceral disease, it is 3 years.

Epstein E, Levin D, Croft J, et al. Mycosis fungoides: survival, prognostic features, response to therapy, and autopsy findings. *Medicine.* 1972;51:61–72.

6. What is parapsoriasis?

    The skin diseases included under this diagnosis are poorly understood and encompass a morass of confusing terms. Parapsoriasis is a term that means like psoriasis. Parapsoriasis and CTCL can appear identical in terms of the rash on the skin.

    Small-plaque parapsoriasis is characterized by chronic, well-marginated, mildly scaly, slightly erythematous, and round to oval skin lesions measuring less than 4 to 5 cm in diameter. The long axes of the lesions are arranged in a parallel configuration, and the lesions occur on the trunk and proximal extremities in a pityriasis rosea–like pattern. The lesions have been likened to fingerprints and reported under the descriptive term of *digitate dermatoses*. This form of parapsoriasis does not progress to lymphoma.

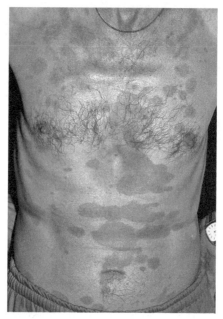

Fig. 45.1 Mycosis fungoides, patch-stage, on the trunk of a 45-year-old man. (Courtesy Fitzsimons Army Medical Center teaching files.)

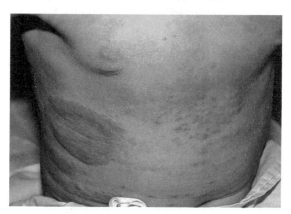

Fig. 45.2 Mycosis fungoides on the trunk of an 8-year-old boy demonstrating both patch-stage mycosis fungoides and plaque-stage mycosis fungoides. (Courtesy John L. Aeling Collection.)

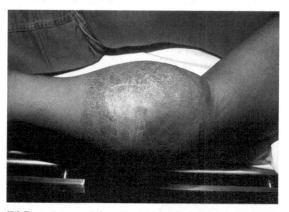

Fig. 45.3 Tumor-stage mycosis fungoides of the arm. (Courtesy John L. Aeling Collection.)

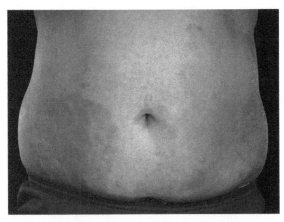

Fig. 45.4 Large-plaque parapsoriasis. The lesion was unresponsive to topical treatment. (Courtesy Fitzsimons Army Medical teaching files.)

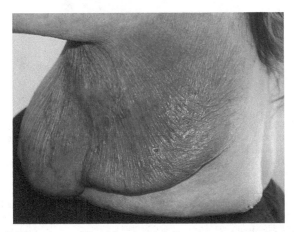

Fig. 45.5 A young woman with granulomatous slack skin, a rare variant of mycosis fungoides.

Large-plaque parapsoriasis presents as palm-sized or larger lesions located most frequently on the thighs, buttocks, hips, lower abdomen, and shoulder girdle areas (Fig. 45.4). The lesions may be pink, red-brown, or salmon-colored. They often have fine scale and show epidermal atrophy with cigarette-paper wrinkling. Some patients may have lesions with a netlike or reticular pattern with telangiectasia and fine scale. This clinical type of lesion is referred to as *retiform parapsoriasis* or *poikiloderma atrophicans vasculare*. Between 15% and 20% of patients with large-plaque parapsoriasis eventually develop MF. Many authorities consider it to be on a spectrum with MF.

Sehgal VN, Srivastava G, Aggarwal AK. Parapsoriasis: a complex issue. *Skinmed.* 2007;6:280–286.

7. What type of skin lesions are seen in patients with mycosis fungoides, the most common CTCL subtype?
Although the classic skin lesions are scaly patches, plaques, and tumors, a wide variety of skin lesions have been reported, such as follicular papules and pustules with or without alopecia (alopecia mucinosa). Bullous, erythrodermic, hypopigmented, hyperpigmented, vasculitic, and hyperkeratotic lesions also have been described.
A rare variant of MF is granulomatous slack skin disease (Fig. 45.5). This disorder is characterized by the slow development of lax erythematous skin that eventually develops large pendulous folds of redundant integument. Histologic examination shows a dense atypical granulomatous infiltrate with destruction and phagocytosis of elastic tissue.

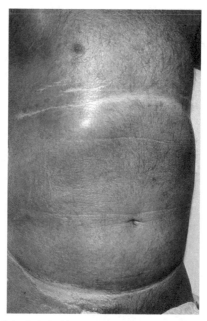

Fig. 45.6 A patient with Sézary syndrome demonstrating diffuse erythema.

8. What are the other subtypes of CTCL?

In addition to MF (60%), there are other CTCL subtypes. Other CTCL subtypes include Sézary syndrome, primary cutaneous CD30-positive lymphoproliferative disorders (primary cutaneous anaplastic large cell lymphoma and lymphomatoid papulosis [LyP]), subcutaneous panniculitis-like T-cell lymphoma, primary cutaneous gamma/delta T-cell lymphoma, primary cutaneous aggressive epidermotropic CD8-positive cytotoxic T-cell lymphoma, and primary cutaneous small/medium CD4-positive T-cell lymphoma.

9. What is Sézary syndrome?

Sézary syndrome is named after the French dermatologist Albert Sézary, who first identified this leukemic variant of CTCL. Sézary syndrome (5%), the second most common subtype of CTCL (Fig. 45.6), presents with the classic triad of erythroderma, lymphadenopathy, and atypical circulating mononuclear cells (Sézary cells). These cells are moderately large mononuclear cells with hyperconvoluted nuclei. The current assessment of peripheral blood involvement. B_0 and B_1 ratings are defined by SCs ($B_0 < 5\%$ SCs; $B_1 > 5\%$ SCs but either less than 1.0 K/μL absolute SCs or absence of a clonal TCR rearrangement, or both), while the current B_2 rating is defined by clonal rearrangement of the TCR in conjunction with any one of the following: (1) >1000 SCs/μL, (2) increased CD4+ or CD3+ population with CD4/CD8 >10, or (3) an increase in CD4+ cells with an abnormal phenotype (i.e., >40% CD4+/CD7-; >30% CD4+/CD26-). However, the finding of circulating Sézary cells must be evaluated in context with the clinical picture and skin biopsy. Severe pruritus, ectropion, nail dystrophy, peripheral edema, alopecia, and keratoderma of the palms and soles are common associated features. The disease tends to wax and wane and generally progresses faster and is more resistant to treatment than the MF subtype.

10. What is the TNM (tumor, nodes, metastasis) classification of mycosis fungoides?

Staging of CTCL involves the evaluation of four disease compartments with clarifications on skin, lymph nodes, and viscera, and the incorporation of the blood rating. Stages IA and IB are determined by the extent of body surface area covered by patches and/or plaques and may have blood involvement. Patients with stage IIA disease have the same skin involvement as stage I plus lymphadenopathy, also with potential blood involvement. Stage IIB is associated with the development of skin tumors, and stage III, with a confluence of erythema covering 80% body surface area. Both stages IIB and III may also have blood or nodal involvement. Stage IIIB is identical to stage IIIA with the addition of low blood tumor burden. Both stages IVA and IVB may involve the lymph nodes or blood, but only patients with stage IVB have visceral involvement. Stage IVA is defined in terms of skin and either blood or nodal involvement and is subdivided into stage IVA_1 and stage IVA_2. Stage IVA_1 is defined by skin and blood involvement, where the blood rating equals 2, with a nodal rating of 0 to 2. Stage IVA_2 is defined in terms of skin and nodal involvement, where the nodal rating equals 3, with a blood rating of 0 to 2.

T (Skin)		N (Nodes)	
T1	Limited patch/plaque (< 10% of total skin surface)	N0	No clinically abnormal LNs
		N1	Clinically abnormal LNs; histopathology Dutch grade 1 or NCI LN0-2 (clone +/-)
T2	Generalized patch/plaque (≥ 10% of total skin surface)		
		N2	Clinically abnormal LNs; histopathology Dutch grade 2 or NCI LN3 (clone +/-)
T3	Tumors		Clinically abnormal LNs; histopathology Dutch grade 3- or
T4	Generalized erythroderma	N3	NCI LN4 (clone +/-)
		Nx	Clinically abnormal LNs, no histopathology info

M (VISCERA)		B (BLOOD)	
M0	No visceral involvement	B0*	No significant blood involvement
M1	Visceral involvement	B1†	Low blood tumor burden
		B2‡	High blood tumor burden

- CD4/CD8 ratio ≥ 10 (setting of an expanded CD4), or CD4+CD7- cells ≥ 40% or CD4+CD26- ≥ 30% of lymphocytes, or other aberrant expression of pan T-cell markers. *LNs*, lymph nodes; *NCI*, National Cancer Center.

Olsen E, Vonderheid E, Pimpinelli N, et al. Revisions to the staging and classification of mycosis fungoides and Sézary syndrome: a proposal of the International Society for Cutaneous Lymphomas (ISCL) and the cutaneous lymphoma task force of the European Organization of Research and Treatment of Cancer (EORTC). *Blood.* 2007;110:1713–1722.

11. How is mycosis fungoides worked up?
See Table 45.1 for the CTCL essential diagnostic workup.

NCCN Clinical Practice Guidelines in Oncology. *Non-Hodgkin's lymphomas.* Version February 2015.

12. How is mycosis fungoides treated?
There are many treatments for MF. Treatments can be classified as skin-directed therapy or systemic therapy. See Table 45.2.

National Cancer Institute. *Mycosis fungoides and the Sézary syndrome treatment.* http://www.cancer.gov/cancertopics/pdq/treatment/mycosisfungoides/healthprofessional/allpages. Accessed December 6, 2006.

13. Describe topical nitrogen mustard (HN_2) therapy.
Mechlorethamine has been known to be active in lymphomas since 1946 and has been utilized as a topical agent since the 1950s. It has been used for years as a topical to treat MF-type CTCL (MF-CTCL). Mechlorethamine, also known as nitrogen mustard or mustargen, was originally dissolved into water, and later, it was compounded into petrolatum-based ointments. The water formulation was done by the patient at home, after which the solution was painted on the skin. Approximately 10% of individuals using the water formulation or compounded ointment developed an allergic

Table 45.1	Recommended evaluation of patients with CTCL
Physical examination	• Examination of the entire skin • Palpation of peripheral lymph node regions • Palpation for organomegaly/masses
Laboratory studies	• Complete blood (CBC) count with Sézary screen • Sézary flow cytometric study • *TCR* gene rearrangement of peripheral blood lymphocytes if Sézary syndrome suspected • Comprehensive metabolic panel • Lactic dehydrogenase (LDH)
Imaging	• Contrast-enhanced CT scan of the neck/chest/abdomen and pelvis or integrated whole-body PET/CT scan
Biopsy	• Biopsy of suspicious skin sites • Dermatopathology review of biopsy

CT, computed tomography; *CTCL*, cutaneous T-cell lymphoma; *PET*, positron emission tomography.

Table 45.2 Treatment of CTCL

Skin-directed	
	• Topical corticosteroids
	• Topical chemotherapy
	◦ Nitrogen mustard (Valchlor)
	◦ Carmustine (BCNU)
	• Topical retinoids: Bexarotene gel (Targretin gel)
	• Phototherapy
	◦ Narrowband ultraviolet B (NBUVB)
	◦ Psoralen with ultraviolet A (PUVA)
	• Radiation therapy
	◦ Total-skin electron beam therapy (TSEBT)
	◦ Site-directed radiation
Systemic	
	• Vorinostat (Zolinza)
	• Bexarotene capsules (Targretin)
	• Denileukin diftitox (Ontak)
	• Alemtuzumab (Campath)
	• Interferon-α (intron)
	• Extracorporeal photochemotherapy
	• Targeted monoclonal antibody therapy (mAb) (single agent)
	◦ Bentuximab vedotin (Adcetris)
	◦ Mogamulizumab (Poteligeo)
	• Chemotherapy (single agent)
	◦ Chlorambucil (Leukeran)
	◦ Cladribine (Leustatin)
	◦ Fludarabine (Fludara)
	◦ Methotrexate (Trexall, Rheumatrex)
	◦ Gemcitabine (Gemzar)
	◦ Pegylated doxorubicin (Doxil)
	◦ Pentostatin (Nipent)
	• Combination chemotherapies
	◦ CHOP
	◦ ESHAP
	◦ EPOCH

BCNU, bis-chloroethylnitrosourea (Carmustine).

reaction, which usually occurred within 3 to 6 weeks after initiation of treatment. Symptoms include reddening, burning, stinging, itching, or blisters, like a poison ivy reaction. The irritation usually subsided with a dose or application frequency adjustment and concomitant use of topical steroids. The Food and Drug Administration (FDA) recently approved the use of mechlorethamine gel (Valchlor) for the treatment of CTCL for patients with early-stage (IA and IB) MF-CTCL, who have received previous skin-directed therapies. The mechlorethamine hydrochloride 0.02% gel was studied in a blinded, multicenter study, observer-blind, active-controlled noninferiority trial; 260 previously treated, early-stage CTCL (IA, IB, IIA) patients were randomized between the gel and a compounded mechlorethamine 0.02% ointment. In the 12-month study, Valchlor resulted in a significant overall response in a majority of patients with stage IA and IB MF-CTCL. Sixty percent of the Valchlor patients (*n* = 119) had an overall response using the Composite Assessment of Index Lesion Severity analysis and 50% of the Valchlor patients had an overall response using the Severity Weighted Assessment Tool analysis. Time to response, local reactions, and withdrawal due to adverse events were higher in the gel arm. The most common adverse reactions were local skin reactions. No systemic side effect has been observed with topical use of Valchlor.

Lessin SL, Duvic M, Guitart J, et al. Topical chemotherapy in cutaneous T-cell lymphoma: positive results of a randomized, controlled, multi-center trial testing the efficacy and safety of a novel 0.02% mechlorethamine gel in mycosis fungoides. *JAMA Dermatol.* 2013;149:25–32.
Vonderheid E, Tan E, Kantor A, et al. Long-term efficacy, curative potential, and carcinogenicity of topical mechlorethamine chemotherapy in cutaneous T-cell lymphoma. *J Am Acad Dermatol.* 1989;20:416–428.

14. Is photochemotherapy an effective treatment of mycosis fungoides?
    Yes. In patients with patches and thin plaques, narrowband ultraviolet B (NBUVB) should be preferentially used. Psoralen plus ultraviolet A (PUVA) may be reserved for patients with thick plaques and those who relapse after initial NBUVB therapy.

The response rates to PUVA are at least equal to those with topical nitrogen mustard. Ultraviolet light irradiation required special instruments for whole-skin irradiation of ultraviolet A (UVA) light. Adding psoralens potentiates the effects of UVA light (PUVA). A study from Sweden, where PUVA is the treatment of choice, showed a 50% decrease in mortality from MF after the introduction of PUVA.

NBUVB (311- to 313-nm range) phototherapy has certain advantages over PUVA: no oral premedication is required, eliminating systemic side effects, and long-term skin carcinogenic effects may be decreased. The use of 308-nm excimer laser in the treatment of early MF is beneficial for patients with isolated lesions or lesions in areas that may be difficult to treat because of anatomic location.

Dogra S, Mahajan R. Phototherapy for mycosis fungoides. *Indian J Dermatol Venereol Leprol.* 2015;81(2):124–135. doi:10.4103/0378-6323.152169.

Swanbeck G, Roupe G, Sandström MH. Indications of a considerable decrease in the death rate in MF by PUVA treatment. *Acta Derm Venereol (Stockh).* 1994;74:465–466.

15. What are the major side effects of bexarotene in the treatment of patients with CTCL?

Bexarotene (Targretin) is a synthetic retinoid that selectively activates retinoid X receptors. The drug is given orally at a recommended dose of 300 mg/m^2. Partial response rate (50% improvement) was 67% and complete response occurred in 7% of patients. Like other retinoid drugs, bexarotene is teratogenic and should not be given to pregnant women. In a study of 58 patients with patch- and plaque-stage disease, side effects included hyperlipidemia in 83%, neutropenia in 47%, central hypothyroidism in 74%, and hypercholesterolemia in 47% of patients.

Duvic M, Martin AG, Kim Y, et al. Oral Targretin (bexarotene) capsules are safe and effective in refractory or persistent early-stage cutaneous T-cell lymphoma: results of the phase 2–3 clinical trial. Presented at the American Society of Hematology Annual Meeting; 1999 New Orleans.

16. How does one manage the side effects of bexarotene?

Hypothyroidism caused by bexarotene results in a low thyroid-stimulating hormone level because the drug stops RNA transcription. Central hypothyroidism is managed with levothyroxine replacement. It is recommended that one start and stop levothyroxine and bexarotene together. Measure free thyroxine (T_4) at baseline, at 2 weeks, then monthly. Normalizing free T_4 helps clear plasma lipids.

Hyperlipidemia caused by bexarotene can be managed with lipid-lowering agents. The preferred lipid-lowering agents include atorvastatin (Lipitor), an β-hydroxy β-methylglutaryl-CoA (HMG-CoA) reductase inhibitor (statin), and fenofibrate (TriCor), which acts by increasing lipolysis through activation of lipoprotein lipase. Over the counter fish oil or prescription Lovaza is a combination of ethyl esters of omega 3 fatty acids, principally eicosapentaenoic acid (EPA) and docosahexaenoic acid (DHA), is also used to reduce triglyceride levels in patients on oral bexarotene.

17. Are interferons effective in treating mycosis fungoides?

Yes. Of the interferon group of drugs, recombinant interferon-α has been the most promising. Both complete remissions and partial remissions have been reported. Low-dose treatment protocols are as effective as high-dose protocols and have fewer side effects. The recommended dose is 3 million units, given subcutaneously, three times weekly.

18. Is chemotherapy an effective treatment of mycosis fungoides?

Yes. Both partial and complete remissions can be achieved with both single-drug and multidrug chemotherapy protocols. However, the remissions are short-lived, and no one drug or combination of drugs appears to be superior. Single-agent chemotherapy agents used include chlorambucil (Leukeran), cladribine (Leustatin), fludarabine (Fludara), methotrexate (Trexall, Rheumatrex), gemcitabine (Gemzar), pegylated doxorubicin (Doxil), and pentostatin (Nipent). Combination chemotherapies used include cyclophosphamide, doxorubicin hydrochloride (hydroxydaunorubicin), vincristine sulfate (Oncovin), and prednisone (CHOP), etoposide, methylprednisolone (Solumedrol), high-dose cytarabine, cisplatin (platinum chemotherapy) (ESHAP), and etoposide, prednisone, vincristine (Oncovin), cyclophosphamide and hydroxydaunorubicin hydrochloride (EPOCH).

Kuzel TM. Systemic chemotherapy for the treatment of mycosis fungoides and Sézary syndrome. *Dermatol Ther.* 2003;16(4):355–361.

19. What is extracorporeal photopheresis?

Extracorporeal photopheresis is a treatment in which peripheral blood is exposed in an extracorporeal circuit to UVA following administration of 8-methoxypsoralen. Response rates of 50% to 80% have been observed in CTCL. The mechanism of action is thought to be activation of cellular apoptosis and possible immunomodulatory effects. The treatment is expensive, requires the availability of specialized equipment, and is administered on an outpatient basis in a hospital setting.

Bisaccia E, Gonzalez J, Palangio M, et al. Extracorporeal photochemotherapy alone or with adjuvant therapy in the treatment of cutaneous T-cell lymphoma: a 9-year retrospective study at a single institution. *J Am Acad Dermatol.* 2000;43:263–271.

KEY POINTS: MYCOSIS FUNGOIDES

1. Mycosis fungoides is an indolent CTCL subtype with a median survival of 12 years for patients with patch- or plaque-stage disease.
2. Sézary syndrome is the term applied to the leukemic subtype of CTCL.
3. Management of MF is best accomplished by the involvement of several specialists, such as those in dermatology, dermatopathology/pathology, hematology/oncology, and radiation oncology.

---

20. Are there any other FDA-approved treatments for cutaneous T-cell lymphoma?

Yes. Denileukin diftitox (Ontak) is interleukin-2 (IL-2) conjugated to diphtheria toxin. The drug is given intravenously only to patients whose malignant cells express CD25, the IL-2 receptor. The drug can be associated with significant toxicity, including capillary leak syndrome, acute hypersensitivity–type reactions, hypoalbuminemia, and hypotension. Flulike symptoms for several weeks following infusion are frequently noted. Partial responses are reported in 30% and complete responses in 10% of patients.

Histone deacetylase inhibitors (HDACis) inhibit the deacetylation of histone proteins associated with DNA and nonhistone proteins. The exact mechanism involving the treatment of CTCL is unknown, but DNA microarray studies show that HDACi affects the expression of numerous genes and proteins involved in cell proliferation, migration, and apoptosis. Oral Vorinostat (suberoylanilide hydroxamic acid) targets HDAC class 1 and class 2 enzymes and is FDA approved for the treatment of refractory CTCL, with response rates of 24% to 30%.

Newer targeted monoclonal antibody therapies have been approved. Bentuximab vedotin (Adcetris) is an antibody-drug conjugate designed to target cells expressing CD30. The drug is given intravenously only to patients with CD30-expressing MF as well as CD30+ lymphoproliferative disorders (LyP and primary cutaneous-anaplastic large-cell lymphoma). Mogamulizumab (Poteligeo) is a monoclonal antibody directed against C-C chemokine receptor 4. The drug is given intravenously. Mogamulizumab significantly prolonged progression-free survival for patients with MF and Sézary syndrome. Trials are underway looking into the use of immune checkpoint inhibitors in the treatment of CTCLs.

Gardner JM, Evans KG, Musiek A, et al. Update on treatment of cutaneous T-cell lymphoma. *Curr Opin Oncol.* 2009;21(2):131–137.
Welborn M, Duvic M. Antibody-based therapies for cutaneous T-cell lymphoma. *Am J Clin Dermatol.* 2019;20(1):115–122. doi:10.1007/s40257-018-0402-5.

OTHER LYMPHOMAS AND LEUKEMIAS

21. Outline the Ann Arbor clinical staging system for Hodgkin's disease.
   - **Stage I:** Single lymph node or extralymphatic site.
   - **Stage II:** Two or more lymph node regions on the same side of the diaphragm or nodal involvement with a contiguous extralymphatic site.
   - **Stage III:** Nodal involvement on both sides of the diaphragm, with or without a contiguous extralymphatic site.
   - **Stage IV:** Multiple extralymphatic tissue sites, with or without nodal involvement.
     - **A:** Absence of B symptoms.
     - **B:** Presence of B symptoms (fevers, drenching night sweats, or >10% weight loss over past 6 months).

22. What is a Reed-Sternberg cell?

It is a large cell with two mirror-image nuclei with large distinct nucleoli, often with surrounding halos (owl's eye cells). It is considered to be the malignant cell of Hodgkin's disease, and its presence confirms the histologic diagnosis. The origin of the cell is debated, with marker studies having shown both T- and B-cell immunoenzymatic staining.

23. What are the histologic classes of Hodgkin's disease?
   - **Nodular sclerosis** is the most common type, accounting for 35% of all patients with Hodgkin's disease. It is more common in women and has a relatively good prognosis. It is characterized by a particular type of Reed-Sternberg cell, called the lacunar cell, which is a large cell with a hyperlobulated nucleus and multiple nucleoli surrounded by a clear space (lacunae).
   - **Mixed cellularity** represents a histologic type that is intermediate between lymphocyte-predominance and lymphocyte-depletion types. It is the second most common type. Reed-Sternberg cells are prominent.
   - **Lymphocyte-predominance** type has a diffuse or slightly nodular histologic pattern (popcorn pattern). Reed-Sternberg cells are rare. It is the most common pattern found in young men, and the prognosis is excellent. The anti–CD20 monoclonal antibody, rituximab, which is usually used in NHL, has been shown to produce over a 50% complete response rate for this subtype of Hodgkin's disease.
   - **Lymphocyte-depletion** pattern is characterized by a paucity of lymphocytes and numerous Reed-Sternberg cells or their variants. There is a diffuse fibrotic and a reticular variant of the lymphocyte-depleted subtype. This type tends to occur in older patients, with disseminated involvement and a poor prognosis.

24. Does Hodgkin's disease occur in the skin?

Yes, but very rarely. One series of 1800 cases reported a less than 5% incidence of specific skin lesions in patients with Hodgkin's disease. Many of the early reports of Hodgkin's disease presenting with skin lesions with no nodal involvement probably represent Ki-1–positive, T-cell lymphomas. Nonspecific skin lesions are common and include pruritus, pigmentation, prurigo, ichthyosis, alopecia, and herpes zoster.

Fernandez-Flores A. The early reports on cutaneous involvement of Hodgkin lymphoma. *Am J Dermatopathol.* 2009;31:853–854.

25. How are cells immunophenotyped? What does the CD nomenclature mean?

"CD" stands for *cluster designation* and is a nomenclature for identification of specific cell surface antigens defined by monoclonal antibodies. The procedure can be applied to both formalin-fixed and frozen tissue. It is very helpful in identifying subpopulations of T- and B-cell lymphocytes (Table 45.3).

26. What is lymphomatoid papulosis?

This chronic recurrent skin eruption is characterized by papules and/or nodules that frequently crust or ulcerate and self-heal, often with atrophic scars (Fig. 45.7). There are four histopathologic types. Type A has large Reed-Sternberg–like cells, which are often CD30 (Ki-1) positive. Type B has moderately large atypical cells with cerebriform nuclei similar to the cell type found in MF. These cells are usually CD30-negative. Type C is composed of sheets of cells that resemble the cells of anaplastic T-cell lymphoma. About 15% to 20% of patients with lymphomatoid papulosis will develop a lymphoma. Type D is a newly described variant characterized by epidermotropic atypical lymphocytes with a unique CD8$^+$/CD30$^+$ cytotoxic T-cell immunophenotype.

Cardoso J, Duhra P, Thway Y, et al. Lymphomatoid papulosis type D: a newly described variant easily confused with cutaneous aggressive CD8-positive cytotoxic T-cell lymphoma. *Am J Dermatopathol.* 2012;34:762–765.

Table 45.3 Cells marked by CD antigens	
CD2	T cells (E rosette receptor)
CD3	T-cell receptor
CD4	Helper T cells
CD5	Mature thymocytes, some B-cell subsets
CD7	T cells, natural killer (NK) cells
CD8	T cells, NK cells
CD10	Pre-B cells, lymphoblastic leukemia cells
CD14	Monocytes
CD15	Reed-Sternberg cells, myeloid cells
CD19	Pan-B cells
CD20	Pan-B cells, dendritic cells
CD21	Receptor for complement 2 and Epstein-Barr virus
CD23	Activated B cells, monocytes, eosinophils, and platelets
CD25	Activated T and B cells, monocytes (interleukin-2 receptor)
CD30	Ki-1–related cells, Reed-Sternberg cells, T-cell NHL
CD34	Lymphoid and myeloid precursor cells
CD43	T cells, myeloid cells
CD45	Leukocytes
CD45R	T cells, myeloid cells
CD56	NK cells
CD74	HLA-invariant chain
CD75	Follicular center cells

CD, Cluster designation; *HLA*, histocompatibility locus antigen; *NHL*, non–Hodgkin's lymphoma.

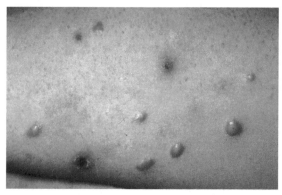

Fig. 45.7 Lymphomatoid papulosis. The lesions occur in crops and self-heal. (Courtesy Fitzsimons Army Medical Center teaching files.)

El Shabrawi-Caelen L, Kerl H, Cerroni L. Lymphomatoid papulosis: reappraisal of clinicopathologic presentation and classification into subtypes A, B, and C. *Arch Dermatol.* 2004;140:441–447.

27. Are CD30-positive cells specific for lymphomatoid papulosis?

No. The monoclonal antibody CD30 (Ki-1) was first described in 1982 with positive staining of Reed-Sternberg cells of Hodgkin's disease. Positive staining was also found in the paracortical cells of reactive lymph nodes. CD30 positivity can be seen in primary T-cell lymphomas, anaplastic large-cell lymphomas, regressing atypical histiocytosis, and occasionally pityriasis lichenoides et varioliformis acuta (Mucha-Habermann disease). CD30-positive primary cutaneous lymphomas have a better prognosis than CD30-negative primary cutaneous lymphomas.

Borchmann P. CD30⁺ diseases: anaplastic large-cell lymphoma and lymphomatoid papulosis. *Cancer Treat Res.* 2008;142:345–365.

28. What is HTLV-1 virus? What is its significance?

Human T-cell lymphotropic virus type 1 (HTLV-1) is a type C retrovirus associated with T-cell lymphoma and leukemia. The virus is endemic in Japan, the Caribbean, and northeastern South America; a few cases have been reported in the United States. It can be transmitted by blood transfusions, intravenous drug abuse, breast feeding, and, less commonly, sexual contact. A small subset of patients who are HTLV-1–antibody positive (<5%) will develop lymphoma or lymphocytic leukemia. The disease is characterized by immunosuppression, lymphadenopathy, cutaneous lesions, and hypercalcemia.

29. Can multiple myeloma present with skin lesions only?

Yes. However, it is extremely rare for myeloma to begin with only skin lesions. Extraosseous lesions in association with osseous myeloma are common, and the skin is one of the extraosseous sites (Fig. 45.8). There are many skin diseases associated with monoclonal gammopathy, including pyoderma gangrenosum, scleromyxedema, scleroderma adultorum, leukocytoclastic vasculitis, collagen-vascular disease, xanthomas, Waldenström's macroglobulinemia, subcorneal pustular dermatosis, pustular psoriasis, and even urticaria. The diagnosis of multiple myeloma is confirmed when there are lytic bone lesions, anemia, hypercalcemia, elevated serum and/or urine monoclonal protein spike, and bone marrow plasma cells exceeding 10%. Subcutaneous myeloma is much more common during late-stage, relapsed disease.

Requena L, Lutzner H, Palmedo G, et al. Cutaneous involvement in multiple myeloma: a clinicopathologic, immunohistochemical, and cytogenetic study of 8 cases. *Arch Dermatol.* 2003;139:475–486.

30. What is pseudolymphoma of the skin?

This term represents several clinical entities that probably have multiple etiologies. Included are lymphocytoma cutis, Spiegler-Fendt sarcoid, lymphadenosis benigna cutis, and Jessner's benign lymphocytic infiltrate. In most cases, the etiology is unknown, although chronic arthropod bite reactions and medications can be an etiologic stimulus in some cases. The lesions present as indolent single or grouped, red or purple nodules or plaques on the head, neck, and upper trunk, and other anatomic sites can be involved (Fig. 45.9). The infiltrate may show either B- or T-cell predominance. Some cases can be difficult to differentiate from lymphoma, and the patient must be followed before a definite diagnosis can be made.

Ploysangam T, Breneman DL, Mutasim DF. Cutaneous pseudolymphomas. *J Am Acad Dermatol.* 1998;38:877–895.

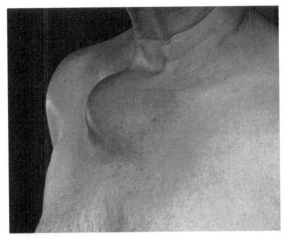

Fig. 45.8 Patient with late-stage multiple myeloma with a large subcutaneous mass of the anterior chest. (Courtesy Fitzsimons Army Medical Center teaching files.)

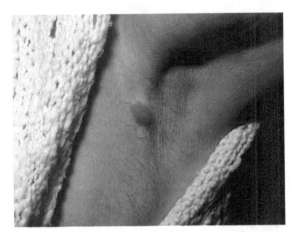

Fig. 45.9 Pseudolymphoma of unknown cause in the axilla of a woman. (Courtesy Fitzsimons Army Medical teaching files.)

31. Can B-cell lymphomas present with skin lesions?

Yes. B-cell lymphomas may be primary and arise in skin or less commonly represent extension of B-cell nodal lymphomas. Cutaneous involvement occurs in greater than 5% of patients with B-cell nodal lymphoma. Primary cutaneous B-cell lymphomas account for approximately 20% to 25% of all primary cutaneous lymphomas. The World Health Organization–European Organization for Research and Treatment of Cancer classification recognizes five subtypes (Table 45.4). Primary cutaneous marginal zone B-cell lymphoma and primary cutaneous follicle center lymphoma (PCFCL) are by far the most common cutaneous B-cell lymphomas.

32. What is primary cutaneous marginal zone B-cell lymphoma?

Primary cutaneous marginal zone B-cell lymphoma is a low-grade lymphoma that may present at any age but it most commonly affects younger adults. The primary lesions are solitary or multiple papules, plaques, or nodules that most commonly affect the proximal upper extremities or trunk (Fig. 45.10). It is composed of small B cells, larger marginal zone B cells (centrocytes), and variable numbers of plasma cells. In Europe, a significant percentage of these cases are associated with *Borrelia burgdorferi* infection; however, this association is not seen in the United States or Asia. Because of the excellent prognosis, treatment options include surgical excision, local radiation, or treatment with Rituximab, a chimeric monoclonal antibody targeted against the pan-B-cell marker CD20.

Jelic S, Filipovic-Ljeskovic I. Positive serology for Lyme disease borrelias in primary cutaneous B-cell lymphoma: a study in 22 patients; is it a fortuitous finding? *Hematol Oncol.* 1999;17:107–116.

Table 45.4 Classification of primary cutaneous B-Cell lymphomas

LYMPHOMA	5-YEAR DISEASE-SPECIFIC SURVIVAL
Primary marginal zone B-cell lymphoma	98%–100%
Primary cutaneous follicle-center lymphoma	95%–98%
Primary cutaneous diffuse large B-cell lymphoma, leg type	38%–74%
Primary cutaneous diffuse large B-cell lymphoma, other	40%–50%
Primary cutaneous intravascular large B-cell lymphoma	65%

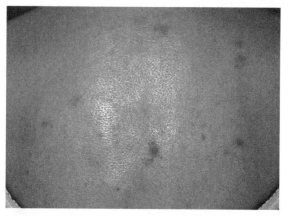

Fig. 45.10 Primary cutaneous marginal zone B-cell lymphoma of the skin presenting as multiple papules and nodules of the trunk of a young adult woman. (Courtesy Fitzsimons Army Medical Center teaching files.)

33. What is primary cutaneous follicle center lymphoma?

PCFCL is a low-grade lymphoma that is most commonly seen in middle-aged adults of both sexes. The primary lesions are solitary or multiple plaques or nodules that most commonly occur on the scalp, forehead, and upper portion of the trunk. Histologically, it is composed of large neoplastic cells (centroblasts) resembling those seen in normal secondary lymphoid follicles. There are also variable numbers of small cleaved cells resembling centrocytes. Treatment of this low-grade lymphoma is highly variable and may include excision of solitary lesions, local radiation, or treatment with **Rituximab**, a chimeric monoclonal **antibody** targeted against the pan-B-cell marker CD20.

Brandenberg A, Humme D, Terhorst D, et al. Long-term outcome of intravenous therapy with rituximab in patients with primary cutaneous B-cell lymphomas. *Br J Dermatol.* 2013;169:1126–1132.

34. What is the most common type of leukemia in adults?

Chronic lymphocytic leukemia. It is the most common cause of specific leukemic skin lesions, which are usually multiple and may present with papules, nodules, plaques, erythema, and, rarely, bullae. This neoplastic proliferation of lymphocytes is usually B cell in origin.

35. Can leukemia present with specific skin lesions?

Yes. Although uncommon, skin infiltration with neoplastic leukemia cells can be a presenting finding and precede the leukemic phase of the disease by several months. This is most common with acute myeloid leukemia (AML). Often, this phenomenon is preceded by a myelodysplastic or myeloproliferative syndrome. The skin lesions may present as greenish, red, or purple papules, nodules, or plaques (Fig. 45.11).

Aractingi S, Bachmeyer C, Miclea J, et al. Unusual specific cutaneous lesions in myelodysplastic syndromes. *J Am Acad Dermatol.* 1995;33:187–191.

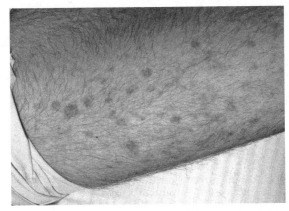

Fig. 45.11 Cutaneous acute myeloid leukemia of thigh demonstrating numerous violaceous papules and plaque. (Courtesy Fitzsimons Army Medical Center teaching files.)

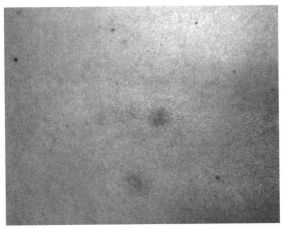

Fig. 45.12 Patient with acute myeloid leukemia and chloroma of the trunk demonstrating characteristic greenish tint. (Courtesy Fitzsimons Army Medical Center teaching files.)

36. What is a chloroma?

A chloroma is an uncommon extramedullary myeloid neoplasm that is also known as cutaneous myeloid sarcoma or cutaneous granulocytic sarcoma that occurs in a minority of patients with AML. It may precede the onset of leukemia or occur at some time during the course of the disease. The name is derived from the Greek word *chloros*, which means green. These tumors often have a distinctive greenish tint because of the presence of myeloperoxidase (Fig. 45.12).

Hurley MY, Gharramani GK, Frisch S, et al. Cutaneous myeloid sarcoma: natural history and biology of uncommon manifestation of acute myeloid leukemia. *Acta Derm Venereol.* 2013;93:319–324.

37. What are some nonspecific skin lesions seen in patients with leukemia?

Nonspecific skin lesions are quite common in patients with all types of leukemia and preleukemia. The most common skin findings are petechiae, purpura, pruritus, papular eruptions, vasculitis, urticaria, herpes zoster, and erythroderma. Approximately 5% to 10% of patients with pyoderma gangrenosum have or will develop leukemia, usually of the myelocytic type. Gingival hyperplasia is a common association with acute myelomonocytic leukemia (French-American-British classification [FAB] subtypes M4 and M5).

CHAPTER 46

UNCOMMON MALIGNANT TUMORS OF THE SKIN

Whitney A. High

ATYPICAL FIBROXANTHOMA/PLEOMORPHIC DERMAL SARCOMA

1. What is an atypical fibroxanthoma (AFX) and what is it relationship to pleomorphic dermal sarcoma (PDS)?

AFX is a malignant neoplasm that occurs chiefly in the elderly, upon sun-damaged skin. These tumors are usually well circumscribed, grow rapidly, and demonstrate an exophytic architecture but are otherwise indistinct (Fig. 46.1A,B). AFX does not invade the deep soft tissue, and in general, it has a favorable prognosis. PDS occurs in a similar population, with cellular morphology similar to AFX, but it manifests more aggressive histological features, such as deep invasion, tumor necrosis, and lymphovascular or perineural invasion. PDS has greater potential for local recurrence and metastasis. Distinguishing AFX from PDS is important due to differences in clinical behavior (see below).

2. What are the histologic features of AFX and PDS?

Both AFX and PDS are dermal processes, without an epidermal connection, but often with an epidermal collarette. The tumor is composed of spindle and slightly epithelioid cells arranged in disordered fascicles, with striking nuclear pleomorphism and hyperchromasia, and numerous mitotic figures, including atypical forms (ring mitoses, tripolar mitoses, etc.). Importantly, as AFX and PDS may be confused with other entities, such as spindle-cell squamous cell carcinoma and desmoplastic/spindle-cell melanoma, immunostains are utilized to exclude other entities. In general, AFX/PDS mark affirmatively with immunostains for CD10, CD68, and procollagen I.

3. What is the clinical course of AFX and PDS?

Despite high-grade cytologic atypia and a malignant histologic appearance, AFX has a favorable prognosis, typically with complete resolution upon extirpation. However, PDS is also managed surgically but is more often associated with local recurrence and even metastatic behavior. PDS can be particularly problematic in persons with immunosuppression, to include chronic lymphocytic leukemia. The metastatic behavior of PDS is problematic for treatment, but the author (W.A.H.) has had success with programmed death protein-1 (PD-1) inhibitors. Attempts to distinguish between AFX and PDS based upon shallow shave specimens are impossible, as depth of invasion is a key determinate. In such cases, full reevaluation will be necessary upon full surgical extirpation.

Griewank KG, Wiesner T, Murali R, et al. Atypical fibroxanthoma and pleomorphic dermal sarcoma harbor frequent NOTCH1/2 and FAT1 mutations and similar DNA copy number alteration profiles. *Mod Pathol.* 2018;31:418–428.

KEY POINTS: ATYPICAL FIBROXANTHOMA AND PLEOMORPHIC DERMAL SARCOMA

- AFX and PDS both present often as a fast-growing nodule on the sun-damaged or radiation-damaged skin of the head, neck, and scalp of older patients.
- Biopsy typically shows high-grade cytologic atypia with impressive pleomorphism and numerous mitoses.
- Distinction between AFX and PDS turns chiefly on more aggressive histological features, such as deep invasion, tumor necrosis, and lymphovascular or perineural invasion seen in PDS. As such, distinction in a shallow shave sampling may not be possible.
- AFX and PDS require surgical intervention to complete eradication, but PDS has a higher likelihood of local recurrence of metastatic disease.

MERKEL CELL CARCINOMA

4. What is a Merkel cell carcinoma (MCC)?

Also known as primary neuroendocrine carcinoma of the skin, MCC is an aggressive skin malignancy. The incidence and mortality of MCC are both increasing. The tumor was originally thought to arise from Merkel cells, which are involved in sensory reception in the skin, but this is not known with certitude and is widely debated.

Kervarrec T, Samimi M, Guyétant S, et al. Histogenesis of Merkel cell carcinoma: a comprehensive review. *Front Oncol.* 2019;9:451.

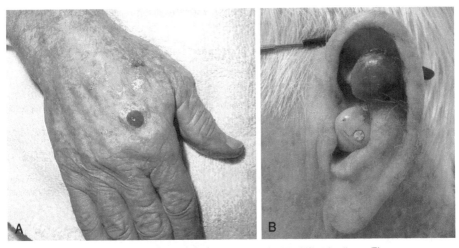

Fig. 46.1 Atypical fibroxanthoma arising on a sun-damaged hand **(A)** and on the ear **(B).**

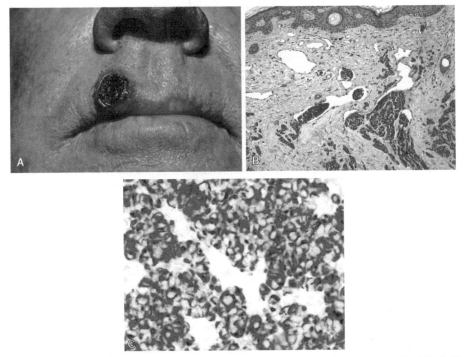

Fig. 46.2 Merkel cell carcinoma. **A,** Ulcerated nodule on the upper lip of an elderly man. **B,** Dermal cords and strands of small basaloid cells with minimal cytoplasm. Note the extension of the tumor into a lymphatic space. **C,** Cytokeratin 20 immunostaining highlights paranuclear/perinuclear dotting. (Panel A courtesy Fitzsimons Army Medical Center teaching files.)

5. Describe the clinical presentation of MCC.

MCC usually presents as a solitary, rapidly growing, painless dermal or subcutaneous nodule with a slight violaceous hue, on the sun-damaged skin of elderly persons. Whites are affected most often. The head and neck (Fig. 46.2A) are high-risk areas, but the extremities and trunk can be involved, on occasion. The mnemonic "**AEIOU + blue**" helps to recollect some of the features of MCC: **A**symptomatic/lack of tenderness; **E**xpanding rapidly; **I**mmune-suppressed persons; **O**lder than 50 years; **U**ltraviolet (UV)-exposed skin, and with a slightly **"blue"** hue.

Adapted by W.A.H. from: Heath M, Jaimes N, Lemos B, et al. Clinical characteristics of Merkel cell carcinoma at diagnosis in 195 patients: the AEIOU features. *J Am Acad Dermatol.* 2008;58:375–381.

6. What is the pathogenesis of MCC?

MCC is rare before the age of 50 years, but the incidence increases sharply after 65 years of age. This suggests an accumulation of pro-oncogenic events, such as:

- **Immunosuppression**—patients with chronic lymphocytic leukemia, HIV, acquired immunosuppression, and organ transplantation have higher incidence of MCC.
- **UV exposure**—most tumors present on sun-exposed areas, and the risk of MCC may be increased by prior psoralen and UV A treatment.
- **Merkel cell polyomavirus (MCV)**—the pathogenic role of MCV is still under investigation. Although MCV infections in humans may be common, the integration of the virus into the genome is not, and this event is strongly associated with MCC and may play a role in the oncogenesis for most, if not all, cases of MCC.

Amber K, Mcleod MP, Nouri K. The Merkel cell polyomavirus and its involvement in Merkel cell carcinoma. *Dermatol Surg.* 2013;39:232–238.
Feng H, Shuda M, Chang Y, Moore PS. Clonal integration of a polyomavirus in human Merkel cell carcinoma. *Science.* 2008;319:1096–1100.

7. Can any other tumors be microscopically confused with MCC?

Yes. MCC is composed of **"small blue (basaloid) cells"** with hyperchromatic nuclei, scant cytoplasm, and numerous mitoses (Fig. 46.2B). It may be confused with metastatic small cell carcinoma of the lung, lymphomas, sweat gland carcinoma, metatypical basal cell carcinoma, metastatic carcinoid tumors, and Ewing sarcoma.

8. How can MCC be distinguished from these other tumors?

MCC often has a characteristic paranuclear/perinuclear "dot" with immunostains for cytokeratins, particularly cytokeratin 20 (Fig. 46.2B, *inset*). Moreover, cytokeratin 20 is not expressed in basal cell carcinoma, lymphomas, or sweat gland carcinoma (Fig. 46.2C). MCC also marked with various neuroendocrine markers, such as synaptophysin, chromogranin A, and neuron-specific enolase. Epithelial membrane antigen (EMA) is also expressed in most MCC, as is CD56. Neurofilament is a useful marker for confirming or refuting the diagnosis of MCC. Electron microscopy may demonstrate the dense core neurosecretory granules seen in MCC but is rarely necessary.

9. How do you treat MCC?

Wide local excision is necessary for MCC. Margins of 1–2 cm are employed, depending upon the clinical size of the lesion. Sentinel lymph node biopsy (SLNB) is recommended for all patients fit for the procedure (remember, MCC is common in the elderly). As with other skin cancers, SLNB is almost always performed at the time surgery for removal of the primary tumor. For patients with uninvolved lymph nodes, the present position of the National Comprehensive Cancer Network is that it is "unclear how to identify patients with MCC most likely to benefit from postoperative radiotherapy." Patients with regional lymph node involvement are often treated with lymph node dissection and/or irradiation. Chemotherapy and immunotherapy may be used for unresectable, metastatic, and recurrent MCC. Current immunotherapies employed in MCC include pembrolizumab and nivolumab (anti-PD-1 agents) and avelumab (an anti-PD-L1 agent).

Bichakjian JCK, Olencki T, Aasi SZ, et al. Merkel cell carcinoma, clinical practice guidelines in oncology. *J Natl Compr Canc Netw.* 2018;16:742–774.

10. Does MCC metastasize, and what is the overall prognosis?

Yes. Up to 75% of patients develop regional lymph node metastases. Distant metastases occur to in 30% to 40%. The prognosis of MCC is related to disease stage, with a 5-year survival rate ranging from 81% in patients with small and localized tumors to 11% in those patients with metastatic disease. More than half of all patients experience recurrence, usually within 1 year of treatment. All patients need close serial surveillance.

KEY POINTS: MERKEL CELL CARCINOMA

- Fast-growing violaceous nodule in sun-damaged skin of elderly Caucasians.
- Characteristic cytokeratin 20–positive paranuclear/perinuclear "dot" upon immunostaining.
- Aggressive malignancy with frequent recurrences and metastases that is treated with surgical intervention, SLNB, or lymph node dissection, and possibly with radiation therapy or chemotherapy/Immunotherapy.

MICROCYSTIC ADNEXAL CARCINOMA

11. What is a microcystic adnexal carcinoma (MAC)?

    MAC is a locally aggressive cutaneous malignancy of sweat duct origin that typically presents as a slow-growing, firm, ill-defined skin-colored or yellow plaque or nodule on the head and neck, most often on the upper lip (Fig. 46.3A). Numbness, paresthesia, burning, discomfort, and rarely pruritus of the affected area may be reported and are caused by a propensity for perineural invasion. Patients are usually Caucasians between 40 and 60 years of age. Because of its innocuous clinical appearance and slow progression, the diagnosis is often delayed.

12. What are the histologic features of MAC?

    The tumor presents as an epithelial tumor without connection to the overlying epidermis and with infiltrative cords and strands with variable keratinization and/or ductal differentiation (Fig. 46.3B). The tumor cells often induce a desmoplastic stroma. Tumor islands become progressively smaller with depth in the dermis. Deep invasion and perineural invasion are characteristic. An adequate biopsy is essential, as a superficial sampling may lead to misdiagnosis. The entity must be distinguished from morpheaform basal cell carcinoma, desmoplastic trichoepithelioma, trichoadenoma, or syringoma.

13. How is MAC treated?

    Micrographic removal (Mohs surgery) is the treatment of choice for MAC. Frequent recurrences, often resulting from perineural invasion, may occur with standard surgical excision. MAC is a locally aggressive malignancy that can infiltrate fat, muscle, cartilage, bone, blood vessels, and nerves, but metastatic disease is rare.

KEY POINTS: MICROCYSTIC ADNEXAL CARCINOMA

- Slow-growing, ill-defined plaque, classically on the upper lip.
- Deeply invasive strands of basaloid cells and ductal structures in a desmoplastic stroma, often with perineural invasion.
- A superficial biopsy may lead to misdiagnosis.

DERMATOFIBROSARCOMA PROTUBERANS

14. What are the clinical presentation and behavior of dermatofibrosarcoma protuberans?

    Dermatofibrosarcoma protuberans (DFSP) is a slow-growing, irregular (often multinodular), ill-demarcated indurated pink plaque, most often on the trunk and extremities of young to middle-aged adults (Fig. 46.4A). DFSP is locally aggressive and may invade deeper tissue, such as fat, fascia, muscle, and bone, but it has a slow growth rate and rarely metastasizes.

15. How does DFSP look like histologically?

    DFSP is characterized as a proliferation of spindle cells in the dermis and subcutaneous fat. The cells form intersecting fascicles (bundles) with a storiform (cartwheel-like) arrangement. Often, DFSP invades the fat, displacing normal adipose and leading to a "honeycomb-like" appearance. The cells are CD34-positive with immunostaining.

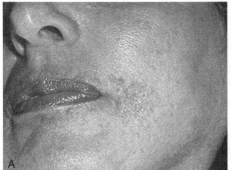 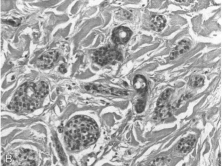

Fig. 46.3 Microcystic adnexal carcinoma. **A,** Middle-aged woman with a typical microcystic adnexal carcinoma of the cheek. She had a past history of radiation for acne vulgaris. **B,** Infiltrative cords and strands of epithelial cells with focal ductal differentiation.

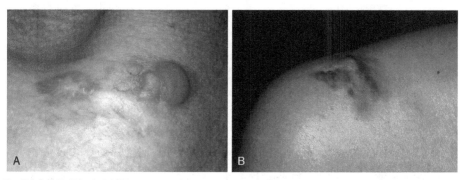

Fig. 46.4 A, Multinodular dermatofibrosarcoma protuberans with atrophic areas on the shoulder of a man. **B,** Bednar tumor on the shoulder of a young woman. (Panel A courtesy David Bertler, MD.)

16. What is a Bednar tumor?

    A Bednar tumor is an uncommon pigmented variant of DFSP (Fig. 46.4B). The pigmentation is due to melanin-containing dendritic cells (melanocytes) that are scattered between the neoplastic spindle-shaped cells. It is not a form of melanoma.

17. What is the chromosomal translocation seen in DFSP?

    Cytogenetic studies in DFSP reveal characteristic translocations of chromosomes 17 and 22, which create a *COL1A1/PDGFB* fusion gene. This results in constitutive expression of the tyrosine kinase, PDGFB, creating a stimulatory loop that drives cell proliferation and fibrosis. This molecular pathway is important because it can be targeted with imatinib, a tyrosine kinase inhibitor.

Noujaim J, Thway K, Fisher C, Jones RL. Dermatofibrosarcoma protuberans: from translocation to targeted therapy. *Cancer Biol Med.* 2015;12:375–384.

18. How is DFSP treated?

    Complete surgical extirpation is the treatment of choice. Micrographic (Mohs) surgery affords the highest cure (>95%). Metastases are rare, but local recurrence is not uncommon, particularly if micrographic removal was not utilized. Imatinib is typically reserved for treatment of unresectable or metastatic DFSP. While the drug may shrink lesions prior to surgery, there is concern that routine preoperative use of imatinib may result in "skip areas" in the tumor.

Serra-Guillén C, Llombart B, Nagore E, et al. Mohs micrographic surgery in dermatofibrosarcoma protuberans allows tumour clearance with smaller margins and greater preservation of healthy tissue compared with conventional surgery. *Br J Dermatol.* 2015;172:1303–1307.

ANGIOSARCOMA

19. What is cutaneous angiosarcoma?

    Cutaneous angiosarcoma is a highly malignant tumor of endothelial cells that typically presents in one of three different clinical situations:

    - Angiosarcoma of the face and scalp in the elderly (most common)
    - Angiosarcoma associated with chronic lymphedema, such as that in the upper extremity following radical mastectomy (Stewart-Treves syndrome)
    - Postirradiation angiosarcoma

20. How does angiosarcoma of the scalp and face present in the elderly?

    It presents as an erythematous or hemorrhagic bruise-like patch on the central face or scalp, which spreads centrifugally and evolves into nodules that bleed easily and ulcerate (Fig. 46.5A). There is extensive infiltration, and tumor size is often underappreciated. Placing the patient's head at a level below the heart ("head-tilt

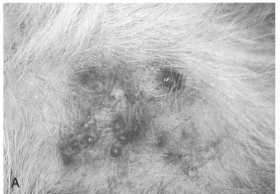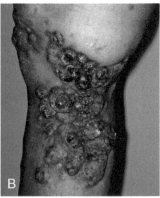

Fig. 46.5 A, Angiosarcoma of the scalp in the elderly. **B,** Angiosarcoma arising on the lower extremity of a patient with chronic lymphedema. (Courtesy Walter Reed Army Medical Center files.)

maneuver") will cause the vascular tumor to become more engorged and violaceous, allowing for better visualization.

21. How does angiosarcoma present in the setting of chronic lymphedema?

Cutaneous angiosarcoma arising in the setting of chronic lymphedema is called Stewart-Treves syndrome. It presents as cutaneous and subcutaneous, firm and violaceous nodules, on a background of nonpitting edema. In the setting of prior mastectomy and lymphadenectomy, it typically occurs, on average, 10 years after the surgical procedure (range 1 to 30 years). Cutaneous angiosarcoma due to lymphedema is less often associated with filarial, congenital, traumatic, or idiopathic causes (Fig. 46.5B).

22. What are the most common clinical scenarios of postirradiation cutaneous angiosarcoma?

The tumor arises in the skin most often after radiation therapy of breast or gynecologic cancer.

23. What are the histologic features of angiosarcomas?

Well-differentiated and poorly differentiated areas may be seen in the same tumor. Well-differentiated areas show an anastomosing network of well-formed, irregular vascular channels, lined by endothelial cells. They exhibit a highly infiltrative pattern, dissecting and splitting collagen bundles. Poorly differentiated areas show large pleomorphic cells with little or no evidence of luminal differentiation and may closely resemble carcinomas, melanoma, or other soft tissue sarcomas, with only subtle vascular lumen formation. Because the histologic features may vary, shallow and small biopsy specimens should be discouraged. Mitotic figures are invariably present. Immunostains, such as ERG, CD31, CD34, factor VIII, and D2-40 are often needed to establish the lineage of the tumor cells.

KEY POINTS: ANGIOSARCOMA

- Three main clinical presentations: (1) face and scalp of elderly; (2) chronic lymphedema or Stewart-Treves syndrome; (3) postirradiation therapy
- Infiltrating cells derived from blood vessels and lining irregular blood-filled spaces
- Aggressive tumors that spread widely and have a high rate of lymph node and systemic metastases

24. What are the clinical course and prognosis for angiosarcoma?

The prognosis in cutaneous angiosarcoma is poor. The 5-year survival rate ranges from 12% to 34%. Metastases to the cervical nodes and hematogenous metastases to the lungs, liver, and spleen can occur, but many patients die as a result of extensive local disease. Early diagnosis and complete extirpation afford the best chance of survival. Because the lesions are often multicentric, extensive, and progress rapidly, management is rarely successful for prolonged durations. Mixed-modality approaches include surgical extirpation, radiation therapy, and adjuvant treatment. Chemotherapy is recommended in cases of systemic disease but is usually not particularly effective.

Shustef E, Kazlouskaya V, Prieto VG, Ivan D, Aung PP. Cutaneous angiosarcoma: a current update. *J Clin Pathol.* 2017;70:917–925.

EPITHELIOID SARCOMA

25. What is an epithelioid sarcoma?

Epithelioid sarcoma is a rare high-grade malignancy of unknown lineage, with both epithelial and mesenchymal differentiation and with no normal cellular counterpart in the skin. It presents as a painless, firm, slow-growing intradermal or subcutaneous nodule, often ulcerated, usually on the distal extremities. The male-to-female ratio is approximately 2:1, and it affects mainly young adults. Epithelioid sarcoma tends to spread through lymphatic channels or along fascial planes, and this may give rise to multiple local nodules. The clinical differential includes mycobacterial or deep fungal infection, squamous cell carcinoma, and other soft tissue sarcomas.

Thway K, Jones RL, Noujaim J, Fisher C. Epithelioid sarcoma: diagnostic features and genetics. *Adv Anat Pathol.* 2016;23:41–49.

26. How is the diagnosis of epithelioid sarcoma established on biopsy?

The diagnosis of epithelioid sarcoma is often challenging, and immunostains are typically necessary. The tumor is composed of malignant eosinophilic epithelioid and spindle cells that are arranged in nodules, with central necrosis. At low power, it may resemble a granulomatous process; however, cellular atypia and tumor necrosis assist in making the correct diagnosis. The tumor cells demonstrate staining with both mesenchymal markers (vimentin and CD34), as well as epithelial markers (keratins and EMA).

Armah HB, Parwani AV. Epithelioid sarcoma. *Arch Pathol Lab Med.* 2009;133:814–819.

27. How are epithelioid sarcomas treated?

Considerable excisional surgery is required. The local recurrence rate has been reported to range from 29% to 77%. Multifocal recurrences are common because the tumor spreads insidiously along the tendons, fascial planes, nerves, and blood vessels. Adjuvant radiotherapy is often used to lower the risk of local recurrence. Amputation is sometimes required. Chemotherapy with ifosfamide and doxorubicin is recommended for metastatic disease.

Jawad MU, Extein J, Min ES, Scully SP. Prognostic factors for survival in patients with epithelioid sarcoma: 441 cases from the SEER database. *Clin Orthop Relat Res.* 2009;467:2939–2948.

28. What are the prognostic factors of epithelioid sarcoma?

The recognized adverse prognostic factors include proximal or axial location, depth of invasion, and nodal involvement. Epithelioid sarcomas spread locally by lymphatic involvement or along fascial planes, resulting in multiple local nodules. Forty-five percent of patients develop metastases, mostly to the lymph nodes and lungs. The overall 5-year survival rates are reported between 32% and 92%.

Chbani L, Guillou L, Terrier P, et al. Epithelioid sarcoma: a clinicopathologic and immunohistochemical analysis of 106 cases from the French sarcoma group. *Am J Clin Pathol.* 2009;131:222–227.

KEY POINTS: EPITHELIOID SARCOMA

- Slow-growing nodule on the distal limbs of young persons.
- Epithelioid and plump spindle cells arranged in nodular aggregates with central necrosis.
- Immunostains demonstrate expression of epithelial and mesenchymal markers.
- Frequent recurrence and high rate of metastasis.

EXTRAMAMMARY PAGET DISEASE

29. What are the clinical features of extramammary Paget disease (EMPD)?

EMPD is a rare cutaneous malignancy most often arising in the perineum, vulva, perianal area, axilla, scrotum, and penis. Clinically, the condition presents as a pruritic, erythematous patch or plaque with sharp irregular border, typically with crusting (Fig. 46.6). The condition is often confused with inflammatory conditions that affect these same areas, such as intertrigo, tinea cruris, or chronic dermatitis, leading to diagnostic delays. Women between 50 and 60 years of age are most commonly affected, but men may develop the condition, as well.

30. What is "primary" and "secondary" EMPD?

Primary EMPD arises in the epidermis without underlying carcinoma. Current evidence supports the Toker cell being the cell of origin for EMPD. Toker cells are found in the mammary line of humans and may represent residua of embryonic development of breast tissue and mammary-like apocrine glands. Although primary EMPD is initially limited to the epithelium, it may slowly progress to an invasive tumor, spreading to the dermis, blood, and lymphatic vessels;

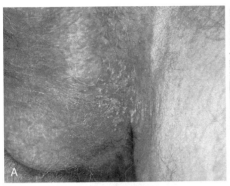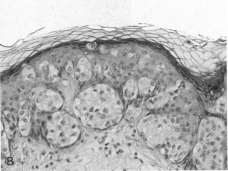

Fig. 46.6 A, Typical extramammary Paget's disease arising in the groin. **B,** Typical large, pale, atypical epithelial cells that demonstrate scattered growth pattern, both as single cells and as small aggregates throughout the epidermis.

in advanced stages, it may produce lymph node or visceral, potentially lethal metastases. Conversely, secondary EMPD is caused by the epidermotropic spread of malignant cells from an underlying adenocarcinoma, usually of genitourinary or gastrointestinal origin.

31. What is meant by "pagetoid" growth?
The term "pagetoid" refers to the scattered spread of atypical cells within the epidermis (Fig. 46.6B). EMPD is not the only disease to demonstrate pagetoid spread, and it may also be seen in mammary Paget disease, squamous cell carcinoma in situ (Bowen disease), melanoma in situ and melanoma, sebaceous carcinoma, and, rarely, Merkel cell carcinoma.

32. How is EMPD treated?
EMPD typically extends well beyond the clinically apparent margins, and a surgical excision with careful margin control is the treatment of choice. However, the tumor can be multifocal, and local recurrences are common. Micrographic (Mohs) surgery offers lower recurrence rates (8% to 26%) when compared to standard surgical excision (30% to 60%). There are reports on radiotherapy, topical imiquimod or 5-fluorouracil, and systemic chemotherapy in patients who were not surgical candidates, in locally advanced or metastatic EMPD, or as adjuvant treatment to surgical excision.

Hendi A, Brodland DG, Zitelli JA. Extramammary Paget's disease: surgical treatment with Mohs micrographic surgery. *J Am Acad Dermatol.* 2004;51:767–773.
Valle L, Deig C, Wright R, High W. An advanced case of extramammary Paget disease: safe and effective treatment in an inoperable elderly patient using extensive en face electron irradiation. *JAAD Case Rep.* 2018;5:72–74.

SEBACEOUS CARCINOMA

33. Where do sebaceous carcinomas occur?
Sebaceous carcinoma is divided into ocular and extraocular forms. Ocular sebaceous carcinoma arises from the meibomian glands (tarsal glands) of the eyelid and is typically more aggressive than extraocular disease. The upper eyelid is most often involved. Sebaceous carcinoma can occur in association with Muir-Torre syndrome, where sebaceous carcinoma, other sebaceous neoplasms, and colorectal and genitourinary carcinoma are associated.

Haber R, Battistella M, Pages C, Bagot M, Lebbe C, Basset-Seguin N. Sebaceous carcinomas of the skin: 24 cases and a literature review. *Acta Derm Venereol.* 2017;97:959–961.

34. How does sebaceous carcinoma present?
Ocular tumors present as firm pink to yellow nodules (Fig. 46.7). Since they may mimic a chalazion, it is important to biopsy persistent or unusual lesions. As sebaceous carcinoma grows, it may spread onto the conjunctiva, where it can be mistaken for keratoconjunctivitis or blepharoconjunctivitis. Extraocular tumors of the head and neck of the elderly can present as a pink to yellow-red nodule.

35. What are the treatment and prognosis?
Treatment is complete surgical removal, and micrographic (Mohs) surgery has a lower recurrence rate than does standard excision. Up to one third of patients with ocular tumors develop metastases to cervical lymph nodes. Ocular

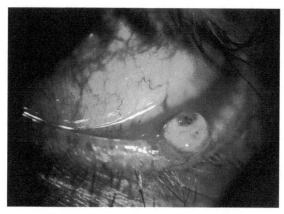

Fig. 46.7 Sebaceous gland carcinoma on the lower eyelid.

sebaceous carcinoma of over 1 cm in diameter if often treated with sentinel lymph node sampling, in addition to excision.

Chang AY, Miller CJ, Elenitsas R, Newman JG, Sobanko JF. Management considerations in extraocular sebaceous carcinoma. *Dermatol Surg.* 2016;42:S57–S65.
Esmaeli B, Nasser QJ, Cruz H, Fellman M, Warneke CL, Ivan D. American Joint Committee on Cancer T category for eyelid sebaceous carcinoma correlates with nodal metastasis and survival. *Ophthalmology.* 2012;119:1078–1082.

LEIOMYOSARCOMA

36. What is leiomyosarcoma?

Leiomyosarcoma is a malignant tumor of smooth muscle. In the skin, it is derived chiefly from the smooth muscle of erector pilorum. The condition is more common in men. The tumor is typically solitary, with a nonspecific appearance, presenting as a red-pink nodule of 0.5 cm to greater than 3.0 cm in diameter. Leiomyosarcoma may be painful. The extensor surfaces of the proximal extremities, and areas of greatest hair distribution, are preferentially affected. Tumors may be ulcerated (Fig. 46.8).

37. What histologic stains help identify leiomyosarcoma?

Masson trichrome is a stain that chemically marks smooth muscle red. Immunostains for smooth muscle actin, muscle-specific actin, calponin, h-caldesmon, and desmin typically mark leiomyosarcoma, as well.

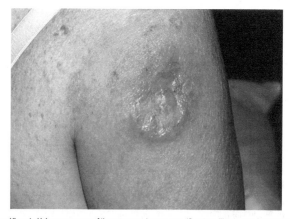

Fig. 46.8 Leiomyosarcoma. Ulcerated leiomyosarcoma of the upper arm in a woman. (Courtesy Fitzsimons Army Medical Center teaching files.)

38. What are the treatment and prognosis?

Wide local excision is utilized, typically with at least a 1-cm margin. Micrographic surgery may also be utilized. It is important to realize that leiomyosarcoma derived from erector pilorum muscle in the skin has an overall favorable prognosis. In fact, for this reason, some authorities refer to the tumor as "atypical intradermal smooth muscle neoplasms" and discourage use of the term "leiomysarcoma." In small lesions, confined to the dermis, it is important not to overtreat the patient. However, admittedly, the prognosis in the condition is related to depth of invasion. In one series, the metastatic rate for dermal tumors was 12% (disease-specific mortality was 6%) and the metastatic rate for subcutaneous tumors was 51% (disease-specific mortality was 40%).

Winchester DS, Hocker TL, Brewer JD, et al. Leiomyosarcoma of the skin: clinical, histopathologic, and prognostic factors that influence outcomes. *J Am Acad Dermatol.* 2014;71:919–925.

Kraft S, Fletcher CD. Atypical intradermal smooth muscle neoplasms: clinicopathologic analysis of 84 cases and a reappraisal of cutaneous "leiomyosarcoma". *Am J Surg Pathol.* 2011;35:599–607.

CHAPTER 47

CUTANEOUS METASTASES

James E. Fitzpatrick and Whitney A. High

1. How often do internal malignancies metastasize to the skin?

Cutaneous metastases from internal malignancies are uncommon, with a reported incidence that varies from less than 1% to over 10%. The largest autopsy study including 7500 patients with internal malignancies demonstrated cutaneous metastases in 9% of patients. Most cases occur late in the course of disease, but cutaneous metastasis may also be the initial presentation of an internal malignancy.

Strickley JD, Jenson AB, Jung JY. Cutaneous metastasis. *Hematol Oncol Clin North Am*. 2019;33:173–197.

2. By what three routes do internal malignancies metastasize to the skin?

Metastases extend by local infiltration or lymphatic or hematogenous spread. Breast carcinoma and oral cancer are the most likely malignancies to directly extend into the skin. It is assumed that the fundamental mechanisms of cutaneous spread are similar to those of metastases to other organs, but this has not been investigated. Rare cases of metastases have been caused by direct inoculation of the skin by invasive procedures, such as surgery (Fig. 47.1).

3. How do malignant cells invade and metastasize?

The genetic and molecular events that allow malignant cells to invade and spread are complex and incompletely understood. Clearly, malignant cells must be able to detach from the bulk of the tumor mass (i.e., downregulate adhesion molecules); adhere to the adjacent matrix via receptors to matrix molecules, such as fibronectin; enzymatically lyse the extracellular matrix to allow movement; and migrate via motility factors, such as hepatocyte growth factor. Once tumor cells gain access to lymphatic spaces or blood vessels, the cells must express adhesion molecules, which allows them to attach to endothelial cells (e.g., CD44). There is also evidence that certain normal tissues produce chemoattractants that may guide malignant cells to a specific site.

Nguyen TH. Mechanisms of metastasis. *Clin Dermatol*. 2004;22:209–216.

4. Why do some patients develop metastatic disease years or decades after initial disease?

Cutaneous metastases can develop years after a primary tumor was diagnosed, and in about 7% of cases, this interval exceeds 5 years. Melanoma and breast carcinoma are the most common tumors to present with delayed skin metastases. It is thought that this occurs because disseminated tumor cells enter dormancy and evade detection and systemic therapy. The mechanisms of dormancy are poorly understood, but stem cell quiescence, extracellular microenvironments, autophagy, genetics, and other mechanisms are thought important. The mechanisms that induce dormant cells to again become proliferative are a focus of research in many laboratories.

5. What is an "in-transit" metastasis?

By definition, an "in-transit" metastasis is a malignancy of cutaneous origin that has spread through a lymphatic vessel to grow more than 2 cm away from the primary lesion, but before it reaches the nearest draining lymph node. This term is most often used in staging melanoma, but it can be used for other primary cutaneous malignancies (e.g., Merkel cell carcinoma). An in-transit metastasis affords a worse prognosis than a primary tumor without such a complication.

Suojävi NJ, Jahkola TA, Virolainen S, et al. Outcome following local recurrence or in-transit metastases in cutaneous melanoma. *Melanoma Res*. 2012;22:447–453.

6. What are the most common cancers that metastasize to the skin in women?

The type of metastatic events observed is impacted by the patient's age, sex, and ethnicity and/or area of the world under study. In a large study done at the Armed Forces Institute of Pathology, in the United States, in the early 1970s, the most common etiologies of cutaneous metastases in women were:

- Breast carcinoma: 69%
- Colon: 9%
- Malignant melanoma: 5%
- Ovary: 4%
- Lung: 4%

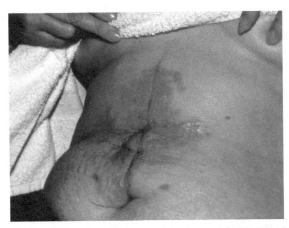

Fig. 47.1 Large eroded plaque of gastric carcinoma that has been implanted into the surgical scar on the abdomen. (Courtesy Fitzsimons Army Medical Center teaching files.)

Because of the rapid increase in the incidence of lung carcinoma and malignant melanoma in women, it is likely that metastatic disease from these two malignancies is now more common than reported in this early study.

7. What are the most common cancers that metastasize to the skin in men?
   In the same study, the five most common causes of skin metastases in men were:
   • Lung: 24%
   • Colon: 19%
   • Malignant melanoma: 13%
   • Oral squamous cell carcinoma: 12%
   • Kidney: 6%
   In a more recent study, malignant melanoma was the most common cause of cutaneous metastases, accounting for 32% of all cases (Fig. 47.2).

8. Do metastases to the skin typically occur in random patterns?
   No. Different tumors demonstrate characteristic patterns of metastases (Table 47.1). A well-known example is ocular malignant melanoma, which frequently metastasizes to the liver. As a rule, cutaneous metastases usually appear in skin near the primary tumor (Fig. 47.3). Most regional metastases are likely spread through the lymphatic system, while distant metastases are more likely to occur via a hematogenous route.

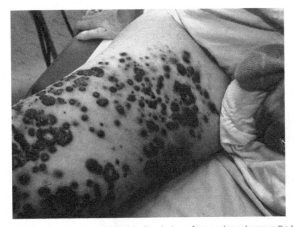

Fig. 47.2 Heavily pigmented metastatic melanoma due to in-transit metastases from a primary tumor on the lower extremity. (Courtesy Rene Gonzalez, MD.)

Table 47.1 Characteristic sites of cutaneous metastases

PRIMARY TUMOR	SITE OF METASTASES
Oral squamous cell carcinoma	Head and neck
Thyroid carcinoma	Neck
Lung	Chest wall
Breast	Anterior chest wall
Renal cell carcinoma	Head
Gastrointestinal carcinoma	Abdomen
Genitourinary carcinoma	Lower abdomen

9. Describe the most common presentations of malignancies metastatic to the skin.

Cutaneous metastases often present as a cutaneous nodule or group of nodules that may be movable or fixed to underlying structures. Less often, cutaneous metastases may present as indurated plaques. Cutaneous metastases may be skin-colored (Fig. 47.4), violaceous, erythematous, or even pigmented (melanoma). The overlying epidermis is typically intact, but large metastatic lesions may be eroded or ulcerated. Clinically, metastatic deposits may mimic epidermoid cysts, lipomas, primary cutaneous malignancies, neurofibromas, scars, pyogenic granulomas, cellulitis, and even dermatitis. For example, metastatic breast carcinoma may present with distinct clinical patterns, such as carcinoma erysipeloides (inflammatory carcinoma; Fig. 47.5), carcinoma telangiectaticum (a variant of inflammatory carcinoma), and carcinoma en cuirasse (a sclerodermoid pattern).

10. What is alopecia neoplastica?

The scalp appears to be a unique site for cutaneous metastasis, and often, cutaneous metastases to the scalp are a presenting sign for internal malignancy. One characteristic clinical presentation is that of an isolated, indurated plaque in the scalp with alopecia (Fig. 47.6). A biopsy of such a site will demonstrate cutaneous metastasis of a visceral malignancy causing a loss of hair follicles. The most common tumors to metastasize to the scalp are those of the breast, lung, and kidney.

11. What is a Sister Mary Joseph's nodule?

It is a nodular umbilical metastatic tumor (Fig. 47.7) named for Sister Mary Joseph, who was the superintendent of St. Mary's Hospital in Rochester, Minnesota, and served as the first surgical assistant to Dr. W.J. Mayo. She is credited with recognizing that patients with this finding had a poorer prognosis.

Davar S, Hanna D. Sister Mary Joseph's nodule. *J Cutan Med Surg.* 2012;16:201–204.

12. Which tumors usually present as a Sister Mary Joseph's nodule?

The four most common tumors to present as a Sister Mary Joseph nodule are stomach (20%), large bowel (14%), ovary (14%), and pancreatic tumors (11%). In about one-fifth of patients, the primary site cannot be determined.

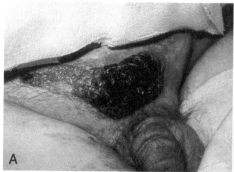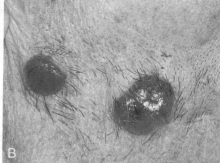

Fig. 47.3 A, Large metastatic nodule of prostate carcinoma. The lower abdomen and pubic area are common sites for metastases of genitourinary cancers. **B,** Lung carcinoma metastatic to the chest wall, which is the most common site. (Courtesy Paul Thompson, MD.)

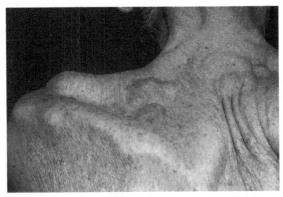

Fig. 47.4 Metastatic adenocarcinoma of the gastrointestinal tract presenting as skin-colored dermal and subcutaneous nodules.

13. Does basal cell carcinoma ever metastasize?

Yes, but only rarely. Basal cell carcinoma is the most common cutaneous malignancy in the United States, with over 1 million new cases per year. It has been estimated that the overall metastatic rate is 0.03%, with most cases occurring as large destructive tumors present for many years. Basal cell carcinoma most often metastasizes to regional lymph nodes followed by the lungs, bones, and skin. The 5-year survival for metastatic basal cell carcinoma is poor, and estimated to be about 10%, but has likely been improved with use of modern biologic therapies including Hedgehog pathway inhibitors, and PD-1 inhibitors.

Spates ST, Mellette Jr JR, Fitzpatrick J. Metastatic basal cell carcinoma. *Dermatol Surg.* 2003;29:650–652.

14. How do you diagnose a cutaneous metastasis?

The diagnosis is best established by doing an excisional, incisional, or punch biopsy and by submitting the specimen in formalin for routine processing. In addition to hematoxylin and eosin (H&E) stains, the pathologist can perform special stains

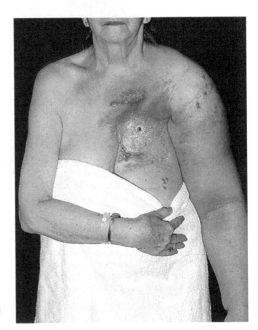

Fig. 47.5 Inflammatory breast carcinoma presenting as an erythematous plaque on the anterior chest wall and red dermal papules on the shoulder.

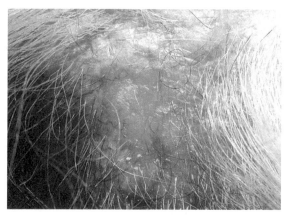

Fig. 47.6 Alopecia neoplastica secondary to metastatic breast carcinoma. On palpation, the lesion was firm and indurated.

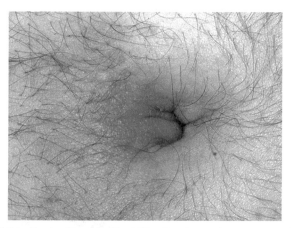

Fig. 47.7 Sister Mary Joseph's nodule of the umbilicus. The primary malignancy was never detected.

mucicarmine for mucin, Fontana-Masson for melanin, or immunohistochemistry studies (prostate-specific antigen for prostate cancer, TTF-1 for thyroid carcinoma, CDX2 for gastrointestinal carcinoma). Problematic cases may require electron microscopy or gene expression profiling. Less often in the skin the tumor specimen is obtained by a fine-needle aspiration.

KEY POINTS: CUTANEOUS METASTATIC TUMORS

1. Approximately 9% of all patients who die from internal malignancy will demonstrate metastatic tumors in the skin.
2. Cutaneous metastasis may be the initial presentation of an internal malignancy.
3. Sister Mary Joseph nodule is a nodular metastatic tumor near the umbilicus.
4. Cutaneous metastasis is usually a poor prognostic indicator.

15. What is the prognosis of a patient with a cutaneous metastasis?
Cutaneous metastasis is usually indicative of a poorer prognosis. It often reflects preexisting widespread internal disease. In one study, the average life expectancy after development of skin metastases was only 3 months, but clearly, the prognosis is dependent upon the primary tumor type and therapeutic options available for a specific disease. Some patients survive for years, and extremely rarely, a patient might (at least in theory) be cured, although this remains unlikely.

SUNSCREENS AND PREVENTION OF SKIN CANCER

Whitney A. High

CHAPTER 48

1. List some important facts about skin cancer.
   - About 90% of nonmelanoma skin cancers are related to ultraviolet (UV) radiation from the sun.
   - More than 5.4 million cases of nonmelanoma skin cancer were treated in over 3.3 million people in the United States during 2012, the most recent year for which data is available.
   - Basal cell carcinoma, a form of nonmelanoma skin cancer, if the commonest cancer of mankind.
   - One in five Americans will develop skin cancer by age 70.
   - Melanoma makes up less than 2% of all skin cancers, but it causes most skin cancer deaths.
   - On average, a person's risk for melanoma doubles if he or she has had more than five sunburns and just one blistering sunburn in childhood or adolescence more than doubles a person's chances of developing melanoma later in life.
   - New melanoma cases diagnosed in 2019 will increase by 7.7%, but the number of melanoma deaths is expected to decrease by 22% in 2019.

Skin Cancer Foundation. Available at: http://www.skincancer.org. Accessed October 11, 2019.

2. How does skin type affect the risk for skin cancer?
   Anyone can get skin cancer, but certain people are at higher risk. The Fitzpatrick Phototyping Scale is used to identify people prone to developing skin cancer. This is a six-tiered scale based on skin color and ability to tan (Table 48.1). Individuals in groups I and II are at highest risk for developing basal and squamous cell carcinomas, and melanoma. Skin types III and IV are less prone to develop basal and squamous cell carcinomas but are still at risk for developing melanoma. Basal cell carcinoma, squamous cell carcinoma, and melanoma are rare in skin types V and VI. If patients in groups V and VI develop melanoma, it usually occurs on acral skin (acrolentiginous melanoma) or on mucosal surfaces, such as in the mouth or genitalia.

3. What are the other risk factors for skin cancer?
   Skin cancer risk factors include family history, cumulative sun exposure, history of blistering sunburns, multiple atypical moles, immunosuppression, and occupational exposures (coal tar, pitch, creosote, arsenic compounds, or radium). Lifetime cumulative sun exposure directly correlates with basal and squamous cell carcinomas risk. Sunburns, particularly in youth, and the number of nevi (moles) and atypical nevi (unusual appearing moles) are related to melanoma risk. One study reported a 2.5- to 6.3-fold increased melanoma risk for a person with a history of three or more blistering sunburns in youth.

4. What body sites are at highest risk for skin cancer?
   - Melanoma occurs most frequently on the chest, shoulders, and back in men and in young women (ages 15 to 29). Melanoma is most often found on the legs of women 30 years of age and older.
   - For both sexes, basal and squamous cell carcinomas develop most often on chronically sun-exposed areas, including the head, neck, shoulders, arms, and hands.

5. What should health care providers teach patients about skin cancer?
   Providers should emphasize two things: 1) prevention and 2) early detection. The most important strategy for preventing skin cancers, including melanoma, is reducing unnecessary exposure to UV light. Unfortunately, some skin cancer risk factors, such as skin color type, are not modifiable. Nearly all skin cancers, even melanoma, are curable when detected early. Early detection of skin cancers is possible through monthly skin self-examination. Patients should be encouraged to examine their entire skin surface on a monthly basis, including the scalp and non–sun-exposed sites, like the buttocks, genitalia, and feet. New or changing lesions should be evaluated by a professional provider.

6. What are warning signs of possible skin cancer?
   - An open sore that does not heal in 3 weeks
   - A spot or sore that persistently itches, burns, stings, crusts, scabs, or bleeds
   - Any "mole" or pigmented lesion that changes in color, size, thickness, texture or develops irregular borders
   - Any skin lesion that appears different or "stands out" from the other lesions on a patient (the so-called "ugly duckling" sign)

Table 48.1 Fitzpatrick Phototyping Scale

SKIN PHOTOTYPE*	UNEXPOSED SKIN COLOR	SUN RESPONSE HISTORY
I	White	Always burns, never tans
II	White	Always burns, tans minimally
III	White	Burns minimally, tans gradually and uniformly
IV	Light brown	Burns minimally, always tans well
V	Brown	Rarely burns, tans darkly
VI	Dark brown	Never burns, tans darkly

*Based on the first 30 to 60 minutes of sun exposure of untanned skin after the winter season.

7. How is UV light classified?

UV light (UV radiation [UVR]) is classified based on wavelength, according to its physical characteristics and biologic effects:
- **UVC: 100- to 280-nm wavelength.** UVC radiation is filtered by atmospheric ozone and does not reach the earth's surface.
- **UVB: 280- to 315-nm wavelength.** Midrange radiation that is incompletely filtered by atmospheric ozone
- **UVA: 315- to 400-nm wavelength.** Longer-wave UVR that is further subdivided into UVA-1 (340 to 400 nm) and UVA-2 (315 to 340 nm). UVA is not filtered by atmospheric ozone, and 150-fold greater amount of UVA reaches the earth's surface, compared to UVB.

8. How do UVA and UVB affect the skin?

UVB penetrates to the basal layer of epidermis and injures skin cells through the formation of DNA thymine dimers and 6-4 photoproducts. If not repaired, these can genetic mutations and lead to altered cell function and skin cancer. UVB is also responsible for causing sunburn.

UVA, being a longer wavelength, penetrates deeper into the skin. UVA damages skin cells predominantly through formation of free radicals. Chronic exposure results in photoaging, such as skin wrinkling, solar lentigines, poikiloderma, telangiectasia, and altered collagen and elastin.

Both UVA and UVB are carcinogenic. Mnemonic: UVB causes sunburn (UV**B** = **B**urn), UVA causes aging (UV**A** = **A**ging).

9. What geographic and environmental factors affect UVR exposure?

At higher altitudes, there is less atmosphere to absorb UVR, and the risk of sunburn is greater. UVR is also stronger near the equator, where the sun's energy strikes the earth most directly. UVR is less intense on overcast days, but it is still present and adds to cumulative skin damage. UVR is reflected off sand, concrete, and snow and this adds to the total UVR exposure. Because UVR is reflected and scattered, shade is not totally protective. Standard window glass blocks UVB, but not UVA.

10. How much does the intensity of UVR exposure increase for every additional 1000 feet of elevation?

The UVR intensity increases about 4% for every 1000 feet of elevation about sea level. This is important to remember on the ski slopes!

11. List the strategies for minimizing UVR exposure.
- Reduce time in the sun. Sun damage is cumulative. Each dose of UVR, large and small, adds up, leading to skin wrinkling, dyspigmentation, and skin cancer.
- Avoid sun exposure between 10 AM and 2 PM (11 AM to 3 PM daylight savings time), when UVR is more intense. Plan outdoor activities for early morning or late afternoon.
- Seek shade and use sun protective clothing. Apply sunscreen to exposed skin.
- Do not use tanning beds. While tanning beds emit primarily UVA, overexposure can still cause skin damage (Fig. 48.1). Tanning beds increase skin aging and cancer risk. There is no such thing as a "healthy tan." Skin tanning is a response to UVR-induced skin injury.

12. What type of clothing and accessories are sun-protective?

Sun-protective clothing and accessories include a hat, UV-blocking sunglasses, a long-sleeved shirt, and long pants. Be sure to choose the correct type of clothing for sun protection. Tightly woven, thick fabrics, with darker color provide for greater protection from UVR. UV-protective fabrics are designated by a UV protection factor that is marketed in specialty clothing.

Milch JM, Logemann NF. Photoprotection prevents skin cancer: let's make it fashionable to wear sun-protective clothing. *Cutis.* 2017;99:89–92.

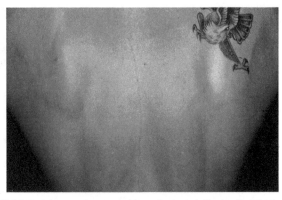

Fig. 48.1 Second-degree sunburn acquired from a tanning bed. (Courtesy David Bertler, MD.)

13. What are sunscreens? What are the different types?
Sunscreens are topical agents that block UVR absorption by the skin. It is tradition to categorize sunscreens as "chemical absorbers" or "physical blockers," depending on the mechanism of action for the active ingredients. "Physical blockers" (like zinc oxide and titanium dioxide) scatter and reflect UVR, while "chemical absorbers" (like avobenzone and oxybenzone) protect against UVR through a photochemical reaction. Sunscreens are available as lotions, creams, pastes, sprays, roll-ons, and gels.

14. Compare the advantages and disadvantages of the physical and chemical sunscreens.
Physical blockers include zinc oxide and titanium dioxide. Advantages are that these agents are inert, do not break down over time, and do not cause contact dermatitis or photodermatitis. These agents block UVA and UVB. The disadvantage of physical blockers is that these agents leave an opaque appearance on the skin.
An advantage of chemical absorbers is that these agents have less opaque appearance on the skin. Newer agents also block both UVB and UVA. Chemical absorbers can cause contact dermatitis and photodermatitis, but the risk is low (0.1% to 2.0%). Another disadvantage of chemical absorbers is that they degrade with UV exposure, requiring reapplication every 2 hours.

15. What are the active ingredients of sunscreens?
See Table 48.2.

16. What factors should be considered in selecting a sunscreen?
    • Desirable sunscreens are broad-spectrum, water-resistant, and with a sun protection factor (SPF) of 30 or greater. "Broad-spectrum" includes protection from UVA and UVB. "Water-resistant" is specified as either 40 minutes or 80 minutes, but even water-resistant sunscreens should be reapplied after swimming or sweating.
    • Avoid sunscreens that contain fragrance, which can lead to contact dermatitis or photocontact dermatitis and can attract insects. Para-aminobenzoic acid (PABA) was an older agent that can cause contact dermatitis, but nowadays nearly all sunscreen products are PABA-free.

17. How is an SPF determined?
Sunscreen SPF is defined as the ratio of the minimal dose of UV light needed to cause redness of sunscreen-protected skin divided by the minimal dose of sunlight needed to cause redness of unprotected skin. SPFs of 15, 30, and 50 effectively reduce UV skin absorption by 94%, 97%, and 98%, respectively.

18. How much sunscreen should be applied? How often should it be reapplied?
Most people apply sunscreen at only ¼ to ½ the concentration at which the SPF is established, and this means that the SPF rating for that sunscreen is not being achieved. Adequately covering the face, arms, legs, and upper torso of an average-sized adult requires 1 ounce of sunscreen, which is enough to fill a shot glass (Fig. 48.2). A smaller person or child needs proportionally less. Sunscreen should be applied evenly to all exposed skin. It should be applied 30 minutes before sun exposure and then reapplied every 2 hours. Sunscreen should be reapplied more often if one is swimming or sweating. Warn patients that reapplication does not double the SPF and to not rely on "redness" as a signal to reapply, as a sunburn does not appear until hours after exposure. Skin damage occurs before a sunburn appears.

19. Can sunscreens be safely used in children?
Yes. Childhood sun exposure increases risk of skin cancer in adulthood, so sun protection in youth is important. Sunscreen is not recommended for infants under 6 months of age for two reasons: (1) infants have immature skin and an increased surface area-to-volume ratio, which increases absorption and the risk of toxicity, and (2) infant skin is

Table 48.2 Active Ingredients Used in Sunscreens

CHEMICAL ABSORBERS	MAXIMUM CONCENTRATION USED (%)	WAVELENGTH BLOCKED
Avobenzone (Parsol 1789)	3	UVA-1, UVA-2
Cinoxate	3	UVB
Dioxybenzone	3	UVA-2, UVB
Ecamsule (Mexoryl SX)	10	UVA-1, UVA-2
Ensulizole	4	UVB
Homosalate	15	UVB
Meradimate	5	UVA-2
Octocrylene	10	UVB
Octinoxate	7.5	UVB
Octisalate	5	UVB
Oxybenzone	6	UVA-2, UVB
Padimate O	8	UVB
Para-aminobenzoic acid (PABA)	15	UVB
Sulisobenzone	10	UVA-2, UVB
Trolamine salicylate	12	UVB
Physical blockers	Maximum concentration used (%)	Wavelength blocked
Titanium dioxide	25	UVA-1, UVA-2, UVB
Zinc oxide	25	UVA-1, UVA-2, UVB

UVA, Ultraviolet A; *UVB*, ultraviolet B.

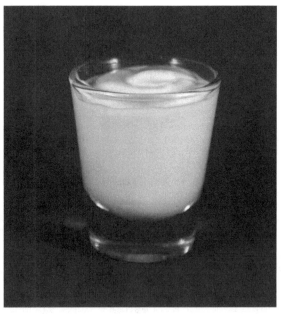

Fig. 48.2 Shot glass of sunscreen, the amount of sunscreen that it takes to cover the face, arms, legs, and torso of a normal-sized adult. (Courtesy James E. Fitzpatrick, MD.)

sensitive to UV damage and sunscreen is not adequate protection—UV light should be avoided entirely. Any child who cannot yet crawl should be protected with long sleeves, long pants, and a hat and should be kept away from direct sunlight. For children over 6 months of age, there are many sunscreen products specially formulated for children, and in general, these formulations focus on physical blockers.

20. **Why are sunglasses included in sun-protection recommendations?**
Sunglasses protect the eyelids, sclera, cornea, and lens from UVR injury. Acute UVR injury of the eye results in sunburn of the eyelids, sclera, and cornea. Chronic sun exposure causes cataracts, ocular melanoma, and skin cancer of periorbital skin. Patients should buy sunglasses that absorb 100% UVA and UVB. Also, a large frame better protects the skin around the eyes.

21. **Are "tan-in-a-bottle" ("sunless tanning") products safe to use?**
Sunless tanning lotions are skin dyes and are safe to use but do not protect the skin from UVR. Therefore, sun-protection measures must be followed by people using self-tanning products.

22. **What is the relationship between UVR, the skin, and vitamin D?**
Humans have three means to obtain vitamin D: 1) cutaneous production with UVB exposure, 2) dietary intake, and 3) vitamin D supplementation. Inactive vitamin D (7-dehydrocholesterol) is contained in epidermal keratinocytes and is converted in the presence of UVB radiation to previtamin D_3. Previtamin D_3 spontaneously isomerizes to vitamin D_3 (3-cholecalciferol). Vitamin D_3 is hydroxylated by the epidermis or liver to 25-hydroxyvitamin D_3, which is further hydroxylated in the kidney to the final active form, 1,25-hydroxyvitamin D_3 (calcitriol). Lesser UVB exposure (latitude, time of day, season, cloud cover, smog) or lesser cutaneous penetration of UVB (clothing, melanin, sunblock) will reduce vitamin D production, making the body more dependent on dietary intake and/or supplementation.

23. **How much sun exposure is necessary to maintain vitamin D levels?**
The amount of sun exposure needed to maintain appropriate vitamin D levels is highly variable and is based on latitude, season, and skin color. Darker skin types need longer exposure to make vitamin D. In the southern United States, short daily UVB exposure (5 minutes for lightly pigmented people and 10 minutes for darkly pigmented people) on a small skin area (face, hands, and arms) will supply ample vitamin D for the body's needs. However, during winter months in northern climes, insufficient UVB reaches the earth's surface to produce adequate vitamin D, even with prolonged exposure to sunlight.

Holick MF. Ultraviolet B radiation: the vitamin D connection. *Adv Exp Med Biol.* 2017;996:137–154.

24. **If sun exposure is restricted, how would one maintain normal vitamin D levels?**
Proper vitamin D levels can be easily maintained by eating a fortified diet. Eggs, beef liver, and oily fish (salmon, catfish, herring, mackerel, and tuna) are excellent sources of vitamin D. Many foodstuffs, such as milk, cereals, and bread, are fortified with vitamin D. Most multivitamins also contain vitamin D. Recommended daily intake from all sources for vitamin D are 400 IU for infants less than 1 year of age, 600 IU for adults less than 70 years of age, and 800 IU for adults greater than 70 years of age. With so many source of vitamin D in the diet, sunscreen use for daily and recreational photoprotection is unlikely to cause vitamin D deficiency.

Passeron T, Bouillon R, Callender V, et al. Sunscreen photoprotection and vitamin D status. *Br J Dermatol.* 2019;181:916–931.

25. **What is proper sunburn treatment?**
Take aspirin or ibuprofen as soon as sunburn is detected to help reduce inflammation and control pain. Cool, wet compresses or tub soaks for 20 minutes, four or five times daily, will help with pain control. Avoid heavy ointments and benzocaine sprays, which can cause skin irritation. Light creams and lotions containing pramoxine will soothe the skin and reduce pain. Because sun-damaged skin is more susceptible to subsequent burns, additional sun exposure should be avoided for the next 1 to 2 weeks.

KEY POINTS: SKIN CANCER RISK FACTORS

1. Skin types I and II
2. Family history of skin cancer
3. History of extensive cumulative sun exposure or blistering sunburns
4. Numerous or atypical moles
5. Immunosuppression

KEY POINTS: ADVERSE EFFECTS OF CHRONIC SUN EXPOSURE

1. Photoaging (wrinkles, dyspigmentation)
2. Precancers (actinic keratoses)
3. Impaired immune surveillance of precancer and skin cancer
4. Cataracts
5. Skin cancers (basal cell carcinoma, squamous cell carcinoma, melanoma)

KEY POINTS: HEALTH BENEFITS OF SOLAR RADIATION

1. Health benefits of solar radiation are few.
2. Skin exposure to ultraviolet B increases vitamin D synthesis.
3. Periodic exposure to the visible spectrum of solar radiation can enhance psychological well-being.
4. The ultraviolet spectrum of solar radiation can be used for the treatment of some skin disorders, such as psoriasis, vitiligo, eczema, and cutaneous T-cell lymphoma.

CHAPTER 49

TOPICAL STEROIDS

Whitney A. High

KEY POINTS: TOPICAL STEROIDS

1. Approximately 2% total body surface area (TBSA) requires one fingertip unit (FTU) or 0.5 g of topical steroid medication. One percent of the patient's TBSA can be estimated as one palmar surface, including the fingers. Approximately 15 g is required to apply a topical medication to all of the skin from the neck down, one time.
2. Provide written instructions *and* demonstration of proper FTU application technique to enhance compliance when using topical steroids. Indicate that *only* low-potency topical steroids should be on thin skin (i.e., face, neck, axilla, inframammary, infrapannus, and groin).
3. Tachyphylaxis can develop with prolonged use of topical steroids. To avoid this, recommend intermittent pulse dosing (i.e., 1 week of "rest" between weekly treatment periods).
4. Monitor the patient for topical corticosteroid side effects, especially potentially irreversible ones (e.g., atrophy, telangiectasia, striae). Steroid-induced skin damage may occur with potent topical steroids and just 1–2 weeks of twice-daily use upon thin skin. Discourage long-term use.
5. If the presumed inflammatory skin disease remains unresponsive, deteriorates, or the morphology changes after topical steroids use, reconsider the diagnosis. Consider also possible contact dermatitis to a component of the topical steroid, bacterial infection, the presence of dermatophytes or yeast, and noncompliance. Further studies such as skin biopsy, bacterial or viral culture, or KOH prep may be warranted.

1. List some common mistakes that are made when prescribing a topical steroid.
   - Incorrect diagnosis or failure to consider coexisting disease(s).
   - Recommending a topical steroid that is too potent or too weak for the skin condition and anatomic site.
   - Prescribing excessive or inadequate amounts of the topical agent.
   - Recommending the wrong vehicle (cream, ointment, solution, etc.).
   - Using the medication for too long or too short a period of time.
   - Use of occlusion.
   - Failure to recognize and monitor for topical steroid side effects.
   - Lack of timely follow-up to reassess the disease and treatment regimen.

2. When were corticosteroids discovered? When were they first used therapeutically?
   - **1935:** Discovery of compound E (cortisone) at by Edward Kendall and Philip Hench.
   - **1948:** First reported use of cortisone and adrenocorticotropic hormone (ACTH) in the treatment of rheumatoid arthritis.
   - **1951:** First report of cortisone and ACTH used in the treatment of inflammatory dermatoses.
   - **1952:** First report of using compound F (hydrocortisone) topically.

   Corticosteroids are synthetic analogs of hormones produced by the adrenal glands, such as cortisone. Since the mid-1950s, there have been numerous modifications of the corticosteroid molecule that have dramatically increased the potency of this topical therapy (i.e., halogenation, esterification, hydroxylation, modification of side chains, and improvements in delivery systems). As the potency of the molecule has increased, so has the likelihood of side effects.

3. Describe the basic steroid nucleus.
   See Fig. 49.1.

4. How is the potency of topical steroid medications determined?
   The human skin blanching assay (also called the vasoconstrictor assay) has been used for nearly 40 years to assess the potency of corticosteroids, particularly as it pertains to commercial formulations and clinical/regulatory purposes. For example, the test has established that identical concentrations of the same drug, but in different vehicles, yields different scores. Many believe the vasoconstrictor assay score correlates with clinical effectiveness, but in truth, it is difficult to compare studies because of a lack of standardization. Moreover, the therapeutic index of a medication does not always correlate with the vasoconstrictor assay or with the clinical outcome.

Hepburn DJ, Aeling JL, Weston WL. A reappraisal of topical steroid potency. *Pediatr Dermatol.* 1996;13(3):239–245.

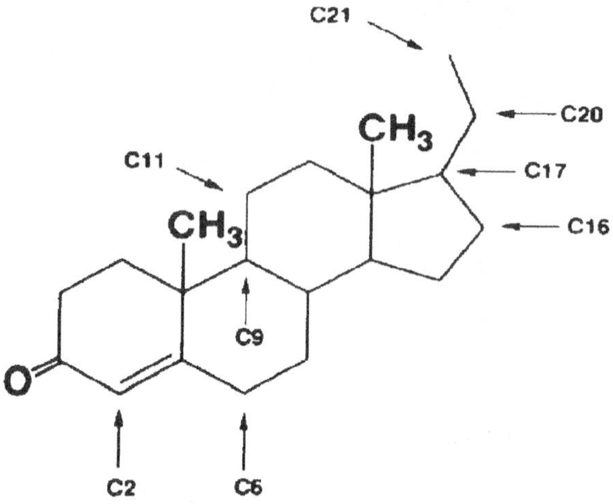

Fig. 49.1 Structure of steroid nucleus.

5. **How do topical steroids inhibit cutaneous inflammation and improve skin disease?**
Topical corticosteroids have multiple mechanism of action that may be further subdivided into antiinflammatory, antimitotic, and immunosuppressive pathways. The antiinflammatory effect of topical corticosteroids consists of vasoconstriction and inhibition of the release of phospholipase A2. Vasoconstriction of blood vessels decreases the delivery of inflammatory mediators to the area. Synthesis of lipocortin, in response to the presence of corticosteroids, inhibits phospholipase A2, thereby decreasing production of prostaglandins and leukotrienes. Corticosteroids decrease release of interleukin-1α, an important proinflammatory cytokine, from keratinocytes. Corticosteroids also translocate to the nucleus of cells, via carrier proteins, and this impacts upon the gene transcription. Transcription of antiinflammatory genes is promoted, and transcription of proinflammatory transcription factors, such as nuclear factor kappa-light-chain-enhancer of activated B cells (NFKB), is inhibited. Lipocortin also has an antimitotic effect on the epidermis. The immunosuppressive effects of topical corticosteroids involve the inhibition of humoral factors involved in the inflammatory response and suppression of the maturation, differentiation, proliferation, and migration of all cells of the immune system.

6. **How are topical corticosteroids classified as to potency?**
In the United States, it is common to classify topical corticosteroids into seven categories of potency: (I) superpotency, (II) high potency, (III) high midpotency, (IV) midpotency, (V) low midpotency, (VI) mildly potent, and (VII) low potency. The authors of this book prefer to rank them into four classes of potency, and this is similar to classification within the United Kingdom, where only "very potent," "potent," "moderate," and "mild" classes exist (Table 49.1).
    It is not necessary to memorize the dozens and dozens of steroid-containing products marketed in the United States; familiarity with one or two preparations in each class is often sufficient.

7. **With so many products available, how does one decide which product to prescribe for a patient?**
A multitude of factors must be considered when prescribing a steroid, including the severity and chronicity of disease being treated, the anatomic site involved, the percentage of body surface involved, the potency of the topical steroid, the vehicle, the frequency of application, potential side effects, and even cost. For example, the thickness of the skin, and hence absorption, may be many orders of magnitude different for the thick palmoplantar skin to the eyelid or genitalia. For this reason, in general, treatment of acral skin requires a potent or superpotent agent, while on the face, and particularly around the eyes, only mild steroids are typically employed. Importantly, if the product is unpleasing in consistency (vehicle), patients may refuse to comply with recommended instructions, thereby jeopardizing therapeutic outcome. See Question 9.

8. **What specific directions should be provided when prescribing super-, high-, and midpotency topical steroids?**
Misuse of strong topical steroids is a danger. Side effects should be well discussed, as should correct application methods. Failure to educate the patient can result in noncompliance or irrational steroid phobia. Timely follow-up should be utilized to judge response and side effects.

Table 49.1 Topical steroid potency*

Group I: Superpotency (Antiinflammatory Activity = 500)
- Clobetasol dipropionate 0.05% (Temovate)
- Betamethasone dipropionate 0.25% (Diprolene)
- Halobetasol propionate 0.05% (Ultravate)
- Diflorasone diacetate 0.05% (Psorcon)

Group II: High Potency (Antiinflammatory Activity = 100 to 500)
- Fluocinonide 0.05% (Lidex)
- Halcinonide 0.05% (Halog)
- Amcinonide 0.05% (Cyclocort)
- Desoximetasone 0.25% (Topicort)

Group III: Midpotency (Antiinflammatory Activity = 10 to 100)
- Fluocinolone acetonide 0.01% to 0.2% (Synalar, Synemol, Fluonid)
- Hydrocortisone valerate 0.2% (Westcort)
- Hydrocortisone butyrate 0.1% (Locoid)
- Triamcinolone acetonide 0.01% to 0.5% (Kenalog, Aristocort)
- Betamethasone valerate 0.1% (Valisone)
- Clocortolone pivalate 0.1% (Cloderm)
- Flurandrenolide 0.05% (Cordran)
- Betamethasone benzoate 0.028% (Benisone, Uticort)
- Mometasone furoate 0.1% (Elocon)
- Diflorasone diacetate 0.05% (Florone, Maxiflor)
- Fluticasone propionate 0.005% (Cutivate)
- Betamethasone dipropionate 0.005% (Maxivate)

Group IV: Low Potency (Antiinflammatory Activity = 1 to 10)
- Hydrocortisone acetate 0.25% to 2.5% (1% is OTC; 0.1% is prescription)
- Desonide 0.05% (DesOwen, Tridesilon)
- Alclometasone 0.05% (Aclovate)
- Prednisolone 0.5% (Meti-Derm)
- Dexamethasone 0.1% (Decadron)
- Methylprednisolone 1% (Medrol)

*The individual steroid molecules can be moved up or down in the potency ranking by changing the vehicle of the topical formulation.
OTC, Over-the-counter.

Directions should specify that the potent topical steroid should *not* be used in areas of thin skin (e.g., face, neck) or in intertriginous locations where skin touches skin (e.g., axilla, inframammary/inguinal folds). Areas with a thinner epidermis lead to greater absorption. Apposition of skin surfaces, or an occlusive dressing also enhances penetration, as well.

Bewley A, Berth-Jones J, Bingham A, et al. Expert consensus: time for a change in the way we advise our patients to use topical corticosteroids. *Br J Dermatol*. 2008;158:917–920.

9. Why is the vehicle important when recommending a topical corticosteroid?
   The vehicle may impact potency, bioavailability, lipid solubility, and the partition coefficient of a product. The vehicle should also be selected based upon the indication, disease severity, the body region treated, and patient preference. Ointments, being occlusive, are often the most potent vehicle, with the greatest penetration. Ointments also contain no preservatives (if there is concern for allergy). This potency pyramid is followed by creams, lotions, solutions, gels, sprays, and shampoos. Interestingly, some of the modern foams are difficult to place upon this schema but can be excellent delivery vehicles. The addition of water to a formulation (present in about anything but an ointment) requires addition of preservatives that may confound an allergic reaction. Compounding, dilution, or addition of ingredients to a proprietary product is often discouraged, as this can affect the uniformity and stability of the active ingredient.

10. Are certain vehicles preferred for certain dermatologic conditions or anatomic sites?
    Ointments work best on chronic, thickened skin lesions. Solutions, gels, sprays, foams, or shampoos are recommended for dermatoses involving hair-covered areas. Creams or lotions are best for intertriginous locations. Gels and sprays can also be used to treat inflammatory lesions on mucosal surfaces.

11. A patient has 8% total body surface area (TBSA) involvement. How much topical steroid should be prescribed for twice-daily application for a 1-week-on and 1-week-off treatment cycle? The patient will return in 4 weeks for follow-up.

    Topical medications are frequently underprescribed or overprescribed, and only a thin layer of medication is necessary. Use the fingertip unit (FTU) application technique and percent of TBSA to calculate the amount needed:
    - 1 FTU equals approximately 0.5 g of medication and will treat 2% TBSA in the average adult.
    - Calculation: (8% TBSA/1 application) × (1 FTU/2% TBSA) × (0.5 g/1 FTU) × 14 days × (2 applications/1 day) = 56 g.
    - Assuming common trade sizes, one 60-g tube should suffice.

        *NOTE: One FTU is the amount of medication expressed from a tube with a 5-mm opening that extends from the distal interphalangeal crease to the tip of the finger (*Fig. 49.2*). One palm size, including fingers, represents 1% TBSA.*

12. How should the FTU application technique be applied to children?

    In children, use the adult FTU method to calculate the amount needed, but then the quantity should be reduced to approximately 25% for less than a 1-year-old child, to 40% for a 1–2-year-old child, to 50% for a 3–5-year-old child, and to 60% for a 6–10-year-old child. However, these are just approximations, and the advice of a pediatric dermatologist should always be heeded.

13. When is combination topical steroid and anti-infective products indicated?

    Combination products are often expensive, and any added benefit may not justify the price. Two often prescribed combination agents are nystatin/triamcinolone (Mycolog II) and clotrimazole/betamethasone (Lotrizone). Clotrimazole and betamethasone in combination is approved by the U.S. Food and Drug Administration for tinea cruris/corporis/pedis in adults and children >12 years of age. However, in younger children and in babies (particularly under the occlusion of a diaper), betamethasone, being fluorinated and potent, can lead to skin atrophy and striae formation. Use of these products is also associated with higher rates of treatment failure and/or recurrence.

Wheat CM, Bickley RJ, Hsueh YH, Cohen BA. Current trends in the use of two combination antifungal/corticosteroid creams. *J Pediatr.* 2017;186:192–195.

14. What is tachyphylaxis and how can it be prevented?

    Resistance to treatment (tachyphylaxis) is a problem with prolonged use of topical steroids, although its clinical prevalence may be debated. Use of topical steroid "holidays," such as intermittent pulse dosing (1 week "on" and 1 week of "rest"), or alternating therapy with nonsteroid treatments (see Questions 28 to 31) should be considered in the setting of chronic skin disease, as this may minimize the onset of topical steroid tachyphylaxis.

Taheri A, Cantrell J, Feldman SR. Tachyphylaxis to topical glucocorticoids; what is the evidence? *Dermatol Online J.* 2013;19:18954.

15. Are topical steroids safe in pregnancy?

    Topical steroids are "Category C" drugs during pregnancy. This means that animal studies show an adverse effect on a fetus, but there are no adequate studies in humans. The potential benefits of a drug may warrant use despite potential risk. A recent systematic review found no association between maternal use of topical corticosteroids of any potency

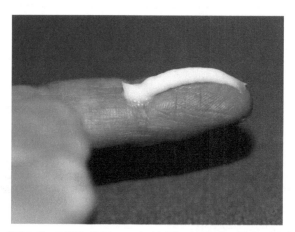

Fig. 49.2 Demonstration of a fingertip unit (FTU), which is approximately 0.5 g of medication. (Courtesy John L. Aeling, MD, Collection.)

and adverse pregnancy outcomes such as mode of delivery, congenital abnormality, preterm delivery, fetal death, and low Apgar score. A probable association between low birth weight and maternal use of potent or very potent topical corticosteroids was identified, particularly when the cumulative dose during pregnancy was large. When prescribing topical steroids to pregnant patients, it is reasonable to limit the body surface area treated, the potency of the steroid applied, and the duration of use.

Chi CC, Wang SH, Wojnarowska F, Kirtschig G, Davies E, Bennett C. Safety of topical corticosteroids in pregnancy. *Cochrane Database Syst Rev.* 2015;26:CD007346.

16. Are topical steroids safe during breast feeding?

    Topical corticosteroids are considered to pose a negligible risk to a breastfeeding infant if precautions are taken to avoid direct contact of the breastfeeding infant with treated areas. Hence, topical steroids should not be applied to the breast or nipple prior to breast feeding.

17. What cutaneous side effects on the epidermis are observed with use of topical steroids?

    Cutaneous side effects are observed with use of topical steroids, and these effects may occur quickly with use of potent topical steroids, especially on thinner skin and intertriginous areas (Table 49.2). For superpotent steroids, thinning of the epidermis can occur with just 7 days of use. After 3 weeks of potent topical steroid use, all layers of the epidermis are reduced in thickness by about one-half. Thinning of the epidermis, particularly the stratum corneum, impairs the barrier function of the epidermis, increasing transepidermal water loss. Thinning of the epidermis can allow telangiectasias (dilated blood vessels) to show through the skin. Pigment production at the dermoepidermal junction may be impaired with use of potent topical steroids, particularly in darker skin types.

18. What cutaneous side effects on the dermis are observed with topical steroids?

    Within 1 to 3 weeks of using superpotent topical steroids, the dermal volume is significantly reduced, chiefly due to decreased fibroblast production of dermal ground substance (hyaluronic acid) and decreased dermal water content. Reduced synthesis of collagen and elastin results in dermal atrophy (Fig. 49.3), skin fragility, striae (Fig. 49.4), telangiectasias, poor vascular support with skin purpura, and decreased wound healing.

19. What are the systemic side effects of topical steroid therapy?

    Superpotent topical steroids are over a thousand times more potent than hydrocortisone. Infants and children may be at greater risk for systemic side effects because of increased surface-to-body ratios compared to adults. Moreover, there may be differences in steroid metabolism, as well.

    Adults can show hypothalamic-pituitary-adrenal (HPA) axis suppression in 3 to 4 days with as little as 7.5 g of superpotent topical steroid daily, but studies show that there is eventual return to baseline adrenal function, despite continued use of topical steroids. It is unusual to see features of hypercortisolism (Cushing syndrome) in an adult patient due to use of topical steroids. Superpotent topical steroids are not recommended for children under age 12 (see Table 49.2).

Levin E, Gupta R, Butler D, Chiang C, Koo JY. Differentiating between physiologic and pathologic adrenal suppression. *J Dermatolog Treat.* 2014;25(6):501–506.

Table 49.2 Topical steroid side effects

LOCAL CUTANEOUS SIDE EFFECTS	SYSTEMIC SIDE EFFECTS
Acne vulgaris, acne rosacea, periorificial dermatitis	Cushing's syndrome
Atypical presentation of skin diseases (i.e., tinea incognito)	Fluid retention
Burning, stinging, erythema, peeling	Growth retardation, failure to thrive
Contact dermatitis	Hypothalamic-pituitary-adrenal (HPA) axis suppression
Delayed wound healing	Hypertension
Dermal atrophy with skin "dents/potholes"	Increased blood sugar
Epidermal atrophy with telangiectasia and purpura	Ocular hypertension, glaucoma, cataracts
Exacerbation of psoriasis with rebound phenomenon	
Exacerbation of skin infections and infestations	
Folliculitis	
Granuloma gluteale	
Hirsutism	
Hypopigmentation	
Skin blanching	
Steroid addiction syndrome	
Striae	
Susceptibility to skin infections	

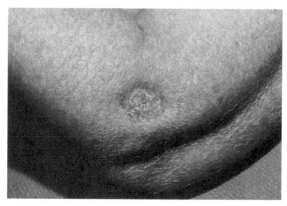

Fig. 49.3 Cutaneous atrophy and slight hypopigmentation from intralesional corticosteroids. (Courtesy Fitzsimons Army Medical Center teaching files.)

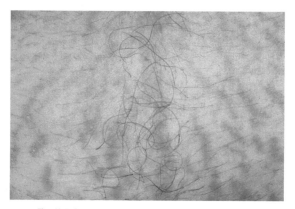

Fig. 49.4 Striae associated with midpotency topical steroid use.

20. Are there topical steroid "addicts?"

Topical steroid "addiction" occurs most often on the face or anogenital skin. Such patients often present with a mild dermatitis that initially responds well to topical steroids. However, once the use of the topical steroid is discontinued, symptoms quickly return and are worse. Thus, the patient is reluctant to discontinue the steroid use despite perpetuation of the syndrome. Patients next complain of burning and stinging of the skin, due to thinning of the stratum corneum and epidermis. Treatment includes discontinuing the topical steroid medication, but the patient should be warned that symptoms will flare and it may take weeks or months to completely clear.

Ghosh A, Sengupta S, Coondoo A, Jana AK. Topical corticosteroid addiction and phobia. *Indian J Dermatol.* 2014;59:465–468.

21. What is perioral (periorificial) dermatitis?

Perioral (periorificial) dermatitis can be caused by inappropriate use of potent topical steroids on the face (Fig. 49.5). It occurs most often in white women with a personal or family history of rosacea. The condition is characterized by inflammatory monomorphic papules and pustules, with erythema and scaling. The condition is located on the perioral skin, and sometimes the perinasal or periocular skin (periorificial). Perinasal disease can be caused by budesonide or other intranasal steroids prescribed for rhinitis/asthma. Most patients respond to discontinuation of potent topical steroids, possibly in combination with a tetracycline-class oral antibiotic for 4 to 6 weeks. Some patients flare when the potent steroid is discontinued, and lower-potency steroids (hydrocortisone 1%), topical antibiotics, and topical nonsteroidal immune response modifiers (pimecrolimus or tracrolimus) may be used as a "bridge" upon discontinuance of potent topical steroids. Patients interested in "zero therapy" (complete discontinuance, without use of any other medications) should be told the condition will flare before improving. The condition may recur.

Peralta L, Morais P. Perioral dermatitis—the role of nasal steroids. *Cutan Ocul Toxicol.* 2012;31:160–163.

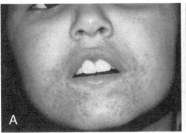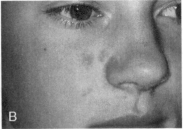

Fig. 49.5 Perioral dermatitis (steroid rosacea). **A,** A prepubertal child with typical perioral dermatitis. **B,** A prepubertal child with perioral dermatitis and steroid vasoconstriction related to a midpotency topical steroid. (Courtesy William L. Weston, MD.)

22. **What is tinea incognito?**

    Topical steroids decrease the inflammatory response, and while they may initially alleviate the symptoms of a dermatophyte infection, by decreasing the body's defense mechanisms, the organism can invade deeper into the follicular structures. This creates an infection that can be difficult to recognize as a superficial fungal infection, hence the term, tinea incognito (Fig. 49.6).

Verma S. Steroid modified tinea. *BMJ.* 2017; 356:j973.

---

23. **Can topical steroid medications cause contact dermatitis?**

    Topical steroids can create an irritant or allergic dermatitis. Irritant reactions are frequent and most often due to propylene glycol, an ingredient in some topical preparations. True allergic contact dermatitis should be suspected when a patient does not respond predictably to appropriate topical steroid management. This phenomenon can be due to the vehicle, preservative, fragrance, or the steroid molecule itself, and there is often cross-reactivity. This is one reason that ointments may be utilized when allergy is suspected, for such preparations commonly contain only the active ingredient and petrolatum, without preservatives. Contact allergies are most common with hydrocortisone, budesonide, and tixocortol and are least common with betamethasone, clobetasol, mometasone, and triamcinolone. Patch testing may be needed to identify the allergen.

24. **Mrs. Jones brings her 9-month-old infant with moderate atopic dermatitis to your office. What topical steroid do you prescribe?**

    Low- to mid-potency steroids should be used in children under age 1. Once-daily application is sufficient, after bathing, with medication use limited to areas of active inflammation. The treatment regimen should include generous skin lubrication, to lessen transepidermal water loss.

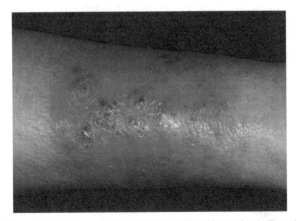

Fig. 49.6 Tinea incognito. Dermatophyte infection with follicular involvement (Majocchi's granuloma) with an atypical presentation being treated with topical corticosteroids. (Courtesy Joanna Burch Collection.)

25. A 40-year-old woman presents with a 5-year history of chronic dermatitis on her palms. Lesions are plaques with abundant scale. What topical steroid do you prescribe?

Super-potent topical steroids should be considered, both because of the severity of the disease and the thicker skin of palmoplantar surfaces, with resultant reduced absorption compared to other anatomic sites. The patient should be transitioned to a topical steroid of lesser potency as the disease improves and the plaques become thinner. Proper lubrication and hand protection from irritants are also important for therapeutic success. Hand moisturizers with 1% dimethicone may serve an important "barrier function" in presenting other noxious agents from irritating the skin. If the patient requires prolonged treatment with high- or superpotency topical steroids, then other regimens, such as phototherapy, should be considered.

26. A 35-year-old woman with moderate psoriasis presents with plaquest upon the scalp, facial, and body. What topical steroid do you prescribe?

In such a situation, more than one topical steroid may need to be prescribed. For the scalp, a high-potency topical steroid lotion or solution would be useful. For the face, a low-potency cream is most appropriate. For the body, a high- or even super-potency ointment would be of utility, with instruction to avoid the intertriginous areas. As her psoriasis improves, the agents of lesser potency may be utilized. Topical steroid "holidays" or alternate treatments (i.e., anthralin, tar, vitamin D analog, phototherapy, methotrexate, biologics) should be considered for difficult chronic cases. For example, for psoriasis, it is not uncommon to use topical calcipotriol on "weekdays" and potent or super-potent topical steroids on "weekends," to avoid constant steroid use and tachyphylaxis or cutaneous steroid side effects.

27. A parent brings a 6-month-old infant with a 2-week history of diaper dermatitis to your office. What topical steroid do you prescribe? Would you recommend other topical therapy?

For the diaper area, a low-potency topical steroid, applied once to twice daily, for only 7 to 10 days. The diaper area is occluded, and this increases the risk of local and systemic side effects (see Table 49.2). Candida infection should be considered for any diaper dermatitis lasting more than three days. Granuloma gluteale is a condition characterized by persistent reddish-purple nodules and plaques in the diaper area. The precise etiology of granuloma gluteale is debated, but most experts feel that topical steroids, candidiasis, and even cloth diapers are involved.

Ramos Pinheiro R, Matos-Pires E, Baptista J, Lencastre A. Granuloma gluteale infantum: a re-emerging complication of diaper dermatitis. *Pediatrics*. 2018;141:e20162064.

28. What are some alternatives to topical steroids?

Calcipotriol/calcipotriene(a form of vitamin D_3), pimecrolimus or tacrolimus (calcineurin inhibitors), and crisaborole (a boron-containing phosphodiesterase-4 inhibitor) represent nonsteroidal topical medications used in inflammatory skin diseases, such as psoriasis and atopic dermatitis. None of these medications have the risk of skin atrophy that occurs with topical steroid use. Studies in atopic dermatitis have shown such agents may be useful in maintenance strategies, even after control has been achieved with topical steroids.

Papier A, Strowd LC. Atopic dermatitis: a review of topical nonsteroid therapy. *Drugs Context*. 2018;3;7.

29. What are the important warnings regarding the topical calcineurin inhibitors?

The topical calcineurin inhibitors, tacrolimus and pimecrolimus, have a black box warning regarding malignancy (skin cancer and lymphoma). This warning is based upon an increased risk of malignancies in renal transplant patients treated with systemic tacrolimus, and mice receiving 47-fold the recommended human dose of topical tacrolimus. Although a recent cohort-based study showed the risk for lymphoma and skin malignancy with topical use appears small, and may even be confounded or subject to causation bias, it is important to counsel patients and parents about this warning. These medications are also not approved for use in children less than 2 years of age, because of concern for systemic absorption in young children with immature immune systems.

Castellsague J, Kuiper JG, Pottegård A, et al. A cohort study on the risk of lymphoma and skin cancer in users of topical tacrolimus, pimecrolimus, and corticosteroids (Joint European Longitudinal Lymphoma and Skin Cancer Evaluation—JOELLE study). *Clin Epidemiol*. 2018; 10:299–310.

30. When prescribing topical calcineurin inhibitors, what are important side effects of use to discuss with the patient?

Topical application of tacrolimus or pimecrolimus may cause a burning sensation (observed in about 50% of patients during clinical trials). Placing the tube of medication in the refrigerator for 15 to 20 minutes prior to skin application (but not storing it in the refrigerator) may diminish this side effect.

31. What is wet wrap therapy and when is it useful?

    Wet wrap therapy is the application of a low- to mid-potency topical steroid to affected areas, which are then wrapped with damp gauze, tubular bandages, or cotton under garments with dry garments placed on top. To avoid chilling the patient (often a child), the damp wraps can be prewarmed in a clothes dryer. Wet wraps are useful for flares of atopic dermatitis and may yield improved control in just a few days. Wet wraps are typically applied once or twice daily, for 5 days to 2 weeks. When using wet wraps, it is important to use only low- to mid-potency topical steroids, as the occlusion of the wrapping increases the potency of the topical steroid.

Copper CA, DeKlotz CMC. Warming up to the idea of wet wraps. *Pediatr Dermatol.* 2017;34:737–738.

CHAPTER 50

FUNDAMENTALS OF CUTANEOUS SURGERY

Misha D. Miller

1. How does one define dermatologic surgery?

   Dermatologic surgery describes procedures involving the skin and/or its appendages. Although many specialties may perform dermatologic surgery, dermatologists receive specific training in treating the skin both medically and surgically. Some dermatologists undergo additional fellowship training in micrographic surgery and dermatologic oncology (MSDO). In this fellowship, a dermatologist focuses on skin tumor extirpation using the Mohs micrographic surgery technique (see Mohs Surgery chapter). Additionally, during the MSDO fellowship, the dermatologist is taught the principals of surgical defect reconstruction (with an emphasis on facial reconstruction) including simple side-to-side closure, flaps, and grafts. Dermatologic surgery also includes cryosurgery, laser treatment of vascular lesions, pigmented skin lesions, and laser skin resurfacing for photodamaged skin. Dermabrasion, chemical peels, sclerotherapy, hair transplantation, liposuction, and soft tissue augmentation are described as types of dermatologic surgery as well.

2. Local anesthetics are divided into two groups. Name these two groups and list their defining characteristics.

   The ester group of local anesthetics is metabolized by plasma pseudocholinesterase and then the kidneys. Some patients have an increased risk of toxicity to ester anesthetics because of inherently atypical forms of plasma pseudocholinesterase. Some examples of ester anesthetics are procaine, chloroprocaine, and tetracaine. The amide group of local anesthetics is metabolized by the hepatic P450 system. Caution must be used when administering an amide anesthetic in a patient with liver failure. Some examples of amide anesthetics include lidocaine, mepivacaine, bupivacaine, and prilocaine.

3. How do local anesthetics work?

   Local anesthetics decrease the sodium permeability of the nerve fiber membrane, thereby lowering the action potential of the nerve fiber and preventing depolarization of the fiber.

4. What should you do if a patient reports a lidocaine allergy?

   Reactions to lidocaine are usually due to an allergy to the methylparaben preservatives found in lidocaine solution. Cutaneous patch testing may be employed to elucidate a true lidocaine allergy versus an allergy to methylparabens. One can also use an ester anesthetic. One percent diphenhydramine or 0.9% normal saline injected in the skin in a very superficial fashion can be used to achieve cutaneous anesthesia.

5. Why is it beneficial to mix lidocaine with epinephrine?

   Epinephrine is a vasoconstrictor and therefore helps to slow systemic absorption of lidocaine. The duration of lidocaine activity is prolonged. Also, epinephrine decreases bleeding at the surgical site, thus aiding in hemostasis and decreasing surgical morbidity.

6. What are the maximum doses of lidocaine?

   5 mg/kg if without epinephrine, 7 mg/kg if mixed with epinephrine.

7. What are the symptoms and signs of lidocaine toxicity and how is it treated?

   See Table 50.1.

8. Can lidocaine and epinephrine be used safely in pregnant patients?

   Lidocaine is defined as a pregnancy category B drug. Studies in pregnant rats and rabbits utilized lidocaine doses up to six times the maximum human doses and there were minimal to no harmful fetal effects. There are no studies in humans. Epinephrine is a pregnancy category C drug. Animal studies have revealed teratogenic effects when epinephrine was administered at 25 times the maximum human dose. No studies in humans have been done. The optimal time to use lidocaine/epinephrine for cutaneous surgery in pregnancy is during the second trimester and in the postpartum period.

Li JN, Nijhawan RI, Srivastava D. Cutaneous surgery in patients who are pregnant or breastfeeding. *Dermatol Clin.* 2019;37(3):307–317.

Table 50.1 Lidocaine toxicity

LIDOCAINE SERUM LEVEL	>5 MCG/ML	5–9 MCG/ML	10 MCG/ML
Symptoms	Circumoral numbness, metallic taste, dipoplia, light headed	Nystagmus, emesis, slurred speech, tremors, seizures	Nystagmus, emesis, slurred speech, tremors, seizures
Intervention	Hold lidocaine	Diazepam, maintain airway	Tx: ACLS

ACLS, Advanced cardiovascular life support

9. What are other circumstances that dictate caution with epinephrine use?
One should use caution when using epinephrine in a patient with uncontrolled hypertension, ischemic heart disease, or a pheochromocytoma. It was once thought that epinephrine should not be used on the digits, the tip of the nose, or the penis for fear of necrosis. Studies have not supported avoiding epinephrine use when operating on these specialty sites.

Chowdhry S, Seidenstricker L, Cooney DS, Hazani R, Wilhelmi BJ. Do not use epinephrine in digital blocks: myth or truth? Part II. A retrospective review of 1111 cases. *Plast Reconstr Surg.* 2010;126(6):2031–2034.

10. Name three common antiseptic solutions used in dermatologic surgery? What are the pros and cons of each skin preparation?
See Table 50.2.

11. What is the difference between a punch biopsy and a shave biopsy?
A biopsy is a sampling of a skin lesion to submit for histopathologic examination to render a diagnosis. A punch biopsy provides a deep sample of tissue, which many times includes epidermis, dermis, and subcutaneous fat. A punch biopsy is useful when the pathologic process is suspected to exist in the dermis or subcutaneous tissues (e.g., alopecia, panniculitis). A shave biopsy is a thin sampling that captures mostly epidermis and some dermis. This technique is best used to sample a sessile lesion or when the pathologic process to be captured is superficial in the skin (Fig. 50.1).

12. What is sampling error?
Sampling error occurs when an area of a lesion or inflammatory process is biopsied that is not representative of the pathologic process. Thus, an incorrect diagnosis is assigned to the specimen. Sampling error is difficult to avoid when a small portion of a large lesion is sampled.

13. What is electrosurgery?
Electrosurgery is the use of an electric current in order to achieve hemostasis, tissue cutting, or the destruction of benign and malignant skin lesions.

14. What is the difference among electrocautery, electrodesiccation, electrofulguration, and electrocoagulation?
- **Electrocautery** uses heat as a surgical tool. A metal tip or wire transfers heat from itself to another surface. This is the safest type of electrosurgery for patients with a pacemaker or a defibrillator.
- **Electrodesiccation** uses high-voltage, low-amperage electric current. Heat is generated when the current meets resistance in the tissue when contact occurs between the electrode tip and the tissue. The result is tissue dehydration. The heat "halo" is wider and deeper than that caused by electrofulguration.

Table 50.2 Skin antiseptics

	ISOPROPYL ALCOHOL	BETADINE	CHLORHEXIDINE
Pros	Fast onset	Broad coverage: microbicidal for gram-positive and gram-negative bacteria, fungi, viruses, protozoa, and yeasts	Broad coverage: microbicidal for gram-positive and gram-negative bacteria, facultative anaerobes, aerobes, and yeast, viruses, and *M. tuberculosis.*
Cons	No residual activity Skin Irritant	Minimal residual activity Must dry to be bactericidal Neutralized by blood	Avoid skin near eyes and tympanic membranes
Adverse effects	Flammable	Hypothyroidism in newborns	Can cause: keratitis, conjunctivitis, otitis

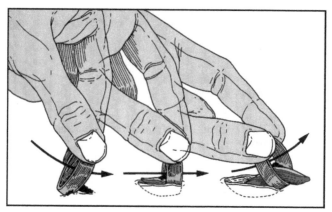

Fig. 50.1 Schematic demonstrating the technique for a shave biopsy of skin. (From Fewkes JL, Cheney ML, Pollack SV. *Illustrated atlas of cutaneous surgery*. New York: Gower Medical Publishing; 1992, with permission.)

- **Electrofulguration** uses a high-voltage, low-amperage electric current to generate a spark that jumps from the electrode tip to the tissue. The result is tissue dehydration and carbonization. There is no contact between the electrode and the tissue, resulting in a smaller heat "halo."
- **Electrocoagulation** uses a low-voltage, high-amperage current to coagulate blood vessels by generating heat in tissue. The patient forms part of the circuit by using a dispersive electrode, which allows for a greater degree of coagulation than either electrofulguration or electrodesiccation.

Meeuwsen FC, Guédon ACP, Arkenbout EA, van der Elst M, Dankelman J, van den Dobbelsteen JJ. The art of electrosurgery: trainees and experts. *Surg Innov.* 2017;24(4):373–378.

15. How does cryosurgery work?
    Cryosurgery is performed with liquid nitrogen (temperature = -195°C). When liquid nitrogen is applied to a cutaneous lesion, ice crystals form in extracellular space, then water leaves cell through osmosis and dehydrates the cell, resulting in cell death. Additionally, water inside the cell freezes and the cell bursts.

16. What is the most destructive way to treat a skin lesion with cryosurgery?
    Fast freeze, slow thaw = most destructive.
    Thaw time is usually twice as long as freeze time.

17. What is the expected natural history of a lesion treated with cryosurgery? What are adverse reactions associated with cryosurgery?
    Natural history: erythema, edema, bullae formation, eschar, then sloughing and resolution.
    Adverse results: severe pain, ulceration, infection, and hyper/hypopigmentation.

18. What are the skin tension lines (RSTLs)? Why are they important?
    The insertion of the underlying musculature into the skin results in a somewhat predictable pattern of skin creases, called RSTLs. Typically, these lines run perpendicular to the long axis of the underlying musculature (Fig. 50.2). Surgical incisions/excisions placed within or parallel to these lines will create the most favorable scar.

19. How do you design an fusiform excision?
    Draw an appropriate margin around the tumor that is to be extirpated. Then make two triangles off of opposite ends of the circle. Conventional teaching is that the length of the fusiform shape should be three to four times as long as the widest part of the defect and that the angle of the apices should be 30 degrees. The fusiform excision should be undermined an equal distance from all edges including the apices.

Zitelli JA. TIPS for a better ellipse. *J Am Acad Dermatol.* 1990;22(1):101–103.

20. Name four Characteristics of suture material that influence your choice of suture?
    - Absorbable vs. nonabsorbable
      - Absorbable suture: broken down by the body over time hydrolysis or enzymatic degradation.

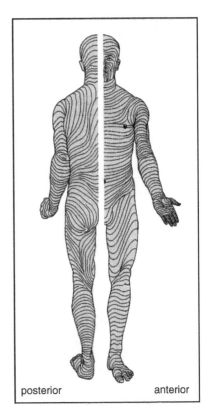

Fig. 50.2 Schematic demonstrating the most likely direction of relaxed skin tension lines. (From Fewkes JL, Cheney ML, Pollack SV. *Illustrated atlas of cutaneous surgery.* New York: Gower Medical Publishing; 1992, with permission.)

posterior   anterior

- Use in the dermis
  - Nonabsorbable suture:
    - Use for long-term tissue approximation
    - Use in the epidermis where it can be removed
- Coefficient of friction: how easily does the suture pass through tissue
  - Poliglecaprone 25, polypropylene (low)
  - Polyglactin 910 (high)
- Memory: ability of a suture material to return to previous shape after deformation
  - Monofilament/one strand: high memory
  - Multifilament/many strands, braided: low memory
- Tensile strength: a measure of the time it takes for suturing material to lose 70% to 80% of its initial strength (the maximum stress that a material can withstand while being stretched or pulled before breaking).
  - Chromic cat gut (low)
  - Polydiaxanone (high)

Dennis C, Sethu S, Nayak S, Mohan L, Morsi YY, Manivasagam G. Suture materials—current and emerging trends. *J Biomed Mater Res A.* 2016;104(6):1544–1559.

21. It is dogma to achieve wound eversion when repairing cutaneous wounds. Does wound eversion lead to a superior cosmetic result?
    This thought is being challenged. A split incision study showed that there was minimal difference in scar appearance (blinded observers and patients) when comparing everted and noneverted cutaneous repairs.

Kappel S, Kleinerman R, King TH, et al. Does wound eversion improve cosmetic outcome? Results of a randomized, split-scar, comparative trial. *J Am Acad Dermatol.* 2015;72(4):668–673.

22. When is it appropriate to close a cutaneous wound with a glue?
    It is appropriate to close a cutaneous wound with a glue:
    - If the wounds has no tension on the skin edges when closed (lacerations)
    - If the patient does not have an allergy to adhesives

23. How can hemostasis be achieved?
    - Holding pressure
    - Topical agents (aluminum chloride, 20% ferric sulfate)
    - Physical hemostat (mesh, foams)
    - Electrosurgery
    - Suture ligation of vessels

24. Name some factors that will complicate achieving hemostasis
    - Patient disease: hypertension, liver failure, clotting disorders (e.g., Von Willebrand disease), thrombocytopenia
    - Medications: aspirin, warfarin, platelet function inhibitors
    - Herbs: vitamin E, fish oil, garlic, evening primrose oil

CHAPTER 51

CRYOSURGERY

Eileen L. Axibal and Mariah R. Brown

1. **What is cryosurgery?**

   Cryosurgery is the controlled application of low temperatures to cause tissue damage. It can be used to treat both benign and malignant skin conditions. With cryosurgery, the degree of tissue damage is controlled in order to destroy the target lesion with minimal damage to normal surrounding tissue.

   Gage AA. History of cryosurgery. *Semin Surg Oncol.* 1998;14:99–109.
   Korpan N. *Atlas of cryosurgery.* Wien: Springer; 2001.

2. **How does cryosurgery cause tissue injury?**

   All parts of the freeze-thaw cycle can cause tissue injury. During freezing, ice crystal formation and vascular thrombosis result in cell dehydration and ischemia, respectively. During thawing, cells undergo swelling and vascular stasis. The most efficient technique employs a rapid freeze and slow thaw. Repetitive short freezes produce more damage than a single long freeze.

   Gage AA, Baust J. Mechanisms of tissue injury in cryosurgery. *Cryobiology.* 1998;37:171–186.

3. **Does sensitivity to cryosurgery depend on cell type?**

   Yes. Different cell types have variable susceptibility to the effects of freezing. Melanocytes are damaged at a much higher temperature ($-5°C$) than keratinocytes ($-25°C$). This differential has implications for the treatment of melanocytic lesions as well as the use of cryosurgery in patients with darkly pigmented skin (i.e., risk of hypopigmentation).

4. **Which agents are used for cryosurgery?**

   The most commonly used cryogen is liquid nitrogen. It is readily available, inexpensive, easy to store, easy to use, and works quickly. Liquid nitrogen is also the coldest cryogen available, with a boiling point of $-196°C$ ($-321°F$). Other cryogenic agents include chlorodifluoromethane, solid carbon dioxide, liquid nitrous oxide, oxygen, and helium, but these tend to be used for anesthesia rather than tissue destruction.

5. **Do you need a lot of expensive equipment to use cryosurgery?**

   No. Compared to other surgical techniques, the amount of equipment needed for cryosurgery is minimal. First, you need a reservoir for the liquid nitrogen. This is normally a 20- to 30-L thermos (Dewar flask). From there, the liquid nitrogen (LN_2) is transferred to smaller containers. For basic cryosurgery, most dermatologists use small, handheld canisters that spray the LN_2 directly onto the skin (Fig. 51.1). There are also various probes, cones, and thermocouple-pyrometer systems to aid in cryosurgery.

6. **What types of skin conditions can be treated with cryosurgery?**

   Benign, premalignant, and malignant lesions can be treated with cryosurgery (Table 51.1). The most common benign lesions treated with cryosurgery are warts, seborrheic keratoses, and molluscum contagiosum. In particular, cryosurgery is one of the most common modalities for treating precancerous actinic keratoses.

   Andrews MD. Cryosurgery for common skin conditions. *Am Fam Physician.* 2004;69:2365–2372.

7. **How is cryosurgery performed?**

   There are several methods to apply cryogens, including contact (cotton-tipped dipstick, cold-instrument) and spray (open, semiopen cone, semiclosed chamber, closed cryoprobe, and intralesional).

   In the dipstick method, various-sized cotton swabs are dipped in LN_2 and touched to the target lesion. Because swabs have poor thermal capacity resulting in rapid cold dispersal, this technique often results in subtherapeutic temperatures. Various surgical instruments, such as hemostats and pick-ups (tweezers), can be used for cryosurgery

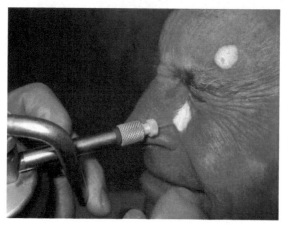

Fig. 51.1 A handheld cryotherapy unit is being used to spray actinic keratoses with liquid nitrogen. Note the cutaneous ice ball that forms in the treated areas.

Table 51.1 Lesions treatable by cryosurgery	
BENIGN	**PREMALIGNANT AND MALIGNANT**
Warts	Actinic keratosis
Molluscum contagiosum	Actinic cheilitis
Acrochordon (skin tag)	Kaposi sarcoma
Seborrheic keratosis	Basal cell carcinoma*
Sebaceous hyperplasia	Squamous cell carcinoma*
Angioma	Lentigo maligna
Pyogenic granuloma	
Chondrodermatitis nodularis helicis	
Lentigines, lentigo simplex, solar lentigo, ephelides	
Mucocele/Myxoid cyst	

*Superficial basal cell carcinoma and squamous cell carcinoma in situ are most amenable to cryosurgery, but other subtypes may be treated in nonsurgical candidates.

of raised or pedunculated lesions. The surgical instrument is submerged in LN$_2$ for 20 to 30 seconds and then the target lesion is grasped with the instrument. It is necessary to use a separate swab or surgical instrument and cup of cryogen for each patient to avoid cross-contamination.

Orengo I, Salasche SJ. Surgical pearl: the cotton-tipped applicator—the ever-ready, multipurpose superstar. *J Am Acad Dermatol.* 1994; 31(4):658–660.
Kuwahara RT, Huber JD, Ray SH. Surgical pearl: forceps method for freezing benign lesion. *J Am Acad Dermatol.* 2000; 43(2 Pt 1):306–307.

The spray technique uses modified thermoses that allow the LN$_2$ to spray out of a nozzle (Fig. 51.1). It is important that the spray tip (or any attachment) is tightly screwed onto the handheld unit because, if it is loose, the force of the liquid nitrogen may propel the attachment. The degree of freezing is dictated by the nozzle size, pressure in the thermos, distance to the lesion, rate and duration of freezing, rate of thawing, and number of freeze-thaw cycles. The spray apparatus can be used for several hours without risk of contamination. It can also be used to treat very large lesions. Some cryosurgeons use cones, chambers, and probes (either external or intralesional) to further control the LN$_2$ tissue destruction.

Torre D. Cryosurgical instrumentation and depth dose monitoring. *Clin Dermatol.* 1990;8(1):48–60.

8. **What pre-cryosurgery techniques can be used to improve the treatment efficacy?**
   Hypertrophic lesions should be debulked with a curette, scissors, or electrosurgery prior to cryosurgery. This allows for sufficient assessment of the margins and improves cold conduction. If a target lesion is bleeding, it needs to be stopped prior to cryosurgery, as blood rapidly increases the local temperature and decreases treatment efficacy.

9. **How are benign skin lesions treated?**
   The basic concept of all cryosurgery is that the depth of freezing is proportional to the width of the area frozen. When cryogen is applied, an ice ball forms in the skin for which the depth of freezing is equal to the radius of the surface freeze. Freezing 1 to 2 mm beyond the lesion with a single freeze-thaw cycle is adequate for most benign lesions, which require a final tissue temperature of $-20°C$ to $-25°C$ for destruction. Warts may be deeper, so either a deeper freeze or multiple smaller freezes can be used. Thick seborrheic keratoses can be frozen lightly and quickly curetted. To avoid causing a scar during the treatment of a benign lesion, it is always better to undertreat at first. It is important to be confident in the clinical diagnosis when treating benign lesions. If you are uncertain about whether a lesion is benign or not, or if it does not resolve with cryosurgery, a biopsy should be performed to provide a histologic diagnosis.

Jester DM. Office procedures: cryotherapy of dermal abnormalities. *Prim Care.* 1997; :269–280.

10. **How do you treat malignant lesions?**
    When treating skin cancers, it is important that the cryosurgical technique is adequate in destroying the malignant cells. Most importantly, the clinical margins of the lesion should be identified. Second, you must know the histology of the cancer to be sure cryosurgery is appropriate. Third, you must have equipment that ensures you reach a temperature of $-50°C$ to $-60°C$ beyond the peripheral extent and depth of the cancer. Malignant lesions require longer freeze times than do benign lesions. Most malignant tumors require at least a 30-second freeze with two freeze-thaw cycles. When performing such treatments, the cryosurgeon may need to provide local anesthesia, as it can be quite painful. Repeat biopsies after cryosurgery can histologically confirm the resolution of the tumor.

Graham GF. Cryosurgery in the management of cutaneous malignancies. *Clin Dermatol.* 2001;19:321–327.
Kuflik EG. Cryosurgery for skin cancer: 30-year experience and cure rates. *Dermatol Surg.* 2004;30(2 Pt 2):297–300.

KEY POINTS: CRYOSURGERY

1. Cryosurgery can be used for benign, premalignant, and, less commonly, malignant lesions.
2. Avoid scarring when treating benign lesions. Consider a biopsy if there is no response.
3. Counsel patients on the normal course of healing for a lesion treated with cryosurgery.

11. **Is cryosurgery a preferred method for the treatment of cutaneous malignancies?**
    Cryosurgery is not considered first-line therapy for the treatment of cutaneous cancers. The technique has become less prevalent over time due to the absence of histologic confirmation of clear margins, postoperative morbidity, suboptimal scarring, and the need for specialized cryosurgery probes. As a result, many dermatologists reserve cryosurgery for malignant lesions under special circumstances. In particular, patients who cannot tolerate conventional surgery due to health comorbidities may be candidates for cryosurgery.

Thissen M, Nieman F, Ideler A, Berretty PJ, Neumann HA. Cosmetic results of cryosurgery versus surgical excision for primary uncomplicated basal cell carcinomas of the head and neck. *Dermatol Surg.* 2000;26:759–764.

12. **What cutaneous malignancies can be treated with cryosurgery?**
    Basal cell carcinoma (BCC) and squamous cell carcinoma (SCC) can both be treated with cryosurgery. Cryosurgery is usually reserved for the superficial variant of BCC and SCC in situ. More aggressive histologic variants and invasive tumors of BCC and SCC are best treated by other modalities, unless the patient cannot tolerate surgery. The lentigo maligna subtype of melanoma in situ has also been treated with cryosurgery, either alone or in conjunction other treatment modalities, due to its superficial nature and the sensitivity of melanocytes to freezing. Cryosurgery is not an appropriate therapy for invasive melanoma.

Neville J, Welch E, Leffell DJ. Management of nonmelanoma skin cancer in 2007. *Nat Clin Pract Oncol.* 2007;4:462–469.
McLeod M, Choudhary S, Giannakakis G, Nouri K. Surgical treatments for lentigo maligna: a review. *Dermatol Surg.* 2011;37(9):1210–1228.
Bassukas ID, Gamvroulia C, Zioga A, Nomikos K, Fotika C. Cryosurgery during topical imiquimod: a successful combination modality for lentigo maligna. *Int J Dermatol.* 2008;47(5):519–521.

13. Are there contraindications to cryosurgery?

People with cold-related conditions such as cryoglobulinemia, cryofibrinogenemia, pernio, cold urticaria, and Raynaud's disease should not be treated with cryosurgery. Patients with heavily pigmented skin should be treated with caution because they are more likely to heal with dyspigmentation, due to the sensitivity of melanocytes to freezing.

14. What are the complications of cryosurgery?

After cryosurgery, the wound is allowed to heal by itself (second intention). A normal cryosurgery wound may blister (Fig. 51.2), ooze, form an eschar, and take 1 to 6 weeks to heal. Complications are uncommon and include hypopigmentation > hyperpigmentation, large bullae, dysesthesia due to damage to superficial sensory nerves, and secondary infection. Rarely, hypertrophic scars and keloids may form. Alopecia (if treating hair-bearing areas), nail dystrophy (if treating near the nail matrix), and notching of the ear or nose (if treating near cartilage) have been reported. Before performing cryosurgery, the normal course of healing and the potential risks of the procedure should be discussed with the patient.

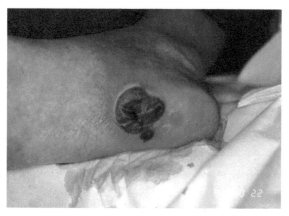

Fig. 51.2 Hemorrhagic blister with oozing due to aggressive cryotherapy of a wart. (Courtesy Fitzsimons Army Medical Center teaching files.)

CHAPTER 52

MOHS SURGERY

Eileen L. Axibal, Misha D. Miller, and Mariah R. Brown

1. What is Mohs surgery?

   Mohs micrographic surgery is a surgical technique used to remove skin cancer. During Mohs surgery, the dermatologist acts as both the surgeon and the pathologist. The goals of Mohs surgery are to completely remove the skin cancer and to maximize conservation of normal tissue, resulting in high cure rates, optimal cosmesis, and preservation of function. Mohs surgery is recommended as first-line treatment for the majority of skin cancers that are aggressive and/or arising in high-risk patients and anatomic locations.

2. How was Mohs surgery developed?

   Dr. Frederic Mohs (1910–2002), of the University of Wisconsin, developed a tumor extirpation technique for skin cancer in the late 1930s. Initially, Mohs micrographic surgery involved chemically fixing in vivo cancerous tissue with zinc chloride paste. This tissue was then excised and systematically mapped, and frozen sections were examined under the microscope. The process was repeated if necessary to remove any residual malignancy until a completely tumor-free plane was achieved. Using the zinc chloride paste, each stage of Mohs took 24 hours, and the process was quite painful. In the early days, Mohs surgeons only removed the skin cancers and allowed the resultant defects to heal in over time (second intention healing), rather than performing surgical reconstruction.

   Mohs FE. Chemosurgery: a microscopically controlled method of cancer excision. *Arch Surg.* 1941;42(2):279–295.

3. Is Mohs surgery still performed with the zinc chloride chemical paste?

   No. The Mohs technique has evolved to use fresh-frozen tissue methods. In the 1970s, the use of frozen sections alone in Mohs surgery was shown to have comparable cure rates to the use of zinc chloride paste. The elimination of zinc chloride paste allowed Mohs surgery to take place in a single day and avoided the pain associated with paste application. In addition, using only frozen sections made it possible for reconstruction of the Mohs defect to occur on the same day as tumor removal. Today, Mohs surgery is performed as a single-day, outpatient procedure and most commonly consists of tumor removal and pathology analysis followed by surgical defect reconstruction.

   Stegman SJ, Tromovitch TA. Fresh tissue chemosurgery for tumors of the nose. *Eye Ear Nose Throat Mon.* 1976;55(2):26–30, 32.
   Stegman SJ, Tromovitch TA. Modern chemosurgery—microscopically controlled excision. *West J Med.* 1980;132(1):7–12.

4. What tumors can be treated with Mohs surgery?

   The majority of tumors treated with Mohs surgery are basal cell carcinoma (BCC) and squamous cell carcinoma (SCC), as these make up greater than 95% of skin cancers. However, Mohs surgery can also be used for melanoma (discussed later) and more rare cutaneous tumors. Less common tumors that have been demonstrated to have high cure rates with Mohs surgery (90% to 100%) include:
   - Dermatofibrosarcoma protuberans (DFSP)
   - Microcystic adnexal carcinoma
   - Merkel cell carcinoma
   - Sebaceous carcinoma
   - Extramammary Paget's disease
   - Atypical fibroxanthoma
   - Malignant fibrous histiocytoma
   - Desmoplastic trichoepithelioma
   - Leiomyosarcoma
   - Angiosarcoma
   - Other adnexal carcinomas: primary cutaneous mucinous carcinoma, trichilemmal carcinoma, hidradenocarcinoma, eccrine porocarcinoma, squamoid eccrine duct tumor, pilomatrical carcinoma, and spiradenocarcinoma.

   Thomas C, Woods G, Marks V. Mohs micrographic surgery in the treatment of rare aggressive cutaneous tumors: the Geisinger experience. *Derm Surg.* 2007;33:333–339.

5. What tumors are the best candidates for Mohs surgery?

Mohs micrographic surgery is especially advantageous in treating skin cancers in areas where tissue sparing is of paramount importance. These anatomic locations include the face, neck, scalp, hands, feet, and genitalia. Mohs surgery is also ideal for high-risk tumors in any anatomic location. High-risk tumors include those that are recurrent, large, histologically aggressive, or arising in individuals with immunosuppression or genetic diseases predisposing to skin cancer. Cure rates with Mohs surgery are 99% and 97% for primary, low-risk BCC and SCC, respectively. Cure rates are lower for recurrent or high-risk tumors.

6. Is Mohs surgery appropriate for all BCCs and SCCs?

BCC and SCC are epidemic in the United States. Excisional surgery, electrodesiccation and curettage, cryosurgery, radiation therapy, topical chemotherapy, photodynamic therapy, and oral chemotherapy are other treatment modalities available for treating skin cancers. Each treatment has a different cure rate, side effect profile, and cosmetic outcome and should be tailored to the specific patient and tumor. The use of Mohs surgery should be limited to the indications outlined in Question 5, due to the time and expense of the procedure.

Kauvar AN, Cronin Jr T, Roenigk R, Hruza G, Bennett R. Consensus for nonmelanoma skin cancer treatment: basal cell carcinoma, including a cost analysis of treatment methods. *Dermatol Surg.* 2015;41(5):550–571.

Kauvar AN, Arpey CJ, Hruza G, Olbricht SM, Bennett R, Mahmoud BH. Consensus for nonmelanoma skin cancer treatment, part II: squamous cell carcinoma, including a cost analysis of treatment methods. *Dermatol Surg.* 2015;41(11):1214–1240.

7. What are the Appropriate Use Criteria for Mohs surgery?

In 2012, the Mohs Appropriate Use Criteria (AUC) were developed to guide clinicians as to whether or not a specific tumor should be treated with Mohs micrographic surgery. The AUC was developed to help prevent overutilization of Mohs surgery. Two hundred seventy clinical scenarios were included in the published document, which included the input from multiple experts in the field of dermatology. The AUC algorithms can be found at http://www.aad.org/education/appropriate-use-criteria/mohs-surgery-auc or by downloading the Mohs AUC mobile app. The AUC stratify tumors based on:

- Patient characteristics
- Location
- Recurrent/nonrecurrent
- Size
- Histologic subtype.

Connolly SM, Baker DR, Coldiron BM, et al. AAD/ACMS/ASDSA/ASMS 2012 Appropriate Use Criteria for Mohs micrographic surgery: a report of the American Academy of Dermatology, American College of Mohs Surgery, American Society for Dermatologic Surgery Association, and the American Society for Mohs Surgery. *Dermatol Surg.* 2012;38(10):1582–1603.

8. Is Mohs surgery appropriate therapy for malignant melanoma?

The use of Mohs surgery for melanoma varies among practitioners. Many dermatologic surgeons perform Mohs surgery on melanoma in situ, particularly the lentigo maligna variant, as the poorly defined margins of the tumor make it a good candidate for the technique. Some surgeons perform Mohs surgery on melanocytic tumors with fresh-frozen sections alone, but the majority perform immunohistochemical stains such as Melan-A (MART-1) to better highlight the atypical melanocytes. The use of Mohs for invasive melanoma remains more controversial. Multiple studies have reported 5-year cure rates with Mohs surgery for invasive melanoma as being equivalent or better than those seen with standard wide local excision. However, some practitioners feel that fresh-frozen tissue does not allow adequate assessment of melanocytic tumors. Modifications of the Mohs technique, such as "slow Mohs" with rushed permanent en face paraffin sections, have been advocated as a way to perform staged tissue-sparing surgery without fresh-frozen sections.

Hui AM, Jacobson M, Markowitz O, Brooks NA, Siegel DM. Mohs micrographic surgery for the treatment of melanoma. *Dermatol Clin.* 2012;30:503–515.

Etzkorn JR, Sobanko JF, Elenitsas R, et al. Low recurrence rates for in situ and invasive melanomas using Mohs micrographic surgery with melanoma antigen recognized by T cells 1 (MART-1) immunostaining: tissue processing methodology to optimize pathologic staging and margin assessment. *J Am Acad Dermatol.* 2015;72(5):840–850.

Valentin-Nogueras SM, Brodland DG, Zitelli JA, González-Sepúlveda L, Nazario CM. Mohs micrographic surgery using MART-1 immunostain in the treatment of invasive melanoma and melanoma in situ. *Dermatol Surg.* 2016;42(6):733–744.

9. How is Mohs surgery performed?

Mohs surgery is performed in the outpatient setting. Patients are advised that the procedure may last an entire day. After informed consent is obtained, the tumor site is identified, measured, and photographed. Local anesthetic is then infiltrated into the surgical site. The majority of surgeons perform Mohs as a clean rather than sterile procedure. Prior to taking the Mohs layer, many surgeons will debulk the cancer with a curette or scalpel to better delineate its dimensions. A saucer-shaped piece of tissue is then excised with a beveled angle at the peripheral margin. This piece of tissue includes the area of skin cancer with a small rim of normal tissue—the size of the margin is tailored to each specific tumor. The specimen is then sectioned into manageable pieces (if needed) and oriented with ink. Using an anatomic drawing of the site, a map is drawn to precisely label the area from which the tumor is taken. The tissue is then submitted to the Mohs histotechnician, who prepares the frozen tissue sections. When the frozen tissue slides are completed, the Mohs surgeon examines the slides under the microscope to assess for residual tumor. If tumor is identified, the map is used as a guide to obtain additional tissue layers only from the areas of positivity until a tumor-free plane is reached. Between stages of Mohs surgery, the wound is covered with a temporary dressing and the patient waits in a comfortable area. Various steps of the procedure are illustrated in Fig. 52.1 using an apple model.

Chung VQ, Bernardo L, Jiang SB. Presurgical curettage appropriately reduces the number of Mohs stages by better delineating the subclinical extensions of tumor margins. *Dermatol Surg.* 2005;31(9 Pt 1):1094–1099.
Davis DA, Pellowski DM, Hanke WC. Preparation of frozen sections. *Dermatol Surg.* 2004;30:1479–1485.
Benedetto PX, Poblete-Lopez C. Mohs micrographic surgery technique. *Dermatol Clin.* 2011;29(2):141–151, vii.

10. How does Mohs histology differ from standard tissue processing?
    Using a scalpel, Mohs sections are taken with a 30 to 45 degree beveled edge at the peripheral margin. This technique allows the peripheral and deep margins to be flattened into the same plane of sectioning during tissue processing. Mohs sections are processed in a horizontal fashion, cutting through the tissue block from the true surgical margin up toward the skin surface. This horizontal "en face" processing allows for visualization of 100% of the surgical margin. If residual tumor is identified, the location of the tumor is marked on a schematic of the defect that will then serve as a map that guides further tissue resection until a tumor-free plane is achieved. Standard tissue excision is performed with a 90-degree angle of excision. The tissue is processed using a technique known as "bread loafing," which involves embedding the tissue vertically and evaluating a few (usually one to three) random "slices" of tissue throughout the tissue block. Bread loafing is estimated to examine less than 0.1% to 1% of the total histologic margin and can result in false-negative results. Because the Mohs surgeon removes, maps, and interprets the tumor tissue, the chances of errors in orientation or interpretation are also reduced during Mohs surgery versus standard excision.

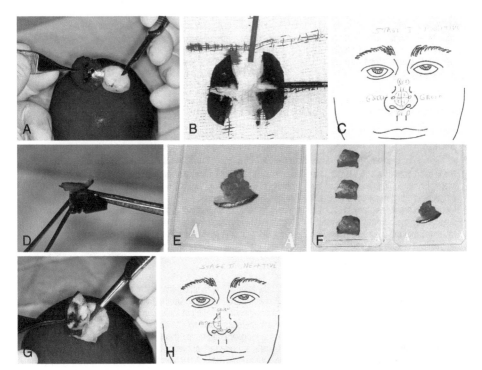

Fig. 52.1 Apple model with tumor. **A,** Cancerous tissue is excised with the blade beveled. **B,** Tissue is sectioned and color coded. **C,** Anatomic map is labeled. **D** to **F,** Horizontal frozen sections are obtained to allow examination of the entire excision margin. **G** and **H,** Residual tumor is excised until the margins are clear.

van der Eerden PA, Prins ME, Lohuis PJ, Balm FA, Vuyk HD. Eighteen years of experience in Mohs micrographic surgery and conventional excision for nonmelanoma skin cancer treated by a single facial plastic surgeon and pathologist. *Laryngoscope.* 2010;120:2378–2384.
Abide JM, Nahai F, Bennett RG. The meaning of surgical margins. *Plast Reconstr Surg.* 1984;73(3):492–497.

11. What are the potential complications of Mohs surgery?
Overall, the rate of complications in Mohs surgery is very low—a large, multicenter, prospective study of more than 20,000 Mohs surgery patients demonstrated a 0.72% complication rate. The rate of serious complications was only 0.02%. Potential complications include pain, bleeding, infection, sensory or motor nerve damage, functional impairment, and tumor recurrence. Many of the complications from Mohs surgery result from the reconstruction of the surgical defect rather than the Mohs procedure itself.

Alam M, Ibrahim O, Nodzenski M, et al. Adverse events associated with Mohs micrographic surgery: multicenter prospective cohort study of 20,821 cases at 23 centers. *JAMA Dermatol.* 2013;149:1378–1385.

12. What histologic stains are used in Mohs surgery?
The majority of Mohs surgeons stain their fresh-frozen tissue with hematoxylin and eosin (H&E), the most common stain used in paraffin-fixed sections. Some Mohs surgeons use toluidine blue, a stain that is particularly useful for highlighting BCC, but this has become less common. The most common immunohistochemical stain used by Mohs surgeons is a Melan-A (MART-1) stain, used to highlight melanocytic cells in lentigo maligna and other melanocytic tumors. Other immunohistochemical stains that can be used include CD-34 for dermatofibrosarcoma protuberans and cytokeratin stains for SCC (AE1–AE3—high-molecular-weight keratins) and Paget's disease (cytokeratin 7).

Stranahan D, Cherpelis B, Glass L, Ladd S, Fenske NA. Immunohistochemical stains in Mohs surgery: a review. *Dermatol Surg.* 2009;35:1023–1034.
Silapunt S, Peterson SR, Alcalay J, Goldberg LH. Mohs tissue mapping and processing: a survey study. *Dermatol Surg.* 2004;30:961.

13. How are the defects created in Mohs surgery repaired?
The precision of Mohs surgery allows for maximum preservation of normal tissue, but the surgical defects created during Mohs surgery often require repair. Some defects may be allowed to heal by themselves (second intention healing), but this should be limited to smaller, shallow defects on concave surfaces. The majority of Mohs defects will need to be reconstructed using elliptical primary closures, flaps, or skin grafts (Fig. 52.2). Reconstruction after Mohs surgery is performed using sterile technique, although there has been some shift toward using clean technique based on recent studies. Mohs surgeons, especially those who have completed fellowships, are experienced in aesthetic reconstruction.

Mehta D, Chambers N, Adams B, Gloster H. Comparison of the prevalence of surgical site infection with use of sterile versus nonsterile gloves for resection and reconstruction during Mohs surgery. *Dermatol Surg.* 2014;40:234–239.

KEY POINTS: MOHS SURGERY

1. Mohs micrographic surgery is the controlled, serial, microscopic removal of skin cancer resulting in high cure rates.
2. Mohs micrographic surgery allows for maximum preservation of uninvolved tissue and, consequently, results in smaller defects compared to conventional tumor excision protocols.
3. Mohs micrographic surgery is indicated for basal cell and squamous cell carcinomas arising on the face and other sites where the maximal preservation of normal skin and cosmesis is an important goal.
4. Mohs micrographic surgery is also indicated for skin cancers in all sites that are large, recurrent, histologically aggressive, or rare (such as dermatofibrosarcoma protuberans and microcystic adnexal carcinoma).

14. Who performs Mohs surgery?
The Accreditation Council for Graduate Medical Education currently accredits fellowship training in Micrographic Surgery and Dermatologic Oncology, formerly Procedural Dermatology. During fellowship, physicians who have completed a residency in dermatology receive comprehensive training in Mohs surgery and all aspects of cutaneous oncology. The period of training is typically 1 year and there are currently 77 training centers in the United States. Many dermatologists know the basic techniques of Mohs surgery and employ them in their practices. However, when patients require more extensive surgery, they usually are referred to a fellowship-trained Mohs surgeon. Board certification in Micrographic Dermatologic Surgery was approved in 2018, and the exam will become available in the next few years.

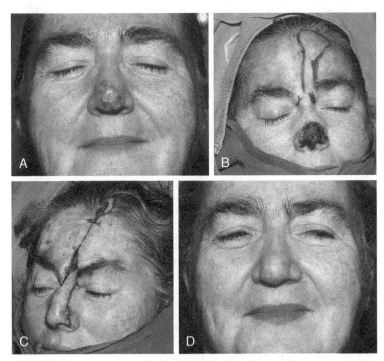

Fig. 52.2 A, Preoperative basal cell carcinoma of the nasal tip. **B,** Defect of the nose following Mohs micrographic surgery. Paramedian forehead flap is designed. Note preservation of cartilaginous skeleton. **C,** Paramedian forehead flap is attached to reconstruct the nose. The forehead defect is closed. The pedicle is divided at 2 weeks. **D,** Long-term results.

15. What are the advantages and disadvantages of Mohs surgery?

Mohs surgery allows for the targeted removal of tumors while sparing the greatest amount of normal tissue. Mohs surgery has the highest cure rate of any technique used to treat skin cancer. It also spares the patient the risks of general anesthesia and allows the removal of the tumor and reconstruction of the surgical defect to occur in a single day. Mohs surgery is limited to cutaneous tumors that have contiguous spread, and Mohs frozen sections are designed for margin control of tumor, rather than assessments such as tumor depth or identification of inflammatory conditions. For large tumors, surgeons may be limited by the maximal allowable dosage of local anesthesia, although this is uncommon. The procedure can be time consuming, and the long days can be difficult for some patients. While Mohs surgery may be more expensive than other modalities for treating skin cancer, some studies have demonstrated Mohs to be quite cost effective due to its high cure rates and bundling of tumor excision and reconstruction.

Ravitskiy L, Brodland DG, Zitelli JA. Cost analysis: Mohs micrographic surgery. *Dermatol Surg.* 2012;38:585–594.

CHAPTER 53

LASERS IN DERMATOLOGY

Steven E. Eilers and David J. Goldberg

1. What does the term "laser" stand for?

Laser is an acronym for "**L**ight **A**mplification by **S**timulated **E**mission of **R**adiation."

Herd RM, Dover JS, Arndt KA. Basic laser principles. *Dermatol Clin.* 1997;15:355–372.

2. What does "stimulated emission of radiation" mean?

Stimulated emission is a complicated phenomenon of physics, first described by Albert Einstein. Atoms must be in an excited state (an electron is in an elevated orbit). Normally, adding a photon with energy equal to the energy between orbits would raise this electron to a higher orbit. Instead, in special circumstances found in laser systems, two photons are released from the atom, and the electron returns to its lower, resting state. These two photons are then able to enter two other atoms with excited electrons, allowing rapid multiplication of photons in a process similar to a chain reaction. This process accounts for the stimulated emission of radiation used in the acronym *laser*.

3. How is the light amplified in the laser system?

The laser system uses an optical resonator to amplify and orient the light. This is a cylindrical chamber filled with the laser medium. There are mirrors on each end and an absorptive lining. The photons of light are reflected between the mirrors. The lining will absorb any light that is not perfectly parallel. These parallel photons continue to enter additional atoms, producing more photons by stimulated emission. By this process, the laser light is amplified. One end of the optical resonator has a mechanism to release the light periodically from the chamber.

4. What types of medium are used in laser systems?

The ability of an atom to be used in a laser system is a complicated function of quantum mechanics and the physical characteristics of the lattice in which it is constructed. The basic requirement of any medium is to be able to support a population inversion so that there may be stimulated emission. Some types of lasers include the following:

- **Solids:** Ruby crystal: composed of aluminum oxide (Al_3O_2) with scattered atoms of chromium (Cr) replacing some aluminum atoms in the crystal lattice
- **Gases:** Carbon dioxide (CO_2). Excimer (xenon chloride)
- **Dyes:** Fluorescent liquid dye (often rhodamine)
- **Other:** Electrical diodes

5. What are the special features of laser light?

Laser light is unique because of three inherent features:

- **Coherence:** Coherence is the property that represents a uniform wave front, that is, the peaks and valleys of the waves are aligned as the light exits the laser, which allows the light to be in phase and focused to very small areas. This also allows the energies to be additive.
- **Monochromaticity:** This means all light waves have the same wavelength. Some lasers produce more than one wavelength of light, but these are predictable and the laser still produces only those specific wavelengths of light expected by the laser medium used.
- **Collimation:** This means that all of the light exiting the laser is parallel and will not diffuse over distances.

6. Why is monochromatic light useful?

Many lasers target specific chromophores, which are biologic structures with a specific absorption spectrum. Two common chromophores are hemoglobin within the red blood cell and melanin within melanosomes. The absorption spectrum is the amount of light absorbed at various wavelengths. The idea is to match a peak absorption wavelength with the wavelength of the laser (Fig. 53.1).

7. What are the four interactions treated skin will have with laser light?

Reflection: 4%–7% of light is reflected from the skin due to differences between the refractive index of air and the stratum corneum.

Scattering: Light bounces off of fibers and particles, diffusing into the surrounding skin and limiting depth of penetration.

Transmission: Light does not interact with the skin or particles and passes through the tissue.

Absorption: The desired effect, light is absorbed by its intended target.

Anderson RR, Parrish JA. The optics of human skin. *J Invest Dermatol.* 1981;77:13–19.

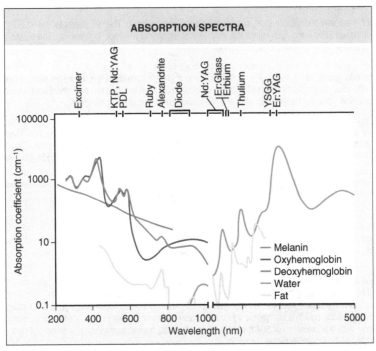

Fig. 53.1 Absorption spectra. The heterogeneous absorption spectra of chromophores allow selective photothermolysis to work. *Er*, Erbium; *KTP*, potassium titanyl phosphate; *Nd*, neodymium-doped; *PDL*, pulsed dye laser; *YAG*, yttrium aluminum garnet; *YSGG*, yttrium scandium gallium garnet. (From Sakamoto FH, Avram MM, Anderson RR. Lasers and other energy-based technologies—principles and skin interactions. In: Bolognia JL, Schaffer JV, Cerroni L, eds. *Dermatology*. 4th ed. Philadelphia: Elsevier; 2018.)

8. What is selective photothermolysis?
   The theory of selective photothermolysis assumes the laser light will pass through tissue until it targets a specific chromophore with an absorption spectrum corresponding to the wavelength of the laser. The target then absorbs the light, generating heat in the target tissue. The spread of heat is determined by the thermal relaxation time (TRT) of the tissue. This is the amount of time necessary for 50% of the peak heat to diffuse out of the target. It is important for the laser pulse duration not to exceed the TRT of the target or the heat will diffuse into surrounding tissue, causing damage and possibly scarring. Thus, the TRT depends on the actual size of the target. The smaller the target, the shorter the TRT, and thus the need for shorter laser pulse durations.

Anderson RR, Parrish JA. Selective photothermolysis: precise microsurgery by selective absorption of pulsed radiation. *Science*. 1983;220:524–527.

9. What is an ablative laser?
   An ablative laser vaporizes tissue. Different lasers cause different types of ablative reactions. Erbium (Er):yttrium aluminum garnet (YAG) lasers, due to their very high water absorption, cause almost pure ablation with very little collateral thermal heating. CO_2 lasers have less water absorption and therefore deliver less pure ablation and have more collateral heating. This heat causes thermal damage in a positive and negative manner. An example of a positive effect is collagen contraction and new collagen stimulation. Other positive effects of CO_2 lasers are sealing of blood vessels leading to less bleeding and sealing of nerve endings leading to less pain. An example of a negative effect is hypopigmentation due to inadvertent melanocyte damage. Scarring from laser procedures is usually due to excessive collateral heating.

10. What is a nonablative laser?
    Most lasers are capable of delivering laser energy in a nonablative or nonvaporizing manner. Pulsed dye lasers, long-pulsed alexandrite, and neodymium-doped (Nd):YAG and many diode lasers deliver energy so as not to ablate tissue. The only lasers that truly ablate are those listed earlier and are used to remove tissue in a physical manner. The entire concept of selective photothermolysis is the ability to deliver energy in a nonablative manner.

Alexiades-Armenakas MR, Dover JS, Arndt KA. The spectrum of laser skin resurfacing: nonablative, fractional, and ablative laser resurfacing. *J Am Acad Dermatol*. 2008;58:719–737.

11. **What is Q-switching?**

Q-switching is a way of obtaining short, powerful pulses of laser radiation. The "Q" stands for the "quality" factor of the optical resonator. There are many electrical, mechanical, or optical methods to Q-switch. The pulses generated by Q-switching are in the nanosecond (10^{-9}) range.

12. **Are there lasers with even shorter pulses than Q-switched lasers?**

There are now lasers that deliver pulses in the picosecond (10^{-12} second) range. There are several new lasers with 350- to 900-psec ranges that are used for tattoo removal. In addition to tattoo removal, there are new protocols using the picosecond pulse for treating pigmented lesions, melasma, and skin rejuvenation.

13. **What is a fractional laser?**

Fractional lasers deliver short pulses of laser that are separated by space on the surface of the skin. These lasers may either be nonablative, leaving a column of heat-damaged skin, or ablative, leaving a column of true ablation. This will be discussed in detail in a later question. The concept of fractional lasers was first proposed by Dr. Rox Anderson.

Manstein D, Herron GS, Sink RK, Tanner H, Anderson RR. Fractional photothermolysis: a new concept for cutaneous remodeling using microscopic patterns of thermal injury. *Lasers Surg Med.* 2004;34(5):426–438.

14. **How are the types of dermatologic lasers classified?**

The lasers are usually classified by the laser medium that generates the light, the specific wavelength of laser light, the length of the laser pulse, and the uses of the laser (Table 53.1).

15. **What lasers have historic interest but are seldom used?**

The argon laser (488 nm, 514 nm) was one of the first dermatologic lasers. This is seldom used because of scarring issues. The krypton laser generates dual wavelengths: 520-nm (green) and 568-nm (yellow) light. The continuous-wave thermal nature of the laser caused too much surface heating. Copper vapor lasers generate dual wavelengths of 511 nm (green light) and 578 nm (yellow light). These lasers are not currently used. There was a pulsed dye pigment lesion laser with a wavelength of 504 nm. This laser effectively treated surface pigmentation but was mechanically unsound and is no longer available (Table 53.2).

16. **What are the basic features of the carbon dioxide (CO_2) laser?**

The CO_2 laser emits radiation at 10,600 nm, in the far-infrared region. All water in tissue absorbs this wavelength of light, and this absorption is not dependent on selective absorption by any biologic tissue. As the water absorbs energy, the temperature rapidly rises, vaporizing the tissue. The amount of tissue damage is related to the energy setting and the amount of time the laser impacts on the target. There is some true ablation of tissue and this is surrounded by a zone of thermal damage. This area of thermal damage is used in resurfacing by causing immediate collagen contraction and later collagen remodeling.

The standard delivery system for the CO_2 laser is an articulated arm, which comprises a series of rigid tubes with mirrored joints capable of rotating in all directions. The CO_2 laser light is invisible and therefore must use a helium-neon laser as an aiming beam. The CO_2 laser operates in a range between 1 and 30 W of power. The mechanical pulses are set between 0.01 and 0.1 seconds, but the laser may also operate in a continuous-wave mode. CO_2 lasers are usually used in a focused or defocused mode, the former for high-intensity use, such as cutting, and the latter for low-power destructive uses.

There are now many fractional CO_2 lasers designed to reduce the side effects of CO_2 laser ablation (Table 53.3).

17. **What are some uses for the standard carbon dioxide laser?**

Treatment of warts has been the hallmark of CO_2 laser therapy. Large plantar and periungual warts are effectively treated. The main advantage of CO_2 laser treatment in these larger warts is the ability to decrease the bleeding during the laser excision and a slight decrease in scarring. Any benign lesion may be removed using CO_2 laser, but this is not a common method used in dermatology. CO_2 lasers in a high-power focused mode are very effective at surgical cutting, especially in patients on anticoagulants or those with other bleeding disorders.

Olbricht SM. Use of the CO_2 laser in dermatologic surgery. *J Dermatol Surg Oncol.* 1993;19:364–369.

18. **How is the CO_2 laser used for resurfacing?**

Historically, the ultrapulsed CO_2 laser effectively removed the top layers of the epidermis and caused collagen contraction in the superficial dermis. This combination of effects allows the treatment of moderate facial wrinkles and sun damage. This procedure is still the most effective for laser resurfacing but is seldom used because of very prolonged healing and many side effects.

Fractional CO_2 laser resurfacing dramatically reduces the healing time and side effects but may not have as much overall effect as with fully ablative lasers.

Table 53.1 Types of lasers

LASER MEDIUM	WAVELENGTH	PULSE DURATION	USES
Carbon dioxide	10,600 nm	msec	Destruction of benign growths Ablative skin resurfacing
Er:YAG	2940 nm	msec	Pure tissue ablation Treatment of fine wrinkles and acne scars
Pulsed dye	577–600 nm	msec	Vascular lesion removal Nonablative skin resurfacing Scar improvement Lentigines Wart removal Treatment of rosacea Reduction of poikiloderma of Civatte
Nd:YAG laser (Q-switched)	1064 nm	nsec	Black, blue tattoos Lentigines Nonablative laser resurfacing
Nd:YAG laser (long-pulsed)	1064 nm	msec	Hair removal Vascular lesions Skin tightening
KTP laser (Q-switched)	532 nm	nsec	Red tattoos
KTP laser (long-pulsed)	532 nm	msec	Vascular lesions Lentigines
Alexandrite laser (Q-switched)	755 nm	nsec	Green tattoos Lentigines
Alexandrite laser (long-pulsed)	755 nm	msec	Hair removal Lentigines Vascular lesions
Ruby laser (Q-switched)	694 nm	nsec	Black, blue tattoos
Ruby laser (long-pulsed)	694 nm	msec	Hair removal
Diode laser	810 nm	msec	Hair removal
Diode laser	1350–1450 nm	msec	Nonablative skin resurfacing

Er, Erbium; *KTP*, potassium titanyl phosphate; *Nd*, neodymium-doped; *YAG*, yttrium aluminum garnet.

19. What precautions must be used with the CO_2 laser?

The main precaution with the CO_2 laser is smoke evacuation. During the procedure, the laser generates a large amount of smoke that may harbor viral particles. Studies have suggested the presence of live viral particles or genetic material of human papillomavirus, hepatitis viruses, and human immunodeficiency virus. Adequate vacuum devices and surgical masks are a must for use with this laser. The CO_2 laser will also burn any cloth or paper that it contacts; therefore, appropriate fire precautions must be observed. Clear plastic or glass eyewear is adequate to protect the eyes from this wavelength of laser light. Patients having skin resurfacing with CO_2 or Er laser should be treated both before and immediately after the laser treatment with anti–herpes simplex medication.

Table 53.2 Lasers of historic interest only

LASER MEDIUM	WAVELENGTH	PROBLEMS
Argon	488 nm, 512 nm	Scarring
Krypton	520 nm, 568 nm	Scarring
Copper vapor	511 nm, 578 nm	Ineffective
Pulsed pigment	504 nm	Mechanical nightmare

Table 53.3 Carbon dioxide lasers
10,600-nm light
Energy absorbed by water
Nonspecific vaporization of tissue
Used for tissue destruction
Used for laser resurfacing of moderate wrinkles
May be used for surgical cutting

20. **What are the basic features of the Er:YAG laser?**

YAG crystals are composed of **y**ttrium and **a**luminum in a **g**arnet crystal matrix. The Er:YAG crystal has some of the atoms of yttrium replaced with Er atoms. The laser output is at 2490 nm. This wavelength is absorbed by water 10 times better than the 10,600-nm light of CO_2 lasers. This more efficient effect leads to little collateral damage to surrounding collagen and more efficient ablation of tissue. The clinical result is less effect on wrinkles but a smoother, faster-healing resurfacing procedure. By itself, the Er:YAG laser has been used to treat mild facial sun damage, some sun damage on necks and hands, and acne scarring. In treating scars, the laser has the ability to plane down the edges of acne scars. Er:YAG lasers are also often used as a fractional device to decrease the healing time and side effects (Table 53.4).

Goldberg DJ, Cutler KB. The use of the erbium: YAG laser for the treatment of class III rhytids. *Dermatol Surg.* 1999;25:713–715.
McDaniel DH, Lord J, Ash K, Newman J. Combined CO_2/erbium:YAG laser resurfacing of perioral rhytides and side-by-side comparison with carbon dioxide laser alone. *Dermatol Surg.* 1999;25:285–293.

21. **What are pulsed dye lasers?**

The most common pulsed dye lasers use a flashlamp to energize the laser. The active medium is a fluorescent dye, often rhodamine. This will generate a wavelength between 200 and 700 nm. The older vascular lesion pulsed dye lasers used either 577 or 585 nm as the preferred wavelength, corresponding to a small peak in the oxyhemoglobin absorption spectrum in an area that does not have much competition from melanin. Newer pulsed dye lasers usually set the laser at 595 nm. The flashlamp generates pulses with a duration from 350 μsec up to 40 msec.

22. **What is the flashlamp pulsed dye laser used to treat?**

The pulsed dye lasers may be the most effective lasers in treating thin, lightly colored port wine stains, especially those in children. These lesions have been treated without scarring in children as young as 1 month of age. Increasing the wavelength to 595 nm theoretically allows the treatment of many port wine stains that were resistant to treatment with the shorter wavelengths. Pulsed dye laser treatment is effective for facial telangiectasias, cherry angiomas, infantile hemangiomas, poikiloderma of Civatte (a mottled vascular condition on the necks of adults), warts, scars, and possibly stretch marks. Leg veins less than 1 mm in diameter are also effectively treated with pulsed dye lasers using a pulse duration of up to 20 msec. One of the newer pulsed dye lasers even has a handpiece to treat pigmented lesions. This is a compression handpiece designed to physically compress out the blood, thereby removing one of the competing chromophores of this wavelength. This leaves the laser energy able to treat the remaining melanin targets. A 585-nm pulsed dye laser at very low fluences (2.5 to 3.0 J/cm^2) has been shown to be very effective at treating acne vulgaris. This low-level laser light triggers an increase of transforming growth factor (TGF)-β that stimulates an anti-inflammatory response.

Fitzpatrick RE, Lowe NJ, Goldman MP, Borden H, Behr KL, Ruiz-Esparza J. Flashlamp-pumped pulsed dye laser treatment of port-wine stains. *J Dermatol Surg Oncol.* 1994;20:743–748.
Hsia J, Lowery JA, Zelickson B. Treatment of leg telangiectasia using a long-pulse dye laser at 595 nm. *Lasers Surg Med.* 1997;20:1–5.

23. **What is nonablative resurfacing and how does a pulsed dye laser accomplish this?**

Theoretically, gentle heating of the superficial dermal layer will stimulate the production of new collagen. This helps to fill in fine wrinkles on the face. There is some controversy about this procedure, but most patients think it is helpful. Pulsed dye lasers at low to moderate fluences (nonpurpuric settings) are used for this nonablative resurfacing. The low

Table 53.4 Er:YAG lasers
2490-nm light
Energy absorbed by water (10 times CO_2)
Used for pure tissue ablation (no collateral heating)
Treatment of fine wrinkles and acne scars

Er, Erbium; *YAG,* yttrium aluminum garnet

fluences help to stimulate collagen production. Many other lasers and intense pulsed light (IPL) machines are also purported to be effective.

Goldberg DJ. Nonablative resurfacing. *Clin Plastic Surg.* 2000;27:287–292.
Omi T, Kawana S, Sato S, et al. Cutaneous immunological activation elicited by a low-fluence pulsed dye laser. *Br J Dermatol.* 2005;153 (suppl 1):57–62.

24. **What are the disadvantages of the pulsed dye laser?**
    The pulsed dye lasers are not very useful in treating thicker vascular lesions, because the short pulse duration is not usually sufficient to damage the target vessels without increasing the power to a level that could lead to generalized damage and scarring. There may be significant post-treatment purpura that takes 7 to 10 days to resolve. This purpura results from the explosive optical-acoustic pulse generated by the pulsed dye lasers. This is a cosmetic problem that limits the use of the laser in some patients. The newer pulsed dye lasers are able to treat lesions without purpura by using longer pulse durations in the range of 10 msec (Table 53.5).

25. **What is an Nd:YAG laser?**
    The Nd:YAG laser uses an yttrium-aluminum-garnet crystal in which neodymium has been dispersed into the crystal. The standard wavelength of light emitted is 1064 nm, which is in the near-infrared spectrum. The light from these lasers may be passed through a potassium-titanyl-phosphate (KTP) crystal to double the frequency, halving the wavelength to 532 nm, in the green spectral region. These lasers are usually referred to as KTP lasers. Nd:YAG lasers may be long-pulsed in the 3- to 100-msec pulse duration range or Q-switched with pulses in the 5- to 50-nsec pulse range.

26. **How are the long-pulsed Nd:YAG (1064-nm) lasers used?**
    The long-pulsed Nd:YAG laser (at 1064 nm) has been used for hair removal in dark-skinned patients (Fitzpatrick types IV to VI). This laser has also been used for hair removal in tanned patients, but I would recommend avoiding laser treatments with recently tanned skin. These long-pulsed lasers are also very useful for treating vascular lesions including leg veins and larger vessels on the nose. Long-pulsed Nd:YAG lasers have also been reported to help with skin tightening.

27. **How are the long-pulsed KTP lasers used?**
    This laser is primarily used to treat red vascular lesions. Red vessels on the face respond the best. Leg veins do not appear to respond well to these lasers. The primary advantage over pulsed dye lasers is the lack of purpura after treatment.

Goldberg DJ, Meine JG. A comparison of four frequency-doubled Nd:YAG (532 nm) laser systems for treatment of facial telangiectases. *Dermatol Surg.* 1999;25:463–467.
Massey RA, Katz BE. Successful treatment of spider leg veins with a high-energy, long-pulse, frequency-doubled neodymium:YAG laser (HELP-G). *Dermatol Surg.* 1999;25:677–680.

28. **How are the Q-switched Nd:YAG lasers used?**
    The Q-switched Nd:YAG lasers are primarily used to remove tattoos. The 1064-nm laser effectively removes black, blue-black, and blue tattoo pigment. This laser has also been useful in treating dermal pigmented lesions such as nevus of Ota and nevus of Ito. The 532-nm laser effectively removes red tattoo pigment. The 532 Q-switched Nd:YAG laser is also used for removal of brown lesions such as lentigines, nevus of Ota, and café-au-lait spots. Q-switched Nd:YAG and Q-switched ruby lasers are very popular in Asia for laser toning to decrease pigmentation (Table 53.6).

29. **What is the alexandrite laser?**
    Alexandrite crystal, a rare gemstone, is named after the Russian tsar Alexander II. The most sensational feature about this stone, however, is its surprising ability to change its color. Green or bluish-green in daylight, alexandrite turns a soft shade of red, purplish-red, or raspberry red in incandescent light. An alexandrite laser is a solid state laser in which

Table 53.5 Pulsed dye lasers
585–600 nm
Main target, oxyhemoglobin
Alternative target, epidermal melanin
Alternative target, dermal collagen
Used to treat vascular lesions
Used to treat scars, warts, sebaceous hyperplasia
Nonablative wrinkle removal

Table 53.6 Nd:YAG lasers

LASER	MODE	USES
Nd:YAG, 1064 nm	Long-pulsed	Hair removal Blood vessels, nose Leg veins Skin tightening
Nd:YAG, 1064 nm	Q-switched	Black, blue tattoos Nevus of Ota
KTP, 532 nm	Long-pulsed	Facial telangiectasias
KTP, 532 nm	Q-switched	Red tattoos Epidermal pigmentation

KTP, Potassium titanyl phosphate; *Nd*, neodymium-doped; *YAG*, yttrium aluminum garnet.

chromium ions (Cr^{-3}), at the amount of 0.01% to 0.4%, are embedded in a $BeAl_2O_4$ crystal. Chromium ions are contaminants in the crystal. Both Q-switched and flashlamp-pumped alexandrite lasers are available. These lasers deliver a wavelength of 755-nm light.

30. **How are the alexandrite lasers used?**
    The Q-switched alexandrite laser is effective in removing green and black tattoo pigment. This laser has also been used to remove brown macules. The long-pulsed alexandrite laser is the gold standard for laser hair removal. Dark hair in Fitzpatrick types I to IV skin is very effectively removed. The long-pulsed laser has been reported to effectively remove leg veins that are 1 to 2 mm in diameter and blue in color. The 755-nm alexandrite laser is now used commonly for resistant port wine stains. This laser has recently also been reported to effectively treat brown lentigines on the face and hands (Table 53.7).

Alster TS. Q-switched alexandrite laser treatment (755 nm) of professional and amateur tattoos. *J Am Acad Dermatol*. 1995;33:69–73.
Ash K, Lord J, Newman J, McDaniel DH. Hair removal using a long-pulsed alexandrite laser. *Dermatol Clin*. 1999;17:387–399.

31. **What is the ruby laser?**
    The ruby laser has an active medium of aluminum oxide (Al_2O_3) that has been chromium-doped, meaning that some of the aluminum (Al^{+3}) atoms have been replaced with chromium (Cr^{+3}) atoms. This laser emits a wavelength of 694 nm that is in the red visible light spectrum. These lasers may be Q-switched or long-pulsed.

32. **How are the ruby lasers used?**
    The Q-switched ruby laser light is well absorbed by black, blue, and green tattoo pigment. The Q-switched ruby lasers have also been used in treating some dermal pigmentation abnormalities such as nevus of Ota. The long-pulsed ruby laser has been used primarily for laser hair removal (Table 53.8).

Taylor CR, Gange RW, Dover JS, et al. Treatment of tattoos by Q-switched ruby laser. *Arch Dermatol*. 1990;126:893–899.
Williams RM, Christian MM, Moy RL. Hair removal using the long-pulsed ruby laser. *Dermatol Clin*. 1999;17:367–372.

33. **What is a diode laser?**
    Diode lasers use microscopic chips of gallium arsenide or other semiconductors to generate coherent light. The energy of the light is generated by the differences between energy levels within the semiconductor. The wavelength may be varied to a wide spectral range. The high energy of medical lasers is generated by stacking arrays of the diodes. The advantage of the diode lasers is lower cost, a wide range of wavelengths, and smaller lasers.

Table 53.7 Alexandrite lasers

LASER	MODE	USES
755 nm	Q-switched	Tattoos (green, black) Brown spots
755 nm	Long-pulsed	Hair removal Leg veins (1–2 mm blue) Brown spots

Table 53.8 Ruby lasers		
LASER	**MODE**	**USES**
694 nm	Q-switched	Tattoos (black) Nevus of Ota
694 nm	Long-pulsed	Hair removal

34. **How are the diode lasers used?**
The 810-nm diode lasers are primarily used for hair removal and, occasionally, for treatment of vascular lesions. The 1320-nm diode lasers have been used for nonablative laser resurfacing and treatment of acne scarring. The 1450-nm diode lasers have been used for nonablative laser resurfacing, treatment of acne scarring, and the treatment of active acne (Table 53.9).

35. **What is the excimer laser and what is it used for?**
The excimer laser is a Xenon Chloride 308 nm laser. It is primarily used to treat psoriasis and vitiligo by inducing localized immunosuppression. Psoriatic plaques have been shown to need lower cumulative doses of ultraviolet B (UVB) and clear in half the time compared to conventional UVB phototherapy. Vitiligo has demonstrated impressive improvement with the excimer laser.

Bónis B, Kemény L, Dobozy A, Bor Z, Szabó G, Ignácz F. 308 nm UVB excimer laser for psoriasis. *Lancet.* 1997;350:1522.

36. **How are the Picosecond lasers used?**
The picosecond lasers have a pulse duration that is in the picosecond range. Picosecond lasers have been shown to be more effective than Q-switched lasers to clear tattoos and require fewer treatment sessions. The picosecond Alexandrite 755 nm and Nd:YAG 1064 nm treat black, blue-black, blue, and dark brown tattoo ink, and the Alexandrite 755 nm can also remove green tattoo ink. The picosecond Nd:YAG 532 nm can remove red, orange, yellow, and purple tattoo ink. The picosecond lasers can also be used for pigmented lesions, melasma, skin rejuvenation, and acne treatment (Table 53.10, Fig. 53.2).

37. **What are nonablative fractional lasers, and why are they used?**
The Fraxel (Reliant Technologies, Palo Alto, CA) was the first fractional laser. This was a nonablative 1550-nm Er-doped fiber laser that generated what was termed microscopic treatment zones. Being nonablative, the epidermis is thought to remain intact. Within the area of the thermal damage, there is heat-coagulated tissue termed microepidermal necrotic debris that is exfoliated through the intact epidermis. The theory is that melanin and elastic tissue will be removed, and the thermal injury will lead to collagen stimulation.
Since this first laser, there have been many nonablative lasers with a variety of wavelengths and theoretical mechanisms. These include 1410-nm, 1540-nm, and a combination of 1440- and 1320-nm light. These lasers are purported to treat acne scars, surgical scars, and facial photodamage, including fine rhytids and dyschromia, melasma, and striae distensae. Table 53.11 lists the nonablative fractional lasers.

Narurkar VA. Nonablative fractional laser resurfacing. *Dermatol Clin.* 2009;27:473–478.

Table 53.9 Diode lasers		
WAVELENGTH	**PULSE DURATION**	**USES**
532 nm	10–150 msec	Vascular lesions
810 nm	10–1000 msec	Hair removal Vascular lesions
1320 nm	20 msec	Nonablative resurfacing Acne scarring
1450 nm	3 msec	Nonablative resurfacing Acne scarring Acne treatment

Table 53.10 Pico lasers

WAVELENGTH	TYPE	COMPANY	NAME	USES
532, 1064, 694 nm	Nd:YAG, Ruby	Quanta System	Discovery Pico	Pigmented lesions, tattoo removal
532, 755, 785, 1064 nm	Nd:YAG, Alexandrite, Ti-sapphire	CynoSure	Picosure, Picosure FOCUS, PicoWay	Pigmented lesions, tattoo removal, skin rejuvenation, acne treatment
532, 670, 1064 nm	Nd:YAG	Cutera	Enlighten	Pigmented lesions, tattoo removal, skin rejuvenation
532, 585, 650, 1064 nm	Nd:YAG	Lumenis	PiQ04	Pigmented lesions, tattoo removal
532, 585, 595, 650, 1064 nm	Nd:YAG	WONTECH	Picocare	Pigmented lesions, tattoo removal
755 nm	Alexandrite	WONTECH	Picowon	Pigmented lesions, tattoo removal
532, 1064 nm	Nd:YAG	Lutronic	PICO+4	Pigmented lesions, tattoo removal, skin rejuvenation

Nd, **Neodymium**-doped; *YAG*, yttrium aluminum garnet.

38. What are ablative fractional lasers, and how are they used?

Ablative fractional lasers fire a vaporizing pulse into the skin forming a column of tissue ablation. The fractional lasers spread the pulses out using a variety of scanning devices. The theory of these fractional ablative lasers is to markedly reduce the healing time by spreading out the pulses, leaving normal epidermis between the pulses. As with nonfractional laser pulses, Er:YAG is more purely ablative than CO_2. The latter uses the surrounding tissue heating to help collagen contraction and remodeling. The first ablative fractional laser used was a 2940-nm (Er:YAG) laser called

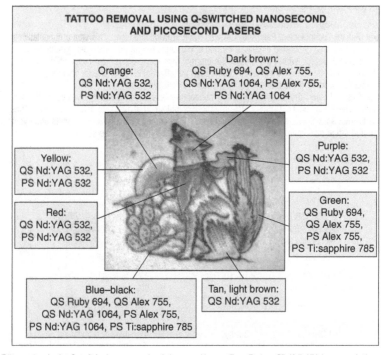

Fig. 53.2 Tattoo removal using Q-switched nanosecond and picosecond lasers. (From Zachary CB, Kelly KM. Lasers and other energy-based therapies. In: Bolognia JL, Schaffer JV, Cerroni L, eds. *Dermatology*. 4th ed. Philadelphia: Elsevier; 2018.)

Table 53.11 Nonablative fractional lasers

NAME	TYPE	WAVELENGTH
Fraxel re:fine	Single-mode fiber	1410 nm
Affirm	Nd:YAG	1320 nm/1440 nm
Lux1440 Fractional	Nd:YAG	1440 nm
Lux1540 Fractional	Er:glass	1540 nm
Fraxel re:store	Erbium fiber	1550 nm

Nd, Neodymium-doped; *YAG*, yttrium aluminum garnet.

PIXEL. This has been joined by other Er:YAG fractional devices and many CO_2 10,600-nm fractional lasers. There is even a diode 532-nm ablative fractional laser.

Fractional lasers are primarily used for cosmetic purposes. They help with mild to moderate facial rhytids, hyperpigmentation, and lentigines and are very effective in helping acne scarring. Table 53.12 lists the ablative fractional lasers.

Brightman LA, Brauer JA, Anolik R, et al. Ablative and fractional ablative lasers. *Dermatol Clin.* 2009;27:479–489.

39. What is an intense pulse light machine?

IPL is a system that uses a flashlamp to generate a high-energy pulse of noncoherent light. The spectrum usually runs from about 550 to 1200 nm. This light, having a wide spectrum, is then subjected to "cutoff" blocking filters to give specific starting wavelengths to each handpiece.

Raulin C, Greve B, Grema H. IPL technology: a review. *Lasers Surg Med.* 2003;32:78–87.

Table 53.12 Ablative fractional lasers

WAVELENGTH	TYPE	COMPANY	NAME
2940 nm	Er:YAG	Alma	PIXEL
2940 nm	Er:YAG	Cynosure	Affirm
2940 nm	Er:YAG	Focus Medical	NaturaLase Er
2940 nm	Er:YAG	Fotona	Dualis XS
2940 nm	Er:YAG	Fotona	Venus-i
2940 nm	Er:YAG	Palomar	Lux2940 Fractional
2940 nm	Er:YAG	Sciton	ProFractional
2790 nm	Er:YSGG	Cutera	Pearl Fractional
10,600 nm	CO_2	Alma	Pixel CO2
10,600 nm	CO_2	Candela	QuadraLASE
10,600 nm	CO_2	Cynosure	Afirm CO2
10,600 nm	CO_2	Eclipse	SmartXide DOT
10,600 nm	CO_2	LaseringUSA	MiXto XS
10,600 nm	CO_2	Lumenis	UltraPulse
10,600 nm	CO_2	Lutronics	eCO2
10,600 nm	CO_2	Solta Medical	Fraxel re:pair

Er, Erbium; *YAG*, yttrium aluminum garnet.

40. What are IPL machines used to treat?

The wide range of available wavelengths allows the IPLs to be very versatile. They have been used for hair removal, treatment of vascular lesions, treatment of pigmented lesions, and nonablative resurfacing. IPL machines have a base platform that delivers the energy to the handpiece. These handpieces now have not only pure IPL but also a variety of laser handpieces. These deliver many different wavelengths based on the different handpieces.

41. Are there any risks for intense pulse light use?

As with all of the lasers that have been discussed, there may be risks of hypopigmentation and hyperpigmentation with the IPL machines. Any delivery of high energy may rarely be associated with scarring.

42. Why is radiofrequency used in dermatology?

Radiofrequency (RF) energy is used to reduce fat, treat wrinkles, and treat acne scars. Unipolar RF and bipolar RF are used for circumferential fat reduction and cellulite treatments. Fractional RF is used in a treatment called Sublative to treat wrinkles, especially periorbital and acne scars. This may be the best available treatment for the latter condition.

Fitzpatrick RE, Geronemus R, Goldberg D, Kaminer M, Kilmer S, Ruiz-Esparza J. Multicenter study of noninvasive radiofrequency for periorbital tissue tightening. *Lasers Surg Med.* 2005;33:232–242.

43. Are there any risks with radiofrequency treatments?

There is some discomfort associated with this treatment when treating fat. RF does not see a color target and therefore may be used in all skin colors.

44. What are microwaves and how are they used?

Microwaves are between radiowaves and infrared light on the electromagnetic spectrum. MiraDry is a product that uses microwaves to treat hyperhidrosis (excessive sweating) via both eccrine and apocrine sweat gland thermolysis. The microwaves induce heat in water over fat and the subcutaneous tissue is protected while targeting the deeper dermis. The upper dermis protected with cooling (Fig. 53.3).

45. What is ultrasound used for?

Ultrasound is now used for fat cell destruction and skin tightening. Some machines use nonfocused devices and one now has a pulsed focused device. This technology has been shown to be helpful in destroying fat cells and tightening collagen. The Zimmer Gentle Pro uses painless shockwaves to help treat erectile dysfunction.

Hruza GJ, Taub AF, Collier SL, Mulholland SR. Skin rejuvenation and wrinkle reduction using a fractional radiofrequency system. *J Drugs Dermatol.* 2009;8:259–265.
Laubach HJ, Makin AR, Barthe PG, Slayton MH, Manstein D. Intense focused ultrasound: evaluation of a new treatment modality for precise microcoagulation within skin. *Dermatol Surg.* 2008;34:727–734.

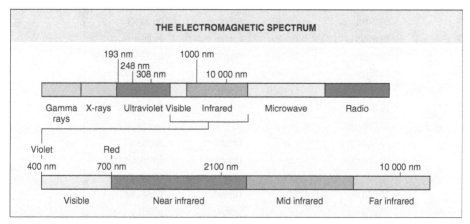

Fig. 53.3 The electromagnetic spectrum. The visible component is only a small portion of the spectrum. (From Sakamoto FH, Avram MM, Anderson RR. Lasers and other energy-based technologies—principles and skin interactions. In: Bolognia JL, Schaffer JV, Cerroni L, eds. *Dermatology.* 4th ed. Philadelphia: Elsevier; 2018.)

KEY POINTS: LASERS IN DERMATOLOGY

1. The wavelengths of common lasers are as follows: KTP, 532 nm; pulsed dye, 585 nm; ruby, 684 nm; alexandrite, 755 nm; diode, 810 to 1450 nm; Nd:YAG, 1064 nm; Er:YAG, 2490 nm; and carbon dioxide, 10,600 nm.
2. The carbon dioxide and the Er:YAG lasers are used for tissue ablation.
3. The pulsed dye laser is the gold standard for treatment of vascular lesions, but the KTP, Nd:YAG, and alexandrite lasers are also useful.
4. The long-pulsed alexandrite laser is the gold standard for laser hair removal, but the long-pulsed Nd:YAG and the long-pulsed ruby lasers are also used.
5. The Picosecond or Q-switched alexandrite and the Picosecond or Q-switched 532-nm Nd:YAG lasers are the gold standards for treatment of brown spots. The long-pulsed alexandrite is becoming very popular for this purpose.
6. Black tattoos are removed with the Picosecond or Q-switched 1064-nm Nd:YAG, the Picosecond or Q-switched alexandrite, and the Picosecond or Q-switched ruby lasers. Green tattoo pigment is removed only by the Picosecond or Q-switched alexandrite laser. Red tattoo pigment is removed only with the Picosecond or Q-switched 532-nm Nd:YAG laser.

CHAPTER 54

THERAPEUTIC PHOTOMEDICINE

Colby C. Evans

1. What is phototherapy?

   Phototherapy is the use of nonionizing electromagnetic radiation (usually in the ultraviolet [UV] range, but also extending into the visible light range) to treat cutaneous disease (Fig. 54.1).
   - Broadband ultraviolet B (BBUVB): 290 to 320 nm
   - Narrowband ultraviolet B (NBUVB): 311 nm
   - Xenon chloride (excimer) laser: 308 nm
   - Ultraviolet A (UVA): 320 to 400 nm
   - UVA-1: 340 to 400 nm
   - Psoralen plus UVA light (PUVA): 320 to 400 nm
   - Blue light in Soret band: Approximately 400 to 410 nm
   - Intense pulsed light and broadband light: 300 to >2000 nm

2. What diseases can be treated with phototherapy?

   See Table 54.1.

Gambichler T, Breuckmann F, Boms S, Altmeyer P, Kreutzer A. Narrowband UVB phototherapy in skin conditions beyond psoriasis. *J Am Acad Dermatol*. 2005;52:660–670.

---

3. How does traditional phototherapy work?

   Immunomodulation locally, and possibly systemically, is the primary mechanism of action of phototherapy. Effects on keratinocyte proliferation and differentiation are likely secondary to the immunomodulatory effects, which include:
   - T-cell apoptosis ($CD8^+$ in epidermis, $CD4^+$ in dermis)
   - Inhibition and depletion of antigen-presenting cells (Langerhans cells in epidermis, dermal dendritic cells in dermis)
   - Release of immunosuppressive cytokines (interleukin [IL]-10 and IL-4); reduced expression of tumor necrosis factor-α, interferon-γ, IL-12, IL-23, IL-17, IL-22 locally
   - Photoisomerization of trans-urocanic acid to cis-urocanic acid (which suppresses cellular immune responses, such as antigen presentation by Langerhans cells)
   - Upregulation of CD95L (Fas ligand that binds to the Fas receptor on T cells inducing apoptosis).

     As a result, the T-helper cell 1 and 17 (Th1/Th17) inflammatory pathways are suppressed, shifting the immune response toward the Th2 profile. IL-18, IL-8, IL-1β, and IL-6 are additional inflammatory mediators that may be suppressed.

Walters IB, Ozawa M, Cardinale I, et al. Narrowband (312-nm) UV-B suppresses interferon gamma and interleukin (IL) 12 and increases IL-4 transcripts: differential regulation of cytokines at the single-cell level. *Arch Dermatol*. 2003;139:155–161.

Johnson-Huang LM, Suárez-Fariñas M, Sullivan-Whalen M, Gilleaudeau P, Krueger JG, Lowes MA. Effective narrow-band UVB radiation therapy suppresses the IL-23/IL-17 axis in normalized psoriasis plaques. *J Invest Dermatol*. 2010;130:2654–2663.

---

4. How is phototherapy administered?

   It is usually administered in a physician's office or treatment center, or patients may purchase certain phototherapy units (usually ultraviolet B [UVB]) and treat themselves at home. Distance from the treatment center may lead to poor adherence due to time and inconvenience of travel, so patients should be appropriately selected for in-office or home treatment. Home- and office-based phototherapy appears to be similar in both effectiveness and cost, while patients prefer home treatment. Patients receive a controlled dose of UV light while standing in a booth lined with high-output UV light bulbs (Fig. 54.2). The initial UV light exposure is determined by assessing the patient's skin type and history of burning or by establishing the minimal erythema dose (MED). Phototherapy can also be combined with other treatments, as in oral retinoids with PUVA (RePUVA), which can lower the necessary dose of both treatments, or combining low-dose NBUVB, with tofacitinib which has been shown to repigment vitiligo. Phototherapy combined with etanercept or adalimumab may result in better clearance than either treatment alone.

Weng QY, Buzney E, Joyce C, Mostaghimi A. Distance of travel to phototherapy is associated with early nonadherence: a retrospective cohort study. *J Am Acad Dermatol*. 2016;74(6):1256–1259.

ELECTROMAGNETIC SPECTRUM

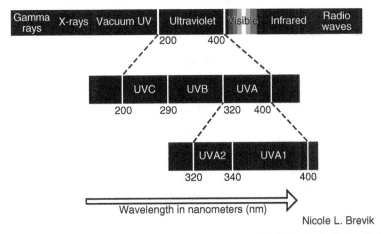

Nicole L. Brevik

Fig. 54.1 Electromagnetic spectrum. *UV*, ultraviolet; *UVA*, ultraviolet A; *UVB*, ultraviolet B; *UVC*, ultraviolet C. (Courtesy Nicole L. Brevik.)

Koek MB, Buskens E, van Weelden H, Steegmans PH, Bruijnzeel-Koomen CA, Sigurdsson V. Home versus outpatient ultraviolet B phototherapy for mild to severe psoriasis: pragmatic multicentre randomised controlled non-inferiority trial (PLUTO study). *BMJ*. 2009;338:b1542.
Kim SR, Heaton H, Liu LY, King BA. Rapid repigmentation of vitiligo using tofacitinib plus low-dose, narrowband UV-B phototherapy. *JAMA Dermatol*. 2018;154(3):370–371.
Armstrong AW, Bagel J, Van Voorhees AS, Robertson AD, Yamauchi PS. Combining biologic therapies with other systemic treatments in psoriasis: evidence-based, best-practice recommendations from the Medical Board of the National Psoriasis Foundation. *JAMA Dermatol*. 2015;151(4):432–438.

5. Compare the induction phase, maintenance phase, and tapering phase for various forms of phototherapy.
   Induction phase:
   - BBUVB: Daily or three times weekly treatments, increasing approximately 10% each treatment until pink or therapeutic level reached.
   - NBUVB: Three times weekly, increasing approximately 10%–20% each treatment until pink or therapeutic level reached.
   - UVA-1: Daily or three times weekly, usually set at a standard dose depending on condition being treated. High-dose regimens (130 J/cm^2), medium-dose regimens (30 to 50 J/cm^2), and low-dose regimens (20 J/cm^2) can used.
   - PUVA: Two to three times weekly, increasing 0.5 to 1 J/cm^2 each treatment until pink or therapeutic level reached.
   The induction phase is continued until clearing of skin lesions is noted, the patient has burning, or the end point is reached. Periods of remission with NBUVB and PUVA may last for weeks to months even after treatment is stopped.
   Maintenance phase:
   - BBUVB: Ranges from three times weekly to once every other week.
   - NBUVB: Taper to between once weekly to once every other week.
   - UVA-1: Once weekly to once every other week.
   - PUVA: Once every other week to once monthly.
   Tapering phase:
   Decreasing frequency of treatments over a period of 1 to 2 months until the patient is completely tapered off therapy or enters maintenance therapy. If flaring of disease occurs after discontinuing therapy or during maintenance therapy, the frequency can be increased or the induction phase restarted. Long-duration treatment is often required for vitiligo, where the most benefit can be expected on the head and neck.
   Note: The tanning effect may significantly decrease after 2 weeks, and the potential for burning patients with treatments spaced greater than every 2 weeks is much higher. Therefore, exercise caution and consider decreasing dose if greater than 2 weeks have elapsed since the last treatment.

Bae JM, Jung HM, Hong BY, et al. Phototherapy for vitiligo: a systematic review and meta-analysis. *JAMA Dermatol*. 2017; 153(7):666–674.

Table 54.1 Diseases treated with phototherapy

DISEASE	PHOTOTHERAPY TYPE	EFFECTIVENESS	EVIDENCE
Psoriasis	Broadband UVB	++	+++
	Narrowband UVB	+++	+++
	PUVA	+++	+++
	308-nm laser	+++	++
	595-nm laser	+	+
Vitiligo	Broadband UVB	++	++
	Narrowband UVB	+++	+++
	PUVA	+++	+++
	308-nm laser	+++	++
Cutaneous T-cell lymphoma (mycosis fungoides)	Broadband UVB	+	+
	Narrowband UVB	+++	++
	PUVA	+++	+++
	UVA-1	+	+
Parapsoriasis	Broadband UVB	+	—
	Narrowband UVB	+++	+
	PUVA	+++	++
Atopic dermatitis	UVA	++	++
	Broadband UVB	+	+
	Narrowband UVB	++	++
	PUVA	++	+
	UVA-1	++	++
Polymorphous light eruption	Broadband UVB	+	+
	Narrowband UVB	++	+
	PUVA	+++	++
	UVA	+	+
Actinic prurigo	Broadband UVB	+	+
	Narrowband UVB	++	+
	PUVA	++	+
Chronic actinic dermatitis/actinic reticuloid	Narrowband UVB	+	+
	PUVA	+	+
Pityriasis rosea	Broadband UVB	+	+
	Narrowband UVB	++	+
	PUVA	++	
Pityriasis lichenoides	Broadband UVB	++	+
	Narrowband UVB	++	+
Nummular dermatitis	Broadband UVB	+	+
	Narrowband UVB	++	+
	PUVA	++	+
Dyshidrotic eczema	UVA-1	+	+

Table 54.1 Diseases treated with phototherapy (*Continued*)

DISEASE	PHOTOTHERAPY TYPE	EFFECTIVENESS	EVIDENCE
Lichen planus	Broadband UVB	+	+
	Narrowband UVB	+	+
	PUVA	+	+
Graft-versus-host disease	Narrowband UVB	+	+
	PUVA	++	++
HIV-associated pruritus	UVB	+	+
	UVA	+	+
Pruritus associated with renal failure	Broadband UVB	++	+
	Narrowband UVB	−	−
	PUVA	−	−
Pruritus associated with polycythemia vera	UVA/B	+	+
	Narrowband UVB	+	+
	PUVA	+	+
Seborrheic dermatitis	Narrowband UVB	+	+
	PUVA	+	+
Acquired perforating disorders	UVB	+	+
	Narrowband UVB	+	+
Morphea/progressive systemic sclerosis	UVA-1	++	+++
	PUVA	++	+
	Narrowband UVB	+	+
Systemic lupus	UVA-1	+	++
Lichen sclerosus	UVA-1	+	+
Nephrogenic systemic fibrosis	UVA-1	+	+
Solar urticaria	Broadband UVB	+	+
	Narrowband UVB	+	+
	UVA	+	+
	PUVA	++	+
Cutaneous mastocytosis	PUVA	++	+
	UVA-1	+	+
	Narrowband UVB	+	+

−, Not effective or not studied; +, case reports; ++, small studies; +++, controlled studies or strong evidence.
PUVA, psoralen + UVA; *UVA*, ultraviolet A; *UVB*, ultraviolet B.

6. What advantages does narrowband UVB have over broadband UVB?
   NBUVB utilizes a TL-01 light source emitting UV light almost exclusively at 311 to 312 nm, which is near the most effective action spectrum for induction of T-cell apoptosis and suppression of dendritic antigen presenting cells in inflammatory skin diseases such as psoriasis. The absence of other wavelengths of UV light decreases side effects (erythema, carcinogenesis, photoaging) without sacrificing efficacy. Unlike BBUVB, suberythemogenic doses are effective.

7. What advantages does narrowband UVB have over PUVA? PUVA or UVB?
   Oral psoralens have many potential side effects, including:
   • **Gastrointestinal**: nausea, vomiting
   • **Neurological**: dizziness, headache, insomnia, depression and anxiety

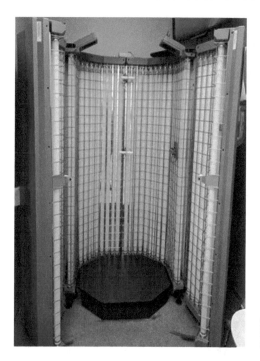

Fig. 54.2 Typical ultraviolet booth demonstrating banks of bulbs. Most modern ultraviolet booths deliver either both ultraviolet B (UVB) and ultraviolet A or deliver narrowband UVB.

- **Systemic**: hepatotoxicity, drug interactions, allergic reactions, narrow window of phototherapy treatment after taking medication (1 to 2 hours), variability of tissue response depending on medication absorption and distribution (which is time sensitive)
- **Cutaneous**: photoallergic reactions, PUVA keratoses, PUVA lentigines, PUVA pain, transient nail pigmentation, photo-onycholysis, facial hypertrichosis, lichenoid eruptions, photosensitivity for 24 hours (even through windows), substantially increased risk of melanoma and other skin cancers including genital skin cancer
- **Ophthalmologic**: risk of cataracts, need for special glasses and avoid natural sunlight after taking medication for 24 hours.

PUVA can be provided with the psoralens applied topically, either as a cream or in a bath. This process may reduce the risks of some systemic side effects but is often impractical for routine use. PUVA has been shown more likely to induce complete remission in cutaneous T-cell lymphoma (CTCL) (mycosis fungoides) compared to UVB (73.8% vs. 62.2%).

Patients in all types of phototherapy should wear appropriate eye protection and cover their genitals, as phototherapy is a known risk factor for genital squamous cell carcinoma.

NBUVB does not carry most of these side effects and has not demonstrated increased carcinogenicity thus far in humans, and the efficacy is similar. However, increased carcinogenicity has been noted in rats with NBUVB, and long-term follow-up is not yet available.

Laube S, George SA. Adverse effects with PUVA and UVB phototherapy. *J Dermatol Treat.* 2001;12:101–105.
Phan K, Ramachandran V, Fassihi H, Sebaratnam DF. Comparison of narrowband UV-B with psoralen-UV-A phototherapy for patients with early-stage mycosis fungoides: a systematic review and meta-analysis. *JAMA Dermatol.* 2019;55:335–341.
Weischer M, Blum A, Eberhard F, Röcken M, Berneburg M. No evidence for increased skin cancer risk in psoriasis patients treated with broadband or narrowband UVB phototherapy: a first retrospective study. *Acta Derm Venereol.* 2004;84(5):370–374.
Douglawi A, Masterson TA. Penile cancer epidemiology and risk factors: a contemporary review. *Curr Opin Urol.* 2019;29(2):145–149.

8. What is targeted laser phototherapy?

An excimer (XeCl) laser, which emits a wavelength of 308 nm (near the NBUVB wavelength of 311 nm), is effective in treating individual psoriatic plaques and patches of vitiligo (Fig. 54.3). Supererythemogenic doses, from 6 to 8 MEDs, are used on individual psoriasis plaques for 8 to 12 treatments and may induce months of remission. It is advantageous in that it avoids irradiating healthy, nonlesional skin. It more effectively induces T-cell apoptosis, as well. In psoriasis, it targets individual plaques with higher fluences and reaches deeper T cells and dendritic cells within the dermis. The pulsed dye laser at 585 to 595 nm has also been shown to be efficacious in treating individual psoriatic plaques but appears less effective than the 308-nm excimer laser.

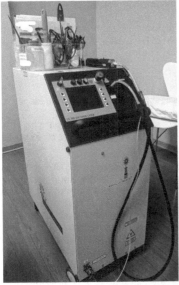
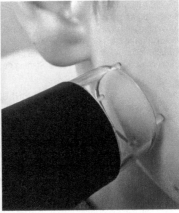

Fig. 54.3 Excimer laser device and handpiece.

Nicolaidou E, Antoniou C, Stratigos A, Katsambas AD. Narrowband ultraviolet B phototherapy and 308-nm excimer laser in the treatment of vitiligo: a review. *J Am Acad Dermatol.* 2009;60:470–477.
Zakarian K, Nguyen A, Letsinger J, Koo J. Excimer laser for psoriasis: a review of theories regarding enhanced efficacy over traditional UVB phototherapy. *J Drugs Dermatol.* 2007;6:794–798.

9. What is UVA-1 phototherapy and why is it used?

UVA-1 is 340- to 400-nm UV light used mainly to treat atopic dermatitis, morphea, and progressive systemic sclerosis. It is less effective than UVB in treating psoriasis, mycosis fungoides, and other inflammatory skin disorders. It has a different mechanism of action:

- Inducing superoxide anion and singlet oxygen–induced T-cell apoptosis.
- Reducing Langerhans cell migration out of the epidermis.
- Decreasing the number of IgE-bearing Langerhans cells and dendritic cells in the epidermis and dermis.
- Decreasing collagen synthesis increasing collagenase I and matrix metalloproteinases in sclerosing disorders of the skin.

UVA-1 penetrates deeper than UVB and appears more effective in cutaneous mastocytosis compared in depleting mast cells from the skin. UVA-1 does not increase viral load in HIV-positive patients. Uniquely, UVA-1 induces immediate (<20 minutes) apoptosis in T cells compared to UVB, which is delayed. UVA-1 can also be used to treat patients with systemic lupus, including subacute cutaneous lupus, unlike UVB which can exacerbate lupus.

York NR, Jacobe HT. UVA1 phototherapy: a review of mechanism and therapeutic application. *Int J Dermatol.* 2010;49:623–630.
Ordóñez Rubiano MF, Arenas CM, Chalela JG. UVA-1 phototherapy for the management of atopic dermatitis: a large retrospective study conducted in a low-middle income country. *Int J Dermatol.* 2018;57(7):799–803.

10. What is the Soret band?

The 400- to 410-nm spectrum of blue light, which is the absorption spectrum of porphyrins. It is an important spectrum in photodynamic therapy (PDT). It is named after Jacques-Louis Soret, who discovered this band in 1883.

11. What is balneophototherapy?

Salt water bathing in combination with UV phototherapy or even natural sunlight (such as patients who visit the Dead Sea to treat psoriasis). Potential mechanisms of action include the following:

- Magnesium salts may decrease antigen presentation in the skin.
- Water-soaked skin allows more UV light to penetrate the skin due to decreased reflectance.
- Possible neuropsychiatric influence (relaxation, vacation, decreased stress).

Use of natural sunlight alone to treat skin disease is called *heliotherapy* and is generally discouraged due to lack of monitoring, lack of targeted treatment, and the risk of skin cancer.

12. **What do minimal erythema dose (MED) and minimal phototoxic dose (MPD) mean and why are they important?**
    Minimal erythema dose (UVB and UVA) and minimal phototoxic dose (PUVA), which represent the lowest dose that produces erythema (sunburn reaction) of the skin. The MED varies depending on the method of phototherapy and skin type.
    - UVA: 20 to 40 J/cm^2 (maximum erythema noted within 12 hours of treatment)
    - BBUVB: 20 to 40 mJ/cm^2 (within 24 hours)
    - NBUVB: 200 to 400 mJ/cm^2 (48 to 72 hours)
    - PUVA: 4 to 15 J/cm^2 (48 to 72 hours)
    - BBUVB is approximately 1000 times more erythemogenic than is UVA. Note that UVA is measured in J/cm^2 and UVB is measured in mJ/cm^2

        MED/MPD testing may be helpful, as it allows the clinician to start phototherapy at a higher dose, achieving quicker responses with fewer treatments. Starting doses based on skin type as more convenient but less precise.

13. **What is Goeckerman therapy?**
    Goeckerman therapy, named in honor of Dr. William H. Goeckerman, who developed it in 1925, is UVB phototherapy used in combination with topical coal tar to treat psoriasis. The therapy is administered by having patients apply crude coal tar or tar derivatives to the skin and removing the excess tar before exposure to UVB. After treatment, the patient takes a bath or shower to remove any remaining tar or scale. With each visit, the dose of UVB administered is gradually increased, with the treatment being administered three or more times per week for 3 to 4 weeks or longer. This extremely safe treatment can be supplemented with topical corticosteroid preparations or descaling agents. Patients may stay in remission for 12 to 18 months or longer. Long remission rates and relative safety have made this the therapy of choice in many psoriasis treatment centers. Disadvantages include its inconvenience, messiness of the tar, and need for numerous office visits.

14. **What are the most common acute UVB phototherapy side effects?**
    The most common acute side effect is a sunburn-like effect within 24 to 48 hours of treatment manifested by erythema and tenderness of the skin. When this occurs, therapy is usually withheld until the erythema fades, and the amount of UVB administered is usually reduced at the next treatment session. Patients who fail to wear eye protection that blocks UVB may develop corneal burns. Occasionally, patients with psoriasis may experience temporary pustular flares of psoriasis during treatment. Topical preparations used in conjunction with UVB phototherapy, such as emollients and tar, may produce a folliculitis. This complication can be prevented by instructing the patient to apply topical preparations in a downward fashion to prevent follicular irritation. A severe blistering burn is rare when UVB is properly administered and may be associated with *Koebner's isomorphic phenomenon*, resulting in psoriatic plaques in the burned area of skin.

15. **What are the most common long-term UVB phototherapy side effects?**
    Long-term side effects include skin cancer and skin aging (dermatoheliosis). The exact risk of skin cancer has not been determined, but it is greater in patients with fair skin, a family history of skin cancer, or who use other therapies associated with a risk of producing skin cancer (i.e., PUVA, cyclosporine). Patients with prolonged UVB therapy and other risk factors should have periodic skin examinations to detect early skin cancers. Thus far, NBUVB has not been associated with increased cancer risk.

16. **What is PUVA phototherapy?**
    PUVA is an acronym for psoralen and UV light, type A. It involves the combined use of a prescription psoralen (methoxsalen or trioxsalen) and long-wave UV light (UVA). PUVA therapy for psoriasis was approved by the Food and Drug Administration in 1982 and became one of the treatments of choice for many adult patients with extensive patch- and plaque-type psoriasis and mycosis fungoides prior to the advent of NBUVB. The psoralen usually is administered orally (sometimes topically) and followed by exposure to UVA light. While UVA is most commonly delivered in booths, special portable units are also available to treat the hands, feet, and scalp (Fig. 54.4). PUVA has declined in popularity in the United States as it has been replaced by safer effective treatments like NBUVB and biologic therapy for psoriasis.

17. **What are psoralens?**
    Psoralens are a subclass of drugs that belong to a group of compounds called furocoumarins, which are derived from the fusion of a furan with coumarin (Fig. 54.5). Psoralens are natural constituents in a large variety of medicinal plants (e.g., limes, lemons, figs, parsnips). The two psoralens that are used therapeutically in the United States are methoxsalen and trioxsalen. Methoxsalen (8-methoxypsoralen [8-MOP]) is a naturally occurring photoactive plant substance found in the seeds of *Amnii majus*, a plant that grows wild along the Nile delta. Methoxsalen is absorbed from the upper gastrointestinal tract and metabolized by the intestine and liver. Ninety percent is excreted within 24 hours, with the major portion being excreted in the urine. Trioxsalen is a synthetic psoralen usually reserved for the treatment of vitiligo.

18. **How do the psoralens work?**
    Psoralen compounds by themselves do not affect the skin in the absence of UVA, but in the presence of UVA (320 to 400 nm), they are potent photosensitizers. Ninety minutes after oral ingestion, absorption of UVA photons photochemically links DNA by forming cycloadditive products between the intercalated psoralen and the pyrimidine bases of cellular DNA. These psoralen-DNA cross-links cause a decrease in the rate of epidermal DNA synthesis, which some authorities believe to be the primary mechanism of action of these agents. Irradiation of psoralens also induces the formation of reactive oxygen species that can damage both cell membranes and organelles, as well as activate arachidonic acid metabolism. There is considerable evidence that PUVA therapy has a direct effect on the

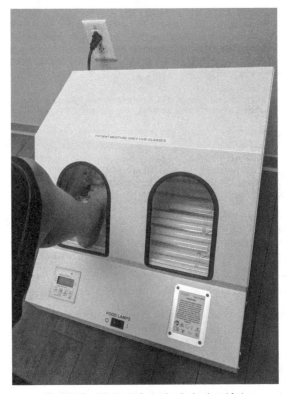

Fig. 54.4 Specialized units for treating the hands and feet.

cutaneous immune system, and some authorities feel that this may be more important in terms of the therapeutic effect. The induction of T-cell apoptosis, decreased function of antigen-presenting cells, and altered cytokine profile is likely the most important component of PUVA therapy.

19. Are there contraindications to using PUVA?
    Contraindications include:
    - history of psoralen hypersensitivity reactions
    - photosensitive diseases including lupus erythematosus
    - porphyria
    - xeroderma pigmentosum
    - albinism
    - history of malignant melanoma
    - pregnancy
    - aphakia (absence of a lens may produce retinal damage).
      PUVA should be used with caution in patients with fair skin, a history of previous ionizing radiation, history of multiple skin cancers, cataracts, immunosuppression, uremia, or renal failure. Patients with disabilities that may disallow standing for prolonged periods in the treatment cabinet may not be able to receive phototherapy.

20. What is bath PUVA?
    The patient is immersed for 15 minutes in a bathtub containing five 10-mg capsules of methoxsalen dissolved in the water. Topical methoxsalen gradually loses its photoactivity, and the patient should ideally be treated with the standard

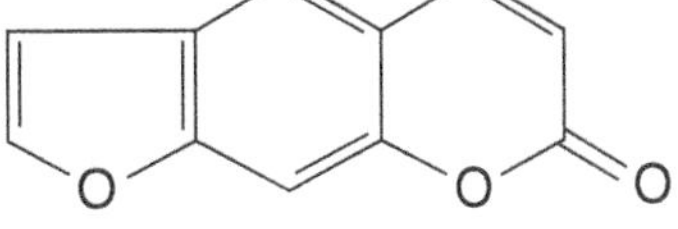

Fig. 54.5 Molecular structure of furocoumarin from plants of the *Psoralea* genus.

UVA light treatments within 15 minutes after immersion. Bath PUVA therapy using trimethylpsoralen, which is more hydrophobic than 8-MOP, has been used for more than 30 years in Sweden and Finland, with no observed increase in the number of skin cancers. It is also useful for patients who are not able to tolerate oral methoxsalen because of nausea, and for children under 15 years of age. Hand and foot dermatoses are uniquely suited for this type of therapy. Disadvantages include the time required, falls in the bath environment (especially for elderly patients), expense, and requirement to sanitize the facilities between patients.

Coven TR, Murphy FP, Gilleaudeau P, Cardinale I, Krueger JG. Trimethylpsoralen bath PUVA is a remittive treatment for psoriasis vulgaris. Evidence that epidermal immunocytes are direct therapeutic targets. *Arch Dermatol.* 1998;134:1263–1268.

KEY POINTS: THERAPEUTIC PHOTOMEDICINE

1. Phototherapy is used to treat many inflammatory skin diseases, is safe and effective, has relatively low cost, and provides another tool for the dermatologist to treat patients.
2. NBUVB is now the phototherapy treatment of choice for psoriasis, vitiligo, and possibly mycosis fungoides (patch stage) and atopic dermatitis given its superior efficacy to broadband UVB and decreased side effects compared to oral PUVA.
3. Phototherapy exerts its effects primarily through immunomodulation (T-cell apoptosis within the epidermis and dermis, and suppression/depletion of Langerhans cells within the epidermis).
4. Photodynamic therapy utilizes aminolevulinic acid, which is converted to protoporphyrin IX in keratinocytes, and when illuminated with blue or red light is activated, producing phototoxic products and free radicals that induce cellular apoptosis.
5. PUVA is the acronym for psoralen and UVA.
6. Treatment with PUVA is associated with an increased risk of skin cancer, including squamous cell carcinoma and malignant melanoma.
7. RePUVA is the combination of a retinoid (e.g., acitretin) and PUVA, which may allow lower doses of both treatments to be used.

21. What is RePUVA?

RePUVA treatment uses an oral retinoid (usually acitretin) and PUVA in combination. Studies suggest that this therapeutic combination offers a practical way to clear psoriasis (with an overall response rate of 73%) with less cumulative UVA exposure than PUVA alone. Additionally, RePUVA can be successfully applied in patients resistant to standard PUVA. Patients receiving acitretin plus PUVA clear 40% faster than those treated with PUVA alone, even though the UVA dose is reduced by 50%. Most commonly, the oral acitretin is begun 7 to 10 days before the first PUVA treatment, and the two therapies are given concurrently until maximal clearing occurs. The acitretin is usually discontinued, and the patient is maintained on PUVA for about 2 months. Retinoids may also be used in combination with BBUVB and NBUVB (known as ReUVB).

22. What is photopheresis?

Photopheresis, also known as extracorporeal photochemotherapy (ECP), is a form of apheresis therapy. First introduced for the treatment of CTCL, it has since been evaluated in studies and randomized trials as a potential treatment for autoimmune diseases, solid organ transplant rejection, and graft-versus-host disease (GVHD). ECP involves discontinuous leukapheresis by centrifugation, followed by exposure of the buffy coat lymphocytes to UVA light in a special unit about 2 hours after the administration of methoxsalen. Following exposure of the lymphocytes to UVA, the photoirradiated cells are reinfused into the patient. The procedure is done on two consecutive days at 4-week intervals. The adverse side effects are usually minimal; patients may experience nausea and about 10% develop a transient fever after reinfusion. Iron deficiency anemia is a known risk of treatment.

Sanford KW, Anderson J, Roseff S, McPherson RA. Iron deficiency anemia in patients undergoing extracorporeal photopheresis for cutaneous T-cell lymphoma. *Lab Med.* 2019;50(1):29–33.

23. Which diseases have been treated with extracorporeal photopheresis?

Photopheresis is used for the treatment of CTCL (mycosis fungoides). It is most effective in the erythrodermic variants (Sézary syndrome) that involve greater than 25% of the body surface. The response rate in this group of patients is about 64%. Photopheresis has also been successfully used in treating graft vs. host disease without altering the frequency of regulatory T cells. Lack of response to photopheresis in GVHD is associated with increased transplant-related mortality. Photopheresis, as a form of immunotherapy, has also been tried on other T cell–mediated diseases, such as pemphigus vulgaris, chronic Lyme arthritis, psoriatic arthritis, and progressive systemic sclerosis.

Zic JA. Photopheresis in the treatment of cutaneous T-cell lymphoma: current status. *Curr Opin Oncol.* 2012;24(suppl 1):S1–S10.

Gandelman JS, Song DJ, Chen H, et al. A prospective trial of extracorporeal photopheresis for chronic graft-versus-host disease reveals significant disease response and no association with frequency of regulatory T cells. *Biol Blood Marrow Transplant.* 2018;24 (12):2373–2380.

Sakellari I, Gavriilaki E, Batsis I, et al. Favorable impact of extracorporeal photopheresis in acute and chronic graft versus host disease: Prospective single-center study. *J Clin Apher.* 2018;33(6):654–660.

24. How is PDT used in dermatology?

PDT is a two-step process. A photosensitizing agent is topically applied to the patient's skin, followed by illumination with a light source of the proper wavelength. Aminolevulinic acid is used most often in the United States and is converted to protoporphyrin IX by keratinocytes. Keratinocytes lack the final enzyme in the heme synthesis pathway, and the process ends with protoporphyrin IX, which is photosensitizing, particularly in the Soret band (400 to 410 nm). Porphyrins used in combination with blue (415 to 425 nm) or red (600 to 700 nm) light are the most common forms of PDT. Smaller absorption peaks are also noted around 585 to 595 nm, which correlates with the pulsed dye laser absorption spectrum. Cancer cells and precancerous cells derived from keratinocytes (actinic keratoses, squamous cell carcinomas, basal cell carcinomas) accumulate porphyrins at higher concentrations than normal keratinocytes and are more susceptible to the phototoxic effects of the treatment. Treatment of actinic keratoses with PDT may be more cosmetically acceptable than traditional treatments like cryotherapy. In acne, *Propionibacterium acnes* is susceptible to both blue light alone and to porphyrin-induced injury. The sebaceous glands in the skin accumulate significant amounts of porphyrin and are very susceptible to injury by PDT. When used in combination with the pulsed dye laser at 585 to 595 nm or red light–emitting diodes, deeper penetration into the sebaceous gland is achieved and a better therapeutic outcome is noted when treating acne. After three monthly treatments, acne may stay in remission for up to 1 year. PDT has been tried for many other skin conditions, including cosmetic improvement, prurigo nodularis, and disseminated superficial actinic porokeratosis. It can be quite painful, especially with long incubation times of the photosensitizer. The use of a microneedle roller can reduce incubation times from 1 hour to 20 minutes with similar efficacy. Other pretreatments have also been shown to increase photosensitizer uptakes, including curettage, microdermabrasion with abrasive pads, microneedling with dermarollers, and ablative fractional laser.

Petukhova TA, Hassoun LA, Foolad N, Barath M, Sivamani RK. Effect of expedited microneedle-assisted photodynamic therapy for field treatment of actinic keratoses: a randomized clinical trial. *JAMA Dermatol.* 2017;153(7):637–643.

Bay C, Lerche CM, Ferrick B, Philipsen PA, Togsverd-Bo K, Haedersdal M. Comparison of physical pretreatment regimens to enhance protoporphyrin IX uptake in photodynamic therapy: a randomized clinical trial. *JAMA Dermatol.* 2017;153(4):270–278.

25. What is blue light phototherapy?

Some degree of jaundice is common in newborns and is seen in up to 50% of infants between the second and fourth day of life. Before birth, bilirubin is conjugated and excreted chiefly by the placenta; however, after birth, this function shifts to the neonatal liver. Transient neonatal hyperbilirubinemia is the result of insufficient activity of the conjugative hepatic enzyme glucuronyl transferase. Phototherapy with blue light (430 to 490 nm) is an effective means of preventing hyperbilirubinemia by producing a photoproduct called photobilirubin, which is nontoxic. In the treatment of hyperbilirubinemia, phototherapy should be considered at serum bilirubin levels of 222 to 260 mmol/L, after considering other clinical factors. Blue light phototherapy alone is also used to treat acne vulgaris. *P. acnes* is susceptible to blue light (415 to 425 nm) and is significantly reduced in number within the pilosebaceous unit with treatment. Improvement in acne has been reported.

CHAPTER 55

RETINOIDS

Brian J. Abittan and Gary Goldenberg

KEY POINTS

1. Retinoids are structural or functional analogs of vitamin A (retinol).
2. In dermatology, topical tretinoins are mainly used in the treatment of acne vulgaris, psoriasis, and photoaging.
3. Oral retinoids are mostly used to treat severe acne, cutaneous T-cell lymphoma, and psoriasis.
4. Oral retinoids require strict monitoring, specifically due to their teratogenicity.

1. What are retinoids?
   Retinoids are structural or functional analogs of vitamin A (retinol). Vitamin A is a fat-soluble vitamin. It is obtained directly from our diet (liver) or produced from carotenoids, a pigmented precursor found in yellow vegetables (carrots). The role of retinoids in cutaneous biology was discovered by S. Burt Wolbach, who noted that vitamin A–deficient animals had altered keratinization. This finding led von Stuettgen and Bollag to treat skin disorders with various forms of vitamin A.

2. How do retinoids work at the molecular level?
   Vitamin A influences cells by binding to nuclear retinoic acid receptors (RARs) and other retinoid X receptors (RXRs) leading to downstream biological effects. These nuclear receptors contain three isotypes (α, β, and γ). Different retinoids vary in their individual affinity for these receptors, accounting for the variety of pharmacologic effects produced by different retinoids. Additionally, various tissues have distinct expressions of receptor subtypes, allowing regulation of vitamin A by altering the concentration of these binding proteins.

3. What are the different categories of retinoids used in the treatment of skin disorder?
   There are three generations of synthetic retinoids. First-generation retinoids are nonaromatic, second-generation are monoaromatic, and third-generation are polyaromatic. See Table 55.1.

4. Which retinoids are prescribed for the treatment of skin disorders?
   Oral and topical formulations of retinoids are used in the treatment of skin disorders. Oral synthetic formulations available in the United States are isotretinoin, acitretin, and bexarotene. Etretinate has been taken off the market and is no longer available in the United States. There are multiple Food and Drug Administration (FDA)–approved topical retinoids currently available. Tretinoin, all trans-retinoic acid, is a natural metabolite of vitamin A and the most bioactive topical retinoid. Tazarotene (synthetic vitamin A analog), alitretinoin (9-cis retinoic acid), and adapalene (receptor selective retinoid analog) are other topical options. See Table 55.2.

5. Are there any retinoids used in topical over-the-counter products?
   There are currently no over-the-counter (OTC) products available with tretinoin as the active ingredient. However, adapalene is now available OTC. While this is the first prescription-strength retinoid available OTC, studies have shown it to be less efficacious than tretinoin. Additionally, multiple other formulations, mostly used in topical rejuvenation and antiaging products, are also available OTC.
   Retinol, an alcohol formulation of vitamin A, and retinal, an aldehyde formulation, are both well tolerated and commonly used in OTC cosmeceuticals. However, they are significantly less potent than tretinoin. Retinyl esters (retinyl palmitate and retinyl acetate) are also commonly used in OTC products. It is important to note that these formulations must be enzymatically converted into their active form, retinoic acid, before they are able to bind to retinoid receptors. As such, these formulations are susceptible to oxidation and less effective than prescription retinoids.

6. What are the clinical indications for topical tretinoin?
   The FDA has approved topical tretinoin for the treatment of acne, psoriasis, cutaneous T-cell lymphoma, kaposi sarcoma, mottled facial pigmentation, and dermatoheliosis. In clinical practice, however, topical tretinoin has been used to treat many other dermatologic conditions. See Table 55.3.

7. What are the main side effects of topical tretinoin?
   The most commonly experienced side effect from the use of topical tretinoin is skin irritation, or "retinoid dermatitis," characterized by erythema and peeling/scaling. These reactions can be mitigated by decreasing the concentration, frequency, or duration of application and increasing as tolerated. Additionally, the use of moisturizers is helpful as well. Alternatively, avoiding the areas most frequently involved (perioral) is another option. Many patients do report a decreased tolerance to ultraviolet exposure. As such, patients should be counseled on proper sun protection. Allergic contact dermatitis to topical tretinoin is rare.

Table 55.1 Retinoid classes

Retinoids	
First generation	- Tretinoin - Isotretinoin - Alitretinoin
Second generation	- Acitretin - Etretinate
Third generation	- Bexarotene - Tazarotene - Adapalene

Table 55.2 Prescription retinoids

TOPICAL PREPARATIONS	ORAL PREPARATIONS
Tretinoin (All-trans Retinoic Acid) Retin-A (0.025%, 0.05%, 0.1% cream; 0.025% gel; 0.05% liquid) Retin-A Micro (0.04%, 0.1% gel microsphere) Renova (0.02%, 0.05% emollient cream) Altreno (0.05% lotion) Avita (0.025% cream and gel) Atralin (0.05% gel) Refissa (0.05% cream)	**Isotretinoin (13-cis-Retinoic Acid)** Multiple brands (10, 20, 30, and 40 mg capsules) **Acitretin** Soriatane (10 and 25 mg capsules) **Bexarotene** Targretin (75-mg capsules)
Tazarotene Avage (0.1% cream) Tazorac (0.05%, 0.1% gel) Alitretinoin (9-cis-Retinoic Acid) Panretin (0.1% gel)	
Adapalene (Retinoid-Like Drug) Differin (0.1% gel, solution, cream, pledgets) Epiduo (also contains benzoyl peroxide)	

Generic drugs appear as bold terms in the list.

Table 55.3 Dermatologic uses of topical retinoids

FDA-APPROVED INDICATIONS	SELECTED NONAPPROVED APPLICATIONS
Acne vulgaris (tretinoin, tazarotene, adapalene) Dermatoheliosis/photoaging (tretinoin, tazarotene) Psoriasis (tazarotene) Kaposi sarcoma (alitretinoin) Cutaneous T-cell lymphoma (bexarotene)	Acanthosis nigricans Actinic keratoses Fox-Fordyce disease Ichthyoses (e.g., ichthyosis vulgaris, lamellar ichthyosis) Keloids and hypertrophic scars Keratosis follicularis (Darier's disease) Keratosis pilaris Lichen planus (cutaneous and oral) Linear epidermal nevus Melasma (chloasma) Nevus comedonicus Porokeratosis Pityriasis rubra pilaris Postinflammatory hyperpigmentation Psoriasis Reactive perforating collagenosis Rosacea Striae distensae (stretch marks) Verruca plana (flat warts) Wound healing

FDA, Food and Drug Administration.

8. Is topical tretinoin safe to use during pregnancy or when nursing?

To date, there are no studies showing congenital disorders caused by the use of topical tretinoin during pregnancy. Systemic absorption of topical tretinoin has been shown to be negligible. A retrospective British trial did not reveal teratogenic effects on babies born to women who used topical tretinoin during pregnancy. Nevertheless, due to the theoretical risk and lack of high-quality trials, many physicians prefer recommending alternatives during pregnancy. Similarly, it is recommended for nursing mothers to avoid topical tretinoin, as quality data is lacking.

9. What is the main mechanism of action of tretinoin in acne vulgaris?

While not fully understood, there are likely multiple mechanisms that topical tretinoin impacts. Tretinoin is believed to normalize follicular epithelium proliferation and differentiation. This results in the dislodging of microcomedones, decreasing obstruction of the pilosebaceous unit.

Consequently, topical tretinoin is a very effective treatment for comedonal acne. Topical tretinoin is also thought to block multiple inflammatory pathways seen in acne vulgaris.

10. How should topical tretinoin be used to treat acne vulgaris?

Topical tretinoin is usually prescribed for once-daily use. It should be used at night to prevent photodegradation. One small pea-size application of tretinoin should be enough to cover the entire face. It should be applied to clean, dry skin. Patients concerned about dry skin may start with applications every third night and progress to every other night and nightly as tolerated. Furthermore, it is crucial to moisturize consistently. We often recommend leaving tretinoin for 20–30 minutes, before applying any other products. Additionally, some patients may choose to avoid applying to areas where they are experiencing irritant reactions, or "retinoid dermatitis." Additionally, when applying multiple topical medications, it is best to space them to avoid side effects that may be cumulative. This can be done by applying other preparations in the morning or spacing them out in the evening.

11. Is the formulation of a topical retinoid important?

Yes. Topical retinoids are available in different concentrations and formulations (lotions, creams, gels, solution). Selection of the proper formulation and vehicle is crucial to optimizing results and minimizing side effects. Gels, which are more drying, are often used in patient with oily skin. Cream vehicles provide emollients, which is useful is patients with dry skin. Solutions are very effective vehicles for delivery as well. Patient preference should also be taken into account, which will often ensure the highest rate of compliance.

12. Is topical tretinoin cream really useful in treating photo-induced wrinkles?

Absolutely! There have been multiple studies that have shown the consistent use of topical tretinoin can improve wrinkles and improve dyspigmentation. It is important to remind patients that clinical improvement is usually apparent only at 3–6 months. As such, consistent long-term application is necessary.

13. Is there clinical evidence that topical retinoids improve melsama?

Yes. Multiple studies have shown the efficacy of topical retinoids for the treatment of melasma, solar lentigines, and postinflammatory hyperpigmentation. Additionally, there are also data to support the use of topical tretinoin in a fixed, triple combination therapy consisting of hydroquinone 4%, tretinoin 0.05%, fluocinolone acetonide 0.01% for the treatment of melasma.

14. What are the clinical indications for tazarotene?

Tazarotene is used to treat acne and mild-moderate psoriasis. Tazarotene is a prodrug that is rapidly converted by skin esterases to tazarotenic acid, the active metabolite. If has a high affinity for RAR receptors (including RAR-γ, the primary receptor for keratinocytes) and no affinity for RXR. Tazarotene comes in 0.05% and 0.01% formulations.

15. What are the clinical indications for alitretinoin?

Alitretinoin (9-cis-retinoic acid) is a naturally occurring retinoid that binds to all RAR and RXR receptors. Topical alitretinoin 0.1% is currently approved for the treatment of kaposi sarcoma in the United States. Of note, irritant dermatitis was seen in approximately 75% of patients using alitretinoin. In other countries, oral alitretinoin is used to treat refractory chronic hand eczema.

16. What dermatologic conditions are treated with isotretinoin?

Oral isotretinoin is used to treat acne and other disorders of keratinization. Previously, isotretinoin was reserved for patients with only the most severe or recalcitrant forms of cystic or nodular acne vulgaris. However, recently its use has been expanded to include patients with moderate acne that have failed other treatments, or patients who show signs of scarring.

Isotretinoin has also been used to treat severe lichen planus, severe cases of rosacea, hidradenitis suppurativa, Darier disease, pityriasis rubra pilaris, various forms of ichthyosis, and other rare conditions. See Table 55.4.

17. What is the mechanism of action of oral tretinoin in acne vulgaris?

The complete mechanism of action of isotretinoin has still not been fully elucidated. However, it is likely successful in the treatment of acne because it mediates the pathogenesis of all four known causes of acne: propionibacterium acne colonization, follicular hyperkeratosis, increased sebum secretion, and inflammation. Isotretinoin's strong inhibition of sebum production is probably the most important factor in the treatment of acne. As with topical tretinoin, isotretinoin also reduces microcomedone formation, has antimicrobial properties, and is antiinflammatory as well.

Table 55.4 Dermatologic uses of oral retinoids	
FDA-APPROVED INDICATIONS	**SELECTED NONAPPROVED APPLICATIONS**
Severe recalcitrant acne vulgaris (isotretinoin) Psoriasis (acitretin)	Bazex syndrome Dissecting cellulitis of the scalp Eczema (chronic hand) Eosinophilic pustular folliculitis Hidradenitis suppurativa Ichthyoses Kaposi sarcoma Keratoderma Keratosis follicularis (Darier's disease) Langerhans cell histiocytosis Lichen planus Lupus erythematosus, cutaneous Mycosis fungoides (cutaneous T-cell lymphoma) Nevoid basal cell carcinoma—prevention of basal cell carcinomas Pityriasis rubra pilaris Psoriasis (pustular, erythrodermic) Rosacea Xeroderma pigmentosum—prevention of skin cancers

FDA, Food and Drug Administration.

18. Are there any contraindications to the use of oral isotretinoin?

Isotretinoin is absolutely contraindicated in pregnancy, women trying to conceive, and women breastfeeding. Additionally, patients with hypersensitivity to preservatives in acitretin capsules must also avoid isotretinoin. The most common relative contraindications include leukopenia, hypercholesterolemia/hypertriglyceridemia, hypothyroidism, pseudotumor cerebri, suicidal ideation, and hepatic or renal dysfunction. Lastly, one cannot donate blood while on isotretinoin.

19. How is oral isotretinoin prescribed for acne? What is iPLEDGE?

To prescribe isotretinoin, prescribers and patients must register with iPLEDGE. iPLEDGE is a system in the United States that serves as a pregnancy risk reduction program. In this program, physicians, pharmacies, and patients work together to ensure the safe distribution and monitoring of isotretinoin. In order for isotretinoin to be dispensed to a patient, this system requires monthly counseling, monitoring, pregnancy tests (in females), and a pledge to use two forms of birth control. Failure to comply with all steps will result in the medication being held by pharmacies.

20. How is isotretinoin prescribed for the treatment of acne vulgaris?

Once approved by iPLEDGE, isotretinoin may be prescribed. The dosing is usually initiated at 0.5 mg/kg divided into two doses daily. The dose is often titrated up to 1.0–2.0 mg/kg after 1 month, as tolerated. Treatment duration is generally 15–20 weeks. There are some data showing that a minimum cumulative dose of 120 mg/kg is associated with better outcomes. Recent studies have indicated that dosing as high as 220 mg/kg or more may yield lower relapse rates. For best absorption, isotretinoin should be taken with meals, as it is lipophilic.

21. After starting topical tretinoin and oral isotretinoin for acne vulgaris, the patient reports that his/her acne has worsened. Should he/she immediately discontinue the drug?

Flaring of acne during the early usage of both topical and oral isotretinoin has been reported. Patients should be told to anticipate this prior to initiation of treatment to prevent discontinuation of therapy after a short course. It is crucial to counsel patients on the importance of compliance with tretinoin therapies. Patients should be educated that the benefits of topical tretinoin may not be seen for 6 weeks in some cases. Full results may take 6 months or longer. The effects of oral isotretinoin may take 8 weeks before becoming apparent. Tretinoin has a cumulative effect and must be used consistently.

22. What are the main side effects of oral retinoid therapy?

The most severe side effect of oral retinoid therapy is teratogenicity. Fetal deformities can be severe (cardiovascular, craniofacial, central nervous system [CNS]) and often lead to spontaneous abortion, prematurity, or fetal demise. While there are no reports of male usage of oral retinoids resulting in birth defects, males should be counseled to stop taking oral retinoids while actively trying to have children. Similar to topical retinoids, oral retinoids may cause severe dryness, xerosis, and peeling of the skin. Dryness is often seen involving the lips, eyes, mouth, and nasal mucosa. Alopecia or hair thinning may occur as well, but is generally mild. See Table 55.5.

Bone pain, muscle cramps, and rarely CNS (pseudotumor cerebri) side effects may be seen. Multiple large studies have not shown a connection between inflammatory bowel disease and isotretinoin use. While there has been a correlation suggested between depression and isotretinoin use, meta-analyses have failed to find a link between the two. In patients with a history of depression, it is prudent to discuss this correlation and in some cases confer with the patient's psychiatrist prior to initiating treatment.

Table 55.5 Oral retinoid toxicity	
ACUTE ADVERSE REACTIONS	**CHRONIC ADVERSE REACTIONS**
Mucocutaneous Alopecia (<10%) Cheilitis (>90%) Dermatitis (50%) Pruritus (<20%) Pyogenic granuloma–like lesions in acne vulgaris (rare) Xerosis (>50%)	**Mucocutaneous** Alopecia, persistent (rare) Dry eyes (rare) **Systemic** Osteoporosis Premature epiphyseal closure Skeletal hyperostosis
Laboratory Elevated liver function tests (<10%) Hyperlipidemia (25%) Leukopenia (<10%)	
Systemic Arthralgias (16%) Impaired night vision Mental depression (uncommon) Pancreatitis (rare) Pseudotumor cerebri (rare) Spontaneous abortion Teratogenicity (cardiac, head and neck, CNS)	

CNS, Central nervous system.

Finally, care should be taken to monitor for interactions with other medications used concomitantly. Some of the common medications that require caution and close monitoring include methotrexate (synergistic liver toxicity), doxycycline/minocycline/tetracycline (increase intracranial pressure), alcohol (conversion of acitretin to etretinate and liver toxicity), and vitamin A supplements.

23. What can be done to reduce the dry skin and lips associated with retinoid therapy?
Moisturizing and gentle skin care are a must. Multiple lip balm applications daily usually help prevent cheilitis. Many report Vaseline to be the most effective for this purpose. Recent studies may show that oral omega-3 was effective in decreasing the mucocutaneous side effects of isotretinoin. There have been mixed results in studies regarding the use of vitamin E supplements in reducing cheilitis and dry skin. Finally, as a last resort, decreasing frequency, dose, and duration of treatment can help to minimize unwanted side effects.

24. Can patients treated with oral isotretinoin require a second course of treatment?
Yes. Approximately one-third of patients previously treated with isotretinoin will require a second course. This may be due to inadequate primary treatment course, persistent disease, or relapse. Women who have failed isotretinoin treatment should be evaluated for possible hyperandrogenemia.

25. What are the lab monitoring parameters for isotretinoin and acetretin?
Monthly pregnancy tests for women of child-bearing potential are mandatory in the iPLEDGE system. Baseline monitoring of liver function tests, cholesterol, and triglycerides is recommended. Additionally, routine monitoring of these labs is done by many. The most common lab abnormality seen is hypertriglyceridemia.

26. Are the clinical indications for acitretin the same as isotretinoin?
Not really. Isotretinoin is more effective in follicular diseases (acne vulgaris, rosacea, gram negative folliculitis), while acitretin is used more in psoriasis (pustular psoriasis, psoriasis of the palms and soles, erythrodermic psoriasis). Both have been used in other disorders as well, including ichthyosis and pityriasis rubra pilaris. See Table 55.6.

27. What are the mechanisms of action of acitretin?
The mechanism of action of acitretin is not fully known. Acitretin is the active metabolite of etretinate (no longer available in United States). The key difference between the two is that acitretin is eliminated from the body much quicker, allowing for safer use. Despite weak bonding, acitretin activates all three RAR receptors. Based on the therapeutic response of pustular psoriasis and subcorneal pustular dermatosis, there is a belief that this drug is involved in the modification of neutrophil function.

28. How is acitretin administered for the treatment of psoriasis?
Once baseline laboratory tests have been reviewed and the patient has been counseled, oral acitretin therapy can be initiated. The dosing usually used is 25 to 50 mg/day. Higher dosages are used in select cases, but dose-related side effects become increasingly more likely. Once the patient has responded to treatment (12–16 weeks), a maintenance dose of 25 mg/day or every other day can be employed.

Table 55.6 Dermatologic uses of oral acitretin	
FDA-APPROVED INDICATION	**SELECTED NONAPPROVED APPLICATIONS**
Severe recalcitrant psoriasis	Granuloma annulare, generalized Ichthyoses (e.g., ichthyosis vulgaris) Keratosis follicularis (Darier's disease) Mycosis fungoides (cutaneous T-cell lymphoma) Palmar/plantar pustulosis Pityriasis rubra pilaris Porokeratosis Subcorneal pustular dermatosis

FDA, Food and Drug Administration.

29. What are the clinical indications in dermatology for oral bexarotene?

Oral bexarotene and topical bexarotene are approved for the treatment of cutaneous T-cell lymphoma that has been refractory to at least one systemic agent. It is usually used in combination with other therapies. Bexarotene requires close monitoring for many of the same side effects as other oral retinoids, but also may cause hypothyroidism and hypertriglyceridemia.

FURTHER READING

Akhavan A, Bershad S. Topical acne drugs: review of clinical properties, systemic exposure, and safety. *Am J Clin Dermatol.* 2003;4:473–492.

Baldwin HE, Nighland M, Kendall C, Mays DA, Grossman R, Newburger J. 40 years of topical tretinoin use in review. *J Drugs Dermatol.* 2013;12:638–642.

Bikowski JB. Mechanisms of the comedolytic and anti-inflammatory properties of topical retinoids. *J Drugs Dermatol.* 2005;4:41–47.

Hoffman LK, Bhatia N, Zeichner J, Kircik LH. Topical vehicle formulations in the treatment of acne. *J Drugs Dermatol.* 2018;17(6):6–10.

Kang HY, Valerio L, Bahadoran P, Ortonne JP. The role of topical retinoids in the treatment of pigmentary disorders: an evidence-based review. *Am J Clin Dermatol.* 2009;10:251–260.

Khunger N, Sarkar R, Jain RK. Tretinoin peels versus glycolic acid peels in the treatment of melasma in dark-skinned patients. *Dermatol Surg.* 2004;30:756–760.

Kolli SS, Pecone D, Pona A, Cline A, Feldman SR. Topical retinoids in acne vulgaris: a systematic review. *Am J Clin Dermatol.* 2019;20:345–365.

Saurat J-H, Sorg O. Retinoids. In: Bolognia JL, Schaffer JV, Cerroni L, eds. *Dermatology.* 4th ed. Philadelphia, PA: Elsevier; 2017:2200–2214.

Shalita A. The integral role of topical and oral retinoids in the early treatment of acne. *J Eur Acad Dermatol Venereol.* 2001;15(suppl 3):43–49.

Yentzer BA, McClain RW, Feldman SR. Do topical retinoids cause acne to "flare"? *J Drugs Dermatol.* 2009;8:799–801.

CHAPTER 56

NEONATAL INFECTIONS

Israel David Andrews

1. What are the TORCHES infections in a neonate?
   This acronym stands for several etiologic agents of congenital infections:
   - **T**oxoplasmosis
   - **O**ther (varicella-zoster virus [VZV], parvovirus B19, Zika virus)
   - **R**ubella
   - **C**ytomegalovirus (causes most morbidity and mortality)
   - **H**erpes simplex virus, **H**uman immunodeficiency virus (HIV)
   - **E**nteroviruses, **E**pstein-Barr virus
   - **S**yphilis

Boyer S, Boyer K. Update on TORCH infections in the newborn infant. *Newborn Infant Nurs Rev.* 2004;4:70–80.

---

2. Describe the cutaneous findings in neonatal herpes simplex viral (HSV) infections.
   HSV infection usually presents as grouped vesicles on an erythematous base. These lesions may be present on any part of the skin but are more common on the face, scalp, or buttocks (Fig. 56.1). They may also be generalized or disseminated or occur in the perianal region in a breech-delivered baby. They may also present as aplasia cutis congenita–like skin findings with atrophic areas and scarring.

Corey L, Wald A. Maternal and neonatal herpes simplex virus infections. *N Engl J Med.* 2009;361:1376–1385.

---

3. Is neonatal herpes simplex dangerous?
   Yes. Neonatal herpetic infections are usually severe (especially if lesions are disseminated or the central nervous system [CNS] is involved) and require immediate diagnosis and treatment. The majority of infants with HSV infection acquire it in the perinatal period following contact with infectious genital mucous membrane secretions or herpetic lesions. Even with adequate treatment, the mortality rate approaches 50% in infants with disseminated disease or CNS disease, and the incidence of long-term morbidity is significant.

4. What percentage of herpes-infected neonates display skin or mucosal lesions?
   About 70% of infected infants display lesions shortly after birth, with disseminated disease occurring during the first 2 weeks of life. This includes infants with skin, eye, or mouth disease (40% of all neonatal HSV infections), as well as those with disseminated disease (25%) that includes the skin, of which 77% will manifest with skin lesions. If intrauterine exposure has occurred, lesions are usually present at birth. Fortunately, intrauterine transmission of HSV occurs in fewer than 5% of cases.

   Jacobs RF. Neonatal herpes simplex virus infections. *Semin Perinatol.* 1998;22:64–71.

5. Which is a more common cause of neonatal infection, HSV-1 or HSV-2?
   The majority of neonatal infections are due to perinatally acquired HSV-2 infection.

6. What tests aid in the diagnosis of herpes infections?
   A Tzanck smear (scraping the base of a vesicle followed by staining the material with the Wright stain) can determine the presence or absence of multinucleated giant cells indicative of herpesvirus infections; however, it is unable to distinguish between VZV and HSV (see Fig. 3.5). Viral culture is the most accurate means of diagnosis but can take several days to be processed. HSV polymerase chain reaction (PCR) is both accurate and rapid, with results reported in 12–24 hours, and has become the gold standard in diagnosis. PCR of cerebrospinal fluid is the test of choice to rule in or out CNS involvement, but a Western blot remains the gold standard for serologic assays identifying HSV antibodies and is 99% sensitive and specific.

Strick LB, Wald A. Diagnostics for herpes simplex virus: is PCR the new gold standard? *Mol Diagn Ther.* 2006;10:17–28.

---

7. What is congenital varicella syndrome?
   While the risk of vertical transmission is relatively low, 2%, intrauterine infection with VZV occurring between weeks 8 and 20 may result in congenital varicella syndrome. These infants are born with chorioretinitis, hypoplasia of limbs,

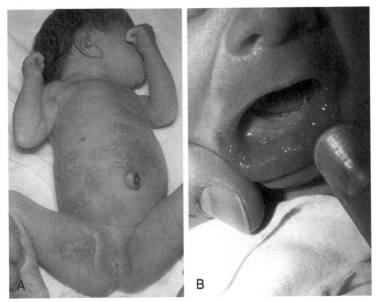

Fig. 56.1 A, Congenital herpes simplex virus infection. **B,** Congenital mucosal herpes simplex virus infection. (Courtesy William L. Weston, MD.)

and/or paresis of the extremities. Cutaneous findings appear scar-like and occur in a dermatomal distribution with underlying tissue atrophy. Maternal herpes zoster during pregnancy does not carry a risk to the fetus.

8. What is the average age of onset of lesions in a neonate exposed to varicella perinatally? When is there an increased risk of mortality?
   The age of onset of varicella lesions is usually within the first 5 to 10 days of life. Neonatal varicella is fatal in about 30% of patients whose mothers developed lesions from 5 days before to 2 days after delivery.

Smith CK, Arvin AM. Varicella in the fetus and newborn. *Semin Fetal Neonatal Med.* 2009;14:209–217.

9. What is the treatment of neonatal HSV and varicella infection?
   Early identification of infection and initiation of therapy are the most important aspects of treatment. Intravenous acyclovir is recommended for varicella and any form of HSV infection (disseminated, CNS, or cutaneous forms). The usual course for HSV infection is 14 to 21 days, the latter is recommended for CNS infection, treatment of neonatal VZV is typically for 10 days. Ophthalmologic examination may be necessary, and adequate isolation precautions must be instituted. For varicella infection, varicella-zoster immune globulin (VZIG) is recommended for cases with evidence of maternal infection 5 days before to 2 days after delivery (given within 48 to 96 hours after exposure). VZIG is not indicated for infants born to mothers with herpes zoster.

10. What is a "blueberry muffin baby"? What is the significance of this diagnosis?
    This term applies to babies exhibiting violaceous or red indurated macules or papules on the face, trunk, or scalp present at birth, or within the first 2 days of life (Fig. 56.2). These lesions represent cutaneous extramedullary hematopoiesis and are seen in congenital rubella syndrome (CRS), toxoplasmosis, cytomegalovirus infection, neuroblastoma, leukemia, erythroblastosis fetalis, and twin transfusion syndrome.

Holland KE, Galbraith SS, Drolet BA. Neonatal violaceous skin lesions: expanding the differential of the "blueberry muffin baby". *Adv Dermatol.* 2005;21:153–192.

11. At what time during pregnancy is there the highest risk of congenital rubella following maternal infection?
    The risk is highest if maternal exposure occurs during the first 12 weeks of gestation, at which point fetal tissue is rapidly developing. The risk of fetal infection is 80%–85% during the first trimester; the majority of these infants suffer from congenital defects. Between the 12th and 20th weeks of gestation, the infection risk drops to 50%, and about one-third of these infants have sequelae.

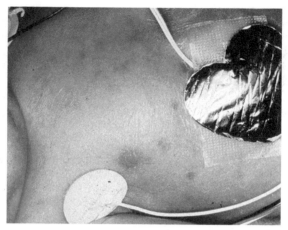

Fig. 56.2 Extramedullary dermal erythropoiesis. Although described as "blueberry muffin" babies, because of the bluish tint in some cases, they can also have red indurated nodules, as seen in this patient. (Courtesy Fitzsimons Army Medical Center teaching files.)

12. List the classic triad of CRS.

The triad consists of congenital cataracts, deafness, and congenital heart malformations.

The syndrome may also include microcephaly, microphthalmia, and intrauterine growth restriction; however, all organ systems are at risk for infection. It is important to follow at-risk infants, as two-thirds of infants with CRS may be asymptomatic at birth. Most will develop sequelae within the first 5 years of life.

13. Are any precautions necessary for infants with CRS at the time of hospital discharge?

Yes. These infants represent potential risks to other pregnant women, as 5% to 10% of affected infants may shed virus for 12 to 18 months.

14. Why is human parvovirus infection important to a pregnant woman?

Human parvovirus B19, the etiologic agent of erythema infectiosum, readily infects erythroblasts and may result in hydrops fetalis and fetal death. This risk is small, with current studies showing a 2% to 9% risk after infection during the first 16 to 28 weeks of pregnancy. Fortunately, about 50% of pregnant women have serologic evidence of prior exposure to parvovirus B19.

Tolfvenstam T, Broliden K. Parvovirus B19 infection. *Semin Fetal Neonatal Med.* 2009;14:218–221.

KEY POINTS: NEONATAL INFECTION

1. The **TORCHES** infections are **t**oxoplasmosis; **o**ther (VZV, parvovirus B19, Zika virus); **r**ubella; **c**ytomegalovirus; **h**erpes simplex virus and HIV; **e**nteroviruses and **E**pstein-Barr virus; and **s**yphilis.
2. Seventy percent of neonates with HSV infection will have cutaneous disease.
3. The classic triad of CRS consists of congenital cataracts, deafness, and congenital heart malformations.
4. Ninety percent of congenital cytomegalovirus (CMV)-infected infants are asymptomatic.
5. Hoarse voice changes in infants might signify human papillomavirus laryngeal infection.
6. Infected and uninfected HIV infants usually cannot be clinically distinguished at birth.
7. Zika virus may be transmitted vertically to the fetus during pregnancy, leading to microcephaly, neurologic sequelae, and fetal loss.

15. Are most infants with CMV infection symptomatic?

No. Ninety percent of congenitally CMV-infected infants are asymptomatic. The other 5% to 10% usually have disease manifested by hepatosplenomegaly, hemorrhagic diatheses, and jaundice. The mortality rate in overtly symptomatic infants is almost 30%. Ten percent to 15% of children born with asymptomatic CMV infection are at risk of developing sequelae, most commonly nonhereditary sensorineural hearing loss.

DeVries J. The ABC's of CMV. *Adv Neonatal Care.* 2007;7:248–255.

16. What cutaneous findings are seen in congenital CMV infection?
    - Petechiae and purpura (as part of the "blueberry muffin baby" syndrome) presenting with papules and/or nodules
    - Maculopapular rash
    - Vesicular eruption (rarely)

Hicks T, Fowler K, Richardson M, Dahle A, Adams L, Pass R. Congenital cytomegalovirus infection and neonatal auditory screening. *J Pediatr.* 1993;123:779–782.

17. What clinical findings are seen in congenital Epstein-Barr virus infection?
    - Micrognathia
    - Cryptorchidism
    - Cataracts
    - Hypotonia
    - Hemolytic anemia
    - Scaly erythematous rash
    - Hepatosplenomegaly
    - Persistent atypical lymphocytosis

18. Describe a clinical presentation of congenital human papillomavirus infection.
    The infant can present with voice changes or a persistent abnormal hoarse cry due to laryngeal papillomatosis acquired during passage through an infected birth canal. The time between rupture of the amnion and delivery is a critical factor in vertical transmission rate. These signs of infection may not be evident for several months to years of age.
    Anogenital warts in young children can also be acquired as a congenital infection, through sexual abuse, or by other postnatal, nonsexual contact with affected adults (Fig. 56.3).

Tenti P, Zappatore R, Migliora P, Spinillo A, Belloni C, Carnevali L. Perinatal transmission of human papillomavirus from gravidas with latent infections. *Obstet Gynecol.* 1999;93:475–479.

19. What is the risk of HIV infection transmission to an infant born from an HIV-positive mother?
    The risk of vertical transmission of HIV from a mother who did not receive intervention is estimated between 13% and 39%. In children born to infected mothers compliant with their antiretroviral medications, and who have a viral load <1.00 copies/mL, the risk of vertical transmission decreases to 1%. The combination of cesarean delivery and antiretroviral therapeutic compliance can decrease this risk to 0.5%. Between 1992 and 2002, the number of pediatric cases of HIV decreased by 90% due to prenatal HIV screening, early initiation of antiretroviral therapy continued through the end of pregnancy, and treatment of newborns for the first 6 weeks of life.

American Academy of Pediatrics, Committee on Infectious Diseases. Herpes simplex, varicella-zoster infections, human immunodeficiency virus, and parvovirus. In: Pickering LK, Baker CH, Kimberlin DW, et al, eds. *Red Book: 2012 Report of the Committee on Infectious Diseases.* Elk Grove Village, IL: American Academy of Pediatrics; 2012:398–408, 774–789, 419–439, 539–541.

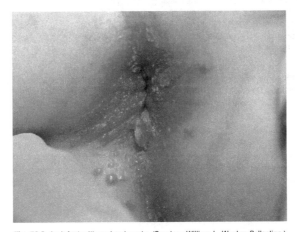

Fig. 56.3 An infant with perianal warts. (Courtesy William L. Weston Collection.)

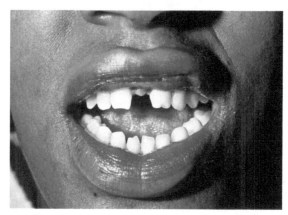

Fig. 56.4 Hutchinson's teeth. Characteristic conical incisors with notching. (Courtesy John L. Aeling Collection.)

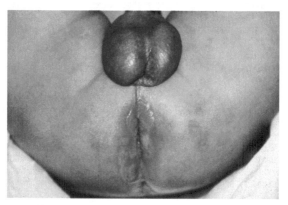

Fig. 56.5 Congenital syphilis demonstrating perianal erosions.

20. What is Hutchinson's triad?

    Interstitial keratitis, Hutchinson's teeth, and eighth nerve deafness. These are common findings in late congenital syphilis. Interstitial keratitis is the most common finding in this triad. It is rare before age 8 and after age 40. Both eyes are usually affected, and the corneal clouding may be spotty or diffuse. Hutchinson's teeth are due to deficient development of the permanent teeth buds and are characterized by conical central incisors with notching of the distal free margin (Fig. 56.4). Eighth nerve deafness usually occurs after interstitial keratitis, is usually bilateral, and is often preceded by tinnitus and vertigo.

21. Are there any other stigmata of late congenital syphilis?

    Bone involvement is common with periostitis of long bones, resulting in thickened and bent tibias (saber shins) and other bony abnormalities. Other stigmata include scarring and wrinkling at the corners of the mouth (rhagades), saddle nose deformity (due to cartilage destruction), Parrot's nodes on the skull, and salt-and-pepper pigmentation of the fundi.

22. What are the physical findings of early congenital syphilis?

    Syphilitic rhinitis is the most important and frequent physical finding in early congenital syphilis. It is characterized by a profuse serous nasal discharge (snuffles) that is teeming with spirochetes (see Fig. 28.7). The inflammatory process leads to eventual cartilage and bone deformity. Other findings include papulosquamous skin lesions, perianal erosions (Fig. 56.5), blistering of the hands and feet, hepatosplenomegaly, meningitis, meningoencephalitis, and osteochondritis. Congenital syphilis is a serious infection that, if untreated, has significant mortality.

23. What is Zika virus and why is it important?

    Zika virus is an emerging tropical disease due to an arthropod-borne flavivirus transmitted by mosquitoes. Currently, there is an ongoing endemic in the Americas, Caribbean, and Pacific. Following an infection from mosquitoes, the virus can be transmitted sexually between individuals and vertically from mother to the fetus causing congenital Zika virus infection. Clinical symptoms present in only 20%–25% of infected adults and are nonspecific. Potential sequelae secondary to congenital infections are highest if infection occurs in the first or second trimester and can include growth restriction, hearing loss, seizures, enlarged cardiac ventricles, microcephaly, intracranial calcifications, and fetal loss. Cutaneous manifestations in adults and infants are nonspecific and women planning to become pregnant should avoid travel to areas where infection is endemic.

World Health Organization. *WHO Statement on the 2nd Meeting of IHR Emergency Committee on Zika Virus and Observed Increase in Neurological Disorders and Neonatal Malformations.* http://www.who.int/mediacentre/news/statements/2016/2nd-emergency-committee-zika/en/.

CHAPTER 57

PEDIATRIC DERMATOLOGY

Grant Plost and Anna L. Bruckner

1. **What is the purpose of a pediatric dermatologist?**
   A pediatric dermatologist specializes in the diagnosis and management of diseases of the skin, hair, and nails in children. The clinical presentation and treatment of skin diseases are often different in the pediatric and adult populations. A pediatric dermatologist has expertise in the management of patients ranging in age from newborns to young adults.

2. **When should you consider a skin biopsy in a pediatric patient?**
   The ability to perform a skin biopsy in the outpatient setting is often limited by the age of the patient and willingness to tolerate a procedure while awake. A skin biopsy should be reserved for situations where there is diagnostic uncertainty and where information gathered from the procedure will change management. A skin biopsy may be helpful in patients who do not respond to empiric or conventional therapy.

3. **List five strategies to make procedures in pediatric patients easier.**
   - Preoperative application of a topical anesthetic can decrease the pain associated with a procedure.
   - Anxiolytic medications can be given to lessen a child's anxiety.
   - The use of vibration or a cold sensation directly on the skin can mitigate the perception of pain.
   - Distraction with talk, music, or a video can help make a patient more comfortable during a procedure.
   - Conscious sedation or general anesthesia may be necessary when a patient cannot otherwise tolerate an in-office procedure with local anesthetics.

NEONATAL

4. **What are congenital melanocytic nevi and what is their associated risk of melanoma?**
   Congenital melanocytic nevi (see Fig. 57.1) are nevi that present at birth or shortly thereafter. They are classified as either small (<1.5 cm), medium (1.5–19.9 cm), or large (≥20 cm) based on the projected size of the nevus in an adult. Small and medium congenital melanocytic nevi are quite common (1 in 100), whereas large congenital pigmented nevi are rare (1 in 20,000). The controversy surrounding these lesions concerns their malignant potential. The lifetime risk for development of melanoma in small and medium congenital melanocytic nevi is less than 1%, while the risk in large congenital melanocytic nevi is less than 5%.

Alikhan A, Ibrahimi OA, Eisen DB. Congenital melanocytic nevi: where are we now? *J Am Acad Dermatol.* 2012;67(4):495.e1–1.

5. **What is dermal melanocytosis?**
   A blue-black patch or patches found in up to 90% of newborns with darker skin types. The most common location is the sacral region (Fig. 57.1), but dermal melanocytosis may occur on any portion of the body. This skin finding typically fades within the first 3 years of life.

6. **Which disease should be considered in a newborn with fragile skin and easy blistering?**
   A child with skin that blisters with minimal trauma should be evaluated for epidermolysis bullosa, an inherited mechanobullous disease. There are multiple subtypes, but clinically there are four important variants: epidermal, junctional, dystrophic, and Kindler Syndrome (see Chapter 6).

7. **What is the most likely diagnosis for a newborn with congenital absence of skin on the vertex of the scalp?**
   Aplasia cutis congenita. This condition may be an isolated finding or associated with ectopic neural tissue, epidermolysis bullosa, or limb defects. Aplasia cutis congenita generally heals by second intention, creating a scar with overlying alopecia.

Browning JC. Aplasia cutis congenita: approach to evaluation and management. *Dermatol Ther.* 2013;26(6):439–444.

8. **What is the most common cause of diaper dermatitis, and what are the treatment strategies?**
   Irritant contact dermatitis due to urine and feces is the most common cause of diaper dermatitis. The treatment consists of application of barrier creams or ointments and frequent diaper changes to minimize exposure to irritants.

Blume-Peytavi U, Kanti V. Prevention and treatment of diaper dermatitis. *Pediatr Dermatol.* 2018;35 Suppl 1:s19–s23.

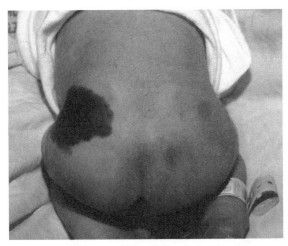

Fig. 57.1 Large blue-gray dermal melanocytosis of the sacral area and dark brown congenital nevus. (Courtesy William L. Weston, MD Collection.)

9. What organism commonly complicates irritant diaper dermatitis?
   Candida albicans. The use of an azole topical antifungal medication is an effective treatment for this secondary skin infection.

Blume-Peytavi U, Kanti V. Prevention and treatment of diaper dermatitis. *Pediatr Dermatol.* 2018;35 Suppl 1:s19–s23.

10. Crusted purpuric papules and a scaly seborrheic-like eruption in the scalp and groin are seen in what serious disease of childhood?
    This constellation of findings suggests Langerhans cell histiocytosis (Fig. 57.2). The disease can vary from a mild skin-limited eruption to a severe, life-threatening, systemic disease. Traditionally, this disease has been treated by pediatric oncologists.

11. What diagnosis and workup should you consider in an infant with annular erythema in a sun-exposed distribution?
    This eruption is consistent with neonatal lupus erythematosus and is confirmed by the detection of maternal autoantibodies to SS-A/Ro and/or SS-B/La. An electrocardiogram should be performed to evaluate for congenital heart block, which can be lethal without intervention.

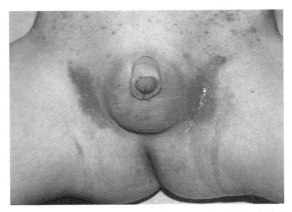

Fig. 57.2 Langerhans cell histiocytosis demonstrating erythematous scale and crusted papules in the groin of a child.

INFANT

12. At what age does atopic dermatitis typically begin?

Atopic dermatitis generally first appears between 3 and 6 months of age. In approximately 90% of patients who develop atopic dermatitis, onset is by 5 years of age.

Eichenfield LF, Tom WL, et al: Guidelines of care for the management of atopic dermatitis: section 1. Diagnosis and assessment of atopic dermatitis. *J Am Acad Dermatol.* 2014;70(2):338–351.

13. What is the natural history of atopic dermatitis?

Infantile atopic dermatitis typically involves the face, neck, and extensor surfaces of the extremities. Childhood and adolescent atopic dermatitis tend to involve flexural areas like the antecubital and popliteal fossae. By adulthood, up to 90% of patients will have resolution of atopic dermatitis.

Eichenfield LF, Tom WL, et al: Guidelines of care for the management of atopic dermatitis: section 1. Diagnosis and assessment of atopic dermatitis. *J Am Acad Dermatol.* 2014;70(2):338–351.

14. Skin-colored to brown macules and papules that become red wheals when stroked (Darier's sign) are diagnostic of what eruption?

Mastocytosis is due to an excess of normal-appearing mast cells in the skin. Subtypes are solitary mastocyoma, maculopapular/urticaria pigmentosa, and diffuse cutaneous mastocystosis. The most common type in children is maculopapular/urticaria pigmentosa (Fig. 57.3). Mastocystosis in children is generally limited to the skin in contrast to adults where involvement of the liver, spleen, bone marrow, and lymph nodes may occur.

Hosking AM, Makdisi J, et al: Diffuse cutaneous mastocytosis: case report and literature review. *Pediatr Dermatol.* 2018;35(6): e348–e352.

15. A child's mother tells you that a rash started at one end of her child's extremity and has now progressed to form a line affecting the entire length of the limb. What is the mostly likely diagnosis?

Lichen striatus, which occurs in children 2 to 12 years old. It characteristically begins at one end of an extremity and can extend to the length of the extremity. It rarely occurs on the torso or face. The appearance of the rash may vary from hypopigmented and macular to thickened and scaly (Fig. 57.4). No treatment is effective, and it disappears spontaneously. The pathogenesis of this unusual dermatosis is unknown.

CHILDHOOD

16. What is the most common cutaneous bacterial infection in children?

Impetigo. This contagious and superficial infection is due to staphylococci (most commonly), streptococci, or a combination of the two organisms.

17. What two organisms are the most common causes of tinea capitis?

Trichophyton tonsurans and *Microsporum canis.*

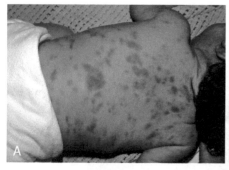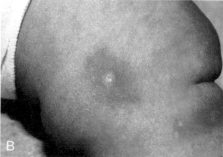

Fig. 57.3 A, Urticaria pigmentosa presenting as ill-defined tan to brownish macules and plaques on the back. **B,** Positive Darier's sign in a lesion of urticaria pigmentosa (wheal and flare of a brown papule after stroking) in a child with multiple lesions. (Courtesy William L. Weston, MD Collection.)

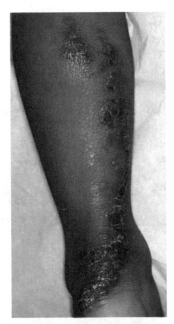

Fig. 57.4 Lichen striatus presenting as hyperkeratotic linear plaque on the lower leg of a child.

18. How is tinea capitis treated?

    Treatment is with oral griseofulvin or oral terbinafine. Oral itraconazole or fluconazole may also be used. Topical antifungals have no role in the treatment of tinea capitis. Some authorities recommend twice-weekly shampooing with 2% selenium sulfide or ketoconazole shampoos as an adjunctive therapy to oral antifungals in order to prevent spread to other children and family members.

19. What hypersensitivity reaction to tinea capitis can be mistaken for a bacterial infection?

    This inflammatory condition is called a kerion. Early treatment is recommended to minimize the risk of scarring alopecia.

20. List four sun protection strategies to prevent sunburn.

    - Try to avoid the sun during the midday when the ultraviolet radiation from the sun is most intense.
    - When outdoors, it is helpful to stay in the shade as much as possible.
    - The use of sun protective clothing, including a wide-brimmed hat, long-sleeved shirts, and sunglasses, is recommended.
    - Application of a broad-spectrum sunscreen with SPF 30 or higher is another useful measure to prevent sunburn. Good consistent sun protection can decrease the risk of developing skin cancers as an adult.

Cestari T, Buster K. Photoprotection in specific populations: children and people of color. *J Am Acad Dermatol*. 2017;76(3S1):S110–S121.

21. Describe the typical clinical presentation of a photosensitive disorder and give three examples of photodermatoses that occur in children.

    Photosensitivity disorders typically manifest as a photo-distributed sunburn-like reaction, with pain, pruritus, or scarring after minimal sun exposure. Polymorphous light eruption (Fig. 57.5), erythropoietic protoporphyria, and systemic lupus erythematosus are three examples.

Chantom R, Lim HW, et al: Photosensitivity disorders in children: part I. *J Am Acad Dermatol*. 2012;67(6):1093.e1–18.

22. Name the inflammatory eruption on the tongue characterized by migratory erythematous patches.

    Geographic tongue (Fig. 57.6).

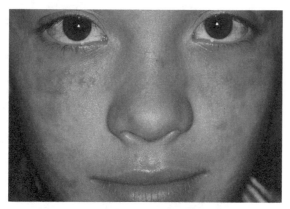

Fig. 57.5 Polymorphous light eruption presenting as erythematous photodistributed papules.

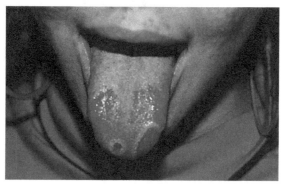

Fig. 57.6 Geographic tongue presenting as migrating annular lesions on the tongue.

23. A child presents with a firm, blue-hued, mobile, subcutaneous nodule on the face. What is the most likely diagnosis?

    Pilomatricoma (Fig. 57.7), which is a benign neoplasm arising from hair follicles. The most common locations are the head, neck, and upper extremities. A characteristic physical exam finding is the "teeter-totter" sign in which downward pressure on one end of a pilomatricoma causes the other end to move upward.

24. A child presents with a red, friable, nodule that frequently bleeds after minor trauma. What is the most likely diagnosis, and what are the treatment options?

    A pyogenic granuloma is a benign neoplasm consisting of lobular proliferations of capillaries. The name is a misnomer because the lesion is neither pyogenic nor granulomatous. The treatment of choice is shave removal, curettage, and electrodesiccation. Other treatment options include pulsed dye laser, topical timolol, and topical imiquimod.

Craig LM, Alster TS. Vascular skin lesions in children: a review of laser surgical and medical treatments. *Dermatol Surg*. 2013; 39(8):1137–1146.

25. What is a spider angioma?

    A small telangiectatic macule radiating from a central arteriole that is commonly seen on sun-exposed skin of children. Treatment with pulsed dye laser is effective although some spider angiomas resolve spontaneously near adolescence.

Craig LM, Alster TS. Vascular skin lesions in children: a review of laser surgical and medical treatments. *Dermatol Surg*. 2013; 39(8):1137–1146.

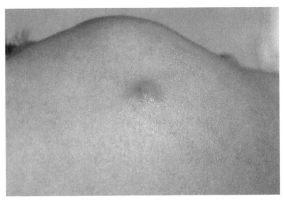

Fig. 57.7 Pilomatricoma presenting as a firm nodule on the cheek of a child.

26. Which is the most common type of vasculitis seen in children?
   Henoch-Schönlein purpura. This is an immunoglobulin A–mediated small vessel vasculitis that most commonly presents with palpable purpura on the lower extremities. Henoch-Schönlein purpura may also involve the gastrointestinal tract, joints, and kidneys.

St John J, Vedak P, et al: Location of skin lesions in Henoch-Schönlein purpura and its association with significant renal involvement. *J Am Acad Dermatol.* 2018;78(1):115–120.

27. Name four common causes of acquired hair loss in children and explain how to differentiate them clinically.
   • Alopecia areata is an autoimmune disorder that presents with round, smooth patches of hair loss.
   • Tinea capitis is a fungal infection of the hair follicles that manifests with scale and broken hairs.
   • Hair pulling is a form of traction alopecia characterized by irregularly shaped patches of alopecia with hairs of varying lengths.
   • Telogen effluvium is a self-limited alopecia that presents with diffuse shedding of hair in response to a stressor.

28. A child presents with a congenital, linear, yellow plaque on the scalp with alopecia. What is the most likely diagnosis, and how do you counsel the patient and family?
   Nevus sebaceous is a congenital hamartoma of the skin that most commonly occurs on the head and neck. During puberty, the birthmark develops a papillomatous surface. A nevus sebaceus can develop secondary tumors, most of which are benign. An excision of the birthmark is curative.

Idriss MH, Elston DM. Secondary neoplasms associated with nevus sebaceus of Jadassohn: a study of 707 cases. *J Am Acad Dermatol.* 2014;70(2):332–337.

29. What are the four cutaneous findings seen in tuberous sclerosis?
   • Hypomelanotic ("ash-leaf") macules
   • Connective tissue nevi (shagreen patch)
   • Facial angiofibromas
   • Periungual fibromas

30. How many café-au-lait macules must be present on a child to fulfill part of the diagnostic criteria for neurofibromatosis type 1?
   Six or more café-au-lait macules of at least 5 mm in diameter before puberty or at least 15 mm in diameter after puberty.

31. What is the diagnosis and treatment for a girl presenting with painful, white, atrophic plaques of the genitalia and perineum?
   Lichen sclerosus, an inflammatory disease of the anogenital skin that occurs in children and adults. In children, the presentation may include purpura and erosions that can be misdiagnosed as child abuse. The first-line treatment is high-potency topical corticosteroids, which alleviate symptoms and prevent the development of scars, strictures, and squamous cell carcinoma.

Tong LX, Sun GS, et al. Pediatric lichen sclerosus: a review of the epidemiology and treatment options. *Pediatr Dermatol.* 2015;32(5):593–599.

Adolescent

32. Describe the characteristic physical exam findings of acne vulgaris.

Acne vulgaris presents with a combination of noninflammatory open and closed comedones with or without inflammatory papules, pustules, nodules, and cysts. The typical distribution involves the face, chest, and back.

33. Explain how the management of comedonal acne differs from the treatment of nodulocystic acne.

Topical retinoid creams are the mainstay of treatment of comedonal acne because they are comedolytic and prevent new acne from forming. Isotretinoin, a systemic retinoid, is the treatment of choice for nodulocystic acne and recalcitrant acne. Early treatment of nodulocystic acne is important to prevent scars. In general, treating acne in adolescents can improve self-esteem.

Zaenglein AL, Pathy AL, et al. Guidelines of care for the management of acne vulgaris. *J Am Acad Dermatol.* 2016;74(5):945–973.e33.

34. What is the diagnosis and management for the papulopustular facial eruption often associated with inappropriate topical corticosteroid use?

Periorificial dermatitis consists of monomorphic erythematous papules and pustules in a perioral, periorbital, and perinasal distribution. Treatment consists of discontinuation of topical corticosteroids and the use of topical or oral antibiotics.

35. A young boy presents with pruritic, scaly, erythematous plaques on the plantar feet associated with hyperhidrosis. What is the most likely diagnosis?

Juvenile plantar dermatosis (Fig. 57.8), which is thought to be a variant of irritant contact dermatitis. Management consists of topical antiperspirants and topical corticosteroids. Juvenile plantar dermatosis typically spares the interdigital spaces in contrast to tinea pedis.

36. What is the most likely diagnosis in a child with 1–2-mm keratotic papules symmetrically distributed on the cheeks, proximal arms, proximal legs, and buttocks?

Keratosis pilaris. This asymptomatic rash is caused by plugging of the hair follicles and is associated with xerosis cutis and atopic dermatitis. Treatment is challenging but regular use of moisturizers and/or keratolytic agents can be helpful.

37. Name three conditions that are often misdiagnosed as tinea corporis and explain how to differentiate them.

Nummular dermatitis, granuloma annulare, and the herald patch of pityriasis rosea. Tinea corporis presents as annular scaly plaques with central clearing. Nummular dermatitis manifests as "coin-shaped" plaques with confluent scale and crust. Granuloma annulare is characterized by non-scaly, annular plaques with central clearing. The herald patch of pityriasis rosea is a solitary, oval, scaly plaque that precedes a generalized eruption.

38. Which pediatric variant of psoriasis in children is often triggered by streptococcal pharyngitis?

Guttate psoriasis, which presents as small, scaly, "drop-like" papules and plaques on the trunk and extremities. Some patients have spontaneous resolution while others progress to plaque-type psoriasis, the most common type of pediatric psoriasis.

Eichenfield LF, Paller AS, et al. Pediatric psoriasis: evolving perspectives. *Pediatr Dermatol.* 2018;35(2):170–181.

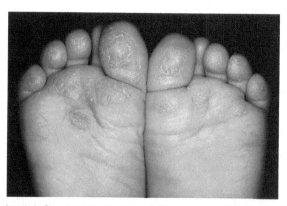

Fig. 57.8 Juvenile plantar dermatosis. Characteristic hyperkeratosis and shiny appearance, with tendency to affect the ball of the foot and the toe pads. (Courtesy Fitzsimons Army Medical Center teaching files.)

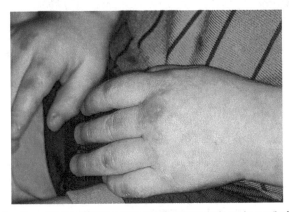

Fig. 57.9 Dermatomyositis. Note Gottron's papules, which present as purple papules over the finger joints.

39. Psoriasis in children tends to involve which two anatomic locations more frequently than in adults?
    Face and anogenital region.

Eichenfield LF, Paller AS, et al. Pediatric psoriasis: evolving perspectives. *Pediatr Dermatol.* 2018;35(2):170–181.

40. Describe the rash associated with juvenile dermatomyositis.
    Violaceous and telangiectatic erythema of the malar cheeks, eyelids (heliotrope rash), shoulders, and upper chest (shawl sign) is common in dermatomyositis. There are often periungual telangiectasias and violaceous, flat-topped papules on the knuckles (Gottron papules) (Fig. 57.9). Juvenile dermatomyositis more commonly presents with calcinosis cutis and, unlike adult disease, is rarely related to internal malignancies.

KEY POINTS: PEDIATRIC DERMATOLOGY

1. Infantile atopic dermatitis typically involves the face, neck, and extensor surfaces of the extremities, while childhood and adolescent atopic dermatitis tend to involve flexural areas.
2. Tinea capitis requires oral antifungal therapy.
3. Consistent sun protection during childhood can decrease the risk of developing skin cancers in adulthood.
4. Common causes of hair loss in children are alopecia areata, tinea capitis, hair pulling, and telogen effluvium.
5. Tuberous sclerosis and neurofibromatosis are two important genetic disorders in which skin findings are often the presenting feature.
6. Early treatment of nodulocystic acne with isotretinoin is important to prevent scarring.
7. Guttate psoriasis is more common in childhood than in later life.

CHAPTER 58

GERIATRIC DERMATOLOGY

Colby C. Evans and Whitney A. High

"If I'd known I was gonna live this long, I'd have taken better care of myself."
—Eubie Blake, American composer, on reaching the age of 100 years

1. How common are skin disorders in elderly persons?

Skin diseases appear more common in the geriatric population than the general population. This may be due to intrinsic skin aging and senescence, immune dysfunction, polypharmacy, and even cognitive and physical impairments that impact personal hygiene. One study revealed that 40% of Americans between the ages of 65 and 74 years had a skin disease significant enough to warrant treatment by a physician. Patients older than 74 years are even more likely to develop significant skin diseases.

Beauregard SA, Gilchrest BA. Survey of skin problems and skin care regimens in the elderly. *Arch Dermatol.* 1987;123:1638–1643.
Farage MA, Miller KW, Berardesca E, et al. Clinical implications of aging skin: cutaneous disorders in the elderly. *Am J Clin Dermatol.* 2009;10:73–86.

2. What is intrinsic aging of the skin?

Aging of the skin is divided into intrinsic aging and extrinsic aging (Table 58.1). Intrinsic aging refers to changes with the passage of time that are due to normal maturity and senescence, and it occurs in all persons. Classically, intrinsic aging was considered unpreventable, but there is renewed interest in the role of antioxidants, such as vitamins C and E, in preventing or slowing intrinsic aging. Research in this area is still in its infancy, and well-designed, controlled long-term studies are still lacking.

Gragnani A, Cornick S, Chominski V, et al. Review of major theories of skin aging. *Adv Aging Res.* 2014;3:265–284.

3. What is extrinsic aging of the skin?

Extrinsic aging of the skin refers to those changes due to external agents. The most important extrinsic factor in aging is cumulative ultraviolet (UV) light exposure. These cutaneous changes caused by sunlight are referred to collectively as **dermatoheliosis.** Skin aging attributable to UV light includes skin wrinkles, "leathery" skin, thinned skin, dyspigmented skin, telangiectasias, and skin fragility ("tearing" and "solar purpura"). Other extrinsic agents that accelerate aging of the skin include smoking and environmental pollutants.

Bonté F, Girard D, Archambault JC, et al. Skin changes during ageing. *Subcell Biochem.* 2019;91:249–280.

4. How does aged skin vary from younger skin under the microscope?

Under the microscope, aged skin demonstrates a flattening of the dermal–epidermal junction with loss of the normal rete ridge pattern (see Fig. 58.1A). There are fewer junctional melanocytes and Langerhans cells. The dermis in aged skin demonstrates fewer fibroblasts, fewer mast cells, fewer blood vessels, depigmentation of hair, loss of hair follicles, and fewer sweat glands.

5. Why does skin "wrinkle" with age?

The answer is complicated, because some authorities recognize as many as five different subtypes of wrinkles. Mots wrinkles on photoprotected skin are fine wrinkles (glyphic wrinkles) that represent accentuation of normal skin markings due to focal skin thinning with fewer keratinocytes. This appears to be intrinsic to aging (Fig. 58.2). Deeper wrinkles in photodamaged skin demonstrate a groove in the epidermis that is associated with solar elastosis (solar damaged elastic tissue) that protrudes on both sides of the groove. These deeper wrinkles are due to extrinsic aging, primarily resulting from UV light. The amount of collagen, elastin, and ground substance also decreases in aged skin, and this may contribute to skin wrinkling, as well.

6. Does smoking cigarettes accelerate skin aging?

Smoking is an important extrinsic factor that accelerates skin aging. This conclusion is supported by epidemiologic studies, animal studies, and in vitro studies. Biochemically, smoking increases the production of tropoelastin and matrix metalloproteinases that degrade collagen and elastic fibers. This leads to abnormal elastotic material. Avoidance of premature aging is an important reason not to smoke!

Morita A, Torii K, Maeda A, et al. Molecular basis of tobacco smoke–induced premature skin aging. *J Investig Dermatol Symp Proc.* 2009;14:53–55.

Table 58.1 Age-related changes in the skin

INTRINSIC AGING	EXTRINSIC AGING (PRIMARILY ULTRAVIOLET LIGHT)
Decrease in corneocyte adhesion	Altered keratinocyte maturation (xerosis)
Slight decrease in epidermal thickness with flattening of rete pegs	Freckles (ephelides)
Decreased number of eccrine sweat glands	Solar lentigo
	Guttate hypomelanosis
Decreased numbers of hair follicles	Wrinkling
Canities (gray hair)	Elastosis (yellowish skin)
Thinning and ridging of nails	Telangiectasia
Decreased dermal collagen (decreases 1% per year)	Senile purpura
Decreased number of dermal elastic fibers	Venous lakes
Decreased dermal ground substance	Comedones
Loss or increase in subcutaneous fat (site dependent)	

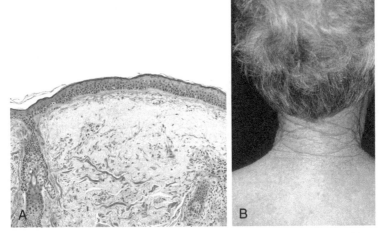

Fig. 58.1 A, Severe solar elastosis. The pale, light blue-gray material in the superficial dermis has largely replaced the normal highly eosinophilic collagen bundles. Also note the loss of the normal rete pegs in the epidermis (hematoxylin and eosin [H&E]). **B,** Cutis rhomboidalis nuchae. Severe solar elastosis and wrinkling of the posterior neck secondary to sun exposure that clearly demarcates from more–normal-appearing skin that is less sun-damaged.

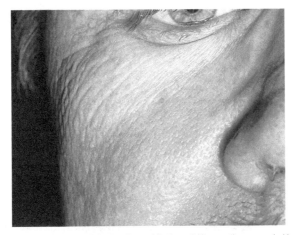

Fig. 58.2 Large, coarse wrinkles due primarily to photoaging. Some of the fine wrinkles near the eye are glyphic wrinkles and are intrinsic to aging.

7. What is solar elastosis?

Solar (actinic) elastosis refers to abnormal degradation of elastotic fibers in the shallow due to UV light exposure (Fig. 58.1A). These abnormal elastotic fibers are apparent as a blue/grey amorphous material, and these fibers mark with elastic tissue stains. Electron microscopy indicates that these solar damaged fibers are similar, but not identical, to normal elastic fibers. Research suggests solar elastosis is due to ultraviolet A (UVA) damage to fibroblasts that yields overproduction and accumulation of elafin, which binds to elastic fibers, making them resistant to normal degradation by elastase. Clinically, large aggregates of solar-damaged elastic fibers impart a yellow color to the skin of older persons. Solar elastosis is often most easily appreciated in the posterior neck, where it is termed *cutis rhomboidalis nuchae* (Fig. 58.1B).

Pain S, Berthélémy N, Naudin C, et al. Understanding solar skin elastosis-cause and treatment. *J Cosmet Sci*. 2018;69:175–185.

8. What is Favre-Racouchot syndrome?

Favre-Racouchot syndrome is a form of extreme extrinsic skin aging characterized by the presence of marked solar elastosis and comedones on the lateral and inferior periorbital areas (Fig. 58.3). Severe cases may demonstrate cysts. While it is most often due to excessive UV radiation, it has also been associated with smoking and with ionizing radiation. The reason for the regional presentation is not well understood, but it has been suggested that the fibroblasts around the hair follicles are damaged by the radiation and no longer produce normal elastic tissue. This predisposes to dilatation of the hair follicles, resulting in comedones and cysts. Most cases can be successfully treated with topical tretinoin cream and comedonal extraction.

Sutherland AE, Green PJ. Favre-Racouchot syndrome in a 39-year old female following radiation therapy. *J Cutan Med Surg*. 2014;18:72–74.

9. What are so-called "liver spots" or "age spots?"

Liver spots/age spots are known by the more proper medical terms solar lentigo. Clinically, solar lentigines (plural) are macular (flat), tan to brown lesions located on sun-exposed skin. The dorsum of the hands, forearms, and face are often affected. These lesions having nothing to do with the liver and are instead the result of accumulated UV damage. Under the microscope, solar lentigines demonstrate elongation of the epidermal rete with modestly increased melanocytes at the dermoepidermal junction, which produce excess melanin. Solar lentigines may be removed with a light liquid nitrogen freeze, with chemical peels, with combination 2% mequinol/0.01% tretinoin, or with lasers that treat pigment. Over-the-counter bleaching cream (1%–2% hydroqunione) or prescription (4% hydroquinone) bleaching cream may lighten lentigines, but with modest sunlight they often recur.

Bolognia JL. Aging skin. *Am J Med*. 1995;98(1A):99S–103S.

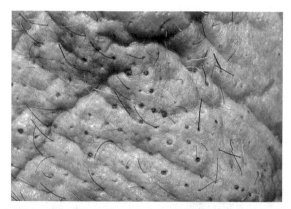

Fig. 58.3 Nodular elastosis with comedones. Numerous comedones in characteristic location associated with background of solar elastotic skin.

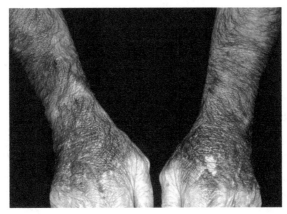

Fig. 58.4 Severe senile purpura on the dorsum of the hands and forearms of an elderly patient.

10. Why do elderly patients often develop bleeding into the skin on the dorsum of the hands and the forearms?
These lesions, referred to as solar purpura (Bateman purpura), are common. One study of patients over age 64 years found solar purpura in 9% of patients examined. Solar purpura typically measure 1 to 5 cm and are sharply circumscribed (Fig. 58.4). Solar purpura occurs upon aged skin that is atrophic and inelastic. It is believed the cumulative solar damage leads to a lesser collagenous support around blood vessels, which results in the loss of normal supporting collagen, and minor trauma leads to rupture of the vessels with intradermal hemorrhage. In support of this theory of solar damage, there is often lateralization of solar purpura to the arm that receives more sunlight (e.g., left arm of a taxicab driver).

Joshi RS, Phadke VA, Khopar US, et al. Unilateral solar purpura as a manifestation of asymmetrical photodamage in taxi drivers. *Arch Dermatol.* 1996;132:715–716.

11. Advertisements in newspapers and magazines frequently tout products that "rejuvenate" the skin or make the skin younger. Is there truth to these claims?
Cosmetic products are not under the purview of the Food and Drug Administration, and such claims are rarely supported by scientific rigor. Two medications proven to improve solar damage are tretinoin and glycolic acid. Both substances have been shown in well-controlled scientific studies to increase collagen production to make wrinkles less noticeable, but the results of these topical treatments are modest and take months or even years of use to foment. Chemical facial peels, laser therapy (laser skin resurfacing), injection of skin fillers, and facelifts may also be used by cosmetic and facial plastic surgery experts to instill a more youthful appearance. Prevention of untoward extrinsic aging by minimizing sun exposure through sun avoidance, sun-protective clothing, and broad-spectrum sunscreen is important. Abstinence from tobacco products is also useful.

12. What is the difference between superficial, medium, and deep chemical peels?
The depth of injury produced varies among these different peels. There are variations in technique, but for typical chemicals used in peels the depth of injury is as follows:
Superficial depth peel (stratum granulosum to superficial papillary dermis)
- Trichloroacetic acid (TCA) 10% to 30%
- α-Hydroxy acid 30% to 70%

Medium depth peel (papillary to upper reticular dermis)
- trichloroacetic acid 35% to 50%
- trichloroacetic acid "combination peels" (e.g., TCA + dry ice, etc.)

Deep depth peel (midreticular dermis)
- Phenol

13. Are some sunscreens better than others in preventing wrinkles caused by photodamage?
It is thought that UV-induced deep wrinkles are attributable to both UVA and UVB wavelengths. Broad-based sunscreens that block both UVB and UVA should be the most efficient in preventing wrinkling.

14. What inflammatory skin diseases are most common in the elderly?
- Xerosis (dry skin)
- Dermatophytosis (see Chapter 30)
- Contact dermatitis (see Chapter 9)

- Stasis dermatitis
- Seborrheic dermatitis (see Chapter 8)
- Rosacea

Farage MA, Miller KW, Berardesca E, et al. Clinical implications of aging skin: cutaneous disorders in the elderly. *Am J Clin Dermatol.* 2009;10:73–86.

15. Why are elderly patients prone to xerosis (dry skin)?

    Xerosis is the most common geriatric dermatosis, with up to 50% of the elderly affected, and it is a frequent cause of pruritus ("dry skin is itchy skin"). Xerosis is more common in the elderly because of less optimal maturation and adhesion of keratinocytes, and this results in rough skin that is characterized by fine white scale. Diminished eccrine function and lesser sebaceous gland lipids may also likely play a role. Asteatosis, which literally means "without oil," is really a misnomer because this is not the primary cause of dry skin. Regardless, it has been well established the transepidermal water loss increases with age, making correct bating and moisturizer use important to the elderly.

Roskos KV, Guy RH. Assessment of skin barrier function using transepidermal water loss: effect of age. *Pharm Res.* 1989;6:949–953.

16. What is the best way to treat xerosis?

    Xerosis is aggravated by low ambient humidity (dry climates and forced-air heated homes), as well as irritants, such as soaps. Xerosis can be improved by increasing ambient humidity (a humidifier) and by using mild synthetic soaps. Most patients also benefit from use of an emollient. The most effective emollients contain lactic acid or a lactate salt, but these are expensive. The effectiveness of emollients is improved by applying them immediately to the skin after bathing, when the skin is well hydrated. In the elderly, improvement of xerosis should be addressed, even when other dermatologic conditions are present.

Berger TG, Shive M, Harper GM. Pruritus in the older patient: a clinical review. *JAMA.* 2013;310:2443–2450.

17. How common is chronic venous insufficiency in the geriatric population?

    Epidemiologic studies show an incidence of chronic venous insufficiency in the elderly that approaches 6%. The economic impact of this condition is enormous; the estimated total cost for treatment of chronic venous insufficiency the United States is $3 billion per year, or up to 2% of the total health care budget of all Western countries.

Davies AH. The seriousness of chronic venous disease: a review of real-world evidence. *Adv Ther.* 2019;36:5.

18. Explain the pathogenesis of chronic venous insufficiency.

    Chronic venous insufficiency is venous hypertension secondary to valvular incompetence in the superficial, perforator, or deep veins of the leg. The most severe disease is produced by valvular insufficiency of deep veins. This insufficiency may be the consequence of hereditary factors, prolonged standing, or prior episodes of venous thrombosis that damage valves. Chronic venous hypertension may manifest as edema, varicosities, brown pigmentation secondary to hemosiderin (hemosiderosis), superficial neovascularization, dermatitis, and venous ulcers (Fig. 58.5). Obesity is a separate risk factor for the development of chronic venous insufficiency.

19. How should you manage chronic venous insufficiency?

    Reducing venous pressure is the goal of therapy. This may be achieved with elevation of the legs, active exercise, supportive stockings, sclerotherapy of select perforator veins, or other surgical treatment. Surgical options depend upon the side but typically include ligation and stripping of the saphenous vein, ligation of incompetent perforators, or valve replacement. Stasis dermatitis, if present, is treated with mild to moderate corticosteroids and many of the physical therapies already discussed (elevation, compression hose, etc.). Oral antibiotics may be used if a secondary infection is present. Venous ulcers require complex wound care management.

Eberhardt RT, Raffetto JD. Chronic venous insufficiency. *Circulation.* 2014;130:333–346.

20. What are arterial ulcers?

    Arterial ulcers are cutaneous ulcers due to a partial or complete occlusion of an artery. The most common cause is progressive narrowing by peripheral atherosclerosis, or less often the ulcers are due to cholesterol emboli. Other manifestations of peripheral atherosclerosis include claudication, atypical leg pain, and gangrene. Patients with severe peripheral atherosclerotic disease are also more likely to have cardiovascular comorbidities.

Davies MG. Critical limb ischemia: epidemiology. *Methodist Debakey Cardiovasc J.* 2012;8:10–14.

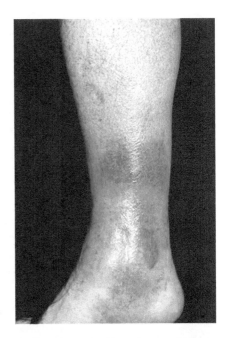

Fig. 58.5 Chronic venous insufficiency manifesting as marked erythema and edema, often called stasis dermatitis.

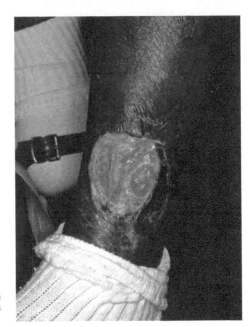

Fig. 58.6 Large deep, round, sharply demarcated arterial ulcer on the anterior leg due to a cholesterol embolus. (Courtesy Fitzsimons Army Medical Center teaching files.)

21. What are the typical characteristics of arterial ulcers?
  • Marked pain (typically more painful than the ulcers caused by chronic venous insufficiency)
  • Tend to occur over bony prominences
  • Sharply demarcated and round (Fig. 58.6)
  • Frequently expose deep structures such as tendons or muscle
  • The base of the ulcer may be dry and contain necrotic debris; granulation tissue less common (compared to other ulcers)

22. **What is rosacea? How does it present?**

Rosacea is a common skin condition that may affect up to 12% of the geriatric population. The pathogenesis is poorly understood, but it is known that patients with rosacea have increased blood flow to the skin and are more likely to demonstrate infestation with *Demodex folliculorum*, a human oil mite. Rosacea affects chiefly the forehead, cheeks, nose, and chin. The three forms of cutaneous rosacea are erythematotelangiectatic, papulopustular, and rhinophymatous. While typically one of these three patterns predominates in a particular patient, mixed forms exist.

KEY POINTS: GERIATRIC DERMATOLOGY

1. Forty percent of Americans between the ages of 65 and 74 years have had a cutaneous disease significant enough to warrant treatment by a physician.
2. Aging of the skin may be divided into intrinsic aging (normal maturity and senescence) and extrinsic aging (external factors such as UV light).
3. Xerosis (dry skin, asteatosis) is the most common geriatric dermatosis and a frequent cause of pruritus.

23. **Is rhinophyma related to alcohol abuse?**

Rhinophyma is a clinical variant of rosacea that presents as severe sebaceous gland hyperplasia of the nose, which may distort its contour. W.C. Fields, a comedian active in the 1920s and 1930s, is perhaps the most well-known celebrity with severe rhinophyma. The lay public often assumes that people with rhinophyma are alcohol abusers, but studies have not demonstrated increased alcohol use in patients with rhinophyma. Patients with rosacea and rhinophyma demonstrate prominent flushing after consumption of alcohol, and this flushing has been incorrectly perceived as being the cause of rhinophyma.

Fink C, Lackey J, Grande DJ. Rhinophyma: a treatment review. *Dermatol Surg.* 2018;44:275–282.

24. **Name the most common types of skin tumors seen in the elderly.**
    - **Benign tumors:** Seborrheic keratoses, cherry hemangiomas, nevi, acrochordons, sebaceous hyperplasia
    - **Premalignant tumors:** Actinic keratoses, Bowen's disease
    - **Malignancies:** Basal cell carcinoma, squamous cell carcinoma

Dewberry C, Norman RA. Skin cancer in elderly patients. *Dermatol Clin.* 2004;22:93–96.

25. **What are seborrheic keratoses?**

Seborrheic keratoses are common, benign epidermal growths of the skin. In patients over 64 years of age, the incidence of these growths is 88%. The pathogenesis is uncertain, but recent evidence suggests the seborrheic keratinocytes are derived from the most superficial part of the hair follicle and are not derived from the epidermis, as was previously thought. Lesions typically begin appearing during middle age, or later, and increase over time. Seborrheic keratoses may be located on any cutaneous surface, other than the palms and soles, but are often found on the face and trunk. Clinically, the lesions present as tan, brown, gray, or black, sharply demarcated, exophytic papules that appear "stuck on." The surface often has an irregular contour or pebbly surface, but it may be verrucous or smooth (Fig. 58.7).

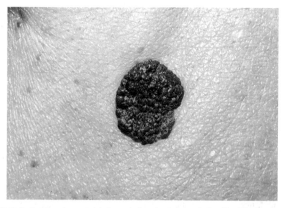

Fig. 58.7 Seborrheic keratosis. Typical deep-brown to black exophytic seborrheic keratosis with a "stuck-on" appearance. This is the most common benign cutaneous growth of the elderly.

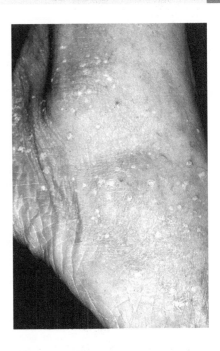

Fig. 58.8 Typical stucco keratosis manifesting as small white or white-gray scaly papules with "stuck-on" appearance.

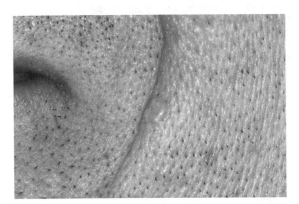

Fig. 58.9 Sebaceous hyperplasia. Typical, small, yellowish-white, symmetrical papule with central depression. (Courtesy Fitzsimons Army Medical Center teaching files.)

26. What are stucco keratoses?

Stucco keratoses are a variant of seborrheic keratoses that present as 1- to 4-mm gray to white scaly papules. This type of keratosis is often located on the arms and lower legs (Fig. 58.8).

27. What is sebaceous hyperplasia?

Sebaceous hyperplasia is the most common benign sebaceous neoplasm. Lesions present in middle age and increase in the elderly. They present as asymptomatic, solitary or multiple, yellow or yellow-white papules that demonstrate a central dell (Fig. 58.9). Increased numbers of lesions are seen in patients with *Muir-Torre syndrome* (sebaceous gland tumors associated with internal malignancy) and in transplant patients, particularly those on cyclosporine. Treatment, if desired, typically focuses upon electrodesiccation, pulse dye laser, or shave removal.

Bader RS, Scarborough DA. Surgical pearl: intralesional electrodesiccation of sebaceous hyperplasia. *J Am Acad Dermatol.* 2000;42:127–128.

28. A 70-year-old man presents to your clinic with the sudden onset of hundreds of seborrheic keratoses. Is there any reason for concern?

The sign of Leser-Trélat is the sudden appearance of a large number of seborrheic keratoses and it may be the harbinger of an underlying malignancy. About one-third of patients with the sign of Leser-Trelat also present with acanthosis nigricans, another cutaneous marker of possible visceral malignancy. The most common associated cancer is gastric adenocarcinoma. The sign is controversial, and the condition is not always a paraneoplastic phenomenon.

Husain Z, Ho JK, Hantash BM. Sign and pseudo-sign of Leser-Trélat: case reports and a review of the literature. *J Drugs Dermatol.* 2013;12:e79–e87.

29. Describe the methods for treating seborrheic keratoses.

Not all seborrheic keratoses must be treated, and many health plans do not pay for treatment because the lesions are benign. Patients may desire that seborrheic keratoses be removed, for cosmetic reasons or because of associated pruritis. Cryotherapy with liquid nitrogen is quick and effective. Seborrheic keratoses can also be removed by curettage or shave biopsy. Shave biopsies are typically performed when the lesion has an unusual clinical appearance and a skin malignancy, such as squamous cell carcinoma or melanoma, is within the differential diagnosis. Seborrheic keratoses can also be treated with the topical application of α-hydroxy acids or potent formulations of hydrogen peroxide (40% H_2O_2).

Kao S, Kiss A, Efimova T, et al. Managing seborrheic keratosis: evolving strategies and optimal therapeutic outcomes. *J Drugs Dermatol.* 2018;17:933–940.

30. An elderly man presents with a soft blue papule on the helix of his ear and he is concerned about melanoma. What is the likely diagnosis?

The differential diagnosis of a soft blue papule on the ear might include a blue nevus, a melanoma, a traumatic tattoo, and a venous lake. The diagnosis of a venous lake can be established by compression of the papule, which will collapse the lesion (Fig. 58.10). Removal of pressure will allow it to refill. Venous lakes are dilated veins that have lost normal elasticity of the vessel wall. Such lesions are usually 1 to 5 mm in diameter and are usually located on sun-exposed surfaces, such as the lips, ears, and face of the elderly. One epidemiologic study of elderly persons found venous lakes in 12% of those examined. Venous lakes require no treatment but can mimic melanoma and may become painful when thrombosed. Treatment, if desired, may utilize saucerization/excision, carbon dioxide laser, radiotherapy infrared coagulation, or injection of sclerosing agents.

Poonia K, Kumar A, Thami GP. Intralesional radiofrequency treatment for venous lake. *Int J Dermatol.* 2019;58:854–855.

31. What is the future of geriatric dermatology?

One hundred years ago, only 2% of the U.S. population was over 65 years of age. By 1980, this percentage was 11%, and, by the year 2030, it is estimated that this faction will be 20%, or more. Given the high incidence of significant dermatologic diseases in the elderly, all health care providers need to familiarize themselves with the diagnosis, prevention, and treatment of skin diseases in the geriatric population.

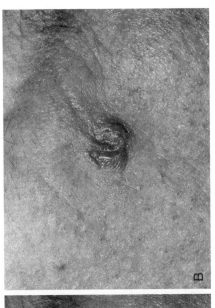

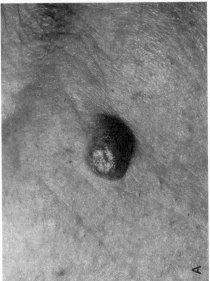

Fig. 58.10 **A,** Venous lake presenting as dark blue–violaceous papule on the cheek. **B,** Same venous lake demonstrating collapse after compression.

CHAPTER 59

DERMATOSES OF PREGNANCY

Misha D. Miller

SPECIFIC DERMATOSES OF PREGNANCY

1. Name four pregnancy-specific dermatologic disorders.
   - Polymorphic eruption of pregnancy (PEP)
   - Pemphigoid gestationis
   - Atopic eruption of pregnancy
   - Intrahepatic cholestasis of pregnancy (ICP)

Ambros-Rudolph CM, Müllegger RR, Vaughan-Jones SA, Kerl H, Black MM. The specific dermatoses of pregnancy revisited and reclassified: results of a retrospective two-center study on 505 pregnant patients. *J Am Acad Dermatol.* 2006;54(3):395–404.

2. What is polymorphic eruption of pregnancy?
   Polymorphic eruption of pregnancy or PEP (also known as pruritic urticarial papules and plaques of pregnancy, or PUPPP) has an incidence of 1 in 160 pregnancies and is most common in primigravidas. Excessive maternal weight gain and pregnancy with multiple gestations have also been associated with the development of PEP. The onset of PEP is usually in the late third trimester or sometimes postpartum. The pruritic, erythematous papules and plaques are usually first seen in the abdominal striae (stretch marks) and then spread to the chest, trunk, and extremities. The papules and plaques typically spare the palms, soles, face, and mucous membranes. Large vesicles or bullae are uncommon, although pinpoint vesicles may be seen (Fig. 59.1).

Vaughan Jones S, Ambros-Rudolph C, Nelson-Piercy C. Skin disease in pregnancy. *BMJ.* 2014;348:g3489.

3. Does PEP have any associated morbidity?
   The pruritus associated with PEP can be very uncomfortable for the mother. There are no fetal sequelae. The skin lesions and pruritus associated with PEP usually spontaneously resolve within 1 or 2 weeks after delivery.

4. How is PEP treated?
   Topical corticosteroids and oral antihistamines are the most common methods of treatment. However, the efficacy of oral antihistamines in treating the pruritus of PEP is questionable. Systemic corticosteroids are used in severe cases.

Bechtel MA. Pruritus in pregnancy and its management. *Dermatol Clin.* 2018;36(3):259–265.

5. From which dermatosis of pregnancy must PEP be differentiated?
   Pemphigoid gestationis. It may be difficult to clinically differentiate PEP from pemphigoid gestationis.

6. What is pemphigoid gestationis?
   Pemphigoid gestationis (also called herpes gestationis or gestational pemphigoid) is an autoimmune subepidermal bullous disorder of pregnancy that may start in the second trimester, the third trimester, or in the postpartum period. The skin lesions are characterized by urticarial papules and plaques, which then progress into painful bullae. The lesions of pemphigoid gestationis initially present periumbilically (Fig. 59.2A) and then spread to involve the trunk and extremities (Fig. 59.2B), usually sparing the face.

Kushner CJ, Concha JSS, Werth VP. Treatment of autoimmune bullous disorders in pregnancy. *Am J Clin Dermatol.* 2018;19(3):391–403.

7. What are the antigens associated with the development of pemphigoid gestationis?
   Bullous pemphigoid antigen 2 (BPAG2) is a 180-kDa transcellular glycoprotein that is part of the hemidesmosome (a structure that binds epithelial cells to the basement membrane of the epidermis). Immunoglobulin G (IgG) binds to BPAG2 and triggers the classic complement pathway leading to a deposition of C3 along the basement membrane zone (Fig. 59.3). Deposition of complement along the basement membrane zone leads to a recruitment of inflammatory cells, particularly eosinophils. This cascade ultimately leads to a release of proteolytic enzymes that cleave portions of the epidermis from the dermis.

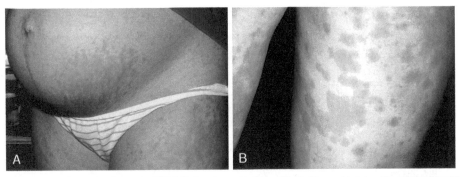

Fig. 59.1 Polymorphic eruption of pregnancy (PEP). **A,** Erythematous papules in the striae of a 21-year-old primigravida woman. **B,** Urticarial papules and plaques that are not associated with striae on the thighs of a woman with PEP.

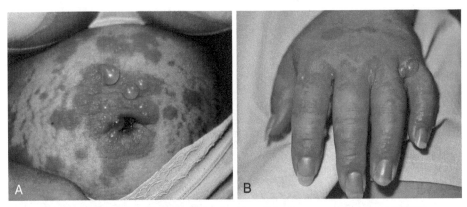

Fig. 59.2 Pemphigoid gestationis. **A,** Umbilical urticarial plaques and tense blisters in a woman with pemphigoid gestationis. **B,** Intertriginous area between fingers demonstrating tense blisters. This is another commonly affected site in pemphigoid gestationis. (Courtesy Fitzsimons Army Medical Center teaching files.)

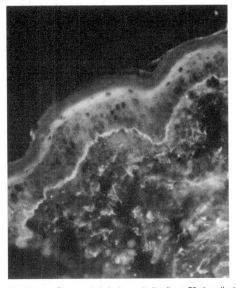

Fig. 59.3 Pemphigoid gestationis. Direct immunofluorescent study demonstrating linear C3 along the basement membrane zone. Less commonly, linear immunoglobulin G is also seen.

KEY POINTS: PEMPHIGOID GESTATIONIS

1. Pemphigoid gestationis is an autoimmune disease that occurs during pregnancy and it is characterized by IgG_1 antibodies directed at BPAG2 (BP180) in the basement membrane zone.
2. Direct immunofluorescent study demonstrates linear C3 and/or IgG along the basement membrane zone and is the test of choice to establish the diagnosis.
3. The primary lesions of pemphigoid gestationis consist of urticarial plaques and/or blisters.
4. The umbilical area is preferentially affected in pemphigoid gestationis and can be a clue to the diagnosis.
5. Neonates of mothers with pemphigoid gestationis may be premature, may demonstrate a lower birth weight, and may occasionally demonstrate transient blisters, but are otherwise healthy.

8. Which human leukocyte antigen (HLA) types have been associated with pemphigoid gestationis?
   HLA-DR3 and HLA-DR4.

Kushner CJ, Concha JSS, Werth VP. Treatment of autoimmune bullous disorders in pregnancy. *Am J Clin Dermatol.* 2018;19(3):391–403.

9. Compare PEP and pemphigoid gestationis.
   See Table 59.1.

High W, Hoang MP, Miller MD. Pruritic urticarial papules and plaques of pregnancy with unusual and extensive palmoplantar involvement. *Obstet Gynecol.* 2005;105(5):1261–1264.

10. What is atopic eruption of pregnancy?
    Atopic eruption of pregnancy is classified to include eczema of pregnancy, prurigo gestationis, and folliculitis of pregnancy. According to the retrospective study by Ambros-Rudolph et al., it is the most common dermatosis of pregnancy, with a prevalence of 50.7%. In this study 20% of the patients were known to have preexisting atopic dermatitis, but 80% of the patients reviewed experienced symptoms de novo during pregnancy. It is known to start early in pregnancy, in the first or second trimesters. The skin lesions are erythematous, excoriated papules, plaques, or

Table 59.1 Compare and contrast polymorphic eruption of pregnancy and pemphigoid gestationis

	POLYMORPHIC ERUPTION OF PREGNANCY	PEMPHIGOID GESTATIONIS
Clinical presentation	Pruritic erythematous papules and plaques Initial lesions present in the abdominal striae, spreading to the trunk and extremities; vesicles may be present Usually spares the palms and soles	Urticarial papules, plaques, and blisters Initial lesions start periumbilically and spread to the trunk and extremities The palms and soles are commonly involved
Direct immunofluorescence	Occasional complement deposition in a perivascular location or in a granular formation along the dermal–epidermal junction	Linear deposition of IgG (25% of the time) and complement (C3) at the dermal–epidermal junction. (see Fig. 59.3)
Fetal sequelae	None	Increased risk of intrauterine growth restriction and prematurity 3%–10% of newborns have lesions of neonatal pemphigoid
Treatment	Topical corticosteroids Oral antihistamines	Topical or oral corticosteroids (prednisone 0.5 mg/kg/day) Oral antihistamines Dapsone, cyclosporine (results are mixed)
Recurrence in future pregnancies	Usually does not recur	Usually recurs in subsequent pregnancies, typically begins earlier in gestation and is often more severe

nodules on the extensor surfaces of the limbs and on the trunk and may appear crusted and eczematous. The treatment involves topical corticosteroids, and the disease usually resolves in the postpartum period. There are no fetal sequelae.

Ambros-Rudolph CM, Müllegger RR, Vaughan-Jones SA, Kerl H, Black MM. The specific dermatoses of pregnancy revisited and reclassified: results of a retrospective two-center study on 505 pregnant patients. *J Am Acad Dermatol.* 2006;54(3):395–404.

11. What is intrahepatic cholestasis of pregnancy?

ICP is characterized symptomatically by an intense pruritus, most often starting on the palms and soles, and then becoming generalized. There are no other dermatologic findings except excoriations. ICP usually occurs in the third trimester of pregnancy. The etiology of ICP is not completely understood, but there is a strong indication that there is interplay between the cholestatic effect of pregnancy hormones (estrogen and progesterone) and genetic susceptibility.

Williamson C, Geenes V. Intrahepatic cholestasis of pregnancy. *Obstet Gynecol.* 2014;124(1):120–133.

12. Are there specific laboratory findings to establish the diagnosis?

Yes. The most specific laboratory derangements are found when measuring bile acids, specifically cholic acid and deoxycholic acid, which may be elevated more than 100 times (upper end of normal: 10 μmol/L). Liver transaminases (aspartate transaminase, alanine transaminase [ALT]) may also be elevated. ALT is thought to be the more sensitive marker, with an increase of 2 to 10 times the upper limit of normal. Bilirubin levels may be elevated, but total bilirubin levels do not often exceed 6 mg/dL. Alkaline phophatase is elevated in pregnancy, and thus is not a good marker to test for ICP.

13. What risks and outcomes are associated with intrahepatic cholestasis of pregnancy?

Traditionally, it has been thought that sudden intrauterine fetal death occurs in 1% to 2% of pregnancies affected by ICP. However, a meta-analysis by Mohan et al. revealed that there is no statistical increase in still birth among pregnant women with intrahepatic cholestasis (IHC). Rather, there is an increased risk of preterm birth, cesarean section, and induction of labor. Other complications include respiratory distress syndrome, meconium staining of amniotic fluid membranes, and premature delivery. The risk of fetal complications increases with bile acid levels greater than 40 μM/ L. There is a risk of vitamin K deficiency and bleeding complications in both the mother and the fetus. The pruritus (maternal) associated with ICP usually resolves within 48 hours to 2 weeks, after delivery.

Mohan M, Antonios A, Konje J, Lindow S, Ahmed Syed M, Akobeng A. Stillbirth and associated perinatal outcomes in obstetric cholestasis: a systematic review and meta-analysis of observational studies. *Eur J Obstet Gynecol Reprod Biol X.* 2019;3:100026.

14. How is cholestasis of pregnancy treated?

See Table 59.2.

Ambros-Rudolph CM, Glatz M, Trauner M, Kerl H, Müllegger RR. The importance of serum bile acid level analysis and treatment with ursodeoxycholic acid in intrahepatic cholestasis of pregnancy: a case series from central Europe. *Arch Dermatol.* 2007;143(6):757–762.
Hepburn IS, Schade RR. Pregnancy-associated liver disorders. *Dig Dis Sci.* 2008;53:2334–2358.

Table 59.2 Treatment regimens of ICP

Ursodeoxycholic acid 15 mg/kg/day	Decreases bile acid concentration
	Aids in transplacental transport of bile acids
S-adenosyl-methionine	Reverses estrogen-induced cholestasis in experimental animals
	Minimally improves bile acid laboratory values and pruritus
	Studies show conflicting evidence regarding the efficacy of this drug
Cholestyramine	Generally not shown to be effective
Dexamethasone	Inhibits placental estrogen synthesis
	Does not improve pruritus or transaminase levels
	Repeated doses may be associated with decreased birth weight and other fetal complications
Delivery	Delivery is the cure for ICP
	Most authors recommend early delivery by 38 weeks (<36 weeks for severe laboratory derangements)

ICP, Intrahepatic cholestasis of pregnancy.

15. What is pustular psoriasis of pregnancy (formerly impetigo herpetiformis)?

Pustular psoriasis of pregnancy is rare and typically presents in the third trimester. This disease is characterized by sterile pustules on an erythematous plaque initially presenting on the flexural and intertriginous areas and then progressing to involve the trunk and remaining surfaces of the extremities. Pustular psoriasis of pregnancy can involve the mucous membranes. There also can be nail involvement, as well as systemic symptoms such as fever and malaise. It is associated with an increased risk of intrauterine growth restriction and stillbirth. It tends to recur earlier in subsequent pregnancies.

Trivedi MK, Vaughn AR, Murase JE. Pustular psoriasis of pregnancy: current perspectives. *Int J Womens Health*. 2018;10:109–115.

16. Are there lab findings associated with pustular psoriasis of pregnancy?

Yes. Associated lab findings include leukocytosis, elevated erythrocyte sedimentation rate, and occasionally hypocalcemia.

17. What is the treatment for pustular psoriasis of pregnancy?

Systemic corticosteroids are the first-line treatment. Some studies have reported good outcomes with cyclosporine and tumor necrosis factor-α inhibitors. The condition resolves with delivery. It is important to be aware of secondary infections of the lesions and then to treat with appropriate antimicrobial medications.

Trivedi MK, Vaughn AR, Murase JE. Pustular psoriasis of pregnancy: current perspectives. *Int J Womens Health*. 2018;10:109–115.

PHYSIOLOGIC SKIN CHANGES IN PREGNANCY

18. List the physiologic skin changes that can occur as a normal part of pregnancy.
- Pigmentary changes
- Hair changes
- Vascular changes
- Connective tissue changes (striae distensae)
- Cutaneous tumors

Kannambal K, Tharini GK. A screening study on dermatoses in pregnancy. *J Clin Diagn Res*. 2017;11(5):WC01–WC05.
Vaughan Jones S, Ambros-Rudolph C, Nelson-Piercy C. Skin disease in pregnancy. *BMJ*. 2014;348:g3489.

19. What are some of the normal pigmentary changes that can be associated with pregnancy?
- Darkening of the nipples, areola, genitalia, axilla, inner thighs, and periumbilical area
- Darkening of the linea alba, which is then referred to as the linea nigra
- Darkening of recent scars
- Melanonychia
- Melasma, which is hyperpigmentation of the face involving the cheeks, nose, or the chin (Fig. 59.4)
- Darkening of ephelides and nevi

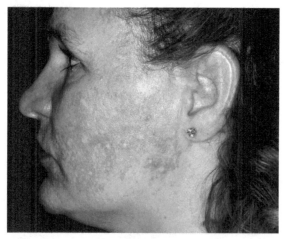

Fig. 59.4 Photodistributed macular hyperpigmentation typical of melasma.

20. **Why do these pigmentary changes occur?**
The exact mechanism is not known, but it is thought that an increase in estrogen, progesterone, and melanocyte-stimulating hormone stimulates melanogenesis.

Barankin B, Silver SG, Carruthers A. The skin in pregnancy. *J Cutan Med Surg.* 2002;6(3):236–240.

21. **How does pregnancy affect patients with melanoma?**
Melanoma is the most common skin malignancy diagnosed in pregnancy. Pregnancy is no longer thought to worsen the prognosis of melanoma, and the survival rates for similarly staged pregnant and nonpregnant individuals are not statistically significant. In advanced cases, melanoma may metastasize to the placenta.

Driscoll MS, Martires K, Bieber AK, Pomeranz MK, Grant-Kels JM, Stein JA. Pregnancy and melanoma. *J Am Acad Dermatol.* 2016; 75(4):669–678.

22. **Is pregnancy associated with changes in hair growth?**
In pregnancy, women experience a prolonged anagen phase, which leads to clinical thickening of the hair. The hairs shift into a telogen phase 1 to 5 months following delivery, and these patients then experience a telogen effluvium. Hirsutism (male pattern facial and body terminal hair growth) may also increase in pregnancy, and usually resolves 6 months postpartum.

23. **List the vascular changes that can occur in pregnancy.**
   • Palmar erythema (Fig. 59.5)
   • Spider angiomas (Fig. 59.6)
   • Varicose veins
   • Hemorrhoids

24. **What factors influence the development of striae distensae (commonly known as "stretch marks")?**
   • Greater degrees of abdominal distention (such as in multiple gestation)
   • High degree of weight gain
   • Genetic predisposition
   • Estrogen, adrenocortical hormone, and relaxin, all of which play a role in connective tissue formation.

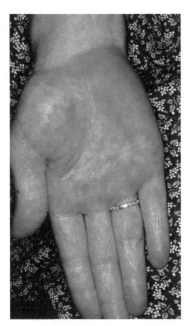

Fig. 59.5 Marked palmar erythema in a pregnant woman.

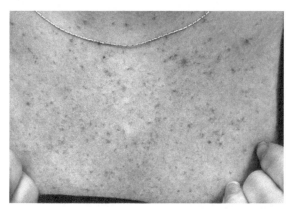

Fig. 59.6 Numerous spider angiomas that appeared on the chest of a pregnant woman. She also developed a pyogenic granuloma of pregnancy on the gingiva. Both types of lesions disappeared following delivery. (Courtesy James E. Fitzpatrick, MD.)

25. Discuss two cutaneous tumors often associated with pregnancy.
    1. **Pyogenic granuloma of pregnancy** (granuloma gravidarum) is a cutaneous tumor consisting of a vascular proliferation, most often of the gingival tissue in pregnant women. These tumors may ulcerate and become painful. Pyogenic granuloma usually spontaneously regresses after pregnancy.
    2. **Molluscum fibrosum gravidarum** are skin tags that develop on the face, neck, axilla, and inframammary areas of pregnant women. They may regress spontaneously postpartum.

Ramos-E-Silva M, Martins NR, Kroumpouzos G. Oral and vulvovaginal changes in pregnancy. *Clin Dermatol.* 2016;34(3):353–358.

26. Do some diseases improve with pregnancy?
    Yes. Examples of such diseases include
    • Psoriasis
    • Rheumatoid arthritis
    • Hidradenitis suppurativa
    • Fox-Fordyce disease
    The regression of psoriasis and rheumatoid arthritis is thought to be related to the suppressed maternal immunity of pregnancy. Improvement of hidradenitis suppurativa and Fox-Fordyce disease is possibly secondary to the decreased apocrine gland activity in pregnancy.

Yang CS, Teeple M, Muglia J, Robinson-Bostom L. Inflammatory and glandular skin disease in pregnancy. *Clin Dermatol.* 2016;34 (3):335–343.

27. Do some mucocutaneous diseases worsen in pregnancy?
    Yes. See Table 59.3.

Table 59.3 Mucocutaneous diseases exacerbated by pregnancy
Infections
Candidal vaginitis
Trichomoniasis
Condyloma acuminatus
Pityrosporum folliculitis
Herpes simplex
Varicella-zoster
Leprosy
Diseases of Altered Immunity
Lupus erythematosus
Systemic sclerosis (renal)
Polymyositis/dermatomyositis
Pemphigus

Table 59.3 Mucocutaneous diseases exacerbated by pregnancy (*Continued*)

Metabolic Diseases
Porphyria cutanea tarda
Acrodermatitis enteropathica

Connective Tissue Disorders
Ehlers-Danlos syndrome (laceration, postpartum hemorrhage)
Pseudoxanthoma elasticum

Miscellaneous Conditions
Erythrokeratodermia variabilis
Mycosis fungoides
Neurofibromatosis
Acquired immunodeficiency syndrome
Hereditary hemorrhagic telangiectasia

CHAPTER 60

DISORDERS OF THE FEMALE GENITALIA

Misha D. Miller

NONNEOPLASTIC EPITHELIAL DISORDERS OF THE VULVA

1. **What is lichen sclerosus (also known as lichen sclerosus et atrophicus)?**

   Lichen sclerosus (LS) (Fig. 60.1) is an inflammatory condition that primarily affects the epidermis and the superficial dermis. The disease process results in thinned or atrophic white papules and plaques of the skin. It is estimated that LS affects 1:60 women. LS primarily affects the anogenital region, but it can also present on the trunk or extremities. LS of the vulva most commonly affects postmenopausal women, but it can also develop in 7% to 15% of prepubertal females.

   Pérez-López FR, Vieira-Baptista P. Lichen sclerosus in women: a review. *Climacteric.* 2017;20(4):339–347.

2. **Describe the clinical signs of LS of the vulva.**

   The characteristic findings associated with LS include white, thinned, crinkled skin (it is frequently described as "cigarette paper" atrophy). Often, there is absorption of the labia minora, fusion of the labia minora to the labia majora, and fusion of the clitoral hood. One also may find vular fissures. The majority of the vagina is usually unaffected; however, a patient may have involvement of the vaginal introitus, leading to stenosis. LS can also simultaneously involve the perianal area, which then forms a "figure-of-eight" pattern.

   Zendell K, Edwards L. Lichen sclerosus with vaginal involvement: report of 2 cases and review of the literature. *JAMA Dermatol.* 2013; 149(10):1199–1202.

3. **What are the symptoms of LS?**

   The most common symptom associated with LS is pruritus. Patients may also report burning, bleeding, and tearing of the vulva or vaginal introitus. If stenosis of the vaginal introitus is present, dyspareunia is often reported.

4. **Is there a need to biopsy LS of the vulva?**

   Yes. Biopsy of the affected site can aid in differentiating LS from other disorders, such as vitiligo (Fig. 60.2) and lichen planus. Hyperkeratotic, ulcerated, or nodular lesions should be sampled to rule out vulvar intraepithelial neoplasia (VIN) or squamous cell carcinoma (SCC) of the vulva. The risk of LS becoming malignant is 4% to 6%.

5. **Are there any other diseases associated with LS?**

   Yes. Research supports that the etiology of LS has a strong autoinflammatory component. Immunoglobulin G (IgG) antibodies targeting the extracellular matrix 1 (ECM-1) protein have been found in 74% of women with LS, as opposed to 7% in controls. Concomitant diseases that may be present with LS include Hashimoto's thyroiditis (12% to 30%), alopecia areata (9%), or vitiligo (6%). Other autoimmune diseases may also be present. Additionally, secondary concomitant infection with yeast or bacteria is common in LS and should be treated accordingly.

   Pérez-López FR, Vieira-Baptista P. Lichen sclerosus in women: a review. *Climacteric.* 2017;20(4):339–347.
   Fistarol SK, Itin PH. Diagnosis and treatment of lichen sclerosus: an update. *Am J Clin Dermatol.* 2013;14(1):27–47.

6. **How does one treat lichen sclerosus?**

   The most widely accepted first-line treatment is use of a high-potency topical corticosteroid, most commonly clobetasol propionate 0.05% ointment. Other therapies used for LS include intralesional corticosteroids (recalcitrant), methotrexate, retinoids, chloroquine, tacrolimus/pimecrolimus, cyclosporine, and photodynamic therapy with topical 5-aminolevulinic acid. LS in children often will resolve at the time of puberty.

   Lee A, Fischer G. Diagnosis and treatment of vulvar lichen sclerosus: an update for dermatologists. *Am J Clin Dermatol.* 2018; 19(5):695–706.

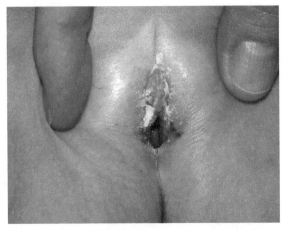

Fig. 60.1 Lichen sclerosus demonstrating typical ill-defined hypopigmentation with wrinkled atrophic appearance that is best visualized near the bottom of the lesion. (Courtesy James E. Fitzpatrick, MD.)

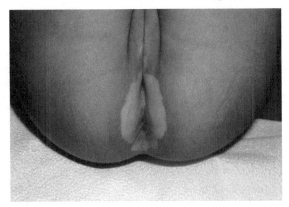

Fig. 60.2 Vitiligo showing characteristic total depigmentation with evidence of atrophy. Notice the typical scalloped margins. (Courtesy Fitzsimons Army Medical Center teaching files.)

7. What is the differential diagnosis of lichen sclerosus of the vulva?
   - Lichen planus
   - Vitiligo
   - VIN
   - Sexual abuse (children)
   - Inverse psoriasis

8. What is lichen planus?
   Lichen planus is an autoimmune inflammatory disorder. The exact pathogenesis is not completely understood, but it is thought to be a T-cell–mediated disorder that results from damage to the epidermal basement membrane secondary to antibodies directed against components of the basal keratinocytes.

9. Are there different variants of lichen planus that affect the vulva?
   Yes. Variants that affect the vulva include erosive lichen planus, papulosquamous lichen planus, and hypertrophic lichen planus. The most common variant found in the vulvar vestibule is erosive lichen planus. This variant is characterized by erosions of the vulvar mucosa, the vaginal introitus, and, often, the vagina. One may also see alterations of the vulvar anatomy similar to that found with lichen sclerosus. Unlike LS, lichen planus more commonly affects the vagina leading to stenosis, synechiae, and scarring. Oral-vulval-vaginal lichen planus may also be seen. One study reported that of the women with oral LP, 75% also had genital involvement.

Andreassi L, Bilenchi R. Non-infectious inflammatory genital lesions. *Clin Dermatol.* 2014;32(2):307–314.
ACOG Practice Bulletin No. 93. diagnosis and management of vulvar skin disorders. *Obstet Gynecol.* 2008;93:1243–1253.

10. **What are the clinical symptoms of vulval lichen planus?**

    Patients most commonly present with complaints of vulvovaginal burning, pruritus, postcoital bleeding, and dyspareunia. Up to 70% of patients also have vaginal lesions. There may be an associated purulent vaginal discharge, and chronic erosions of the vaginal epithelium can lead to the development of extensive adhesions leading to vaginal narrowing and obliteration.

    Lewis FM. Vulval lichen planus. *Br J Dermatol.* 1998;138(4):569–575.

11. **Is lichen planus associated with malignancy?**

    SCC developing in patients with lichen planus has been poorly documented. In patients with SCC developing in a background of vulvar LP, one study found that there is a high rate of inguinal metastasis (~30%), recurrence of SCC even if completely excised, and associated mortality.

    Regauer S, Reich O, Eberz B. Vulvar cancers in women with vulvar lichen planus: a clinicopathological study. *J Am Acad Dermatol.* 2014;71(4):698–707.

12. **How do you treat lichen planus of the vulva?**

    Treatment of lichen planus of the mucosal surfaces, such as the vulvovaginal areas, is very difficult. Potent topical steroids are commonly used, but have mixed results. Other therapies that have been reported include pimecrolimus, tacrolimus, hydroxychloroquine, cyclosporine, and methotrexate.

    Dubey R, Fischer G. Vulvo-vaginal lichen planus: a focussed review for the clinician. *Australas J Dermatol.* 2019;60(1):7–11.

13. **Describe lichen simplex chronicus of the vulva.**

    Lichen simplex chronicus is an end-stage response that results from chronic scratching or rubbing of the skin. The skin becomes thickened, lichenified (exaggeration of the normal skin lines), and will often show excoriations. Any condition that causes pruritus (itching) of the skin, in combination with the patient scratching the involved area, ultimately resuls in the development of lichen simplex chronicus. The primary skin condition is most commonly eczema.

14. **Psoriasis can be present on the vulva. How does it present?**

    Psoriasis of the vulva presents as beefy red symmetrical plaques. The silvery scale associated with psoriatic lesions on other areas of the body is typically absent. A patient may have psoriasis of the inguinal creases, referred to as inverse psoriasis. Skin lesions of psoriasis in this area may be more inflamed and have undergone maceration secondary to friction and moisture. Vulvar pruritus and burning may be prominent symptoms.

15. **How is psoriasis of the vulva treated?**

    Low-potency topical steroids are generally the first line of treatment. Calcipotriene, pimecrolimus, and tacrolimus, although less efficacious, are also used to avoid steroid effects such as atrophy of the more delicate genital skin.

    Beck KM, Yang EJ, Sanchez IM, Liao W. Treatment of genital psoriasis: a systematic review. *Dermatol Ther (Heidelb).* 2018;8(4):509–525.

16. **What are other common causes of vulvar pruritus?**
    - Vulvar contact dermatitis (Table 60.1)
    - Vulvovaginal infections
    - Vulvar malignancy

Table 60.1 Common causes of vulvar contact dermatitis
• Bath soaps
• Feminine hygiene sprays, deodorant sprays
• Fragrance
• Lubricants
• Spermicides
• Semen
• Condoms
• Clothing dyes
• Sanitary pads
• Benzocaine
• Neomycin
• Antifungal creams
• Urine

17. Name some common vulvovaginal infections associated with pruritus?
    - Fungal (candidiasis, tinea cruris)
    - Bacterial vaginosis
    - Trichomoniasis
    - Infestations such as scabies
    - Condylomata acuminata (genital warts)
    - Molluscum contagiosum

18. Compare and contrast condyloma acuminata and molluscum contagiosum.
    See Table 60.2.

VASCULITIC DISEASE OF THE VULVA

19. What is Behçet's disease?
    Behçet's disease (Fig. 60.3) is a chronic relapsing vasculitis of unknown etiology that results in ocular, mucocutaneous, genital, pulmonary, neurologic, gastrointestinal, and articular involvement. Oral and genital lesions are manifested as painful aphthous-like ulcers, and may be the earliest signs of this disease. Behçet's disease is most prevalent along the "silk road," which spans from Japan and China to the Mediterranean Sea (countries such as Turkey), but it is also seen in the United States, though uncommonly. The disease usually presents in the third decade of life.

20. What is the treatment for Behçet's disease?
    - Topical corticosteroids
    - Antibiotic solutions
    - Topical anesthetics
    - Silver nitrate
    For more severe disease:
    - Oral corticosteroids
    - Colchicine
    - Oral antibiotics (benzathine penicillin)
    - Immunosuppressive agents (azathioprine, cyclosporine)
    - Biologic agents (antitumor necrosis factor–α agents, interferon)

Alpsoy E, Akman A. Behçet's disease: an algorithmic approach to its treatment. *Arch Dermatol Res.* 2009;301:693–702.

Table 60.2 Condyloma acuminatum versus molluscum contagiosum

	CONDYLOMA ACUMINATA	**MOLLUSCUM CONTAGIOSUM**
Clinical appearance	Soft fleshy, cauliflower-like papules. Can be very small with a dome shape and thus difficult to differentiate from molluscum contagiosum	Small, dome-shaped, typically flesh-colored papules with a central umbilication when squeezed on the lateral edges
Etiology	Human papillomavirus (HPV) HPV-6 and -11 are responsible for 90% of these lesions	DNA poxvirus—molluscum contagiosum virus (MCV). MCV-1 is most prevalent; MCV-2 is most commonly associated with sexually transmitted molluscum contagiosum
Transmission	Sexually transmitted Highly contagious	Sexually transmitted in adults (this disease is common in children on nongenital skin and is not thought to be sexually transmitted) Highly contagious; known to be spread through fomites (e.g., wet towels, etc.)
Autoinoculation	Yes	Yes
Treatment	Imiquimod Podophyllin Trichloroacetic acid Laser ablation Cryosurgery	Imiquimod Cantharidin Trichloroacetic acid Curettage Laser ablation Cryosurgery Expectant management (many lesions will spontaneously resolve within 2 years)
Vaccine?	Quadrivalent vaccine for immunity against HPV-6, -11, -16, and -18	None

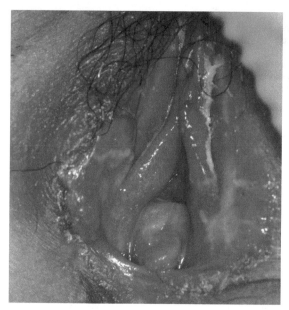

Fig. 60.3 Behçet's disease demonstrating a nonspecific vaginal ulcer. (Courtesy William L. Weston, MD collection.)

NEOPLASTIC DISORDERS OF THE VULVA

21. What is the most common cancer of the vulva?

Ninety percent of vulval cancer are SCC. The remaining 10% of malignancies involving the vulva include melanoma, basal cell carcinoma, Paget's disease, and other rare cancers.

KEY POINTS: DISORDERS OF THE FEMALE GENITALIA

1. LS commonly involves the anogenital area, forming a "figure-of-eight" pattern on the skin.
2. There is a low but present risk (4% to 6%) of squamous cell carcinoma arising in LS.
3. Patients with vulvar lichen planus also commonly have vaginal lesions that may lead to significant morbidity secondary to vaginal adhesions and obliteration.
4. Lichen simplex chronicus is the end-stage result (thickened, lichenified skin) from chronic scratching or rubbing of the skin.
5. The majority of vulvar carcinoma is squamous cell carcinoma.

---

22. Is SCC of the vulva associated with a precancerous state?

Yes. Vulvar intraepithelial neoplasia is the term used to describe dysplasia of vulvar epithelial cells. VIN is further divided into VIN usual type, which is associated with high-risk human papillomavirus (HPV) strains, such as HPV-16 and HPV-18, and differentiated VIN, which is associated with chronic vulvar dermatoses, particularly LS. VIN is associated with vulvar pruritus and burning. The lesion may be described as a raised papule or nodule that is erythematous or white.

Maclean AB, Jones RW, Scurry J, Neill S. Vulvar cancer and the need for awareness of precursor lesions. *J Low Genit Tract Dis.* 2009;13:115–117.

23. How long does it take VIN to progress to SCC of the vulva?

The mean time from the initial diagnosis of VIN to the diagnosis of SCC of the vulva is 4 to 8 years.

24. How does one treat VIN/SCC of the vulva?

VIN is treated mostly with surgical excision or laser ablation if not severe. Using topical imiquimod is also becoming more common. Excision or Mohs micrographic surgery may be used to treat high-grade squamous intraepithelial neoplasia/VINIII. SCC of the vulva is treated surgically, usually by a gynecologic oncologist. Adjuvant therapy may include regional lymphadenectomy, chemotherapy, and radiation.

25. **What is the second most common vulvar malignancy?**

    Melanoma. It is most common in elderly women in the seventh or eighth decade of life. Unlike other cutaneous melanomas that develop in sun-exposed areas, and are thus thought to be related to ultraviolet light exposure, melanomas of the vulva are thought, possibly, to be associated with chronic inflammatory disease, chemical irritants, viral infections (including HPV), and genetic susceptibility.

    De Simone P, Silipo V, Buccini P, et al. Vulvar melanoma: a report of 10 cases and review of the literature. *Melanoma Res.* 2008;18:127–133.

26. **How does melanoma of the vulva present?**

    Patients with melanoma of the vulva present with a pigmented mass of the labia majora, labia minora, or clitoris. Most patients will complain of bleeding, burning or pruritus, and, less often, discharge or ulceration. Some patients may be asymptomatic.

27. **Are melanomas of the vulva more aggressive than other cutaneous melanomas?**

    No. Melanomas found in the vulvar area do not behave differently than melanomas on other areas of the body. Vulvar melanomas tend to be diagnosed at a later stage than other cutaneous melanomas that are on skin that is more visible and examined more frequently than the vulva. The 5-year survival rate is between 36% and 60%.

    Nasu K, Kai Y, Ohishi M, et al. Conservative surgical treatment for early-stage vulvar malignant melanoma. *Arch Gynecol Obstet.* 2010;281:335–338.

28. **What is the treatment of melanoma of the vulva?**

    Traditionally, treatment of vulvar melanoma involves surgical management in the form of a radical vulvectomy with bilateral inguinal–femoral lymph node dissection. However, this disfiguring therapy, which leads to a high rate of morbidity, has not been shown to increase the survival rates or lower the recurrence rate over more conservative management. More conservative surgical treatment includes wide local excision for early-stage disease. The use of adjuvant chemotherapy varies according to the institution.

29. **What is Paget's disease of the vulva?**

    Paget's disease (Fig. 60.4) is a neoplasia of the vulva that consists of adenocarcinoma-type cells that invade the epidermis, the appendages of the skin, and occasionally the dermis. It represents 1% of vulvar neoplasms. However, 25% of the time that extramammary Paget's disease is present, it is associated with an underlying adenocarcinoma

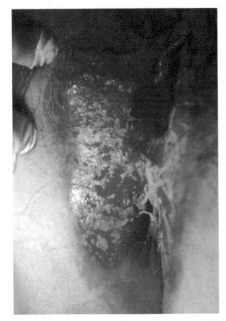

Fig. 60.4 Genital extramammary Paget's disease demonstrating marked erythema with superficial erosions. (Courtesy Whitney A. High, MD.)

(most commonly of the skin adnexa or Bartholin gland) or at a distant site (e.g., the breast, genitourinary system, or the intestinal tract). Thus, it is prudent to search for other possible malignancies if Paget's disease of the vulva is diagnosed.

30. How does Paget's disease of the vulva present?
The most common symptom is pruritus. On examination, there are usually erythematous plaques with white hyperkeratotic areas. Over time, these areas may desquamate.

31. What is the differential diagnosis of Paget's disease?
- Seborrheic dermatitis
- Psoriasis
- Atopic dermatitis
- Tinea cruris
- Candidiasis

32. How does one treat Paget's disease of the vulva?
Surgical excision is the gold standard of treatment. However, clear margins are difficult to obtain. Mohs micrographic surgery, because of the intraoperative margin control, has been shown to have lower recurrence rates when compared to excision. Moreover, recurrence rates after surgical excision are high (up to 58%) in some studies. Other nonsurgical treatments that have been reported include imiquimod, 5-fluorouracil, and laser ablation.

Morris CR, Hurst EA. Extramammary Paget's disease: a review of the literature part II: treatment and prognosis. *Dermatol Surg.* 2020; 46(3):305–311. doi:10.1097/DSS.0000000000002240.

CHAPTER 61

DISORDERS OF THE MALE GENITALIA

Theodore Rosen

1. Circumcision is the most effective treatment in uncircumcised men with Zoon's balanitis.
2. Circinate balanitis is a cutaneous manifestation of reactive arthritis (Reiter's disease).
3. Penile lichen sclerosus and, to a lesser extent, lichen planus may be associated with an increased risk of squamous cell carcinoma.
4. Pearly penile papules are angiofibromas and are not a sexually transmitted disorder.
5. Topical calcineurin inhibitors may prove beneficial for many penile dermatoses, such as psoriasis, when topical corticosteroids are ineffective or not tolerated.

1. **What types of disorders affect the male genitalia?**
   Most any type of skin disorder seen elsewhere can affect the male genitalia, including infections (both sexually transmitted diseases [STDs] and non-STDs), inflammatory dermatoses, cutaneous signs of systemic or metabolic diseases, benign and malignant neoplasms, and exogenous (including factitious) lesions. Male genital lesions should always prompt a complete cutaneous examination, as well as a comprehensive review of systems and past medical history.

   Marcos-Pinto A, Soares-de-Almeida L, Borges-Costa J. Nonvenereal penile dermatoses: a retrospective study. *Indian Dermatol Online J.* 2018;9(2):96–100.

2. **What are some specific disorders to keep in mind when assessing male genitalia?**
   Common sexually transmitted diseases include syphilis, herpes progenitalis, genital warts, scabies, and molluscum contagiosum; much less common in the United States would be granuloma inguinale (donovanosis), lymphogranuloma venereum, and chancroid. Non-STD infections include candida balanitis and Fournier's synergistic gangrene. Psoriasis, seborrhea, and lichen planus (LP) can affect the genitalia, and lichen sclerosus (LS) is common, and Zoon's balanitis and sclerosing lymphangitis are exclusively encountered in this anatomic area. Squamous cell carcinoma (SCC), both in situ and invasive, is the most common malignant tumor, while pearly penile papules (PPPs), angiokeratomas, Fordyce spots, and epidermal cysts are common benign lesions. Penile calciphylaxis, pyoderma gangrenosum, and circinate balanitis may indicate underlying systemic disease. Fixed drug eruption often occurs on the glans.

   Teichman JM, Mannas M, Elston DM. Noninfectious penile lesions. *Am Fam Physician.* 2018;97(2):102–110.
   Heller DS. Lesions and neoplasms of the penis: a review. *J Low Genit Tract Dis.* 2016;20(1):107–111.

3. **How well do penile disorders respond to appropriate therapy?**
   The majority of patients with a dermatological problem involving the penis will complain of a "rash" or a "lesions." Although soreness, pain, burning, or itching may be present in about 20% of patients, many penile dermatoses are asymptomatic. From the time of presentation until 6 months later, some 70% of patients will either be clear or greatly improved, with only about 4%–5% reporting no improvement. In general, therefore, penile skin disorders are largely responsive to appropriate medical or surgical intervention.

   Shah M. Clinical outcomes in a specialist male genital skin clinic: prospective follow-up of 600 patients. *Clin Exp Dermatol.* 2017; 42(7):723–727.

4. **What is Candida balanitis and how is it treated?**
   Balanitis, defined as inflammation of the glans penis, affects 3%–11% of men at some time during their lifetime. *Candida albicans* is one common cause of balanitis, especially in older, obese, and diabetic or immunocompromised/immunosuppressed men. It presents as a pruritic or tender, superficial erythematous erosion, with or without

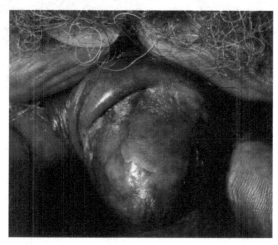

Fig. 61.1 Candida balanitis demonstrates superficial erosion and accumulation of some cheesy debris near the corona.

malodorous, cheesy debris (Fig. 61.1). Culture or stained smear will reveal the etiologic yeast in profusion. Treatment may include either topical imidazole antifungals or oral fluconazole (150 mg once; if severe, 150 mg every 72 hours for three doses). Circumcision may help prevent recurrence.

Morris BJ, Krieger JN. Penile inflammatory skin disorders and the preventive role of circumcision. *Int J Prev Med.* 2017;8(1):32.
Lisboa C, Ferreira A, Resende C, Rodrigues AG. Infectious balanoposthitis: management, clinical and laboratory features. *Int J Dermatol.* 2009;48(2):121–124.

5. What is Zoon's balanitis?

Also known as balanitis circumscripta plasmacellularis and idiopathic lymphoplasmacellular dermatitis, this entity is a chronic, benign inflammatory condition of the glans penis (and/or inner prepuce) affecting middle-aged to elderly uncircumcised men. Classically, Zoon's balanitis has been described as a nontender and nonpruritic, well-circumscribed red-orange plaque containing multiple areas of pinpoint red spots (called "cayenne pepper spots"). Eventually, superficial erosion, accompanied by serous oozing, may ensue. The etiology is unknown. Diagnosis should be verified by biopsy, as the clinical appearance may closely mimic other penile disorders, especially SCC in situ. Classic, well-developed lesions demonstrate a thinned, effaced epithelium with a dense lichenoid plasma cell infiltrate, intermixed with vertically oriented telangiectasia and hemosiderin deposits.

Erdogan BS, Demirkan N, Aktan S, et al. A focus on differential diagnosis of lichen planus and plasma cell balanitis. *J Eur Acad Dermatol Venereol.* 2006;20(6):746–748.
Andreassi L, Bilenchi R. Non-infectious inflammatory genital lesions. *Clin Dermatol.* 2014;32(2):307–314.

6. How can Zoon's balanitis be treated?

Zoon's balanitis may or may not respond to topical therapy, including topical corticosteroids and calcineurin inhibitors. Application of 2% mupirocin ointment three times daily has recently been reported successful. The most reliable treatment is circumcision, given that Zoon's balanitis generally occurs in uncircumcised males. Surgical excision, as well as either CO_2 laser or erbium:YAG laser ablation, are additional potential therapeutic modalities.

Tang A, David N, Horton LW. Plasma cell balanitis of Zoon: response to Trimovate cream. *Int J STD AIDS.* 2001;12(2):75–78.
Albertini JG, Holck DE, Farley MF. Zoon's balanitis treated with erbium:YAG laser ablation. *Lasers Surg Med.* 2002;30(2):123–126.
Pileggi Fde O, Nogueira PL, de Melo Coelho MF, et al. Circumcision as treatment for Zoon's balanitis in an HIV-positive teenage patient. *Int J STD AIDS.* 2013;24(10):837–839.
Lee MA, Cohen PR. Zoon balanitis revisited: report of balanitis circumscripta plasmacellularis resolving with topical mupirocin ointment monotherapy. *J Drugs Dermatol.* 2017;16(3):285–287.

7. What is circinate balanitis?

Circinate balanitis consists of a sharply circumscribed inflammation that characteristically affects the glans penis. Circumcised males present with well-demarcated, erythematous papules that evolve into pustules followed by hyperkeratotic plaques on the glans and/or penile corona. In uncircumcised males, lesions begin as small vesico-pustules on the glans that rupture, leaving painless superficial erosions, which often coalesce to form a serpiginous (or circinate) pattern of moist (rather than hyperkeratotic) plaques. Circinate balanitis is classically associated with reactive arthritis (formerly known as "Reiter's syndrome"), although it may occur separately and may be mimicked by circinate pustular psoriasis of the glans penis or "pseudo–circinate balanitis" or secondary syphilis. Circinate balanitis typically appears concurrently with the other manifestations of this syndrome: urethritis, conjunctivitis, and arthritis.

Singh N, Thappa DM. Circinate pustular psoriasis localized to glans penis mimicking "circinate balanitis" and responsive to dapsone. *Indian J Dermatol Venereol Leprol.* 2008;74(4):388–389.
Wu IB, Schwartz RA. Reiter's syndrome: the classic triad and more. *J Am Acad Dermatol.* 2008;59(1):113–121.

8. What workup is recommended for circinate balanitis, and how is it treated?
   Aside from determining the underlying cause of the reactive arthritis (usually a urethritis or gastroenteritis), a sexually transmitted infection screen is recommended, since syphilis may present with similar features. There is an association between human immunodeficiency virus and reactive arthritis. In equivocal cases, clinical assessment for conjunctivitis and testing for human leukocyte antigen–B27 may corroborate the diagnosis. Circinate balanitis treatment resembles topical treatment of psoriasis, utilizing application of low- to mid-potency topical corticosteroids or calcineurin inhibitors; such treatments are generally effective. Associated reactive arthritis usually responds to systemic therapies employed for psoriasis and psoriatic arthritis, such as methotrexate and tumor necrosis factor-α inhibitors.

de Almeida Jr HL, de Oliveira Filho UL. Topical pimecrolimus is an effective treatment for balanitis circinata erosiva. *Int J Dermatol.* 2005;44(10):888–889.

9. What is balanitis xerotica obliterans?
   Balanitis xerotica obliterans is technically a subset of LS (see below) leading to fibrotic obliteration of the meatal orifice. Sometimes, the term "balanitis xerotica obliterans" (or the abbreviation BXO) is used to designate the disease penile LS. In this chapter, the term "lichen sclerosus" (LS) will be used. LS is about seven times more common in women.

10. What is the clinical appearance of lichen sclerosus? Is it a dangerous condition?
    Although LS is predominantly an adult disease (average age at diagnosis 40–45), it can be encountered in adolescents and children. Initial findings include nonspecific erythematous to hypopigmented macules and thin papules affecting the glans, coronal sulcus, and prepuce. These coalesce and eventuate into well-demarcated white atrophic plaques with prominent follicular plugging. The surface of lesions has a texture resembling crinkled paper or cellophane. Plaques often exhibit purpura, a characteristic that helps differentiate LS from vitiligo (Fig. 61.2). The disease process may be entirely asymptomatic, but more commonly one or more symptoms appear: pruritus, pain, bleeding, or painful erections. Varying degrees of phimosis may occur, leading to urethral obstruction. Thus, incomplete voiding, dysuria,

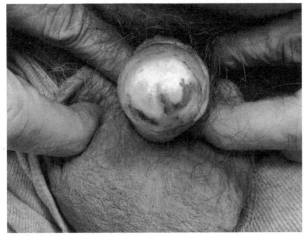

Fig. 61.2 Lichen sclerosus with classic, white-colored atrophy and prominent purpura.

urethral discharge, and urinary retention are possible complications. Urinary dysfunction may be so severe as to cause retrograde urinary reflux, damaging the bladder and leading to obstructive nephropathy. LS is considered a premalignant condition; 4%–10% of patients develop SCC within affected areas.

Celis S, Reed F, Murphy F, et al. Balanitis xerotica obliterans in children and adolescents: a literature review and clinical series. *J Pediatr Urol.* 2014;10(1):34–39.
Yesudian PD, Sugunendran H, Bates CM, et al. Lichen sclerosus. *Int J STD AIDS.* 2005;16(7):465–473.
Clouston D, Hall A, Lawrentschuk N. Penile lichen sclerosus (balanitis xerotica obliterans). *BJU Int.* 2011;108(suppl 2):14–19.
Pietrzak P, Hadway P, Corbishley CM, et al. Is the association between balanitis xerotica obliterans and penile carcinoma underestimated? *BJU Int.* 2006;98(1):74–76.
Powell J, Robson A, Cranston D, et al. High incidence of lichen sclerosus in patients with squamous cell carcinoma of the penis. *Br J Dermatol.* 2011;145(1):85–89.

11. What medical therapies may arrest the progression of lichen sclerosus?

Medical therapy should be attempted first to arrest the progression of this condition. The application of an ultrapotent topical steroid (clobetasol 0.05% or 0.025%, halobetasol 0.05%) has shown to relatively reliably arrest the progression of LS. While there is no difference in the degree of symptomatic relief (itching, pain) between topical calcineurin inhibitors and topical corticosteroids, the former were found to be inferior to corticosteroids in arresting disease progression and in cosmetic improvement in a recent meta-analysis. Once ultrapotent steroid therapy is initiated, it should be continued once or twice daily. It can also be given as a weekend "pulse." The patient should be reevaluated 2 to 3 months later to assess for efficacy, and if the disease enters remission, the frequency of application as well as the strength of steroid may be tapered to maintain a quiescent state.

Chi CC, Kirtschig G, Baldo M, et al. Systematic review and meta-analysis of randomized controlled trials on topical interventions for genital lichen sclerosus. *J Am Acad Dermatol.* 2012;67(2):305–312.
Chi CC, Kirtschig G, Baldo M, et al. Topical interventions for genital lichen sclerosus. *Cochrane Database Syst Rev.* 2011;(12):CD008240.
Edwards S, Bunker C, Ziller F, et al. 2013 European guideline for the management of balanoposthitis. *Int J STD AIDS.* 2014;25(9):615–626.

12. What procedural methods might be used to treat LS?

Surgery is indicated for persistent/resistant disease or if there is clinical suspicion regarding SCC. Circumcision has been shown to ameliorate and in certain cases cure LS, especially in disease confined to the glans and prepuce. Meatoplasty, ureteral dilation, and urethrotomy may improve obstructive disease. Very extensive disease may require glans resurfacing with grafting, while in other cases, excision of all affected areas and extensive reconstruction may be necessary. It is important to note that disease control must be balanced against the patient's desire for sexual and urinary function and acceptable penile cosmesis.

Kirk PS, Yi Y, Hadj-Moussa M, et al. Diversity of patient profile, urethral stricture, and other disease manifestations in a cohort of adult men with lichen sclerosus. *Investig Clin Urol.* 2016;57(3):202–207.
Hartley A, Ramanathan C, Siddiqui H. The surgical treatment of balanitis xerotica obliterans. *Indian J Plast Surg.* 2011;44(1):91–97.

13. What are the physical findings of sclerosing lymphangitis of the penis?

Sclerosing lymphangitis is described as an asymptomatic, "cordlike," firm, translucent to flesh-colored plaque on the coronal sulcus. Extension to the distal penile shaft may occur. A distinguishing characteristic is the seemingly cartilaginous consistency of the lesion on palpation.

Greenberg RD, Perry TL. Nonvenereal sclerosing lymphangitis of the penis. *Arch Dermatol.* 1972;105(5):728–729.

14. In what scenario does sclerosing lymphangitis arise?

Sclerosing lymphangitis is typically found in young, sexually active men between the ages of 20 to 40 years, and within 24 hours of vigorous sexual intercourse or repeated masturbation. An association with sexually transmitted disease is thought to be coincidental rather than etiologic. Sclerosing lymphangitis is typically self-limited, resolving following a period of abstinence from sexual activity. Surgical resection of a persistent lesion may very rarely be required.

Fiumara NJ. Nonvenereal sclerosing lymphangitis of the penis. *Arch Dermatol.* 1975;11(7):902–903.
Rosen T, Hwong H. Sclerosing lymphangitis of the penis. *J Am Acad Dermatol.* 2003;49(5):916–918.
Yap FB. Nonvenereal sclerosing lymphangitis of the penis. *South Med J.* 2009;102(12):1269–1271.

15. What does lichen planus look like on the male genitalia?

LP, an inflammatory disorder of unknown etiology, affects various mucocutaneous sites in about 1% of the general adult population; about one in four LP patients have genital involvement. It is frequently concurrent in both oral and

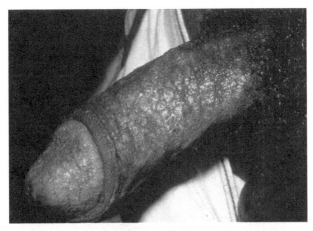

Fig. 61.3 Classic penile lichen planus, with flat-topped, violaceous plaques.

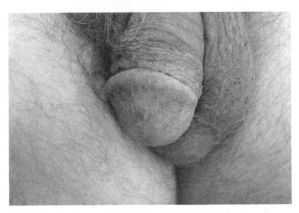

Fig. 61.4 Annular plaque on the glans is a clinical variant of lichen planus in men.

genital sites. The most typical lesion, seen best in circumcised men, is a violaceus, flat-topped leukokeratotic papule. Individual papules may coalesce into larger plaques (Fig. 61.3). Lesions on the glans may assume an annular configuration (Fig. 61.4). In uncircumcised men, lesions are more lacy-white in color and reticulate in distribution. Although much more common on the vulva of women, penile LP may become erosive and painful, thereby resembling Zoon's or candida balanitis, SCC in situ, and fixed drug eruption. Sudden appearance of nodularity, deep ulceration, or induration should suggest evolution into invasive SCC, a rare but reported complication of long-standing genital LP.

Rosen T, Brown TJ. Genital ulcers: evaluation and treatment. *Dermatol Clin.* 1998;16(4):673–685.
Petruzzi M, De Benedittis M, Pastore L, et al. Peno-gingival lichen planus. *J Periodontol.* 2005;76(12):2293–2298.
Hoshi A, Usui Y, Terachi T. Penile carcinoma originating from lichen planus on glans penis. *Urology.* 2008;71(5):816–817.

16. How is lichen planus treated?

Penile LP usually responds well to daily application of mid- to high-potency corticosteroids. Topical calcineurin inhibitors may also be beneficial. Erosive LP has reportedly responded to oral retinoid therapy (acitretin). Some LP patients have coincident viral hepatitis, particularly hepatitis C virus (HCV); in such patients, successful treatment of the underlying viral hepatitis may lead to LP resolution.

Poon F, De Cruz R, Hall A. Acitretin in erosive penile lichen planus. *Australas J Dermatol.* 2017;58(3):e87–e90.
Shengyuan L, Songpo Y, Wen W, et al. Hepatitis C virus and lichen planus: a reciprocal association determined by a meta-analysis. *Arch Dermatol.* 2009;145(9):1040–1047.

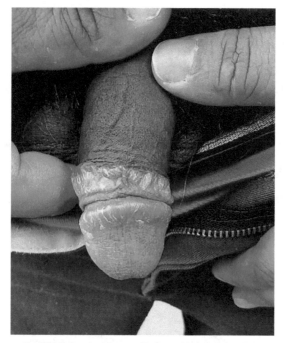

Fig. 61.5 Erythematous plaques with silvery scale, typical of psoriasis.

17. Does psoriasis occur on the genitalia, and how does it appear?

Psoriasis affects 2%–3% of the general population, and some 30%–40% of psoriasis patients have genital involvement. In circumcised men, genital psoriasis closely simulates extragenital disease: erythematous to salmon-colored plaques with overlying silvery scale (Fig. 61.5). In the uncircumcised make, scale is much less prominent and plaques tend to be thinner, with a propensity to weep. Genital psoriasis may well be symptomatic, including the occurrence of itch, pain, general discomfort, stinging, and burning. Genital psoriasis has a significant negative impact on both sexual function and intimate relationships, as well as overall quality of life.

Farber EM, Nall L. Genital psoriasis. *Cutis.* 1992;50(4):263–266.
Meeuwis KA, de Hullu JA, van de Nieuwenhof HP, et al. Quality of life and sexual health in patients with genital psoriasis. *Br J Dermatol.* 2011;164(6):1247–1255.
Meeuwis KA, de Hullu JA, IntHout J, et al. Genital psoriasis awareness program: physical and psychological care for patients with genital psoriasis. *Acta Derm Venereol.* 2015;95(2):211–216.
Yang EJ, Beck KM, Sanchez IM, et al. The impact of genital psoriasis on quality of life: a systematic review. *Psoriasis (Auckl).* 2018;8:41–47.

18. How is genital psoriasis treated?

Application of topical corticosteroids (low to high potency, depending upon response) remains the mainstay of therapy. Topical calcineurin inhibitors (tacrolimus and pimecrolimus) are often quite effective for genital psoriasis but may be irritating. For severe or recalcitrant disease, administration of the biologic drug, ixekizumab, has proven beneficial and is currently Food and Drug Administration (FDA) approved for this indication.

Dattola A, Silvestri M, Bennardo L, et al. Update of calcineurin inhibitors to treat inverse psoriasis: a systematic review. *Dermatol Ther.* 2018;31(6):e12728.
Beck KM, Yang EJ, Sanchez IM, et al. Treatment of genital psoriasis: a systematic review. *Dermatol Ther (Heidelb).* 2018;8(4):509–525.
Ryan C, Menter A, Guenther L, et al. Efficacy and safety of ixekizumab in a randomized, double-blinded, placebo-controlled phase IIIb study of patients with moderate-to-severe genital psoriasis. *Br J Dermatol.* 2018;179(4):844–852.

19. What are pearly penile papules (PPPs) and what do they look like?

PPPs are benign acral angiofibromas, which means that histologically they are composed of fibro vascular stroma with an overlying thickened epithelium. They usually appear as smooth, uniform-sized, dome-shaped papules that are flesh colored to translucent in color. Occasionally, they are elongated rather than dome shaped. They are often arranged in single or double rows along the corona or in the coronal sulcus of the penis There are a few reports of ectopic placement of PPPs along the penile shaft. They are not related to human papillomavirus (HPV) infection and are not contagious. PPPs can be distinguished from external genital warts as the latter are typically "cauliflower" shaped, multilobulated, heterogeneous in appearance, and not limited to the coronal region.

Ackerman AB, Kronberg R. Pearly penile papules. Acral angiofibromas. *Arch Dermatol.* 1973;108(5):673–675.
Hogewoning CJ, Bleeker MC, van den Brule AJ, et al. Pearly penile papules: still no reason for uneasiness. *J Am Acad Dermatol.* 2003; 49(1):50–54.
Korber A, Dissemond J. Pearly penile papules. *CMAJ.* 2009;181(6–7):397.

20. How are PPPs treated?

PPPs are usually asymptomatic and therefore require no treatment. They may regress over time and following circumcision. For cosmetic reasons, some patients still request removal or amelioration. Treatment modalities include gentle cryotherapy, electrodesiccation, and laser ablation using either an erbium:yttrium-aluminum-garnet (YAG), CO_2, or pulsed dye laser. Carefully done, laser therapy typically leads to complete or near complete clearance of PPP with minimal discomfort and few complications.

Agha K, Alderson S, Samraj S, et al. Pearly penile papules regress in older patients and with circumcision. *Int J STD AIDS.* 2009; 20(11):768–770.
Baumgartner J. Erbium:yttrium-aluminium-garnet (Er:YAG) laser treatment of penile pearly papules. *J Cosmet Laser Ther.* 2012; 14(3):155–158.
Sapra P, Sapra S, Singh A. Pearly penile papules: effective therapy with pulsed dye laser. *JAMA Dermatol.* 2013;149(6):748–750.
Maranda EL, Akintilo L, Hundley K, et al. Laser therapy for the treatment of pearly penile papules. *Lasers Med Sci.* 2017;32(1):243–248.

21. What is angiokeratoma of Fordyce and how does it present?

Angiokeratoma of Fordyce is a vascular ectasia of unknown cause. This condition presents, usually in men over age 40, as multiple red-blue or purple dome-shaped, 1- to 6-mm papules. These lesions most characteristically are located on the scrotum but may also appear on the glans and penile shaft, the inguinal folds, the upper thighs, and the lower abdominal wall. Early lesions tend to be soft and compressible while later lesions are firm and keratotic. Angiokeratomas of Fordyce are largely asymptomatic, although irritation, itching, and bleeding may occur sporadically. Lesions affecting the penile shaft, suprapubic skin, and sacrum may be a sign of a genetic disorder, Fabry's disease. This disorder is an X-linked glycosphingolipidosis due to deficient α-galactosidase A activity, caused by pathogenic mutations in the GLA gene. This syndrome consists of angiokeratomas, anhidrosis, renal failure, hypertension, cardiomyopathy, and neurogenic pain; there is pharmacologic therapy available for this rare disorder.

Fordyce J. Angiokeratoma of the scrotum. *J Cut Dis.* 1896;14:81–89.
Gioglio L, Porta C, Moroni M, et al. Scrotal angiokeratoma (Fordyce): histopathological and ultrastructural findings. *Histol Histopathol.* 1992;7(1):47–55.
Hoekx L, Wyndaele JJ. Angiokeratoma: a cause of scrotal bleeding. *Acta Urol Belg.* 1998;66(1):27–28.
Chan B, Adam DN. A review of Fabry disease. *Skin Therapy Lett.* 2018;23(2):4–6.

22. How can angiokeratoma of Fordyce be treated?

Treatment is solely for cosmetic purposes, as the vast majority of angiokeratomas of Fordyce are asymptomatic. Angiokeratomas have been treated successfully with cryosurgery, electrodesiccation, neodymium (Nd):YAG laser, pulsed dye laser, and intense pulsed light. Of the laser/light options, the response seems best to the Nd:YAG unit. As there is evidence that local venous hypertension may play a part in the development of angiokeratomas, some suggest evaluation for causes of scrotal hypertension such as varicoceles or inguinal hernias.

Ibrahim SM. Pulsed dye laser versus long pulsed Nd:YAG laser in the treatment of angiokeratoma of Fordyce: a randomized, comparative, observer-blinded study. *J Dermatol Treat.* 2016;27(3):270–274.
Erkek E, Basar MM, Bagci Y, et al. Fordyce angiokeratomas as clues to local venous hypertension. *Arch Dermatol.* 2005; 141(10):1325–1326.

23. What are median raphe cysts?

Median raphe cysts are relatively rare cysts or canal-like structures which develop from the anomalous fusion of the urethral folds in males.

24. Where are median raphe cysts located and what do they look like?

Median raphe cysts vary from being flesh to blue-colored or translucent structures typically located on the ventral surface of the penis, especially the glans. They do not communicate with the urethra. While this is the most characteristic location, they may occur anywhere from the meatus to the anus. The differential diagnosis includes urethral diverticulum, pilonidal cysts, dermoid cysts, syringomas, steatocystomas, and molluscum contagiosum.

Park CO, Chun EY, Lee JH. Median raphe cyst on the scrotum and perineum. *J Am Acad Dermatol.* 2006;55(suppl 5):S114–S115.
Verma SB. Canal-like median raphe cysts: an unusual presentation of an unusual condition. *Clin Exp Dermatol.* 2009;34(8):e857–e858.

25. What problems may arise from median raphe cysts and how are these cysts treated?

The majority of median raphe cysts are asymptomatic; some may even spontaneously resolve. However, they may cause pain during sexual activity, become infected by cutaneous flora, and be cosmetically distressing. Similar to other cutaneous cysts, simple excision and primary repair are usually curative.

Navalón-Monllor V, Ordoño-Saiz MV, Ordoño-Domínguez F, et al. Median raphe cysts in men. Presentation of our experience and literature review. *Actas Urol Esp.* 2017;41(3):205–209.

Matsuyama S, Matsui F, Yazawa K, et al. Long-term follow-up of median raphe cysts and parameatal urethral cysts in male children. *Urology.* 2017;101:99–103.

26. Which skin cancers are common on the male genitalia?

Penile cancer is rare in the United States, with only 2–3 cases per 100,000 men. Up to 95% of skin cancers encountered on male genital skin are SCCs, and most lesions arise on the glans, on the prepuce, or in the coronal sulcus. Risk factors for the development of SCC include prior HPV infection, presence of LS or LP (especially of long-duration), smoking, older age, poor genital hygiene, being uncircumcised, and the presence of phimosis. There appears to be a bimodal pathway of penile SCC pathogenesis, one HPV related while the other is non–HPV driven. In contrast to other cutaneous sites, basal cell carcinoma is quite rare on genital skin. Melanoma, while not common, should be considered in pigmented lesions, particularly on the glans. Various soft tissue sarcomas may occur, as may metastatic nodules; however, these are uncommon. Invasive penile cancers are typically treated by radical penectomy; however, in selected cases, organ-preserving techniques, including Moh's micrographic surgery and partial penectomy, may be employed, as well as laser ablation or radiation therapy (external-beam and brachytherapy). The precise role and timing of inguinal lymph node dissection are under current investigation.

Heyns CF, van Vollenhoven P, Steenkamp JW, et al. Cancer of the penis—a review of 50 patients. *S Afr J Surg.* 1997;35(3):120–124.

Sánchez-Ortiz R, Huang SF, Tamboli P, et al. Melanoma of the penis, scrotum and male urethra: a 40-year single institution experience. *J Urol.* 2005;173(6):1958–1965.

Mosconi AM, Roila F, Gatta G, et al. Cancer of the penis. *Crit Rev Oncol Hematol.* 2005;53(2):165–177.

Mahesan T, Hegarty PK, Watkin NA. Advances in penile-preserving surgical approaches in the management of penile tumors. *Urol Clin North Am.* 2016;43(4):427–434.

Azizi M, Chipollini J, Peyton CC, et al. Current controversies and developments on the role of lymphadenectomy for penile cancer. *Urol Oncol.* 2019;37(3):201–208.

27. What is erythroplasia of Queyrat?

This is the old name (circa 1911) for penile SCC in situ, currently termed penile intraepithelial neoplasia (PIN). Architectural and cytological features allow further division into several subtypes. PIN most characteristically presents as a sharply demarcated, bright red, and velvety-appearing plaque in older (>40 years of age), often uncircumcised men (Fig. 61.6). These lesions may be anywhere from several millimeters to several centimeters in diameter and favor the glans, urethral meatus, coronal sulcus, and prepuce. Itching and pain occur in up to 50% of patients. Transformation to invasive SCC occurs in 5%–30% of patients. Biopsy is frequently indicated to distinguish PIN from various forms of balanitis and psoriasis.

Gerber GS. Carcinoma in situ of the penis. *J Urol.* 1994;151(4):829–833.

Crispen PL, Mydlo JH. Penile intraepithelial neoplasia and other premalignant lesions of the penis. *Urol Clin North Am.* 2010;37(3):335–342.

Downes MR. Review of in situ and invasive penile squamous cell carcinoma and associated non-neoplastic dermatological conditions. *Clin Pathol.* 2015;68(5):333–340.

28. How is PIN treated?

PIN limited to the prepuce may be treated by circumcision. PIN elsewhere may be treated by simple surgical excision, laser ablation, photodynamic therapy, and topical application of either 5% 5-fluorouracil or 5% or 3.75% imiquimod. Topical therapy (which is off FDA labeled indication) and laser ablation are associated with significant risk of recurrence, and should always be followed by periodic evaluation.

Alnajjar HM, Lam W, Bolgeri M, et al. Treatment of carcinoma in situ of the glans penis with topical chemotherapy agents. *Eur Urol.* 2012;62(5):923–928. doi:10.1016/j.eururo.2012.02.052.

Lucky M, Murthy KV, Rogers B. The treatment of penile carcinoma in situ (CIS) within a UK supra-regional network. *BJU Int.* 2015;115(4):595–598.

Chipollini J, Yan S, Ottenhof SR. Surgical management of penile carcinoma in situ: results from an international collaborative study and review of the literature. *BJU Int.* 2018;121(3):393–398.

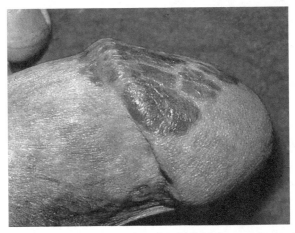

Fig. 61.6 Squamous cell carcinoma in-situ demonstrates velvety, bright red plaques, most commonly on the glans.

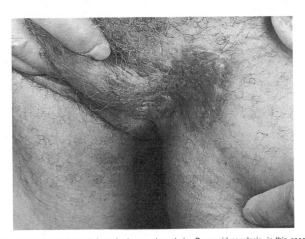

Fig. 61.7 Discrete and confluent pigmented rough plaques characterize Bowenoid papulosis, in this case very extensive.

29. What is Bowenoid papulosis, and does it require treatment?

Although both Bowenoid papulosis (BP) and erythroplasia of Queyrat share the histological finding of SCC in situ, they have different clinical morphologies. BP, seen in somewhat younger men (<40), is characterized by one or more 0.2–3-mm, smooth to verrucous-looking, often pigmented papules. Lesions often aggregate into larger plaques and occur at any or multiple anogenital sites (Fig. 61.7). BP lesions often remain stable, or even regress, over time. They transform into invasive SCC in about 1% of cases. Therefore, treatment can be less aggressive and may include electrodesiccation, liquid nitrogen cryotherapy, and scissors excision.

Nayak SU, Shenoi SD, Bhat ST, et al. Bowenoid papulosis. *Indian J Sex Transm Dis AIDS.* 2015;36(2):223–225.

30. How does invasive SCC differ from PIN?

Due to the usual 6-month delay in seeking care, invasive SCC can assume a wide variety of morphological forms. Intact or ulcerated nodules, fungating neoplasms, or massively destructive lesions may all represent SCC (Fig. 61.8). This is generally considered an aggressive tumor, although prognosis varies considerably depending upon the degree of differentiation, depth of invasion, and involvement of regional lymph nodes. Therapeutic options are discussed above.

Marchioni M, Berardinelli F, De Nunzio C. New insight in penile cancer. *Minerva Urol Nefrol.* 2018;70(6):559–569.

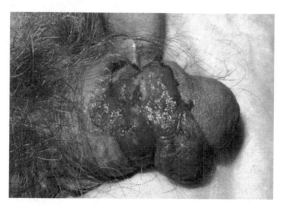

Fig. 61.8 Rock hard, invasive ulceration typical of squamous cell carcinoma.

31. Does fixed drug eruption involve the penis?

The penis, especially the glans, is a preferential site for fixed drug eruption. About 20% of cases involve the male genitalia. Other common locations include trunk, lips, and hands. This eruption begins as a round, red, and edematous plaque, which often progresses to blister formation and thence to erosion. Following resolution, there may remain a circular to oval pigmented to violaceous macule. A single lesion is most common, but multiple or even generalized lesions may be seen. Lesions may be accompanied by mild pain or mild to moderate pruritus. The entire process will be precisely repeated after any subsequent exposure to the same (or a structurally similar) drug or chemical. Fixed drug eruption is classically associated with ingestion of thiazide diuretics, sulfa or tetracycline antibiotics, salicylates, barbiturates, oral contraceptives, and nonsteroidal antiinflammatory drugs. However, the spectrum of agents that can induce this reaction is vast and includes both prescription and over-the-counter medications, chemicals, and plant extracts. Topical steroids may ameliorate any pruritus, but avoidance of the inciting agent is paramount.

Flowers H, Brodell R, Brents M, et al. Fixed drug eruptions: presentation, diagnosis, and management. *South Med J.* 2014; 107(11):724–727.

CHAPTER 62

DISORDERS OF THE ORAL MUCOSA

Robert O. Greer, Jr.

1. **What is the most common form of oral cancer?**
   Squamous cell carcinoma, the most common form of oral cancer, is the sixth most frequent cancer encountered in the United States (Fig. 62.1). Nearly 34,000 Americans are diagnosed with oral cavity squamous cell cancer each year, and if the oropharynx is included, that number increases by another 16,000 cases. More than 370,000 people are diagnosed worldwide. Approximately 10,000 deaths result from oral cavity squamous cell carcinoma in the United States in any one year.

   Siegel, RL, Miller KD, Jemal AJ. Cancer Statistics, 2018. *CA Cancer J Clin*. 2018;68:7–30.

2. **What are the most common risk factors associated with oral squamous cell carcinoma?**
   The most significant risk factors associated with the development of oral squamous cell carcinoma are tobacco and alcohol use, sun exposure, and infection with human papillomavirus (HPV).

   Kumar M, Nanavati R, Modi TG, Dobariya C. Oral cancer: etiology and risk factors: A review. *J Cancer Res Ther*. 2016;12:458–463.

3. **Which human papillomavirus has most often been implicated in the epidemiology of oral cancer?**
   Infection with HPV, a double-stranded epitheliotropic DNA virus with an affinity for skin and mucosa, is a leading reported cause of oral cavity and oropharyngeal cancer. More than 200 numbered strains of HPV exist, 12 of which are considered to be high-risk variants. The most common strain associated with oropharyngeal cancer is HPV-16.

   Cubie H. Diseases associated with human papillomavirus infection. *Virology*. 2013;445:21–34.

4. **What is oral proliferative verrucous leukoplakia?**
   Oral proliferative verrucous leukoplakia (PVL), a form of oral leukoplakia originally described by Hansen in 1985, is characterized by the development of multifocal, progressive, recurrent irregular white patches, plaques, or papillary growths that involve the oral mucosa. The lesions of PVL are indeed true leukoplakias and thus will not scrape off when rubbed vigorously (Fig. 62.2). When viewed microscopically, PVL can display a host of histologic patterns, ranging from simple hyperkeratosis to dysplasia, verrucous hyperplasia, squamous cell carcinoma, and verrucous carcinoma.

   High-risk HPVs, most often HPV-16, have been identified in PVL tissue samples, suggesting that HPV plays a role in lesional development. However, the influence of an infectious agent on the pathogenesis of PVL has not been proven. PVL is far more common in women than men, and the disorder has a peak incidence in individuals between the ages 60 and 70. PVL patients may be smokers or nonsmokers. It has been reported that as high as 90% of patients with PVL will have lesions that harbor *Candida albicans* species. There is some evidence to suggest a possible correlation between DNA aneuploidy, expression of mcm (mini chromosomal protein maintenance) protein, or loss of heterozygosity at locus 9p21 in PVL.

   Upadhyaya JD, Fitzpatrick SG, Mohammed MN, et al. A retrospective 20-year analysis of proliferative verrucous leukoplakia and it's progression to malignancy and association with high-risk human papillomavirus. *Head Neck Pathol*. 2018;11:1–11.

5. **How is oral proliferative verrucous leukoplakia treated?**
   PVL is most appropriately managed by surgical excision and close long-term patient follow-up, although laser ablation and photodynamic therapy have also been employed. Chemopreventive protocols using antifungal agents and high-dose vitamin A have been used in the treatment of PVL, but no long-term prospective longitudinal, well-controlled clinical trials using these agents have been completed.

   Chen, HM, Yu CH, Tu PC, Yeh CY, Tsai T, Chiang CP. Successful treatment of oral verrucous hyperplasia and oral leukoplakia with topical 5-aminolevulinic acid-mediated photodynamic therapy. *Lasers Surg Med*. 2005;37:114–122.

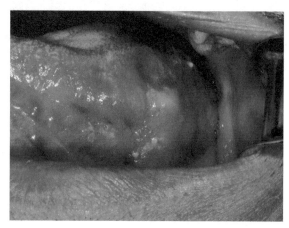

Fig. 62.1 Ulcerated exophytic squamous cell carcinoma of the midlateral tongue.

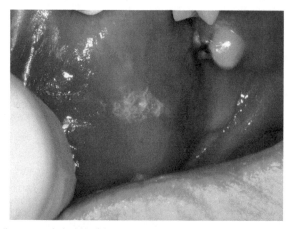

Fig. 62.2 Proliferative verrucous leukoplakia of the buccal mucosa. Note the white corrugated basket weave–like pattern.

6. What is recurrent aphthous ulceration (RAU)?

RAU of the oral cavity is a painful ulcerative disorder characterized by the development of round to ovoid ulcers of the oral mucosa. Lesional ulcers are typically surrounded by an inflammatory halo (Fig. 62.3). Aphthous ulcers can be divided into major, minor, and herpetiform subtypes. Major ulcers are typically 1 cm or more in diameter, whereas minor ulcers typically measure 2 to 8 mm in diameter. Herpetiform ulcers tend to occur in clusters or bunches of small pinpoint ulcers that develop and then coalesce. Most aphthous ulcers will develop on freely movable nonkeratinized oral mucosa. The most common RAU sites are the buccal mucosa, vestibular mucosa, lip mucosa, ventral surface of the tongue, and the soft palatal mucosa. The prevalence of recurrent aphthous ulcers in the oral cavity is thought to be approximately 1 per 100 persons and the disorder is more common in adults than children.

7. How are aphthous ulcers treated?

Table 62.1 describes the most commonly used topical and systemically employed agents for treating recurrent aphthous stomatitis, and the possible use-associated side effects.

Akintoge SO, Greenberg MS. Recurrent aphthous stomatitis. *Dent Clin North Am.* 2014;58:281–297.
Belenguer-Guallar I, Jimenez-Soriano Y, Claramunt-Lozano A. Treatment of recurrent aphthous stomatitis: a literature review. *J Clin Exp Dent.* 2014;6:e168–e174.

8. What is oral lichen planus and how frequently does it occur?

Oral lichen planus (OLP), which typically affects the oral cavity as striated white mucosal lesions, accounts for approximately 9% of all white lesions that affect the oral mucous membranes (Fig. 62.4). While OLP affects people of

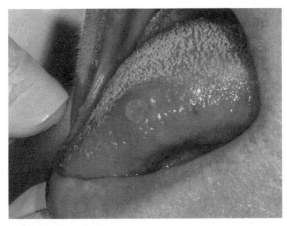

Fig. 62.3 Minor aphthous ulcer of the tongue. The solitary ulcer is covered by yellow proteinaceous debris and marginated by erythema.

Table 62.1 Topical and systemic agents frequently used in the management of RAUs

TOPICAL AGENTS	DOSAGE, EFFICACY, AND POSSIBLE SIDE EFFECTS
Corticosteroids	High-strength formulations preferred
Amlexanox	Typically employed for minor RAUs
Antibiotics	Employed as a rinse for patients with multiple ulcers
Chlorhexidine gluconate	Questionable effectiveness
Systemic Agents Thalidomide	Reserved for rare refractory cases
Dapsone	Immunosuppressive
Pentoxifylline	Efficacy has not been determined
Colchicine	Extreme gastrointestinal toxicity may be seen

RAU, Recurrent aphthous ulceration.

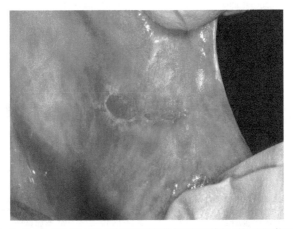

Fig. 62.4 Ulcerative lichen planus of the buccal mucosa. Note the typical radiating striated lichenoid pattern of hyperkeratosis at the margins of the ulcer.

Table 62.2 World Health Organization diagnostic criteria for oral lichen planus	
Clinical criteria	The identification of white papular, reticular, annular, plaque-type lesions that may show gray-white lines radiating from papules.
	Identification of a lacelike network of slightly raised gray-white lines arranged in a reticular pattern.
	The presence of atrophic lesions with or without erosion, and possibly bullae development.
Histopathologic criteria	Identification of thickened ortho- or parakeratinized lesional tissue in sites that are normally keratinized. If the lesional site is normally nonkeratinized, this keratin layer may be quite thin.
	Identification of Civatte or colloid bodies in basal layer epithelium, and the superficial connective tissue.
	Identification of a well-defined bandlike zone of inflammatory cells that is confined to the superficial part of the connective tissue, and consists primarily of lymphocytes.
	Signs of liquefaction degeneration of the basal cell epithelial layer.

Data from Kramer IR, Lucas RB, Pindborg JJ, et al. Definition of leukoplakia and related lesions: an aid to studies on oral precancer. Oral Surg Oral Med Oral Pathol. 1978;46:518–539.

all ethnic groups, women are more commonly affected than men, and most patients will develop the disease between 30 and 60 years of age. The disorder is not limited to the oral cavity and can affect skin, scalp, and nails. OLP is a chronic disease, the etiology of which is not completely understood. Some investigators believe that an immune reaction mediated by a virus such as hepatitis C may be causal, resulting in epithelial basal layer cells being damaged, ultimately resulting in an oral vesicular bullous eruption. Other investigators suggest that psychological disorders, such as stress, allergies, injury, or infection, may be causal factors. Most authorities agree, however, that the disease is a $CD8^+$ T cell–mediated autoimmune disorder.

9. What are the diagnostic criteria for oral lichen planus?
The World Health Organization (WHO) diagnostic criteria for the diagnosis of OLP are listed in Table 62.2.

10. Does oral lichen planus have malignant potential?
The WHO regards OLP as a disease that may evolve to cancer. In published literature reviewed between the years 1985 and 2004, the malignant transformation rate for OLP to squamous cell carcinoma was reported to be between 0% and 5.3%. Greer and colleagues reviewed 588 cases of OLP over a 20-year period in which study patients underwent a minimum of six biopsies and routine long-term diagnostic follow-up. These studies showed a 2.01% transition rate of OLP to squamous cell carcinoma. Most patients with OLP who develop oral squamous cell carcinoma in association with the disease will present with ulcerative, erosive lesions that are often also distinctly papillary. There is a clear female predilection, and the tongue is the favored site for such lesions.

Treatment for OLP is designed to alleviate symptomatology. Medications that can be used to achieve this include topical or systemic corticosteroids, interlesional injections of steroids, tacrolimus, retinoids, and cryosurgery. Tobacco and alcohol use should be discouraged in OLP patients, and patients with high-risk ulcerative and/or papillary-appearing OLP should be screened for HPV infection and lichenoid dysplasia.

Greer RO, McDowell JD, Hoernig G. Oral lichen planus: a premalignant disease. *Pathol Case Rev*. 1999;4:28–34.
Skully C, Carrozzo M. Oral mucosal disease. Lichen planus. *Br J Oral Maxillofac Surg*. 2008;46:15–21.
Giuliani M, Troiano G, Cordaro M, et al. Rate of malignant transformation of oral lichen planus: a systemic review. *Oral Dis*. 2019;25:693–709. doi:10.1111/odi.12885.

11. What is geographic tongue (benign migratory glossitis)?
Geographic tongue is a benign condition of the oral mucous membranes that occurs in approximately 1% to 3% of the population. Females are affected more often than males, and the disorder is most often characterized by the presence of well-demarcated desquamated erythematous zones involving the tongue papilla. These desquamated zones will be marginated by a white border (Fig. 62.5). Lesions tend to be more concentrated along the tip and the lateral borders of the tongue than in other tongue sites. Suggested etiologies include allergies, hormonal disturbances, nutritional deficiencies, psychological factors, juvenile diabetes, and pustular psoriasis.

12. From what does the erythema that is seen clinically in cases of geographic tongue result?
The erythema that is seen in association with geographic tongue is caused by atrophy of the tongue's filiform papilla. Lesions tend to heal or resolve quickly over a 2- to 4-week course and then move on to other sites on the tongue. Patients with geographic tongue can be symptomatic or asymptomatic, although most patients will be asymptomatic. Symptomatic patients will often complain of a burning sensation or sensitivity to hot or spicy foods, toothpaste, or tobacco.

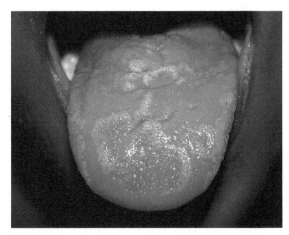

Fig. 62.5 Geographic tongue demonstrating well-demarcated zones of desquamation that are marginated by a white border. (Courtesy James E. Fitzpatrick, MD.)

13. **Can geographic tongue occur elsewhere in the oral cavity?**

    Yes. Geographic tongue can affect other oral mucosal sites, including the buccal mucosa and labial mucosa. When this form of the disease occurs, the disorder is typically known as *ectopic geographic tongue* or *erythema arenata migrans*. Oral erythema arenata migrans has no relationship to the *erythema chronicum migrans* lesions that occur in Lyme disease. The etiology of geographic tongue remains unknown, although stress, infection with *Candida albicans*, and hypersensitivity to certain environmental factors have all been implicated in the etiology of the disorder. Typically no treatment is indicated in patients who have asymptomatic geographic tongue. Occasional application of topical corticosteroids has proven beneficial, for symptomatic patients.

Alikhani K, Khalighinejad N, Ghalaiani P, Khaleghi MA, Askari E, Gorsky M. Immunologic and psychologic parameters associated with geographic tongue. *Oral Surg Oral Med Oral Pathol Oral Radiol.* 2014;118:68–71.

14. **What is mucous membrane pemphigoid?**

    Mucous membrane pemphigoid (MMP), classified as cicatricial pemphigoid in the dermatologic literature, is an autoimmune mucocutaneous disease that is chronic and blister forming. In this disorder, antibodies that are tissue bound become directed against one or more components of basement membrane substance. Benign MMP tends not to be associated with scarring of the mucosa, unlike the scar-prone lesions that affect skin and ocular mucosa. The vast majority of patients with MMP will be in the 50- to 60-year age range, and females are affected more frequently than males at a ratio of 2:1. In addition to eye, oral, and skin lesions, patients can also develop nasal, esophageal, laryngeal, and vaginal lesions.

    Oral lesions typically present as a diffuse erythematous gingivitis that may vesiculate (Fig. 62.6). In the past, the disorder has inappropriately been referred to as *desquamative gingivitis*, although desquamative lesions of the gingiva are clearly not diagnostic of MMP. Other clinical differential diagnoses that should be considered include lichen planus, pemphigus, erythema multiforme, and lupus erythematosus.

15. **How is mucous membrane pemphigoid diagnosed?**

    MMP can be diagnosed by routine hematoxylin and eosin (H&E)–stained evaluation of a biopsy specimen, often in concert with associated direct immunofluorescence studies. Assessment of perilesional tissue is most diagnostic. Lesional blisters, when biopsied, are typically not diagnostic. The lesions of MMP result in subepithelial clefting in which immunoreactants, when viewed with immunofluorescence, will be demonstrable along the basement membrane zone. Deposits of immunoglobulin G (IgG) and C3 are common immunoreactants at the basement membrane zone in 9 out of 10 patients. Rarely, IgA and IgM can also be identified. From a diagnostic standpoint, other disorders, including linear IgA disease, epidermolysis bullosa acquisita, and hemorrhagic bullae, can be confused with benign MMP, both clinically and microscopically. Therefore, a thorough and appropriate clinical and laboratory workup of the patient suspected of having MMP is mandatory.

16. **How is mucous membrane pemphigoid treated?**

    In most instances, MMP is treated using topical corticosteroids or immunosuppressant agents such as cyclophosphamide. Tacrolimus has been employed in the management of MMP as well. The disorder tends to be a chronic, lingering disease that has to be continually monitored and managed with medication.

Xu HH, Werth VP, Parisi E, Sollecito TO. Mucous membrane pemphigoid. *Dent Clin North Am.* 2013;57:11–30.
Saccucci M, DiCarlo G, Bossù M, Giovarruscio F, Salucci A, Polimeni A. Autoimmune diseases and their manifestations on oral cavity: diagnosis and clinical management. *J Immunol Res.* 2018;2018:6061825. doi:10.1155/2018/6061825.

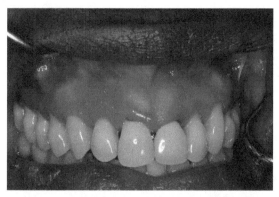

Fig. 62.6 Diffuse generalized erythematous gingiva with erosions characterizes benign mucous membrane pemphigoid. (Courtesy Kentaro Ikeda, DDS.)

17. **What is oral candidiasis?**
   Candidiasis of the oral cavity is a disorder that is most often caused by the fungal organism, *Candida albicans*. Oral candidiasis is by far the most common mycotic infection of the oral cavity, and it has been reported that as high as 50% of individuals harbor the organism in their mouth without evidence of infection.

18. **What factors determine whether or not a patient will develop oral candidiasis?**
   The most important factors that will determine whether or not a patient will develop an oral *Candida* infection are the immune status of the host, the oral mucosal environment, and the strain of *Candida* that is involved. Table 62.3 demonstrates the various clinical forms of candidiasis that can involve the oral cavity.
   The most common form of candidiasis to affect the oral cavity is the pseudomembranous form of the disease. Also known as thrush, this form of the disease will result in white corrugated or milk curd–like plaques that involve the oral mucous membrane (Fig. 62.7). Plaques can be easily removed by scraping the mucosa vigorously with a tongue blade. Individuals who develop pseudomembranous candidiasis will often complain of a burning sensation in the oral cavity or complain of blister-like formations. Identifying short-term lesional blisters can be difficult. Affected individuals are frequently cancer patients on chemotherapy regimens or patients who are immunologically compromised or who are on high-dose antibiotics. Erythematous and hyperplastic forms of the disease are less common than pseudomembranous forms of the disease. The hyperplastic form of the disease, which is often plaque-like, can be confused with dysplasia or oral cancer. Candidiasis that occurs beneath dentures, often referred to as denture stomatitis, is characterized by erythematous mucosa that is sometimes ulcerated and painful.

19. **Is there a form of candidiasis that is related to neoplasia?**
   Some authorities suggest that the chronic hyperplastic form of candidiasis, also referred to as chronic hyperplastic or *leukoplakic candidiasis*, can be a precursor to oral epithelial dysplasia and cancer. However, the difficulty in making such a judgment relates to the fact that it is often not known whether or not dysplastic oral leukoplakia was present to begin with, only to become secondarily infected with *Candida* organisms. Some authorities suggest that since *Candida* organisms are capable of producing cancer-causing nitrosamines, *Candida* can indeed be associated with dysplastic epithelial or cancerous epithelial lesions.

Dineshankar J, Sivakumar K, Karhikegan M, Udayakumar P, Shanmugam KT, Kesavan G. Immunology of oral candidiasis. *J Pharm Bioallied Sci.* 2014;6:S9–S12.

20. **How can a diagnosis of candidiasis involving the oral cavity be established?**
   Most often, a smear or evaluation of a biopsy specimen, both of which can be periodic acid–Schiff stained to demonstrate the nonbranching septate hyphae of *Candida albicans*, can prove diagnostic of the disease.

21. **How is oral candidiasis treated?**
   Oral candidiasis is generally treated with an antifungal agent. The most common agents include nystatin, ketoconazole, and fluconazole. Many additional variations of these drugs, including imidazoles, triazoles, and polyene antifungal agents, are also available for disease management. Recently, management of oral candidiasis using anti-biofilm therapies including biomolecules produced by *streptococcus mutans* has been proposed.

Darling MR, McCord C, Jackson-Boeters L, Copete M. Markers of potential malignancy in chronic hyperplastic candidiasis. *J Investig Clin Dent.* 2012;3:176–181.
Chanda W, Thomson P, Wang W. The potential management of oral candidiasis using anti-biofilm therapies. *Med Hypotheses*, 2017;106:15–18.

Table 62.3 Candidiasis: clinical forms

CLINICAL TYPE	ANATOMIC SITE(S)	SYMPTOMS AND APPEARANCE	ADDITIONAL SIGNIFICANT FACTORS
Angular cheilitis	Angles of mouth	Red, fissured lesions	Immunosuppression can precipitate the disorder
Median rhomboid glossitis	Midline, posterior/dorsal tongue surface	Red, atrophic mucosal zones; may be asymptomatic	Immunosuppression may precipitate the disorder
Chronic multifocal candidiasis	Posterior palate, posterior tongue dorsum, angles of mouth	Red areas, with white associated plaques; burning sensation can occur	Immunosuppression may precipitate the disorder
Chronic atrophic candidiasis (denture sore mouth)	Denture-bearing mucosa of the palate	Erythematous lesions	Denture may be an infective fomite
Endocrine-candidiasis syndromes	Tongue, buccal mucosa, palate	White plaques that are not removable are common	Endocrine disorder may develop after candidiasis
Erythematous candidiasis	Hard palate, buccal mucosa, tongue dorsum	Red macules and a burning sensation are common	Antibiotic therapy and immunosuppression may precipitate the disorder
Leukoplakic candidiasis (hyperplastic candidiasis)	Buccal mucosa, tongue and lip commissures	White plaques or nodular excrescences	May be associated with dysplasia
Mucocutaneous candidiasis	Tongue, buccal mucosa, palate	White plaques and red areas	May be related to idiopathic immune dysfunction
Pseudomembranous candidiasis (thrush)	Buccal mucosa, tongue, palate	Creamy-white removable plaques, burning sensation	Antibiotic therapy and immunosuppression are common causes

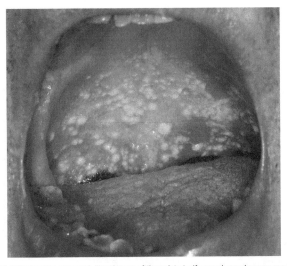

Fig. 62.7 Diffuse white milk-curd–like plaques of the palate typify pseudomembranous candidiasis.

22. What is the most common viral infection encountered in the oral cavity?

The most common viral infection to involve the oral mucous membranes is the herpes simplex virus infection (HSV), existing as HSV-1 (herpes labialis). HSV-2, varicella-zoster virus infection, and human herpesvirus 3 (HHV-3) are much less common, as are Epstein-Barr viral infections and cytomegalic viral infections. HHV-8 infection, most commonly associated with human immunodeficiency virus infection and Kaposi's sarcoma, does occur orally, but not with the frequency of common herpes simplex infections.

Chayavichitsilp P, Buckwalter JV, Krakowski AC, Friedlander SF. Herpes simplex. *Pediatr Rev.* 2009;30:119–129.

23. What are the two clinical forms of herpes simplex infection to affect the oral cavity?

Two forms of herpes viral infections typically affect the oral cavity: primary infections and secondary, or recurrent, infections.

24. What are the clinical features of a primary herpes labialis outbreak?

A common presentation of a primary oral herpes infection is acute herpetic gingivostomatitis. This infection, which occurs most often in children, will result in gingival and mucosal ulcerations and vesicles that arise abruptly in association with chills, fever, nausea, and severe mucosal pain. Gingival lesions will be quite erythematous and boggy, whereas lesions on other mucous membrane surfaces tend to be much more ulcerative in their appearance (Fig. 62.8). Associated eye, genital, and skin involvement may occur. Most cases of primary herpetic gingivostomatitis will resolve within 1 to 2 weeks.

25. Where and why do recurrent (secondary) oral herpes viral infections develop?

Recurrent oral herpes simplex viral infections occur in two primary sites: either as recurrences at the site of primary invasion or inoculation by the virus or in epithelium that has a ganglion associated with it. A high percentage of lesions occur along the vermilion border of the skin and mucosa of the lips. Such lesions are typically known as cold sores or fever blisters. These lesions are commonly triggered by trauma or ultraviolet light, and very often patients will complain of a burning, tender, or itching sensation in the primary site. Recurrent herpetic lesions most often present as 2- to 4-mm vesicles that will rupture within 24 to 48 hours, leaving behind a crusty hemorrhagic surface. Vesicles over time will tend to coalesce. Most recurrences will heal within 7 days to 2 weeks (see Chapter 25 for treatment).

26. Are there unique pathologic findings that are characteristic of oral herpes viral infection?

Microscopically, herpes simplex infections will often demonstrate epithelial cells that show the cytopathic effect of the virus, causing infected cells to demonstrate significant ballooning degeneration. The chromatin in these cells will marginate to the cell periphery, and cells frequently become multinucleate. Affected cells, known as *Tzanck cells*, are characteristic of the infection and are often diagnostic of the process.

Stoopler ET, Alfaris S, Alomar, et al. Recurrent intraoral herpes. *J Emerg Med.* 2016;51:324–325.

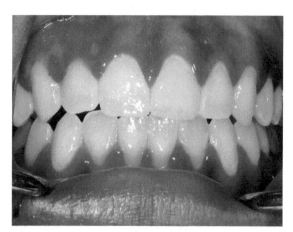

Fig. 62.8 Erythematous and ulcerated gingival lesions characterize primary herpetic gingivostomatitis.

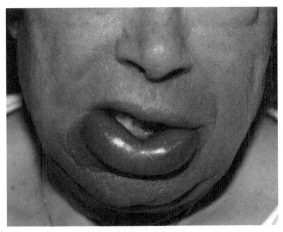

Fig. 62.9 Marked erythema and swelling of the lower lip in a patient with cheilitis granulomatosa.

Table 62.4 Assessment of patients with orofacial granulomatosis	
DISEASE	**SCREENING METHODOLOGY**
Chronic granulomatous disease	Complete a neutrophil nitroblue tetrazolium reduction test if a medical history of chronic infections is noted.
Crohn's disease	Hematologic evaluation for evidence of gastrointestinal malabsorption (e.g., low albumin, calcium, folate, iron, and red blood cell count; elevated erythrocyte sedimentation rate) or leukocyte scintigraphy using ^{99m}Tc-HMPAO (hexamethylpropylene amine oxime); if initial screen positive, recommend esophagogastroduodenoscopy, ileocolonoscopy, and small bowel radiographs.
Sarcoidosis	Serum angiotensin-converting enzyme and chest radiograph to assess for hilar lymphadenopathy.
Tuberculosis	Skin test and chest radiograph required. Acid-fast bacillus (AFB) stains that are negative on biopsy do not rule out mycobacterial infection.

27. What is orofacial granulomatosis?

Orofacial granulomatosis is a term used to define a complex of granulomatous diseases of the orofacial region that are most frequently characterized by swelling of the lips (Fig. 62.9), although other soft tissues in the head and neck region can be involved. These lip swellings are usually accompanied by histologically evident granulomatous disease. The disorders generally included as being associated with orofacial granulomatosis and methods for screening for the disease are listed in Table 62.4.

Alawi F. An update on granulomatous diseases of the oral tissue. *Dent Clin North Am.* 2013;57:657–671.

28. What is Melkersson-Rosenthal syndrome?

Melkersson-Rosenthal syndrome is one of the components of orofacial granulomatosis in which patients develop intraoral lip swelling(s) known as cheilitis granulomatosa. These enlargements can be painful and they may also be associated with tongue enlargement, oral edema, ulcers, and oral papules.

Critchlow WA, Chang D. Chelitis granulomatosa: a review. *Head Neck Pathol.* 2014;8:209–213.

29. Are there specific microscopic findings associated with orofacial granulomatosis?

No diagnostically specific histologic features are associated with this disease. Histologic findings will typically consist of demonstrating aggregates of multinucleated giant cells, histiocytes, and nodular granulomas. Stains for microorganisms are typically negative and foreign material will not be found within disease-associated granulomas.

30. What causes orofacial granulomatosis?

The etiology of the disorder is unknown, although it is believed that the process is an immune reaction to an exogenous or chemotactic stimulus. A delayed hypersensitivity reaction with a predominant Th-1-mediated immune response has been implicated in the etiology of the disease process. The disease has been treated by a host of interventions, including steroid injections, cyclosporine, azathioprine, methotrexate, and other drugs. Surgery is typically not the first intervention of choice, although surgery is sometimes employed in disease management. Occasionally, lesions will undergo spontaneous regression.

31. What are some of the common causes of localized non–melanocytic-related pigmentations involving the oral mucosa?

The placement of dental amalgam fillings, in which amalgam is incorporated into the oral mucosa can cause localized oral pigmentations, as can intentional tattooing, and systemic lead/mercury and bismuth intoxication. In addition, localized pigmentations of the oral cavity can occur from other sources, including melanosis from smoking- and drug-related pigmentations associated with the use of estrogen and chemotherapeutic agents for neoplastic disease.

Tavares TS, Meirelles DP, de Aguiar MCF, Caldeira PC. Pigmented lesions of the oral mucosa: a cross sectional study of 458 histopathological specimens. *Oral Dis.* 2018;24:1484–1491.

32. How do amalgam tattoos typically appear clinically?

Clinically, amalgam tattoos generally appear as localized gray to black/blue lesions that are occasionally raised above the mucous membrane surface (Fig. 62.10). Metallic fragments may show up on radiographs, while biopsied tissue samples will show linear- to granular-appearing aggregates of pigmented foreign material that often surrounds blood vessels and which will be entrapped within foreign body giant cells. Most amalgam tattoos require no treatment. However, when melanoma is considered in the differential diagnosis, a biopsy is mandatory.

33. How are other pigmentations of the oral mucous membrane treated?

Smoker's melanosis is treated by discontinuing the habitual use of tobacco products. Drug-related discolorations of the oral mucosa associated with the use of chemotherapeutic drugs are usually transitory, although they can be disconcerting to the patient. When the offending medication is discontinued, most pigmentations will disappear. Systemic melanotic intoxications that occur from lead, mercury, bismuth, and arsenic are quite rare. Removal of the intoxicating agent, along with supportive care, and the use of chelating agents may prove helpful. However, chelating agents have significant side effects and must be used appropriately.

Alani F. Pigmented lesions of the oral cavity: an update. *Dental Clin North Am.* 2013;57:699–710.

34. What is smokeless tobacco?

Smokeless tobacco (SLT) is a broad, encompassing term used to describe topically applied tobacco products, most often chewing tobacco and snuff. Three types of SLTs are commonly manufactured: loose-leaf chewing tobacco, moist

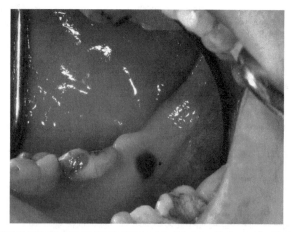

Fig. 62.10 Amalgam tattoo involving the alveolar ridge mucosa. Note how well-circumscribed the lesions appear.

snuff, and dry snuff. In the United States, loose-leaf tobacco is less commonly used than moist snuff. Dry snuff is a fermented and dry-cured form of the product that is now rarely used, but which was at one time commonly inhaled nasally. Colloquially, the oral use of snuff is termed "snuff dipping."

Greer RO. Pathology of malignant and premalignant oral epithelial lesions. *Otolaryngol Clin North Am.* 2006;39:249–255.

35. Can one develop oral lesions from the use of snuff?
    The use of snuff in any of its forms can produce localized or generalized leukoplakic oral lesions that are typically identified and classified as SLT keratoses (STKs). The use of snuff can also cause gingival inflammation, periodontal inflammation, and alveolar bone damage. Tooth abrasion and staining of tooth structure can also occur. Dysplasia and oral cancer have been reported in the literature as a consequence of snuff use; however, most well-documented and properly controlled prospective trials have demonstrated that oral cancer is an exceedingly rare outcome in individuals who use SLT products.
    Sixteen significant prospective experimental and cross-sectional studies of the oral manifestations of SLT use have been done throughout the United States and Europe, and most studies show that oral cancer is a rare consequence of SLT.
    STKs can be categorized and graded clinically into three various classes of lesions defined as grade I, II, or III SKTs. Lesions will present as leukoplakic thickenings of the oral mucosa that may show intervening furrows of normal mucosal color and prominent mucosal wrinkling (Fig. 62.11). Most lesions represent a reactive hyperkeratotic response to an injurious insult from the tobacco product and are not neoplastic.

Greer Jr RO. Oral manifestations of smokeless tobacco use. *Otolaryngol Clin North Am.* 2011;44:31–56.

36. Are there any factors besides the tobacco use itself that predict or determine the risk of an SLT lesion developing into cancer?
    Mucosal infection with HPV, overexpression of the enzyme telomerase, and altered host immune surveillance may play a role in the progression of STKs from simple hyperkeratoses to neoplastic lesions. Nonetheless, in 2009, the International Head and Neck Cancer Epidemiology Consortium examined pooled data from 17 European and American case-controlled studies that included 11,221 cases and 16,168 controls and concluded that "a substantial proportion of head and neck cancers cannot be attributed solely to tobacco or alcohol use alone, particularly for the oral cavity." These studies have led the research community to conclude that HPV infection represents a significant risk factor in the case of tobacco and non–tobacco-associated cancers and that HPV infection may play a role in as high as 20% to 25% of all oropharyngeal cancers.

37. Can smokeless tobacco lesions regress on their own?
    Grade I and grade II STKs often will regress on their own if the tobacco product is discontinued. Grade III lesions regress on their own less frequently, demonstrating less of a regression rate when the tobacco product is discontinued.

Hashibe M, Brennan P, Chuang SC, et al. Interaction between tobacco and alcohol use and the risk of head and neck cancer. Pooled analysis in the International Head and Neck Cancer Epidemiology Consortium. *Cancer Epidemiol Biomarkers Prev.* 2009;18:541–550.

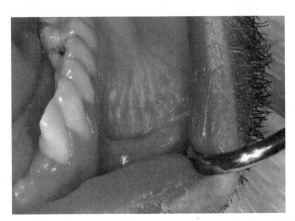

Fig. 62.11 Grade III smokeless tobacco keratosis of the mandibular labial mucosa is characterized by a classic leukoplakic "washboard" appearance.

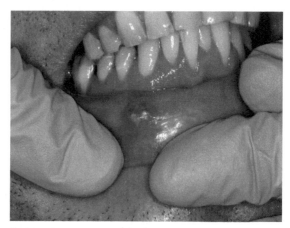

Fig. 62.12 Nodular fluctuant blue- to purple-appearing mucocele of the lower lip.

38. How should patients be counseled concerning the use of smokeless tobacco products?
Tobacco products in any form have significant medical and dental risks, and therefore, patients should be counseled by their physician or dentist regarding the risks associated with using such products, including possible side effects and consequences.

39. Is there any significant clinical difference between lesions known as mucous retention cysts, mucous duct cysts, salivary duct cyst, and mucoceles?
These terms all refer to the many variations on the theme of a typically trauma-induced channel-like mucous-containing cavity that can affect the oral cavity and result in a solitary mucosal swelling, most often of the lip. The fact that multiple terms are used for the same clinical phenomenon relates to whether or not the area of retention of the mucin is epithelially lined or not. In those instances in which the cavity is lined by epithelium, the term *cyst* can be used. In those instances in which there is no true epithelial lining, or in which extravasated mucin simply pools within connective tissue, the term *cyst* is not employed. Most mucoceles will present as slow-growing asymptomatic bluish swellings (Fig. 62.12). Lesions can range from fluctuant to firm on palpation. Cysts that affect the floor of the mouth or the deep floor of the mouth are often referred to as either ranulas or plunging mucoceles.

deMonterio B, Bezerra TM, daSilveria ÉJ, Nonaka CF, da Costa Miguel MC. Histopathological review of 667 cases of oral mucoceles with emphasis on uncommon histopathological variations. *Ann Diagn Pathol.* 2016;21:44–46.

40. What is the treatment for a mucocele?
Mucoceles, due to their chronic nature, are usually treated by surgical excision. Recurrence is in the 3% to 7% range. Most instances of recurrence are related to feeder glands that are not removed at the time of initial surgery. Mucoceles have no malignant potential.

41. How common are irritation fibromas in the oral cavity?
Irritation fibromas are far and away the most common connective tissue lesion to affect the oral cavity. In the truest sense, fibromas are not neoplasms, but are in fact reactive hyperplastic growths. Most tumors will be asymptomatic and develop as a result of localized irritation or trauma. The most common precipitating event is biting of the mucosa. The buccal mucosa is an exceedingly common site for the irritation fibroma as is the lip. Lesions tend to be quite nodular in their appearance (Fig. 62.13) and may become ulcerated if repeatedly traumatized.

42. What are some other differential diagnoses that can be considered for the irritation fibroma?
Differential diagnoses include sclerosing pyogenic granuloma, lipoma, fibrolipoma, tumors of nerve sheath origin, and peripheral ossifying fibroma. The histopathology of these various lesions tends to be quite unique, and thus they can all be easily separated from the common irritation fibroma. Irritation fibromas have no malignant potential.

43. What causes white sponge nevus?
White sponge nevus is a genodermatosis that is inherited in an autosomal dominant fashion. The disorder arises due to a defect in the normal oral mucosal keratinization process. A mutation in keratin-producing genes, particularly keratin 4 and 13, represents the root cause.

Westin M, Rekabdar E, Blomstrand L, Klintberg P, Jontell M, Robledo-Sierra J. Mutations in genes for keratin-4 and keratin-13 in Swedish patients with white sponge nevus. *J Oral Pathol Med.* 2018;47:152–157.

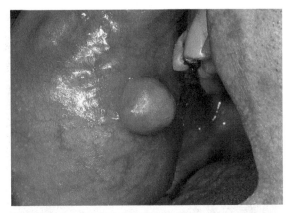

Fig. 62.13 Well-circumscribed nodular "irritation" fibroma of the buccal mucosa.

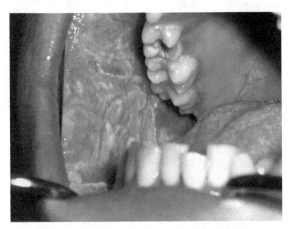

Fig. 62.14 Diffuse white plaque-like lesions of the buccal mucosa in a patient with white sponge nevus.

44. How will white sponge nevus appear clinically?

Most individuals who develop white sponge nevus will present with the condition as children. The disorder will classically present as a hyperkeratotic plaque-like process involving the buccal mucosa (Fig. 62.14), although the tongue, labial mucosa, and palate can be involved, as can the alveolar mucosa.

Lucchese A, Favia G. White sponge nevus with minimal clinical and histological changes: report of three cases. *J Oral Pathol Med.* 2006;35:317–319.

45. Does white sponge nevus have premalignant potential?

White sponge nevus is a benign condition that has no malignant potential and does not require treatment, other than the occasional biopsy that may be necessary to distinguish it from other disorders.

46. What is the cause of nevoid basal cell carcinoma syndrome (Gorlin syndrome) and what are the most significant syndrome components?

The nevoid basal cell carcinoma syndrome is caused by a mutation in the *PTCH* tumor suppressor gene, mapped to chromosome 9q22.3-q31. The syndrome is classically characterized by clinical findings that include multiple odontogenic keratocysts of the jaws, intracranial calcifications, multiple basal cell carcinomas of the skin (Fig. 62.15), vertebral and rib abnormalities, epidermoid cysts of the skin, palmar/plantar pits, and mild ocular hypertelorism as well as a host of other less common features.

Fujii K, Miyashita T. Gorlin syndrome (nevoid basal cell carcinoma syndrome). An update and literature review. *Pediatr Int.* 2014;56 (6):667–674.
Gielen RCAM, Reinders MGHC, Kollinen HK, Paulussen ADC, Mosterd K, van Geel M. PTCH 1 isoform 1b is the major transcript in the development of basal cell nevus syndrome. *J Hum Genet.* 2018;63:965–969.

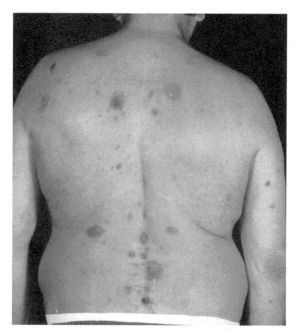

Fig. 62.15 Nevoid basal cell nevus syndrome. Patient with numerous basal cell carcinomas of the back. (Courtesy Fitzsimons Army Medical Center teaching files.)

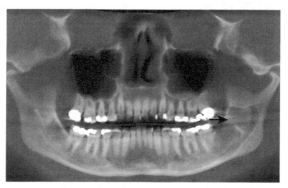

Fig. 62.16 Multiple mandibular odontogenic keratocysts are a characteristic component of the nevoid basal cell carcinoma syndrome. The largest keratocyst is identified by the *arrow*.

47. What are the most significant medical or dental concerns in a patient with nevoid basal cell carcinoma syndrome?

Contrary to popular belief, it is the odontogenic keratocysts that arise in the jaws of patients with basal cell nevus syndrome that are often the most significant and problematic component of the syndrome (Fig. 62.16). These cysts can be locally destructive and quite recurrent, and they have malignant potential. Only rarely do the basal cell carcinomas that are part of the syndrome present a management problem.

CHAPTER 63

SPECIAL CONSIDERATIONS IN SKIN OF COLOR

Misha D. Miller and Whitney A. High

1. **What is "skin of color"?**

   There are many ways to subcategorize humans. Widely recognized racial groups include Africans, African-Americans, Asians, Middle Easterners, Northern Europeans, Native Americans, Pacific Islanders, and Hispanics, to name a few. Even within a racial group, gradations exist with regard to skin pigmentation. Simply put, people with "skin of color" have darker skin tones than those of typical white skin. The term may be used also to reference other shared cutaneous characteristics, such as hair color or quality, or a common reaction pattern to skin insults, all of which may be clinically relevant. By 2044, more than 50% of the U.S. population will be composed of people with skin of color. Accordingly, a solid understanding of the myriad differences in diagnosing and treating persons with skin of color is essential to the competent practice of dermatology.

   Taylor SC, Cook-Bolden F. Defining skin of color. *Cutis*. 2002;69:435–437.

   U.S. Census Bureau. *2008 National Population Projections: Tables and Charts*. https://www.census.gov/data/tables/2008/demo/popproj/2008-summary-tables.html. Accessed September 7, 2020.

2. **How might these ethnic differences impact upon the practice of dermatology?**

   While diversity in the population is increasing, there is concern that the ethnic composition of dermatologists, who spend 12 years in higher education and 20–40 years in clinical practice, may not diversify at the same rate. For example, a 2017 survey found the current ethnic make-up of dermatologists to be 68% white, 15% Asian, 6% black, and 3% Latino; this does not correspond to the ethnic make-up of the general population. Therefore, it is important that practicing dermatologists undergo appropriate education on the skin care practices and concerns of persons with skin of color. In fact, a recent study found that for black patients, even when there was no racial concordance between the dermatologist and the patient, there was increased patient satisfaction when the dermatologist had familiarity with and specialized knowledge of the care of black skin and hair.

   Gorbatenko-Roth K, Prose N, Kundu RV, et al. Assessment of black patients' perception of their dermatology care. *JAMA Dermatol*. 2019;155:1129–1134.

3. **What accounts for differences in color between ethnic and racial groups?**

   Although the number of melanocytes varies within anatomic regions of the body, interestingly, among different races and ethnicities, the actual number of melanocytes in the skin does not vary with skin color. Instead, among variations, it is the amount and distribution of melanin produced that changes. In mammals, two types of melanin are produced by melanocytes, eumelanin and pheomelanin. Eumelanin is a tyrosine-derived dark brown or black pigment. Pheomelanin, derived from a biochemical shunt in the normal melanin production pathway, has a yellow to red-brown hue. Pheomelanin is the predominant pigment produced by those with freckles and red hair. It is also increased in Asian skin, and in women when compared to men. Melanin is packaged in melanosomes, which are membrane-bound vesicles containing a unique scaffolding of matrix proteins. Melanosomes within keratinocytes of white skin are distributed as membrane-bound clusters. In black skin, melanosomes tend to be larger and more diffusely located in the cell. Therefore, the quantity and composition of melanin, as well as melanosome size and distribution, vary considerably within the epidermis, both with ethnicity and with chronic sun exposure, yielding various degrees and hues of pigmentation.

   Thong HY, Jee SH, Sun CC, et al. The patterns of melanosome distribution in keratinocytes of human skin as one determining factor of skin colour. *Br J Dermatol*. 2003;149:498–505.

4. **Do any physiologic differences exist between black skin and that of other racial/ethnic groups?**

   Yes. In truth, the color of "black" skin ranges from light brown to very dark brown/black, and it is difficult to generalize given this tremendous variability. Nevertheless, studies have demonstrated that the stratum corneum of most black skin maintains more layers and is more compact and cohesive than white skin. This finding may explain why black skin tends to manifest a decreased susceptibility to cutaneous irritants. One study demonstrated that black skin had a spontaneous desquamation rate 2.5 times that of white skin, and this may explain why some blacks experience a particular type of xerosis commonly referred to as *ashy skin*. Ashy skin consists of fine white flakes yielding a dry appearance. Other differences in black skin include an increased transepidermal water loss, lower pH, and larger mast cell granules when compared with white skin. Black skin also produces less vitamin D_3 in response to equivalent sunlight, and this has been postulated to possibly represent the driving evolutionary force in development of paler skin as early humans migrated away from the equator. Conflicting data exist regarding differences in resistance, capacitance, conductance, impedance, and skin microflora.

Jablonski NG, Chaplin G. The evolution of human skin coloration. *J Hum Evol.* 2000;39:57–106.
Wesley NO, Maibach HI. Racial (ethnic) differences in skin properties: the objective data. *Am J Clin Dermatol.* 2003;4:843–860.

5. What are the "ashy dermatoses"?

In addition to the term "ashy," used to refer to a characteristic type of xerosis among blacks, there are also "ashy dermatoses," a term that refers most often to a family of conditions observed in Latinos. Other terms, such as "erythema dyschromicum perstans," "lichen planus pigmentosus," and "idiopathic eruptive macular pigmentation," may refer to these same conditions, which maintain overlapping clinical features. Some dermatologists consider these "ashy dermatoses" to be variants of lichen planus (see Chapter 12). Clinically, these ashy dermatoses present as macules or even large patches, with brown to grayish hues of pigmentation with scant erythema. Under a microscope, there is often a subtle lichenoid interface reaction, with underlying pigmentary incontinence in the shallow dermis. While there is not full consensus among dermatologists, it may be the degree of inflammation and the extent of involvement that distinguishes "ashy dermatoses" from frank lichen planus. Unless one practices in Latin America, or among a largely Latino community, it is probably adequate simply to be aware of the disparate viewpoints.

Zaynoun S, Rubeiz N, Kibbi AG. Ashy dermatoses—a critical review of the literature and a proposed simplified clinical classification. *Int J Dermatol.* 2008;47:542–544.
Vega-Memije ME, Domínguez-Soto L. Ashy dermatosis. *Int J Dermatol.* 2010;49:228–229.

6. Are the brown streaks on the nails of people with skin of color always a cause for concern?

No. Pigmented streaks of the nail may be a normal variant in people with skin of color. The condition is called *melanonychia striata*, and it is characterized by longitudinal bands of pigmentation that may vary from light brown to dark black. Multiple bands may be seen within the same nail or, alternatively, several nails may be involved. The cause is unknown, but the rarity of bands in children may indicate that they are a sequela of accumulated trauma. Some studies have revealed that such bands are present in 75% of blacks older than 20 years. Another recent study found that simple racial variation was the most common cause of nail pigmentation in Hispanics as well, although malignancy was a cause in about 6% of cases. In general, solitary bands are of greater concern than are multiple lesions. Close examination of the nail fold may be helpful, assessing for diffusion of pigment into the surrounding skin; however, the absence of this sign does not rule out a more serious condition, such as nail unit melanoma. Other causes of nail pigmentation include drugs such as actinomycin, antimalarials, bleomycin, cyclophosphamide, doxorubicin, 5-fluorouracil, melphalan, methotrexate, minocycline, nitrogen mustard, and zidovudine, to name a few. Laugier-Hunziker syndrome, Addison's disease, hemochromatosis, Peutz-Jeghers syndrome, and vitamin B_{12} deficiency may also cause nail pigmentation.

Dominguez-Cherit J, Roldan-Marin R, Pichardo-Velazquez P, et al. Melanonychia, melanocytic hyperplasia, and nail melanoma in a Hispanic population. *J Am Acad Dermatol.* 2008;59:785–791.
Pappert AS, Scher RK, Cohen JL. Longitudinal pigmented nail bands. *Dermatol Clin.* 1991;9:703–716.

7. Is pigmentation of the oral mucosa in people with skin of color invariably concerning?

No. Pigmentation of the oral mucosa is often subdivided into conditions related to melanin (including racial differences in pigmentation) and non–melanin-associated conditions, such as metabolic conditions or pigmentation related to drugs. Therefore, oral pigmentation in people with skin of color is neither uncommon nor necessarily indicative of a serious condition. Idiopathic, racially related pigmentation of the oral mucosa often involves the gingiva, palate, buccal mucosa, or tongue (Fig. 63.1). The color may vary, but it often has a blue or gray appearance. Symmetry is frequently observed. As always, obtaining an appropriate medical history is important, particularly with respect to the length of time present and any associated symptoms.

Meleti M, Vescovi P, Mooi WJ, et al. Pigmented lesions of the oral mucosa and perioral tissues: a flow-chart for the diagnosis and some recommendations for the management. *Oral Surg Oral Med Oral Pathol Oral Radiol Endod.* 2008;105:606–616.

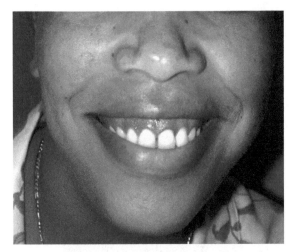

Fig. 63.1 Increased pigmentation of the gingiva in an African American. (Courtesy Whitney A. High, MD.)

8. Are there other areas of the body where hyperpigmentation represents a normal racial variant?
   Hyperpigmented macules of the palms and soles occur in people with skin of color, particularly in those with darker skin types. Such lesions may vary in color from light tan to dark brown. The number of lesions may range from one or two lesions to dozens or more. This potential for natural racial variation must be kept in mind, particularly when one considers other diseases associated with palmoplantar lesions, such as erythema multiforme and secondary syphilis. As acral lentiginous melanoma is the most common form of melanoma occurring in blacks, Asians, and Hispanics, this potentially life-threatening diagnosis must always be considered, and excluded by biopsy where indicated. Other areas with possible increased pigmentation among persons with skin of color include the sclera, the labia and vaginal mucosa, and the glans penis.

Coleman WP III, Gately LE III, Krementz AB, et al. Nevi, lentigines, and melanomas in blacks. *Arch Dermatol.* 1980;116:548–555.

9. What are Futcher lines?
   Futcher's lines, also known as *Voigt lines* or *Futcher-Voigt lines* or *Ito lines*, are areas of abrupt demarcation between lighter and darker pigmented skin. Common locations include the anterior arms, the sternum, and the posterior thighs and legs (Fig. 63.2). There appears to be no appreciable difference in melanin concentration between the adjacent darker and lighter areas when examined by light microscopy. The distribution and symmetry of the lines allow differentiation from other diagnoses, such as whorled nevoid hypomelanosis, incontinentia pigmenti, linear epidermal nevus, or lichen striatus. Interestingly, drug eruptions have, on occasion, affected preferentially the skin on one side of the line, suggesting that the skin in these areas has slightly different embryologic origin, at least with regard to a susceptibility to metabolic insult.

James WD, Carter JM, Rodman OG. Pigmentary demarcation lines: a population survey. *J Am Acad Dermatol.* 1987;16:584–590.
Shelley ED, Shelley WB, Pansky B. The drug line: the clinical expression of the pigmentary Voigt-Futcher line in turn derived from the embryonic ventral axial line. *J Am Acad Dermatol.* 1999;40:736–740.

10. What causes postinflammatory hyperpigmentation?
    Postinflammatory hyperpigmentation represents a residual darkening of the skin as a result of an inflammatory insult, such as lichen planus, lupus erythematosus (Fig. 63.3), or atopic dermatitis (Fig. 63.4). It is most severe in those diseases that result in significant disruption of the basal layer, which allows melanin to escape into the upper dermis, where it is engulfed by macrophages. The resultant hyperpigmentation requires months to years for fading. Treatment includes bleaching creams, such as hydroquinone, tretinoin, and azelaic acid; however, if the pigmentation is significantly deep, topical management does not often augment the body's normal, albeit slow, corrective mechanisms. Bleaching agents containing greater than 4% hydroquinone may cause exogenous ochronosis, with a resultant blue-gray discoloration of the skin. Patients from countries in Africa and Europe may have access to harsh bleaching agents without prescription and should be warned against such use. Disorders such as inflammatory acne, occurring in dark skin types, should be treated early and aggressively, to prevent pigmentary alterations.

Olumide YM, Akinkugbe AO, Altraide D, et al. Complications of chronic use of skin lightening cosmetics. *Int J Dermatol.* 2008;47:344–353.

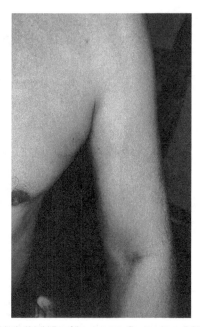

Fig. 63.2 Futcher's (Voigt's) line of the upper arm. (Courtesy James E. Fitzpatrick, MD.)

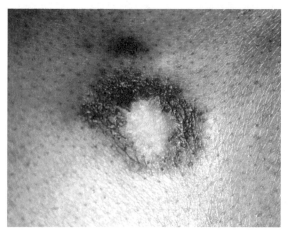

Fig. 63.3 Postinflammatory hyperpigmentation and hypopigmentation in a patient with lupus erythematosus. (Courtesy James E. Fitzpatrick, MD.)

11. What causes postinflammatory hypopigmentation?

Postinflammatory hypopigmentation, another sequela of inflammatory skin disorders in dark skin, is thought to result from impaired transfer of melanosomes from melanocytes to keratinocytes. This occurs in many diseases, such as atopic dermatitis (see Figs. 63.3 and 63.4) and psoriasis. The increased mitotic rate of keratinocytes, as well as the decreased transit time of cells within the epidermis, does not allow enough pigment transfer. After the inflammatory process resolves, pigment typically normalizes over weeks to months.

Nicolaidou E, Katsambas AD. Pigmentation disorders: hyperpigmentation and hypopigmentation. *Clin Dermatol.* 2014;32:66–72.

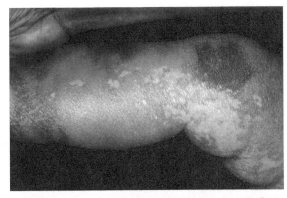

Fig. 63.4 Postinflammatory hyperpigmentation and hypopigmentation in a child with atopic dermatitis. (Courtesy James E. Fitzpatrick, MD.)

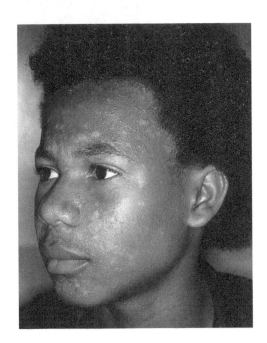

Fig. 63.5 Pityriasis alba, demonstrating hypopigmented macules of the face. (Courtesy James E. Fitzpatrick, MD.)

12. **Is pityriasis alba the same thing as postinflammatory hypopigmentation?**
    Pityriasis alba is seen primarily in children with darker skin types, and it manifests as hypopigmented macules on the face and/or upper arms (Fig. 63.5). The lesions lack a distinct border and may have overlying fine scale. Patients often report a history of atopic dermatitis. Some studies show boys may be preferentially affected. While many consider pityriasis alba to be a mild form of postinflammatory hypopigmentation, it is often considered a separate entity. Although the condition typically resolves with time, brief treatment with low-potency topical corticosteroids and/or generous emollients may be helpful.

Blessmann Weber M, Sponchiado de Avila LG, Albaneze R, et al. Pityriasis alba: a study of pathogenic factors. *J Eur Acad Dermatol Venereol.* 2002;16:463–468.

13. **Is vitiligo more common in patients with darker skin?**
    Vitiligo is a common disorder, affecting 1% to 2% of the world's population. There is no clear racial predisposition for vitiligo; however, the condition is more readily apparent in darker skin (Fig. 63.6). Consequently, people with darker

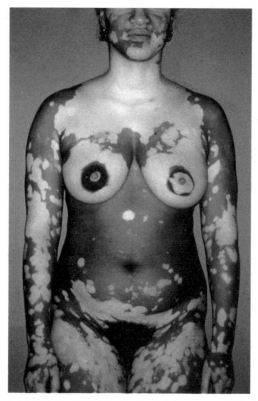

Fig. 63.6 Vitiligo in a black woman demonstrating striking differences in color between normal and affected skin. (Courtesy Walter Reed Army Medical Center teaching files.)

skin types may seek medical attention or manifest with more cosmetically debilitating disease. Also, the tendency for familial inheritance of vitiligo must be considered when conducting prevalence studies. In some societies, particularly Indian culture, there is a social stigma associated with vitiligo that pertains to a historic overlap with the appearance of cutaneous leprosy. In these cultures, patients with the condition, especially young women, may be considered "unfit for marriage," and the sociodynamic aspects of vitiligo must always be carefully considered by the clinician.

Shah H, Mehta A, Astik B. Clinical and sociodemographic study of vitiligo. *Indian J Dermatol Venereol Leprol.* 2008;74:701.
Silverberg NB. Pediatric vitiligo. *Pediatr Clin North Am.* 2014;61:347–366.

14. Why does tinea (pityriasis) versicolor cause hypopigmented spots on darker skin?
    Tinea versicolor, also known as *pityriasis versicolor*, is a common superficial yeast infection caused by the lipophilic organism *Malassezia globosa* and other species in this genus. The typical presentation in darker skin types is that of multiple hypopigmented thin plaques with fine scale distributed over the densely seborrheic skin of the chest, upper back, and proximal upper extremities (Fig. 63.7). The cause of the hypopigmentation is not completely understood; however, extracts from cultured organisms contain dicarboxylic acids that may competitively inhibit tyrosinase, an enzyme important in melanin production. Production of other indoles or tryptophan-based metabolites may also be involved in the resultant hypopigmentation.

Thoma W, Kramer HJ, Mayser P. Pityriasis versicolor alba. *J Eur Acad Dermatol Venereol.* 2005;19:147–152.

15. Why is it more difficult to appreciate erythema in darker skin?
    Erythema, or the amount of visible redness in the skin, is caused by increased blood flow and/or blood vessel engorgement in the dermis with the presence of oxyhemoglobin. If the epidermis is deeply pigmented, the red hues of oxyhemoglobin may be difficult to visualize. For this reason, the interpretation of patch testing for sensitivity to

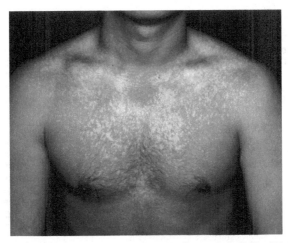

Fig. 63.7 Hypopigmented tinea versicolor on Asian skin. (Courtesy James E. Fitzpatrick, MD.)

cutaneous allergens in black patients is challenging. This is an important point to remember, as many diseases that have erythema as a hallmark, such as seborrheic dermatitis or atopic dermatitis, may present more subtly in a black patient. Cyanosis is also difficult to perceive in a dark-skinned patient for similar reasons.

Ben-Gashir MA, Hay RJ. Reliance on erythema scores may mask severe atopic dermatitis in black children compared with their white counterparts. *Br J Dermatol.* 2002;147:920–925.

16. Can any other generalizations be made about common cutaneous reaction patterns in skin of color?
    In addition to the difficulty in perceiving erythema, there exist other cutaneous reaction patterns more prevalent in darker skin. Papulosquamous diseases, such as psoriasis and nummular eczema, tend to exhibit a more violaceous color, leading to possible confusion with lichenoid conditions. Certain diseases, such as atopic dermatitis or tinea versicolor, may demonstrate a follicular accentuation. Pityriasis rosea may present atypically, with either papular or vesiculobullous forms, in black skin. In addition, some disorders, such as lichen planus and seborrheic dermatitis, have an increased propensity toward formation of annular lesions (Fig. 63.8). The reasons for these observations remain largely unknown.

McLaurin CI. Unusual patterns of common dermatoses in blacks. *Cutis.* 1983;32:352–355, 358–360.

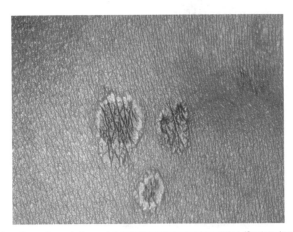

Fig. 63.8 Annular lichen planus, demonstrating central postinflammatory hypopigmentation. (Courtesy James E. Fitzpatrick, MD.)

17. What is the significance of multiple brown papules often seen on the periorbital area, cheeks, and nose?

The condition described is dermatosis papulosa nigra, and it is commonly seen in blacks, particularly black women. They are often referred to colloquially as "flesh moles." In truth, they are not "moles" (nevi) at all and represent a variant of seborrheic keratoses. The lesions tend to increase in number over time and do not typically resolve on their own. They have no malignant potential and are largely a cosmetic concern. Removal may be accomplished by light electrodesiccation (a personal favorite) and/or curettage. Alternatively, lesions may be treated with light application of liquid nitrogen, but care must be taken to avoid permanent hypopigmentation, a sequela of increased risk in persons with dark skin.

18. What is cutaneous sarcoidosis?

Cutaneous sarcoidosis is a granulomatous process of unknown etiology that is more prevalent among blacks, particularly among those in the southern United States, where the incidence is three to four times that of appropriately matched white patients. The cause of the disease is unknown. Cutaneous lesions may occur in association with pulmonary disease or may be present in isolation. Diverse patterns of skin lesions occurring in black patients with sarcoidosis have been observed. Shiny, somewhat waxy papular lesions are the most frequent cutaneous manifestation of sarcoidosis in blacks. When such dermal granulomatous papules are located near the nose, the condition has been referred to as *lupus pernio* (Fig. 63.9), and it may be indicative of a higher association with pulmonary disease. Because of its protean cutaneous manifestations, sarcoidosis should be included in the differential diagnosis of nearly all chronic dermatoses in black patients.

Cutaneous sarcoidosis is a granulomatous process of unknown etiology that is more prevalent among blacks, particularly among those in the southern United States, where the incidence is three to four times that of appropriately matched white patients. The cause of the disease is unknown. Cutaneous lesions may occur in association with pulmonary disease or may be present in isolation. Diverse patterns of skin lesions occurring in black patients with sarcoidosis have been observed. Shiny, somewhat waxy papular lesions are the most frequent cutaneous manifestation of sarcoidosis in blacks. When such dermal granulomatous papules are located near the nose, the condition has been referred to as lupus pernio (Fig. 63.9), and it may be indicative of a higher association with pulmonary disease. Because of its protean cutaneous manifestations, sarcoidosis should be included in the differential diagnosis of nearly all chronic dermatoses in black patients.

High WA. A woman with "keloids" on the nose and restrictive pulmonary disease. *Medscape Dermatol Clin*. September 7, 2004. http://www.medscape.com/viewarticle/488343. Accessed September 7, 2020.

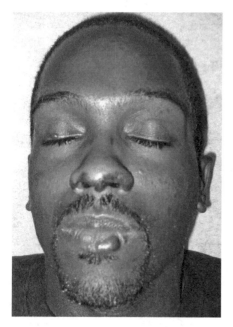

Fig. 63.9 Multiple sarcoidal granulomas along the right eyelid, nasal margin, and lower lip in a patient with sarcoidosis. (Courtesy Whitney A. High, MD.)

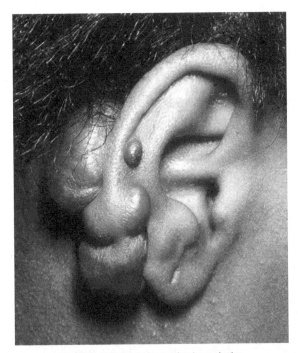

Fig. 63.10 Multiple keloids secondary to ear piercing.

19. What are keloids?

Keloids are benign dermal neoplasms composed of broad collagen bundles (Fig. 63.10). It is believed that they represent an aberrant healing process. In distinction from hypertrophic scars, keloids extend beyond the bounds of the original wound. There exists a distinct tendency toward keloid formation in persons of color. Sites of predilection include the shoulders, mandible, earlobes, presternal area, and deltoid region. Any form of trauma can induce keloids, including thermal injuries, insect bites, acne scars, injection sites, or cosmetic piercings and surgical incisions. Keloids may occur spontaneously, particularly in the central chest area. It is quite possible that such a "spontaneous" keloid represents a reaction to unrecognized trauma. The causal abnormality in the normal healing process is not known with certainty. It appears, however, that genetically predisposed fibroblasts are stimulated to produce abnormally high levels of procollagen messenger RNA, leading to excessive collagen production and secretion. Treatment options have included radiation or pressure therapy, cryotherapy, intralesional corticosteroids or verapamil, interferon, fluorouracil, topical silicone dressings, and laser treatment (either pulsed dye or Nd:YAG). Surgical excision is typically followed by recurrence unless adjunct preventive therapies are employed.

Arno AI, Gauglitz GG, Barret JP, et al. Up-to-date approach to manage keloids and hypertrophic scars: a useful guide. *Burns.* 2014;40:1255–1266.

20. What are "razor bumps"?

The hair follicles of blacks and many other people of color, such as Puerto Ricans, are elliptical, leading to development of tightly curled hair. After shaving, as the hairs regrow, there is a tendency for the sharp end of the curled hair to curve back into the skin. When the hair pierces the skin, it causes an inflammatory reaction, just as one might see with a splinter. This inflammatory reaction leads to the development of pseudofolliculitis barbae. This condition is not normally seen in men who grow beards, because after attainment of a certain length, usually 3 to 6 mm, the hair does not curve back into the skin. Accordingly, the condition is most common among populations required to be clean-shaven, such as black men in the military. Acne keloidalis nuchae represents a similar condition arising on the occipital scalp and/or nuchal area of those with shaved or very tightly cropped haircuts.

Kelly AP. Pseudofolliculitis barbae and acne keloidalis nuchae. *Dermatol Clin.* 2003;21:645–653.

21. How is pseudofolliculitis barbae treated?

Clearly, the definitive treatment is growth of a beard; however, if this is not an option, several techniques may decrease the number of inflamed papules. The beard should be shaved in the direction of growth with a single-edged razor. The skin should *not* be stretched while shaving. Hairs that have clearly recurved into the skin should be released with a sterile needle, but such hairs should *not* be plucked. Some men with this condition may use clippers that purposefully leave short stubble. Others may obtain good results with chemical depilatories. If inflammation is severe, short-term treatment with a low-potency topical corticosteroid may be effective. Laser hair removal, photodynamic therapy, or topical eflornithine represent emerging treatment options for those with intractable disease and a requisite need to maintain a clean-shaven appearance.

Diernaes JE, Bygum A. Successful treatment of recalcitrant folliculitis barbae and pseudofolliculitis barbae with photodynamic therapy. *Photodiagnosis Photodyn Ther.* 2013;10:651–653.

22. Are there other racial differences that may affect the treatment of hair or scalp conditions in blacks?

Blacks have elliptical follicular ostia and tightly curled hair with a small mean cross-sectional area. Asians have round ostia and straight hair with a large mean cross-sectional area. Whites have round to slightly ovoid follicles with an intermediate mean cross-sectional area. Nevertheless, these remain broad generalizations, and the entire racial and genetic make-up of the individual must be considered. The angles of curvature in the spiral structure of black hair yields multiple vulnerable points along the hair shaft, making it relatively fragile and prone to breakage. This structural arrangement also inhibits effective transmission of secreted sebum down the shaft, making the hair drier and less manageable relative to other hair types. For these reasons, the hair of blacks cannot be shampooed as often as that of other racial groups. Daily washing would lead to excessive dryness and hair breakage. A moisturizing conditioner should be used after shampooing. Such differences in hair care must be considered when prescribing treatment for scalp conditions that involve medicated shampoos. When evaluating alopecia, a thorough history of hair-grooming techniques used should be obtained. Specifically, questions about the use of chemical relaxers, permanent hair dyes, curling irons, hot combs, blow dryers, braids, or weaves should be asked, because many of these modalities cause damage to the hair shaft or the scalp. Finally, some unusual forms of alopecia, such as lipedematous alopecia (Fig. 63.11), with associated cotton-batting textural changes of the scalp, are associated nearly exclusively with black women.

High WA, Hoang MP. Lipedematous alopecia. *J Am Acad Dermatol.* 2005;53:S157–S161.
McMichael AJ. Ethnic hair update: past and present. *J Am Acad Dermatol.* 2003;48:S127–S133.

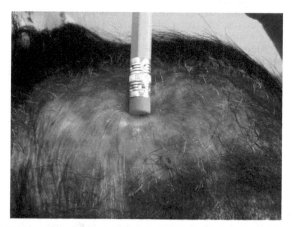

Fig. 63.11 Lipedematous scalp in an elderly black woman, indicated by pressure applied using a pencil, yielding remarkable induration of the skin. (Courtesy Whitney A. High, MD.)

KEY POINTS: SKIN OF COLOR

1. Skin of color, particularly black skin, manifests minor physiologic differences, including a stratum corneum with increased layers and cohesiveness and a decreased ability to synthesize vitamin D_3.
2. Erythema may be more difficult to appreciate on darkly pigmented skin, and this must be considered during clinical examination.
3. Pigmentation of the oral mucosa, benign-appearing palmoplantar macules, or multiple longitudinal pigmented streaks of the nails may represent normal variants in persons with darker skin types.
4. Many cutaneous diseases may present with follicular accentuation or other unusual clinical aspects in persons with darker skin types.
5. Ethnic and cultural differences in skin and hair must be considered in the examination and treatment of persons with skin of color.

23. **Are patients with skin of color particularly susceptible to any life-threatening illnesses?**

    Coccidioidomycosis, also known as San Joaquin Valley fever, is a deep fungal infection caused by *Coccidioides immitis*. It is typically acquired via inhalation of arthrospores and demonstrates occasional hematogenous dissemination to subcutaneous tissues, bone, or skin. Endemic areas include the Sonoran life zone of southern California, Arizona, New Mexico, southwestern Texas, and northern Mexico. It has also been reported in certain areas of South America. Infection occurs equally in both sexes and in all races and ages. For reasons that are not entirely clear, black persons are 14 times more likely to have severe disseminated disease than are Caucasians (Fig. 63.12), and individuals of Filipino descent are 10 times more likely to develop coccidioidomycosis-related meningitis than Caucasians. Further investigation has revealed that certain host genetics, the human leukocyte antigen class II and ABO blood group genes, influence susceptibility to severe coccidioidomycosis. Untreated, nonmeningeal coccidioidomycosis has a 50% mortality rate; therefore, early aggressive treatment with systemic antifungal agents is essential.

Louie L, Ng S, Hajjeh R, et al. Influence of host genetics on the severity of coccidioidomycosis. *Emerg Infect Dis*. 1999;5:672–680.
Pappagianis D. Epidemiology of coccidioidomycosis. *Curr Top Med Mycol*. 1988;2:199–238.

24. **Do any special considerations exist when performing skin surgery on patients with skin of color?**

    Due to the increased risk of pigmentary alterations, hypertrophic scars, and keloids among black patients, any surgical undertaking should be carefully considered with respect to the risks and benefits of the procedure. Because melanocytes are more sensitive to cold injury than keratinocytes, liquid nitrogen can cause permanent loss of pigmentation, and this is generally more noticeable in darker skin types. Treatment of benign growths, such as warts

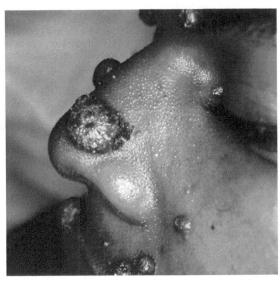

Fig. 63.12 Coccidioidomycosis. Disseminated coccidioidomycosis in a young black soldier. (Courtesy Fitzsimons Army Medical Center teaching files.)

or seborrheic keratoses, with cryotherapy can result, therefore, in permanent loss of pigment, and this modality must be judiciously implemented.

Grimes PE, Hunt SG. Considerations for cosmetic surgery in the black population. *Clin Plast Surg.* 1993;20:27–34.

25. Why is skin cancer less common in skin of color?

Ultraviolet (UV) radiation–induced damage to the DNA of cells in the lower epidermis, including keratinocyte stem cells and melanocytes, is prevented to a greater degree in darker skin, suggesting that the pigmented epidermis serves as an efficient UV filter. In addition, UV radiation–induced apoptosis (programmed cell death) is significantly greater in darker skin, indicating that any damaged cells may be removed more efficiently from the epidermis in skin of color. Together, the combination of decreased DNA damage due to UV radiation and the more efficient removal of damaged cells likely play a critical role in the decreased photocarcinogenesis seen in individuals with skin of color.

Yuji Y, Takahashi K, Zmudska BZ, et al. Human skin responses to UV radiation: pigment in the upper epidermis protects against DNA damage in the lower epidermis and facilitates apoptosis. *FASEB J.* 2006;20:E630–E639.

26. Are there any unique presentations of skin cancer when it does occur in patients with darker skin?

Although skin cancer is decidedly less common in people with skin of color, it is often associated with greater morbidity and mortality. Squamous cell carcinoma (SCC) is the most common skin cancer in blacks and Asian Indians, and it is the second most common skin cancer in Chinese and Japanese. Also, in skin of color, malignancies occur more often upon non–sun-exposed surfaces and the lower extremities. In fact, the most important risk factors for developing SCC in blacks are chronic scarring processes and areas of chronic inflammation. Acral lentiginous melanoma presents more often in persons with skin of color. Other reported risk factors for melanoma in blacks include albinism, burn scars, radiation therapy, trauma, immunosuppression, and preexisting pigmented lesions. Mycosis fungoides, a type of cutaneous T-cell lymphoma, occurs more often in persons with skin of color (see Chapter 45). Because many individuals with dark skin do not believe that they are susceptible to skin cancers, they may delay seeking care for a suspicious lesion, thereby leading to a less favorable prognosis. Public education in ethnic communities regarding the performance of self-skin examination, and the utility of regular visits to a dermatologist when skin conditions exist may lessen the associated morbidity and mortality of skin cancer in these populations.

Gloster HM, Neal K. Skin cancer in skin of color. *J Am Acad Dermatol.* 2006;55:741–760.
Hinds GA, Herald P. Cutaneous T-cell lymphoma in skin of color. *J Am Acad Dermatol.* 2009;60:359–375.

27. List skin diseases or conditions that are often considered more common in persons with skin of color

The diseases listed in Table 63.1, while not all-inclusive, represent many skin conditions thought to be seen with higher frequency in blacks. Some diseases, particularly the tropical infections, may be more common in blacks living outside of the United States. The perception of these diseases being more common in blacks may be related purely to this geographic distribution. Furthermore, such entities may be rarely encountered within the United States but are listed here for completeness.

Table 63.1 Dermatologic conditions more common in skin of color

Acne keloidalis nuchae
Acral lentiginous melanoma
Acropustulosis of infancy
African histoplasmosis
Ainhum
Buruli ulcer
Chancroid
Dermatitis cruris pustulosa et atrophicans
Dermatosis papulosa nigra
Dissecting cellulitis of the scalp
Dracunculiasis (guinea worm)
Filariasis
Granuloma inguinale
Granuloma multiforme

Table 63.1 Dermatologic conditions more common in skin of color (*Continued*)

Hamartoma moniliformis
Infundibulofolliculitis
Juxtaclavicular beaded lines
Kaposi's sarcoma (endemic)
Keloids
Leishmaniasis
Leprosy

Lichen nitidus
Lichen simplex chronicus
Loiasis
Madura foot
Melanonychia striata
Mongolian spots
Nevus of Ito
Nevus of Ota
Onchocerciasis
Papular eruption of blacks
Pityriasis rotunda
Pomade acne
Porphyria cutanea tarda (South African Bantus)
Pseudofolliculitis barbae
Pseudomonas toe web infection
Sarcoidosis
Sickle cell ulceration
Traction alopecia
Transient neonatal pustular melanosis
Tropical ulcer
Trypanosomiasis

CHAPTER 64

CULTURAL DERMATOLOGY

Scott A. Norton, Ali Damavandy, and Whitney A. High

1. A girl from southern India is anemic, and her school performance has declined. On examination, the child has dark, mascara-like makeup around her eyes. You suspect the makeup is the cause of these medical and social problems. What is the name of this traditional Indian eye makeup?
   Kohl is the Punjabi name for the eye makeup. It is also called *kajal* or *surma* in other Indian dialects.

2. What is kohl made from? How did it affect the child?
   Kohl is a fine powder resembling mascara that is applied to the margins of the palpebral conjunctiva. While originally made from antimony sulfide or carbon soot, it is now often adulterated with lead sulfide. Absorption of these lead-based pigments can cause lead poisoning. Use of these lead-based pigments has produced lead toxicity in Indoasian communities in the United Kingdom, leading to a nationwide ban. In the Middle East, a similar traditional eye cosmetics also often contain high levels of lead and can cause lead poisoning.

Centers for Disease Control and Prevention (CDC). Childhood lead exposure associated with the use of kajal, an eye cosmetic from Afghanistan—Albuquerque, New Mexico, 2013. *MMWR Morb Mortal Wkly Rep.* 2013;62(46):917–919.
Al-Ashban RM, Aslam M, Shah AH. Kohl (surma): a toxic traditional eye cosmetic study in Saudi Arabia. *Public Health.* 2004;118:292–298.

3. A Vietnamese child is seen in the emergency department with an earache. On examination, the child has several linear ecchymoses on her back. The physician suspects child abuse, but the interpreter says it is not. What caused the marks on the child?
   Cao gió (pronounced gow yaw), or "coin rubbing," is a traditional Vietnamese medical practice. A traditional healer first applies a liniment and then rubs a metal object upon the patient's skin, usually a coin, forcefully over the area. Petechiae and linear ecchymoses often develop and may be mistaken as evidence of abuse by providers who are unfamiliar with *cao gió*.

Davis RE. Cultural health care or child abuse? The Southeast Asian practice of cao gió. *J Am Acad Nurse Pract.* 2000;12:89–95.
Lilly E, Kundu RV. Dermatoses secondary to Asian cultural practices. *Int J Dermatol.* 2012;51:372–379.

4. An older Chinese man has dozens of uniform round scars on his back that resemble large cigarette burns. The patient is unconcerned about the lesions and indicates that someone did this to him. What ancient Chinese medical practice produces burn scars?
   Moxibustion has yielded the scars.

5. What is moxibustion?
   Moxibustion is derived from the words *moxa* and *combustion*, and it is the practice of igniting medicinal herbs on the skin. Moxa is derived from the species name for wormwood (*Artemisia moxa*), and it is a medicinal herb often used in the practice. When the healer extinguishes the flame, therapeutic properties of the herb supposedly enter the body. A burn scar is the sequelae of moxibustion. Sites utilized for moxibustion are similar to those used in acupuncture. The practice is still taught and utilized in Chinese medicine. Moxibustion was introduced into Europe by the end of the 17th century. In the movie *The Madness of King George*, there is a scene in which his physicians are treating him with moxibustion to cure his "madness." In actuality, it is thought that King George III (1738–1820) suffered from variegate porphyria.

Park JE, Lee SS, Lee MS, et al. Adverse events of moxibustion: a systematic review. *Complement Ther Med.* 2010;18:215–223.

6. In the emergency room, you are evaluating an elderly Iranian woman with an erythematous drug rash when you notice linear well-healed, vertically oriented scars on her back. When you inquire about them, she states they are the result of an old-fashioned medical procedure, employed "back home," when she was a child. What was the procedure?
   Bloodletting ("therapeutic phlebotomy") is a folk-healing procedure that in earlier centuries was considered a treatment option for a wide variety of medical conditions. For example, it was the treatment of choice for pneumonia.

While the practice has persisted longer in certain areas of the world, its efficacy has been disproven for all but a limited number of conditions, such as some forms of porphyria.

Papavramidou N, Thomaidis V, Fiska A. The ancient surgical bloodletting method of arteriotomy. *J Vasc Surg.* 2011;54:1842–1844.
Thomas DP. The demise of bloodletting. *J R Coll Physicians Edinb.* 2014;44:72–77.

7. What is the most common dermatologic side effect of acupuncture?
   A large survey of more than 6300 acupuncture patients in the United Kingdom revealed at least one adverse event in about 10% of procedures. The most common adverse event was bruising and bleeding. There have been reports of abundant petechiae (in one case, resembling meningococcemia) caused by acupuncture needles. Hematomas and ecchymoses often occur. Pyoderma, prolonged anesthesia, needle breakage, burns, itching, argyria, ulcers, postinflammatory hyperpigmentation, foreign body granuloma, and Koebnerization of psoriasis have also been reported. Transmission of HIV, hepatitis virus, parapoxvirus, and atypical mycobacteria has occurred via contaminated acupuncture needles.

Macpherson H, Scullion A, Thomas KJ, et al. Patient reports of adverse events associated with acupuncture treatment: a prospective national survey. *Qual Saf Health Care.* 2004;13:349–355.
Ryu HJ, Kim WJ, Oh CH, et al. Iatrogenic *Mycobacterium abscessus* infection associated with acupuncture: clinical manifestations and its treatment. *Int J Dermatol.* 2005;44:846–850.
Wu JJ, Caperton C. Images in clinical medicine. Psoriasis flare from Koebner's phenomenon after acupuncture. *N Engl J Med.* 2013;368:1635.
Yamashita H, Tsukayama H, Taanno Y, et al. Adverse events in acupuncture and moxibustion treatment: a six-year survey at a national clinic in Japan. *J Altern Complement Med.* 1999;5:229–236.

8. In the emergency room, you are asked to see a Chinese woman to rule out pneumonia. On her back, you identify sharply demarcated purpuric round lesions. Why does this patient have these lesions?
   The ecchymotic lesions on the woman's back are due to "cupping" (Fig. 64.1). Cupping is an ancient therapy that dates back to 1550 BC, in Egypt. It is still often employed in Asia and the Middle East to treat a broad range of ailments, such as respiratory distress (e.g., bronchitis, pneumonia), musculoskeletal problems, neurologic disorders (e.g., migraine headaches), hypertension, and skin conditions (e.g., herpes zoster, acne vulgaris, eczema). Suction is created by mechanical devices (e.g., hand or electrical pumps) or heat (e.g. warmed cups are placed on the skin and allowed to cool). "Wet cupping" is a variation where suction is applied to the skin, and then a small incision is made into the

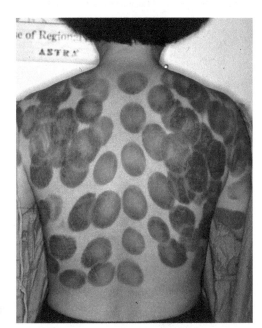

Fig. 64.1 Chinese woman with numerous sharply demarcated hemorrhagic lesions of the back due to cupping therapy. (Courtesy David Bertler, MD.)

purpuric area, with the blood withdrawn by repeating the suction process. Advocates of cupping believe it promotes blood flow.

Lee MS, Kim I, Ernest E. Is cupping an effective treatment? An overview of systematic reviews? *J Acupunct Meridian Stud.* 2011;4:1–4.
Ryu HJ, Kim WJ, Oh CH, et al. Iatrogenic *Mycobacterium abscessus* infection associated with acupuncture: clinical manifestations and its treatment. *Int J Dermatol.* 2005;44(10):846–850.
Wu JJ, Caperton C. Images in clinical medicine. Psoriasis flare from Koebner's phenomenon after acupuncture. *N Engl J Med.* 2013;368 (17):1365.

9. Where did the practice of tattooing start?
   Archaeological evidence shows that tattooing was part of indigenous cultures worldwide. Tattoos were used in ancient Europe, in the Mediterranean region, in the Middle East, in southern Asia, in northern Japan, in the Americas, and throughout the Pacific islands.

Levy J, Sewell M, Goldstein N. A short history of tattooing. *J Dermatol Surg Oncol.* 1979;5:851–856.
Schmid S. Historical essay. *Travel Med Infect Dis.* 2013;11:444–447.

10. What does the word *tattoo* mean?
    Tattoo comes from the pan-Polynesian word *tatau* meaning "to mark." Polynesian tataus were, and still are, richly symbolic, revealing heritage and status.

11. What culture has the most elaborate tattoos?
    The Marquesan Islanders of French Polynesia once applied tattoos to almost the entire body. Hawaiians, Samoans (Fig. 64.2), and Maoris of New Zealand also had extensive tattoos. Today, the practice is experiencing a cultural resurgence among many Polynesian groups. Japanese tattoos (horimono) are often regarded as the most skillful and artistically prepared.

12. Why do sailors have tattoos?
    European sailors adopted the habit of tattooing during voyages to the Polynesian islands in the 18th century. The practice is still associated with the sea-faring occupations.

13. Sailors sometimes have rooster and pig tattoos on their lower legs. Does this have a meaning?
    Yes. Many ethnic groups, cultures, and even subcultures, including sailors, have tattoos with symbolic meanings. Sailors may tattoo a rooster and pig on their lower legs (Fig. 64.3) or feet because these animals do not swim, and there is symbolic belief that if their ship sinks, or they are thrown overboard, the tattoo will get them to land quickly.

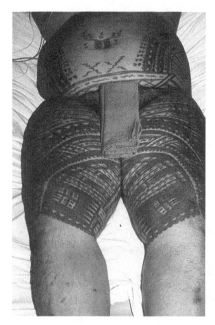

Fig. 64.2 A Samoan man with extensive and elaborate cultural tattoo. The traditional patterns of Polynesian tattoos are distinctive for each island or island group. (Courtesy Scott A. Norton, MD, MPH.)

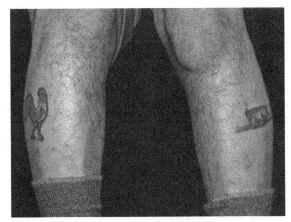

Fig. 64.3 Sailor with tattoos of a rooster and a pig on his legs. (Courtesy Fitzsimons Army Medical Center teaching files.)

Similarly, in sailing, an anchor tattoo symbolizes the wearer has sailed the Atlantic Ocean, or a tattoo of a fully rigged sailing ship symbolizes the wearer has sailed around Cape Horn.

14. Who is the Ice Man? Why are his tattoos so important?
The Ice Man is the name given to the 5200-year-old frozen corpse of a Bronze Age hunter found preserved in the ice of a Tyrolean glacier on the border of Austria and Italy. He had 15 groups of tattoos that are noteworthy because they are neither decorative nor on exposed surfaces. Most of the Ice Man's tattoos are on standard acupuncture sites. Subsequent radiographic examinations of the body indicated traumas at the sites, strengthening the notion that the Ice Man's tattoos served as a form of therapy, akin to acupuncture.

Dorfer L, Moser M, Bahr F, et al. A medical report from the Stone Age? *Lancet.* 1999;354:1023–1025.
Kean WF, Tocchio S, Kean M, et al. The musculoskeletal abnormalities of the Similaun Iceman ("ÖTZI"): clues to chronic pain and possible treatments. *Inflammopharmacology.* 2013;21:11–20.

15. A man from rural Nigeria has small parallel scars on his face. He says that his village doctor made these with a sharp stone when the man was young. What are ritually placed incisions called?
Scarification.

16. Why is scarification performed in some societies?
In some societies, scarification is thought to enhance beauty, provide identification, and/or protect from illness or evil.

17. What is an omega brand?
In the United States, the omega brand is associated with the black college fraternity Omega Psi Phi. While not officially sanctioned by the national office, many men (and "little sisters") have branded a Greek letter "O" on the deltoid or pectoral region. A similar practice is associated with the "Kappas" (Kappa Alpha Psi) (Fig. 64.4) and "Alphas" (Alpha Phi Kappa).

18. Name the familiar dark-red spot placed on the central forehead of Hindu women.
Bindi, kumkum, or tilak.

Kumar AS, Pandhi RK, Bhutani LK. Bindi dermatoses. *Int J Dermatol.* 1986;25:434–435.

19. What dermatologic problems can bindi cause?
The pigments employed (mercuric or lead compounds) can cause allergic contact dermatitis a lichenoid eruption, and contact leukoderma.

20. While on a surfing trip in Fiji, you notice that many of the men have dry, scaly skin. You wonder if there might be a disease outbreak, but the villagers explain the skin problem is called "kani" and it is caused by drinking excessive amounts of "yaqona." What is this?
Kani is the Fijian word for "kava dermopathy," which is an acquired ichthyosiform disorder caused by consumption of kava (or yaqona in Fiji). It yields "crocodile-like" skin. It is not known why the beverage causes this disorder, but it is speculated that kava may interference with cholesterol metabolism in the skin.

Norton SA, Ruze P. Kava dermopathy. *J Am Acad Dermatol.* 1994;31:89–97.

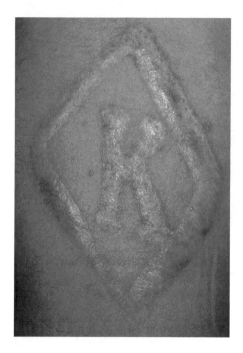

Fig. 64.4 Kappa brand of the college fraternity Kappa Alpha Psi. (Courtesy Fitzsimons Army Medical Center teaching files.)

21. What is kava?

Kava is a beverage made from the roots of *Piper methysticum*, a true pepper found on many tropical Pacific islands. Kava has psychoactive properties and is used socially and ceremonially throughout Micronesia, Melanesia, and Polynesia.

22. During a mission to a refugee camp in southern Africa, you see hundreds of children and adults with a shiny, slightly erosive eruption upon the sun-exposed forearms and neck. What is this eruption called?

Pellagra.

23. Why is pellagra abundant in the refugee camps?

Pellagra is caused by niacin deficiency (a B vitamin). Pellagra can be caused by malnutrition. Outbreaks can occur in refugee camps, orphanages, and prisons. Historically, pellagra occurred among sharecroppers in the early 20th century because their diet was based almost exclusively on corn.

Frank GP, Voorend DM, Chamdula A, et al. Pellagra: a non-communicable disease of poverty. *Trop Doct.* 2012;42:182–184.

24. What is betel nut? Who chews it?

"Betel nut" refers to the fruit of the areca palm (*Areca catechu*) that in some societies is chewed when wrapped in betel leaves (*Piper betle*). Technically, there is no true "betel nut"; "betel" refers to the leaves and the "nut" is actually the areca nut (technically a drupe). The practice is seen among many cultures ranging from Pakistan to Micronesia. It has been estimated that 10% to 20% of the world chews betel nut. Some cultures vary the practice by adding lime, clove, cardamom, catechu, or even tobacco. Men and women alike chew betel nut for mild psychoactive properties of the alkaloids found in the areca nut and the eugenol found in the betel leaf. Immigrants to the United States may continue this practice. Betel leaves have been reported to cause mottled dyschromia of the skin, perhaps as a chemical contact dermatitis.

25. What dermatologic changes are associated with chewing betel nut?

Betel nut chewing stains the teeth, gingiva, and oral mucosa. The color ranges from red to black. Chewers regard the color change as desirable. However, there is an increased risk of oral squamous cell carcinomas among betel nut chewers, attributable to the areca nut and/or lime.

Norton SA. Betel: consumption and consequences. *J Am Acad Dermatol.* 1998;38:81–88.

26. A Somali family is resisting forced deportation because she fears that her daughters will be compelled to undergo circumcision if they return to Mogadishu. What is female circumcision?
Female circumcision is a Western term for several forms of culturally sanctioned surgical procedures performed on female genitalia. It is most prevalent in Muslim nations of North Africa, where perhaps 100 million women have had the procedure. The procedures range from partial clitoridectomy (Sunna circumcision) to total infibulation (or pharaonic circumcision), with removal of the clitoris, labia minora, portions of the labia majora, and suturing that partially closes the vaginal orifice.

Dave AJ, Sethi A, Morrone A. Female genital mutilation: what every American dermatologist needs to know. *Dermatol Clin.* 2011;29:103–109.

27. What are the complications of female circumcision?
Complications of the procedure include infection, hemorrhage, reproductive issues (fetal death), sexual dysfunction (dyspareunia), and psychological scarring (posttraumatic stress disorder, chronic anxiety).

Hardy DB. Cultural practices contributing to the transmission of human immunodeficiency virus in Africa. *Rev Infect Dis.* 1987;9:1109–1119.

KEY POINTS: CULTURAL DERMATOLOGY

1. With increased mobility and immigration, it is important that health care providers understand how different cultural practices impact upon the skin.
2. The sequelae of some cultural practices (e.g., *cao gió*) may be mistaken for child, spouse, or elder abuse.
3. By analogy, some Western "cosmetic" procedures (e.g., breast augmentation, circumcision, fillers, liposuction) might be viewed with distaste from the perspective of a different culture.

28. What is the most common culturally sanctioned alteration of skin in the United States?
Perhaps piercing (of the ear, nose, etc.) is the most obvious answer in the United States.

29. Are there any culturally sanctioned surgical alterations of male genitalia?
Dozens exist, including the religion-associated circumcisions of Judaism, Islam, and the Seventh Day Adventist faith. Many Western societies practice widespread routine circumcision of neonates, even if it is not faith based. Australian aborigines practiced subincision, which is an incision of the distal ventral penis exposing the urethra. Ancient Pohnpeians practiced hemicastration (removal of one testicle) as a manhood rite. Many cultures practice the simple release of the ventral frenulum. Occupational castration (eunuchs), punitive castrations, and gender-altering surgery among transsexuals have received varying degrees of cultural acceptance throughout history.

30. What are artificial penile nodules?
Objects placed permanently under the skin of the prepuce or penile shaft, purportedly to enhance a partner's pleasure during intercourse. Other names include *tancho nodules* and *bulleetus*. The practice is most common in East Asian nations (e.g., Thailand and Philippines). In Japan, members of the yakuza, or Japanese criminal underground, often have artificial penile nodules.

Norton SA. Fijian penis marbles: an example of artificial penile nodules. *Cutis.* 1993;51:295–297.

31. Your cousin is marrying a woman from Mumbai, India. On the wedding day, the bride's hands are painted with an intricately detailed red-brown pigment. What is this called?
The Indian name for this is *mehndi*. It is produced by a semipermanent dye called henna.

32. Describe the use of henna on the skin
Henna is a natural red-brown pigment obtained from the plant *Lawsonia inermis*. It is used to prepare ceremonial body paint used in many Middle Eastern and South Asian societies. Women in these societies often use it to ornamentally paint the palms and soles, especially for celebrations. Henna is now commonly used in a deritualized fashion by Western women.

33. Are there any medical problems associated with henna?
Some people develop irritant contact dermatitis using henna. Henna may also cause hemolysis in glucose-6-phosphate dehydrogenase–deficient individuals after percutaneous absorption. However, most complications occur in "black-henna" preparations that ***do not*** contain henna at all, but instead contain para-phenylenediamine that can induce cutaneous and pulmonary allergic reactions (Fig. 64.5).

deGroot AC. Side-effects of henna and semi-permanent "black henna" tattoos: a full review. *Contact Dermatitis.* 2013;69:1–25.

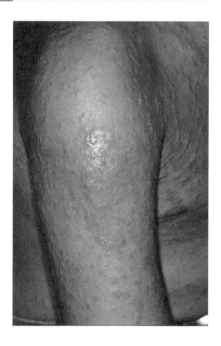

Fig. 64.5 Allergic contact dermatitis to henna tattoo on the arm. The outline of the tattoo is clearly visible. The other skin lesions represent an id reaction (autoeczematization) to the allergic contact dermatitis. (Courtesy William L. Weston, MD, Collection.)

34. Stretched ear lobes ("gauging") are an increasingly common sight on the streets of America. Where did the practice begin and what is its cultural significance and background?
    Ear lobe stretching has a history that dates back centuries and involves many parts of the world. The Maasai tribes of Africa stretched their ear lobes using progressively larger pieces of stone, wood, tusk, and thorn, with larger ear lobes regarded as a sign of age and wisdom. The Huaorani tribe of the Amazon also begin ear lobe stretching in childhood and gradually employ larger stones and pieces of wood. In older age, the Huaorani people remove all piercings and wear their ear lobes in a stretched state. In this country, as people age, enthusiasm for stretched ear lobes sometimes wanes, in particular among those who have adopted the practice from other cultures. This has led to increased need for surgical techniques to return the earlobe to its unstretched state.

Henderson J, Malata CM. Surgical correction of the expanded earlobe after ear gauging. *Aesthetic Plast Surg.* 2010;34:632–633.

35. A 51-year-old Saudi man is noted to have asymptomatic thickening and hyperpigmentation on the forehead, knees, ankles, and dorsa of the feet. What is this condition called?
    This patient has "prayer marks." Prayer marks with this distribution are most common in Muslims who pray for prolonged periods. The changes are due to the repeated and prolonged friction and pressure associated with praying. Prayer marks are not confined to Muslims and may be seen in any religious person who prays for prolonged periods.

Abanmii AA, Al Zouman AY, Al Hussaini H, et al. Prayer marks. *Int J Dermatol.* 2002;43:985–986.

36. A 22-year-old man from India presents with tinea cruris that involves the penis. What most likely accounts for this highly atypical clinical distribution of infection?
    Tinea cruris often involves the inner thighs and spares the penis/scrotum. In this case, the unusual pattern is likely cause by wearing a *langota*, which is a semiocclusive undergarment that is associated with increased involvement of the penis in patients with tinea cruris. At one time, in some parts of India, it was the only type of underwear that men used. In some parts of India, it is still considered to be the garment of choice for various athletic endeavors such as traditional wrestling, martial arts training, and gymnastics. A very similar garment called the *fundoshi* is worn in Japan.

Pandey SS, Chandra S, Guha PK, et al. Dermatophyte infection of the penis. Association with a particular undergarment. *Int J Dermatol.* 1981;20:112–114.

DERMATOLOGIC EMERGENCIES

James E. Fitzpatrick and Whitney A. High

1. **"Dermatologic emergencies" sounds like an oxymoron. Are there dermatologic emergencies?**
   Yes, while perhaps not as ubiquitous as other areas of medicine, there are some dermatologic emergencies. In some of these emergent conditions, the skin is the primary organ affected (pemphigus vulgaris [PV]), while in others, the cutaneous manifestations an important diagnostic clue to a severe underlying condition (meningococcemia). Prompt recognition of dermatologic emergencies is important because these conditions can be morbid or lethal but can be treated successfully, particularly early in the course of the disease.

2. **What are the major groups of dermatologic emergencies?**
   - **Vesiculobullous disorders and drug reactions:** Stevens-Johnson syndrome (SJS), toxic epidermal necrolysis (TEN), drug reaction with eosinophilia and systemic symptoms (DRESS), PV
   - **Serious infections:** acute meningococcemia, Rocky Mountain spotted fever (RMSF), disseminated herpes/zoster in immunocompromised persons
   - **Autoimmune disorders:** acute cutaneous eruption of systemic lupus erythematosus (SLE)
   - **Serious inflammatory conditions:** desquamative erythroderma, acute pustular psoriasis (of von Zumbusch), pustular psoriasis of pregnancy (impetigo herpeticum)
   - **Environmental/exogenous disorders:** heat stroke, child abuse, elderly abuse

VESICULOBULLOUS DISORDERS AND DRUG REACTIONS

3. **How does toxic epidermal necrolysis differ from the Stevens-Johnson syndrome or erythema multiforme major?**
   While not without controversy, it is now most widely accepted that SJS and TEN exist on a spectrum.
   SJS—skin lesions limited to less than 10% of the body surface area with two mucosal membranes affected in 92% to 100% of patients.
   SJS/TEN "overlap" syndrome—skin involvement of greater than 10% but less than 30% of body surface area
   Toxic epidermal necrosis—full-thickness leads to sloughing of greater than 30% of the body surface area and mucous membranes are involved in nearly all cases.
   Because SJS and TEN have different prognoses and variations in treatment and therapy, it is important to differentiate between them (Table 65.1). The diseases can usually be distinguished by their clinical presentation (Fig. 65.1), histologic findings, and course.

Mockenhaupt M. Stevens-Johnson syndrome and toxic epidermal necrolysis: clinical patterns, diagnostic considerations, etiology, and therapeutic management. *Semin Cutan Med Surg.* 2014;33:101–116.

---

4. **How do you treat Stevens-Johnson syndrome?**
   Discontinuation of any offending medication is always a cornerstone of therapy. However, since SJS appears to be immunologically mediated, it may respond to systemic corticosteroids and/or cyclosporine. Extremely mild presentations of SJS may not require systemic therapy, at all, if the offending medication is promptly discontinued. Patients with more severe SJS, especially with involvement of the oral mucosa, which interferes with eating and fluid intake, may be treated with a short course of high-dose systemic corticosteroids to abort the disease.

5. **How do you treat toxic epidermal necrolysis?**
   In addition to discontinuing the suspected drug(s), patients should be treated as burn patients with transfer to a burn unit, or an intensive care unit if a burn unit is not available. This will allow for appropriate supportive care to maintain fluid balance, monitor for infection, and prevent adult respiratory distress syndrome. Therapies that have been used or advocated include systemic corticosteroids, intravenous immunoglobulin (IVIG), plasmapheresis, cyclosporine, biologics, and a variety of other immunosuppressive drugs. The effectiveness of any of these therapies remains controversial, and without strong evidence. Most recently, the use of IVIG, associated with great expense, has been cast into doubt. There is limited evidence that cyclosporine has both a beneficial mortality benefit and a relatively safe side effect profile.

Gilbert M, Scherrer LA. Efficacy and safety of cyclosporine in Stevens-Johnson syndrome and toxic epidermal necrolysis. *Dermatol Ther.* 2019;32:e12758.

Table 65.1 Clinicopathologic features of toxic epidermal necrolysis (TEN) versus Stevens-Johnson syndrome (SJS)

	TEN	SJS
Maximal intensity	1–3 days	7–15 days
Skin pain	Severe	Minimal
Mucosal involvement	Mild	Severe
Lesional pattern	Diffuse erythema, exfoliation*	Annular and targetoid lesions
Skin histology	Few inflammatory cells	Numerous inflammatory cells
Prognosis	Poor	Excellent

*Many authorities require more than 30% exfoliation of the total body surface.

6. With appropriate therapy in a burn unit, what is the overall mortality of TEN?
   In a systematic review of numerous studies from burn units, the overall mortality was 30% in burn centers. The medical literature suggests that the mortality rate of patients with TEN in non–burn centers is approximately 45%. SCORETEN represents a validated instrument to predict prognosis in SJS/TEN that uses (1) patient age, (2) the presence of an associated malignancy, (3) heart rate, (4) serum blood urea nitrogen (BUN), (5) detached or compromised body surface area, (6) serum bicarbonate, and serum glucose.

Torres-Navarro I, Briz-Redón Á, Botella-Estrada R. Accuracy of SCORTEN to predict the prognosis of Stevens-Johnson syndrome/toxic epidermal necrolysis: a systematic review and meta-analysis [published online ahead of print December 3, 2019]. *J Eur Acad Dermatol Venereol.* 2019.

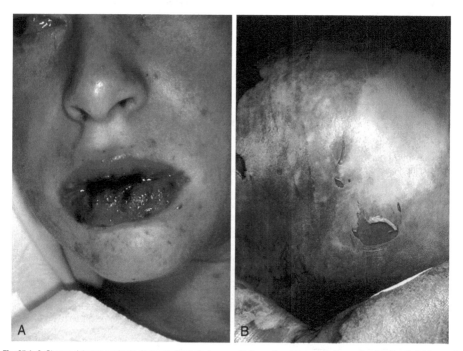

Fig. 65.1 **A,** Stevens-Johnson syndrome demonstrating typical mucosal inflammation of the mouth, lips, and conjunctiva. **B,** Fatal case of captopril-induced toxic epidermal necrolysis showing violaceous discoloration with sheets of epidermis peeling away from the skin. (Courtesy James E. Fitzpatrick, MD.)

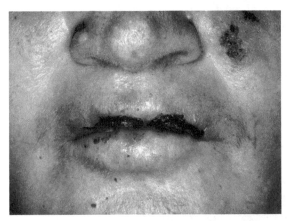

Fig. 65.2 Pemphigus vulgaris demonstrating erosive lesions of the lips and left cheek. (Courtesy James E. Fitzpatrick, MD.)

7. What is pemphigus vulgaris?

PV is a serious blistering disease that most often affects middle-aged persons (Fig. 65.2). It usually first presents with mouth ulcerations (60% of cases), but it can involve blistering of the skin in bulk, particularly above the waist. PV may present acutely, and in severe cases it may resemble TEN or SJS. Early recognition is important because pemphigus can be fatal, if untreated, and current therapies, including prednisone, other immunosuppressive agents, and even rituximab, are highly effective.

8. Describe Nikolsky sign and its relationship to pemphigus vulgaris.

PV involves only the upper layers of the epidermis; the blisters in this condition are fragile, and patients may present with only superficial ulcers. Because of blister fragility, in pemphigus, one can apply lateral pressure with a finger to the intact skin around a lesion, causing the upper layer of the skin to become detached. This is called the Nikolsky sign. It occurs in pemphigus and other superficial blistering disorders and it is distinguishing from deeper blistering diseases (like bullous pemphigoid), where Nikolsky sign is usually absent.

9. How is pemphigus vulgaris treated?

Since pemphigus is an autoimmune blistering disorder, therapy is designed to decrease production of autoantibodies and to reduce the resultant inflammatory response. Initial therapy often focuses on high-dose corticosteroids (~1 mg/kg initial dose), adjusted higher or lower depending on the clinical response. Other immunosuppressive medications, such as azathioprine, cyclophosphamide, and mycophenolate mofetil, may be used as "steroid-sparing" agents. Recently, rituximab has been approved for use in PV, and it is often used in conjunction with corticosteroids, due to a delayed response. Many authorities (including one of these authors—W.A.H.) believe rituximab may be the treatment of choice for most PV.

Atzmony L, Hodak E, Dgalevich M, et al. Treatment of pemphigus vulgaris and pemphigus foliaceus: a systemic review and meta-analysis. *Am J Clin Dermatol.* 2014;15:503–515.

10. What is DRESS syndrome?

DRESS stands for **d**rug **r**ash with **e**osinophilia and **s**ystemic **s**ymptoms, and it can be a life-threatening reaction. The condition is characterized by a morbilliform cutaneous eruption, fever, enlarged lymph nodes, leukocytosis with eosinophilia, and liver or kidney involvement. Typical drugs that induce this reaction include anticonvulsants, allopurinol, and sulfa drugs. The syndrome usually develops several weeks (3–6 weeks) after drug initiation and can persist and/or recur for long periods, even after the drug has been stopped. The delayed onset of DRESS, weeks after drug initiation, is different from the typical more abrupt onset of SJS/TEN. Therapy of DRESS includes high-dose corticosteroids and/or cyclosporine.

11. What is drug-induced antineutrophil cytoplasmic antibody (ANCA)–associated vasculitis?

Drug-induced ANCA-associated vasculitis (AAV) is an entity that has only recently been recognized. These patients, typically drug addicts, present with purpura, ecchymoses, and thrombotic vasculopathy and generalized malaise. The condition seems related to levamisole, an antihelminthic drug, which has been used to cut cocaine. It is now estimated that about 70% of all the cocaine used in the United States now contains levamisole. Ergot, a history of cocaine use should be elicited when the diagnosis is suspected.

Marquez J, Aguirre L, Muñoz C, et al. Cocaine-levamisole-induced vasculitis/vasculopathy syndrome. *Curr Rheumatol Rep.* 2017;19:36.

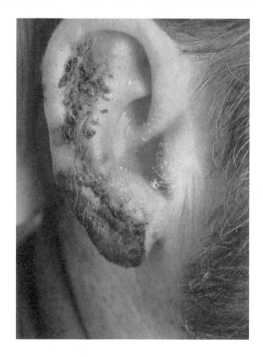

Fig. 65.3 Purpuric hemorrhagic lesions on the ear of patient using levamisole-cut cocaine. (Courtesy Whitney A. High, MD.)

12. **How is the diagnosis made?**
   A clinical picture of purpura and ecchymotic areas coupled with laboratory findings that can include agranulocytosis, thrombocytopenia, and ANCA-positive vasculitis is often present. A gas chromatography–mass spectroscopy analysis of the blood within 48 hours of levamisole exposure will be positive.

13. **Is there any clinical picture that is more common in levamisole-induced vasculitis?**
   Widespread purpura is common, but earlobe involvement is particularly suggestive (Fig. 65.3).

14. **Why is it important to recognize this entity?**
   AAV caused by levamisole will resolve over time, so long as the levamisole exposure ceases. This diagnosis should be considered to avoid unnecessary aggressive management, so long as avoidance can be employed.

INFECTIOUS DISEASES

15. **Are any dermatologic emergencies infectious in origin?**
   Infectious dermatologic emergencies include bacterial infections (necrotizing fasciitis, tularemia, meningococcemia), viral infections (disseminated herpes/varicella infection), rickettsial infections (RMSF), and fungal infections (mucormycosis).

16. **Can emergent infections be differentiated by their cutaneous presentations?**
   Yes, although few cutaneous findings in emergent infections are truly pathognomonic. Infections that involve the skin can be organized generally by the appearance of the primary lesion (Table 65.2). Major cutaneous patterns of presentation include:
   - **Petechial/purpuric papules** (chronic gonococcal septicemia, meningococcemia [Fig. 65.4], subacute/acute bacterial endocarditis, and RMSF)
   - **Vesicular** (neonatal herpes simplex, Kaposi's varicelliform eruption)
   - **Pustular** (disseminated candidiasis)
   - **Maculopapular** (hepatitis B, Lyme disease)
   - **Diffusely erythematous** (staphylococcal scalded skin syndrome).

17. **What is Rocky Mountain spotted fever?**
   RMSF is a rickettsial disease caused by *Rickettsia rickettsii*, a bacterium that is transmitted to humans by ticks of the *Dermacentor* genus. In 2017, there were 6248 cases of SFR reported in the United States. Despite the name, referencing the Rocky Mountains, the disease most common in the southeastern and south-central United States. It may be seen as far north as Canada, and as far south as South America.

Table 65.2 Diagnostic signs in dermatologic infectious emergencies

Petechial/Palpable Purpura
Neisseria gonorrhoeae septicemia
Neisseria meningitidis septicemia
Acute/subacute bacterial endocarditis (*Staphylococcus aureus*, streptococci)
Rickettsia rickettsii (Rocky Mountain spotted fever)
Rickettsia prowazekii (louse-borne typhus)
Borrelia sp. (relapsing fever)
Hemorrhagic fevers (dengue, Rift Valley, Congo-Crimean, Korean)
Cytomegalovirus (viral hepatitis)
Hepatitis B virus
Yellow fever
Rubella
Plasmodium falciparum (malaria)

Violaceous Skin Discoloration
Infectious gangrene
Necrotizing fasciitis
Mucormycosis

Purpura Fulminans (Purpura Secondary to Disseminated Intravascular Coagulation)
Neisseria meningitidis
Streptococcus spp.
Escherichia coli
Salmonella typhi
Bacteroides fragilis
Other enteric gram-negative organisms
Hemorrhagic fevers
Vibrio vulnificus

Vesicular
Neonatal herpes simplex virus
Disseminated vaccinia

Pustular
Staphylococcal endocarditis/sepsis
Disseminated candidiasis
Herpes simplex virus
Corynebacterium diphtheriae

Diffuse Erythema
Toxic shock syndrome

Maculopapular Eruptions
Viral infections
Rickettsial infections
Spirillum minor (rat-bite fever)
Disseminated fungal infections
Toxoplasma gondii
Tularemia
Leptospirosis

Annular Erythema
Lyme disease (*Borrelia burgdorferi*)

18. How does Rocky Mountain spotted fever present?
One to two weeks after the bite of infected tick, patients usually develop a nonspecific prodrome that includes fever, chills, muscle pain, headache, and generalized malaise. Later signs and symptoms include abdominal pain, joint pain, and a petechial eruption that usually begins as acral red macules that progress to cover the trunk over 6 to 96 hours and become petechial and hemorrhagic (Fig. 65.5). About 15% of patients never develop cutaneous findings.

19. How important is it to make an early diagnosis of RMSF?
Untreated RMSF may have a 30% mortality, but with appropriate antibiotic treatment (doxycycline), the mortality is less than 2%. Most deaths are due to delayed diagnosis and treatment. In general, an antibiotic should be initiated based

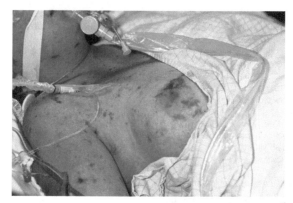

Fig. 65.4 Palpable purpura and ecchymoses in a patient with meningococcemia. (Courtesy William L. Weston, MD, Collection.)

upon the clinical suspicion and to avoid a fatal delay in treatment. Definitive diagnostic methods are too delayed to be of use. It is important to realize the tick will be attached or brought in by the patient in just 20% of cases.

20. What is the differential to consider in hemorrhagic lesions other than infection?
   • Coagulation abnormalities, such as idiopathic thrombocytopenia, disseminated intravascular coagulation (with purpura fulminans), and clotting factor deficiencies
   • TEN can present with petechial lesions
   • Vasculitides, such as leukocytoclastic vasculitis (LCV) secondary to an underlying collagen vascular disease, or polyarteritis nodosa
   • Drug-induced AAV
   • Ergot poisoning

21. What causes necrotizing fasciitis (necrotizing soft tissue infections)?
   Necrotizing fasciitis has been recognized in the modern medical literature since the American Civil War, but it has received much attention in the lay press as "flesh-eating Strep." However, it is important from the outset to recognize that the disorder is not caused by only streptococcus, and it can be caused by a variety of gram-positive and gram-negative organisms, and in fact, it can be polymicrobial. The bacterial infection is rapidly progressive, often over hours, destroying muscle and subcutaneous tissues. Loss of a limb or death may occur if the condition is not diagnosed and treated early in its course.

22. Describe the clinical presentation of necrotizing fasciitis
   In necrotizing fasciitis, the bacteria usually enter through a surgical or traumatic wound and move along fascial planes, destroying vessels and tissue. Within the first 48 hours, the involved area, which is initially erythematous, indurated, and painful, becomes a dusky blue, indicating impaired blood flow (Fig. 65.6). Because there is significant

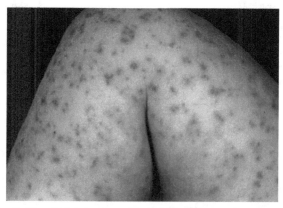

Fig. 65.5 Rocky Mountain spotted fever. Well-developed purpuric lesions on the lower leg. (Courtesy Fitzsimons Army Medical Center teaching files.)

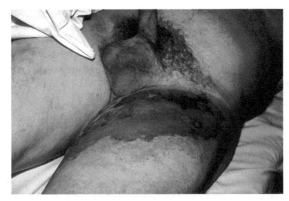

Fig. 65.6 Necrotizing fasciitis. The typical well-demarcated, dusky purpuric lesion is caused by thrombosis of the involved vessels.

thrombosis, a biopsy usually results in little or no bleeding, and this may be a useful diagnostic sign, when present. Extensive surgical debridement and aggressive systemic antibiotics are necessary to prevent demise.

23. Can other cutaneous infections mimic necrotizing fasciitis?
Necrotizing fasciitis is an infectious gangrene that rapidly progresses to destroy skin, subcutaneous tissue, and muscle. Other types of gangrene have cutaneous findings similar to those of necrotizing fasciitis:
- *Staphylococcus aureus* and, occasionally, gram-negative organisms can cause progressive bacterial synergistic gangrene. This disease presents with a dusky erythematous discoloration of the skin followed by deep ulceration.
- Gas gangrene or clostridial gangrene, caused by the anaerobe *Clostridium perfringens*, can follow a penetrating or crush wound, yielding a tender, painful, edematous, white area that often becomes bronze with cutaneous blistering. Occasionally, when one palpates the area, crepitation or a crackling sensation is noted due to gas formation in tissue. As with necrotizing fasciitis, timely diagnosis and treatment are necessary to prevent significant morbidity and mortality.

24. Are there any parasitic "emergencies" that have cutaneous manifestations?
Cysticercosis cutis, a cestoidal infection due to the larval form of the pork tapeworm, *Taenia solium*, can lead to an emergent presentation. Typically, *Taenia* eggs enter the stomach from the intestine via reverse peristalsis, and they develop into oncospheres that penetrate the stomach wall and enter the circulation. The organism becomes lodged in internal organs, such as the heart, brain, muscles, lungs, and eye. Brain involvement can lead to seizures. They also move to the subcutaneous tissues and develop into cysts that contain cysticercus larvae. Lesions are usually numerous and can become calcified, as evidenced by radiographs. Multiple subcutaneous cysts in a patient with unexplained neurologic signs or symptoms can point to this diagnosis.

25. Do mycobacterial infections cause any dermatologic emergencies?
Most mycobacterial infections are relatively chronic and do not constitute emergencies. However, when patients with leprosy undergo treatment, a "reversal reaction" may occur due to changes in immune status. Type I reversal reactions are seen in people with tuberculoid disease, and this results in in acute inflammation of involved areas that may place pressure on affected nerves, resulting in permanent motor and sensory damage to the area. The lack of sensory input and resultant trauma over years lead to severe disfigurement of the extremities. Treatment consists of high-dose prednisone tapered over weeks. A type II reversal reaction (erythema nodosum leprosum) can occur in those with lepromatous disease, and it may leave the patient feeling unwell, but it does not typically result in nerve damage. Type II reactions are treated with prednisone, clofazimine, and sometimes thalidomide.

AUTOIMMUNE DISORDERS

26. What collagen vascular diseases may become dermatologic emergencies?
- Acute cutaneous and bullous SLE
- Dermatomyositis
- LCV (necrotizing venulitis)
- Still's disease
- Neonatal lupus erythematosus (NLE)

27. What are the cutaneous findings in acute and bullous SLE?
The cutaneous findings of acute SLE are most common on the sun-exposed areas of the skin. The eruption consists of an evanescent erythema that is especially evident over the malar area of the face, producing the characteristic "butterfly rash." The erythema lasts hours to days and can resolve without residua. In a significant number of patients, the acute erythema can evolve into discoid lupus erythematosus, which is a chronic scaling eruption with scarring.

In bullous SLE, the patients present with tense vesicles or bullae, usually in sun-exposed sites. These are important presentations because both may be associated with severe internal disease.

28. **How does neonatal lupus erythematosus (NLE) present?**
It is an acute self-limited disease that gradually improves over 1 to 2 months, as maternal antibodies disappear. Cutaneous findings include diffuse superficial erythema and scaling that are often most apparent in the malar area of the face ("racoon eyes") but can occur anywhere. Neonates frequently have other systemic findings, such as those seen in SLE: anemia, thrombocytopenia, jaundice, and hepatosplenomegaly with abnormal liver function tests. Another prevalent finding is atrioventricular heart block, which can be permanent.

29. **Why are prompt recognition and treatment of NLE important?**
Frequently, NLE eruptions are misdiagnosed as infectious in origin. This subjects the infant to the unnecessary risks of systemic antibiotics, while the presence of heart block may be missed, and appropriate systemic treatment (steroids) for the other NLE problems is delayed.

KEY POINTS: DERMATOLOGIC EMERGENCIES

1. Dermatologic emergencies do exist, and some do have characteristic skin findings.
2. Recognition of specific skin signs and the early diagnosis of emergent skin disorders can be lifesaving.
3. Skin signs of TEN include diffuse and severe skin tenderness and "cayenne pepper" nonblanching erythema that evolves into widespread blistering and superficial ulcers.
4. Recognition of the skin signs of necrotizing fasciitis is crucial to patient survival. These signs include systemic toxicity; localized painful induration; well-defined, dusky blue coloration; and lack of bleeding in the area when incised.

30. **Why is dermatomyositis considered an emergency?**
Dermatomyositis can develop rapidly with significant morbidity and rarely mortality. Skin findings in this disease can predate significant muscle involvement and be quite helpful in early diagnosis and treatment, especially in children. The skin findings that are helpful in diagnosis are
- **Gottron papules**—erythematous to violaceous papules occurring over the dorsa of the distal interphalangeal and proximal interphalangeal joints of the hands
- **Gottron sign**—erythematous to violaceous streaking upon the tendons of the arms
- **Shawl sign/Holster sign**—violaceous erythema on the shoulders/outer hips, respectively
- **"Heliotrope" erythema**—violaceous erythema of the eyelids
- **Periungual erythema**—erythema and ragged cuticles surrounding the proximal nail fold

31. **What is leukocytoclastic vasculitis?**
LCV is a group of diseases that cause acute neutrophilic inflammation, fibrin deposition, and damage to the small vessels of the dermis. The condition was formerly known as "hypersensitivity vasculitis," and it can occur due to a variety of perturbations of homeostasis, such as medications, infections, connective tissue disease, or cryoglobulinemia. Henoch-Schonlein purpura is a type of LCV with a characteristic clinical presentation and with disease mediated by immunoglobulin A antibodies. LCV of all forms typically yields "palpable purpura," chiefly on the lower extremities. Cutaneous lesions of LCV usually resolve without sequelae, but internal organ involvement, particularly kidney involvement, can be seen in some cases. The differential diagnosis of LCV should include infections that cause palpable purpura, such as meningococcemia.

32. **What are the skin signs of Still disease?**
The diagnosis of Still disease can be perplexing because a significant number of these patients (25% to 30%) do not present with arthritis but with an evanescent eruption, spiking fever, leukocytosis, lymphadenopathy, and splenomegaly. Despite also being referred to as "juvenile rheumatoid arthritis," not all cases of Still disease present in children, and serologic tests for rheumatoid factor are almost always negative; hence, this nosology is not favored. The disease can be rapidly progressive, with severe bone and joint destruction and growth retardation. The rash, which occurs in 25% to 40% of patients, can be present for months to years before the arthritis. The eruption is typically fleeting, lasting up to 24 hours, and usually occurs in conjunction with fever. The rash may be diffuse with truncal accentuation and consists of coral-salmon red, flat macules to slightly elevated papules. Usually patients with Still disease have massive elevations in serum ferritin. Treatment for this disease usually consists of systemic steroids. Other immunosuppressive drugs have also been used successfully.

INFLAMMATORY CUTANEOUS DISORDERS

33. **Why is pyoderma gangrenosum a dermatologic emergency?**
Pyoderma gangrenosum (PG) is an example of a *neutrophilic dermatosis* because, histologically, such disorders have large dermal infiltrates of neutrophils. It can be a dermatologic emergency because of rapid progression leading to severe local tissue destruction. PG is frequently misdiagnosed, by patients and physicians, as an infectious process, particularly as a brown recluse spider bite. However, in PG, surgical procedures or any mechanical debridement of

acute lesions must be strictly avoided as it leads to progression of the disease (called "pathergy"). Because of pathergy, even blood draws should be combined and minimized in persons with PG. Therefore, it is imperative to recognize and treat these lesions correctly and early to avoid massive tissue destruction and loss. PG is more common in persons with a history of inflammatory bowel disease, rheumatoid arthritis, autoimmune hepatitis, and leukemia/lymphoma.

34. **How does PG present?**
Clinically, lesions of PG begin as a small papule/pustule that enlarges to form an ulcer. The ulcer has a necrotic center that may erode through the subcutis and down to muscle, tendons, and fascia (Fig. 65.7). The intact epidermis at the borders of the lesion is erythematous and may have a violaceous hue and a characteristic "undermined" edge. Typically, lesions of PG are extremely painful, and the extreme nature of the pain and tenderness may be a characteristic clue. Again, while PG may occur sporadically (~50% of cases), the condition is associated with several systemic diseases, inflammatory bowel disease, rheumatoid arthritis, and leukemia/lymphoma.

35. **Under what circumstances do childhood vascular anomalies become dermatologic emergencies?**
Infantile capillary hemangiomas (ICHs) can lead to a dermatologic emergency. ICH lesions can be present at birth (approximately 20%) but more often develop over the first several weeks of life. There is a rapid growth phase, during which ICH rapidly enlarges, before eventual regression. Most often, these tumors represent only a cosmetic problem, but if an ICH occurs around the eyes or in the oral cavity (Fig. 65.8), it can cause morbidity or even mortality. Some ophthalmologists suggest that even a few days of obstructed vision in a newborn can impair normal visual development. Therefore, an ICH that intrudes upon an infant's visual field should be treated aggressively. Likewise, enlarging ICH of the upper aerodigestive tract can result in acute emergent situations and must be treated early in their course. In rare cases, large hemangiomas can also produce high-output cardiac failure.

36. **How are hemangiomas treated?**
Oral propranolol and sometimes oral prednisone are treatments often employed for ICH. Interventions for ICH, such as surgery, laser, or radiofrequency ablation, are used only for high-risk lesions, by skilled experts, under urgent situations. Laser therapy is also used for lesions that persistently bleed.

37. **Is acne fulminans a dermatologic emergency?**
Although most acne is not an emergency condition, acne fulminans, with severe scarring (and resultant psychosocial problems), and even systemic systems, can be an emergency. Acne fulminans usually occurs in teenage boys, but there are cases reported in girls. The eruption is characterized by rapid suppuration of large, highly inflamed nodules

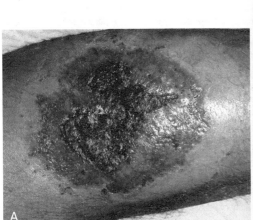
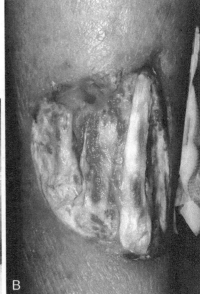

Fig. 65.7 Pyoderma gangrenosum. **A,** Classic lesion demonstrating characteristic undermined border. **B,** Older lesion without an active edge. Note that the depth of the ulcer exposes underlying tendons. (Courtesy James E. Fitzpatrick, MD.)

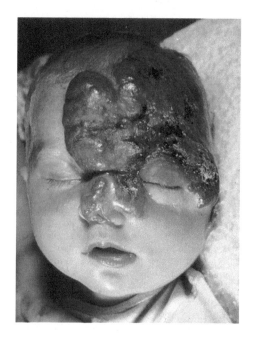

Fig. 65.8 Infantile hemangioma. Rapidly growing infantile hemangioma occluding the orbital space and nasal cavity. (Courtesy Fitzsimons Army Medical Center teaching files.)

and plaques, resulting in ragged ulcerations, and scarring of the chest, back, and, less commonly, face. Often attendant with the cutaneous symptoms are fever, leukocytosis, arthralgias, and myalgias, suggesting a systemic upregulation of the immune system.

38. **What is the treatment for acne fulminans?**
   Treatment for this condition focuses on oral retinoids (13-cis-retinoic acid) to treat the acne, and oral steroids to quell inflammation. Paradoxically, in persons with significant acne, the use of oral retinoids without coadministered oral steroids can induce acne fulminans in the first month of treatment, and providers who use this medication should be aware of this potential side effect.

39. **Are there drug eruptions that are dermatologic emergencies?**
   Most drug eruptions are relatively transient and consist of a morbilliform or macular erythema, perhaps with pruritus, but without other signs or symptoms. On occasion, drug eruptions can be more serious and present as a diffuse exfoliative erythroderma "red man/woman syndrome." In these cases, patients have erythroderma (>98% of the body erythematous) with pruritus and scaling. In addition to drug reactions, other causes of erythroderma such as flares of psoriasis, atopic dermatitis, and lymphoma must be excluded. Other types of drug-induced processes that can present as dermatologic emergencies include SJS, TEN, severe LCV, and severe urticaria/angioedema.

40. **What is Kawasaki disease and how does it present?**
   Kawasaki disease (KD) is an acute febrile illness of young children (often <5 years old) characterized by vasculitis of medium-sized arteries, including the coronary arteries. This latter feature can even lead to coronary artery aneurysms (CAAs) and death. CAAs develop in about 25% of untreated cases of KD, and the risk is greatly diminished with appropriate treatment, making early recognition of the disease important. Features of KD include:
   - Conjunctival congestion
   - Oropharyngeal lesions (mucosal injection, strawberry tongue, fissured lips)
   - Hand and foot erythema
   - Exanthem.

   These aforementioned findings, along with lymphadenopathy, constitute minor criteria for KD. Four of five minor plus the major criterion of fever >38.3°C are necessary for diagnosis of KD. Hand and foot erythema may be accompanied by edema followed and acral desquamation about 2 weeks after onset. The exanthem is a generalized macular erythema.

Vervoort D, Donné M, Van Gysel D. Pitfalls in the diagnosis and management of Kawasaki disease: an update for the pediatric dermatologist. *Pediatr Dermatol.* 2018;35:743–747.

41. **How do you treat Kawasaki's syndrome?**

    High-dose aspirin during the febrile phase (100 mg/kg/day), in addition to intravenous gammaglobulin (IVIG—400 mg/kg/day for 3 to 4 days).

ENVIRONMENTAL DISORDERS

42. **Is heatstroke considered a dermatologic emergency?**

    White heatstroke is not necessarily a "dermatologic problem," exclusively, it does have characteristic skin findings that assist in making a quick diagnosis. In a heatstroke victim, the skin is erythematous, hot, but dry, without perspiration. These findings, in association with unconsciousness, should alert one to the diagnosis. Prompt intervention is necessary to prevent death or severe central nervous system (CNS) damage.

43. **What are the cutaneous signs of child abuse?**

    Child abuse causes morbidity and mortality, as well as lasting psychological damage. Its prompt recognition is of paramount importance. Cutaneous signs of child abuse include:
    - **Bruising and abrasions:** These lesions are usually present in patterns or in areas not consistent with the history or trauma from common childhood accidents (Fig. 65.9).
    - **Burns with unusual patterns:** Examples include cigarette burns that appear randomly over the body or "dunking" scald injuries, with distinct borders and even a "doughnut" pattern on the buttock area when the skin is pressed against a cooler tub surface.
    - **Generalized wastage and dermatitis:** These are due to neglect and malnutrition.
    - **Traumatic alopecia:** This alopecia demonstrates hemorrhage, irregular outlines, and/or hematoma formation.
    - **Bite marks of adults:** These can be distinguished from a child's mouth by width.

44. **What are skin signs of senior/elderly abuse?**

    With the rising population of elderly persons in skilled care environments, senior/elderly abuse is becoming a more prevalent issue. Admittedly, the situation is complicated because elderly persons with dementia may sometimes make

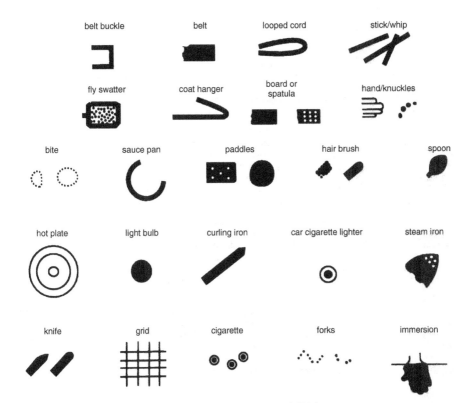

Fig. 65.9 Various cutaneous patterns of child abuse.

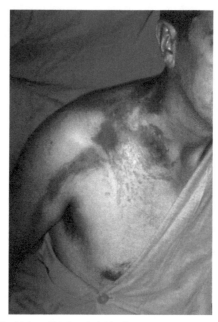

Fig. 65.10 Lightning strike skin burn. Note the whorled fernlike pattern characteristic of this type of burn injury.

false accusations. Unfortunately, there are times when seniors with dementia are being abused by care providers. Physical abuse in elderly persons may include unexplained injuries, like burns, bruises, new/unexplained scars, broken bones, sprains, or dislocations. Signs of excessive use of restraints, like rope marks on wrists, should be noted. Moreover, any nonconsensual sexual contact is sexual abuse, and warning signs of this may include bruises on the breasts or genitals, unexplained vaginal or anal bleeding, or dermatologic ailments (condyloma, syphilis, etc.) that lack an appropriate history or context.

45. **What are the skin signs of a lightning strike?**
Lightning strikes produce some characteristic skin findings. In addition to burn wounds at entry and exit points, the skin of patients struck by lightning can exhibit a swirled or fern-like pattern of erythema called "Lichtenberg figures" (Fig. 65.10). If there is doubt of the etiology, a skin biopsy often yields pathognomonic findings. It is important to diagnose this type of injury because unrecognized injury to the fascia and muscles may be present. The process must be recognized, and the degree of damage fully assessed, with the patient treated for arrhythmias, shock, fluid/electrolyte imbalances, and peripheral and CNS damage.

46. **What are the cutaneous findings in cholesterol emboli?**
Cholesterol emboli can present anywhere in the body, but cutaneous manifestations usually occur on the lower extremities. The condition can occur spontaneously, but often cholesterol emboli to the skin arise after angiography, when trauma to aortic plaques dislodges cholesterol and places it in circulation. Clinically, patients with cholesterol emboli present acutely with well-demarcated areas of cyanosis or livedo reticularis on the feet and lower legs, caused by emboli impairing the circulation. These areas can progress to necrotic changes and painful ulcers.

47. **How are cholesterol emboli diagnosed?**
On biopsy, cholesterol crystals in the lumens of vessels are diagnostic. An ideal skin biopsy would be an excision, and step sections may be necessary as atheromatous emboli are often focal and difficult to locate in histologic sections. It is helpful to auscultate carefully over major vessels of the abdomen and lower extremities, after the patient has exercised to increase the heart rate. Recognition of this disorder is important because in affected patients, often, other organ systems are involved, especially the kidneys. Further angiographic studies should be limited to those absolutely required, and treatment of any underlying hyperlipidemia should be initiated.

CHAPTER 66

OCCUPATIONAL DERMATOLOGY

Leslie A. Stewart and Matt Zirwas

1. What is the most common type of skin disease due to workplace exposures?

   Contact dermatitis accounts for more than 90% of occupational skin disease (OSD). The most common location of job-related contact dermatitis is the hands. It has been historically accepted that 80% of the contact dermatitis cases are irritant (Fig. 66.1), while 20% are allergic (Fig. 66.2). Recent studies challenged this teaching, with up to 40% of work-related skin diseases being allergic contact dermatitis (ACD). However, pure ACD in the occupational setting remains uncommon because an element of irritant contact dermatitis (ICD) is often present. Data from the Bureau of Labor and Statistics show that OSD accounted for 16.5% of all occupational illness in 2005. Some have estimated the true number of cases to be 10 to 50 times higher than that due to underreporting and underdiagnosis. The "standard" patch test screens for only approximately 75% of common allergens, so additional specialized testing with industrial chemicals to which the worker is exposed is often warranted. Testing should only be done with known materials in accepted concentrations.

Lushniak BD. Occupational contact dermatitis. *Dermatol Ther.* 2004;17:272–277.

Sasseville D. Occupational contact dermatitis. *Allergy Asthma Clin Immunol.* 2008;4:59–65.

2. List some other types of occupational skin diseases and give examples of their causes.
   - Folliculitis or acne (e.g., due to greases and oils)
   - Chemical-related depigmentation (e.g., due to germicidal phenolic detergents)
   - Lichen planus (e.g., from photographic developing agents)
   - Granulomas (e.g., due to silica or beryllium dust)
   - Infections (e.g., a dentist contracting herpetic whitlow from a patient with oral herpes)
   - Photodermatoses (e.g., due to celery psoralens in agricultural workers)
   - Contact urticaria (e.g., due to raw foods in food service workers)

3. Are there risk factors for the development of OSD?

   Personal history of atopic dermatitis is a significant risk factor for OSD. Other preexisting skin diseases with compromised epidermal barriers, such as xerosis or nummular eczema, can predispose a person to contact dermatitis because of enhanced absorption of irritants and allergens through the skin. Poor personal hygiene plays a role if patients neglect to wash off irritating and sensitizing chemicals, prolonging contact time. Yet, overwashing is perhaps a more common problem. The use of harsh soaps and frequent wetting/drying cycles induce chapping and compromises the barrier function of the skin. Use of gloves after washing the hands increases the irritation if residual cleanser exists upon the skin surface. Environmental factors are also important. In hot and humid climes, workers may perspire, which can solubilize particulate matter, enhancing its penetration into the skin. Sweat can also leach out allergens, such as chromates from leather shoes, inducing an ACD. Conversely, low temperature and humidity cause chapping of the skin, which can lead to ICD. Certain "wet work" jobs also are more likely to be associated with OSD, such as healthcare workers, hairdressers, and housekeepers.

Hamnerius N, Svedman C, Bergendorff O, Björk J, Bruze M, Pontén A. Wet work exposure and hand eczema among healthcare workers: a cross-sectional study. *Br J Dermatol.* 2018;178:452–461. https://doi.org/10.1111/bjd.15813

Belsito D. Occupational contact dermatitis: etiology, prevalence, and resultant impairment/disability. *J Am Acad Dermatol.* 2005;53:303–313.

Rietschel RL, Mathias CG, Fowler Jr JF, et al. A preliminary report of the occupation of patients evaluated in patch test clinics. *Am J Contact Dermatol.* 2001;12:72–76.

4. My patient has a hand dermatitis that appeared to begin at his job. Does this mean he has an occupationally related skin disease?

   Not necessarily. Just because a patient has a rash, and he or she works, does not mean it is job-related skin disease. To help make that determination, investigators have outlined seven criteria to be assessed. Four out of the seven criteria should be present for reasonable medical probability that the skin issue pertains to work:
   1. Is the eruption consistent with a contact dermatitis? It should look like an eczematous dermatitis and not like other disorders (i.e., vasculitis).
   2. Are there occupational exposures to possible irritants or allergens? There should be known documented irritating or sensitizing compounds to which the patient has been exposed at work.

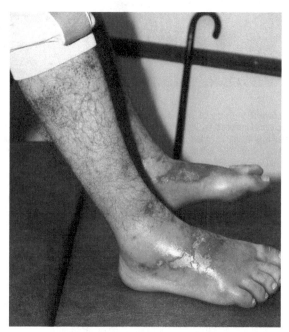

Fig. 66.1 Acute toxic insult–form of irritant contact dermatitis in a cement worker who developed cement burns from fresh cement getting into his boots.

3. Is the anatomic location of the eruption consistent with the exposure a worker would obtain on the job? For example, a worker may handle a chemical daily and break out with dermatitis only on his back. This is not consistent with an OSD because he should have developed an eruption where he contacted the compound the most, namely his hands.
4. Is the onset and time course of the eruption consistent with contact dermatitis? ACD is a delayed reaction (occurring 48 to 72 hours after exposure), while irritant reactions may be immediate or delayed. Contact dermatitis is not, for example, consistent with a worker's one-time exposure to a chemical when a rash occurs 3 months after that one incident.
5. Are nonoccupational exposures excluded as a possible cause of the dermatitis? Hobbies, second jobs, and household contactants should be pursued as possible sources of contact dermatitis.

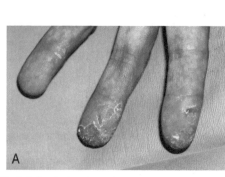
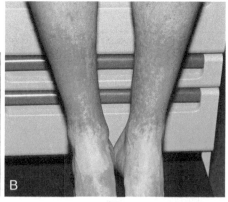

Fig. 66.2 Chronic allergic contact dermatitis. **A,** A case in an orthodontist who was allergic to nickel and to the glutaraldehyde used to sterilize his instruments. Note how the scaling dermatitis can mimic irritation. **B,** This patient developed sensitization to chromium, which was used to tan the leather in his work boots. The dorsal foot distribution is typical for a shoe contact dermatitis.

6. Does the eruption improve away from work? Work-related eruptions tend to improve when a worker is away from his job, although sometimes the same allergens and irritants may be found at home. Also, approximately 25% of workers with an OSD have a chronic and persistent dermatitis despite leaving their job and therapeutic intervention, and improvement does not occur when the worker is away from his place of employment.
7. Does patch testing reveal a likely causative agent? If a positive patch test reveals a likely allergen source with which the worker had contact, it is useful for pointing to the job exposure as the problem. However, patch tests must be interpreted within the context of the patient's history and physical examination. A positive test does not necessarily mean the allergen is responsible for the patient's current dermatitis, because it could be unrelated sensitization. The patch test reaction must always be assessed for its relevance to the present eruption.

Mathias CGT. Contact dermatitis and workers' compensation: criteria for establishing occupational causation and aggravation. *J Am Acad Dermatol.* 1989;20:842–848.

5. **How do I find out what a worker is exposed to on the job?**
By law, employers must provide their employees information regarding all possible workplace exposures. Information sheets, known as a Material Safety Data Sheet (MSDS), have information about a particular product, including any hazardous ingredients it contains in concentrations greater than 1%. MSDS sheets also list the manufacturer name and phone number, which may prove useful to contact the company to inquire about cutaneous allergens present in the final product in concentrations less than 1%. Dermatology and occupational medicine textbooks may also provide lists of allergens and irritants that are more likely with a particular occupation. On occasion, a more in-depth investigation may require a visit to the place of employment to observe the worker performing duties, note the general working conditions, gauge the protective measures employed, and investigate other contactants the patient might have overlooked.

KEY POINTS: OCCUPATIONAL DERMATOLOGY

1. Contact dermatitis is the most common form of OSD.
2. Irritants cause 75% of occupationally induced contact dermatitis, while allergens are responsible for 25%.
3. Hands are the most frequent site of OSD.
4. OSD can be chronic, but early diagnosis and treatment improve prognosis.
5. Treatment includes allergen and irritant avoidance, protective clothing, moisturizers, and topical steroids.

6. **What are some typical workplace irritants and allergens?**
   - **Irritants:** Water, soaps and detergents, solvents, particulate dusts, food products, fiberglass, plastics, resins, oils, greases, agricultural chemicals, and metals. Of note, irritating compounds can be allergenic, and allergenic compounds can be irritating.
   - **Allergens:** Preservatives and fragrances in hand soaps supplied at workplace (e.g. methylisothiazolinone, fragrance), metals (e.g., nickel), germicides (e.g., formaldehyde, glutaraldehyde), plants (e.g., poison ivy; see Fig. 66.3), rubber additives (e.g., thiurams), organic dyes (e.g., para-phenylenediamine in hair dye), plastic resins (e.g., acrylics and epoxies), and first-aid medications containing neomycin.
      Table 66.1 summarizes the possible contactants associated with common occupations.

7. **What is the prognosis of an occupational skin disease?**
In general, workers with occupational hand dermatitis fare poorly. Only about 25% have complete remission, 50% have periodic recurrences, and 25% have chronic persistent dermatitis, despite a change in jobs and therapeutic intervention. Reasons for persistent dermatitis include failure to diagnose and remove a sensitizer responsible for ACD, continued exposure to nonspecific irritants at home and work, continued inadvertent allergen exposure, and secondary sensitization (e.g., to preservatives contained in moisturizers and/or topical steroids provided as treatment). Early diagnosis can be important in preventing chronic OSD. Studies have shown that delay of diagnosis for more than 1 year and continual exposure are crucial factors in chronicity. In addition, sensitization to chromate in cement has a particularly poor long-term prognosis, even if the individual stops working with cement.

Belsito DV. Occupational contact dermatitis: etiology, prevalence, and resultant impairment/disability. *J Am Acad Dermatol.* 2005;53:303–313.
Warshaw E, Lee G, Storrs FJ. Hand dermatitis: a review of clinical features, therapeutic options, and long-term outcomes. *Am J Contact Dermatol.* 2003;14:119–137.
Hald M, Agner T, Blands J, Ravn H, Johansen JD. Allergens associated with severe symptoms of hand eczema and a poor prognosis. *Contact Dermatitis.* 2009;61(2):101–108.

8. **Will gloves prevent occupational skin disease?**
No. There is a widespread misconception that gloves provide a virtual guarantee of safety. Although gloves are recommended on a routine basis to protect against environmental insults, they are a considerable cause of contact dermatitis themselves. Irritant dermatitis occurs because patients sweat beneath their gloves, and gloves may occlude

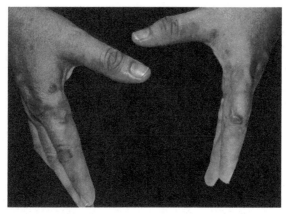

Fig. 66.3 Bullous allergic contact dermatitis in a florist due to cutting and handling carnations. (Courtesy Fitzsimons Army Medical Center teaching files.)

any residual allergen, or yield an irritant effect upon the skin. ACD occurs commonly with rubber gloves containing the chemicals thiuram, mercaptobenzothiazole, and carbamates, which are "rubber accelerator" chemicals used to speed up the vulcanization process. Some allergens can penetrate various glove materials and become trapped against the skin. For example, acrylics, formaldehyde, glutaraldehyde, and epoxy resins all penetrate latex gloves (Fig. 66.4).

9. How do you treat an occupationally related skin disease?
Remove the allergen and as many irritants as possible from the work and home environment. Allergens must be substituted with less sensitizing alternatives. For example, vinyl gloves can be used in place of rubber gloves. Patients must be instructed to avoid excessive water exposure and frequent hand washing, although in many occupations this is not practical. Constant wetting and drying can lead to chapping, which makes any hand dermatitis worse. Hands can be protected from the elements by using cotton glove liners to absorb perspiration, beneath a proper protective glove for the job. Moisturizers should be used immediately after wetting hands, or whenever they appear dry and scaling. Topical corticosteroids are the mainstay of therapy for occupational contact dermatitis, with systemic steroids reserved for acute and/or severe situations. Other medications used for severe or chronic OSD include cyclosporine, methotrexate, topical tacrolimus, and phototherapy. With treatment and hand protection, many workers can return to work despite a hand dermatitis. Job change should be considered in patients whose OSD is causing a severe decrease in quality of life, even despite all reasonable attempts to eliminate exposure to irritants and allergens. Most workers suffer financial and social consequences from changing occupations and do best with environmental modifications that allow a return to the same job.

10. How can occupationally related skin disease be prevented?
It is far easier to prevent ODS than it is to treat it. The basic aim of prevention is to identify risk and eliminate or at least to minimize it. Substitution of a nontoxic agent for a toxic agent is ideal. For example, highly allergenic biocides in cutting oils can be replaced by other preservatives. Modification of production processes may be an acceptable

Table 66.1 Selected occupations and their possible contactants

OCCUPATIONS	IRRITANTS	ALLERGENS
Construction workers	Cleansers, solvents, cement, dirt	Chromium (cement, leather boots), rubber chemicals (gloves), epoxy resin (adhesives)
Hairdressers	Shampoo, water, permanent wave solutions	Para-phenylenediamine (hair dyes), formaldehyde (shampoos), fragrances (shampoos and cosmetics), glyceryl monothioglycolate (permanent hair wave solutions)
Housekeepers	Cleansers, disinfectants, water	Rubber chemicals (gloves), fragrances, and preservatives (cleaning and disinfectant solutions)
Healthcare workers	Soap, water, gloves, disinfectants	Rubber chemicals (gloves), glutaraldehyde (cold sterilizer for instruments), preservatives (skin care products)
Machinists	Metal chips, cutting oils, solvents, soaps, greases	Metals, rubber, fragrances, and preservatives in cutting oils

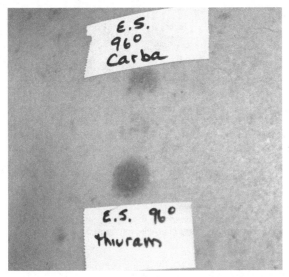

Fig. 66.4 Positive patch test reactions to the rubber accelerators thiuram and carbamates found in rubber gloves in a healthcare worker.

alternative when substitution of an allergen cannot occur. Screens or filters can be used to prevent chemical splashes, or hand tools can be used to retrieve items from irritating compounds. Prompt hand washing, using appropriate materials and technique, should be encouraged, and frequent application of moisturizers and barrier creams should be encouraged. Personal protective equipment, including aprons, boots, visors, sleeves, and gloves, must be adapted to specific situations and exposures. All personnel must be educated regarding hazardous exposures and must have ongoing preventive training, especially if a task or process is modified. Workers and health/safety specialists should be on the lookout for early signs of dermatitis including erythema, scaling, fissuring, maceration, and skin thickening in order to identify and promptly treat OSD early and to prevent chronicity.

Nicholson P, Llewellyn D, English JS. Evidence-based guidelines for the prevention, identification and management of occupational contact dermatitis and urticarial. *Contact Dermatitis.* 2010;63:177–186.

11. **How do disability and workers compensation work?**
    Disability refers to a loss of ability to perform important functions, regardless of if the loss was caused by work or is unrelated to work. It can be permanent (for example, a burn on the hands that leads to scarring that prevents bending the fingers) or temporary (severe psoriasis that is expected to improve with therapy), and complete (for example, severe congenital ichthyosis that prevents almost all daily activities) or partial (for example, sensitivity to sunlight that requires avoidance of going outdoors during daylight). In summary, any disability can be:
    1. Permanent complete disability
    2. Temporary complete disability
    3. Permanent partial disability
    4. Temporary partial disability
       All U.S. citizens have disability insurance through the Social Security system. Individuals who apply to Social Security for disability pay will have their medical records reviewed by a Social Security administrator to determine the qualification and type. Employers or individuals can also purchase private disability insurance that provides for additional income, beyond that provided by Social Security, should they become disabled.
       Workers compensation is insurance that employers purchase to cover medical costs and replace lost wages due to an injury that occurs at work, regardless of cause. Workers compensation systems differ from state to state. In some states, all employers purchase workers compensation insurance through a state agency, while in other states, employers purchase insurance through private insurers. Similar to disability, when a worker is injured, a claim is filed and the insurance company or state agency reviews medical/employment documentation to determine that an injury was caused by a workplace accident or exposure.

CHAPTER 67

PSYCHOCUTANEOUS DISEASES

Quinn Thibodeaux and John Y.M. Koo

KEY POINTS

1. Up to 40% of all dermatologic patients have an associated psychiatric comorbidity.
2. Patients with cutaneous dysesthesia can present with many different complaints, but treatment is based on whether the symptoms are primarily pruritic or primarily painful.
3. When evaluating skin lesions that are self-inflicted, understanding the patient's underlying motivation is essential for accurate diagnosis and treatment.
4. Patients with Morgellons present with a wide spectrum of ego-involvement, and maintaining a good doctor–patient relationship is paramount to successful treatment.
5. Dermatologists should not shy away from prescribing psychotropic medications and should make themselves familiar with the medications commonly used in psychodermatology.

1. What are the different categories of psychocutaneous disorders?
   - **Primary psychiatric disorders with dermatologic manifestations:** In these conditions, the primary pathology is psychological in nature. Patients have no inherent issues with their skin, hair, or nails—all physical findings are self-induced. Examples include delusions of parasitosis, dermatitis artefacta, trichotillomania, dysmorphophobia, and neurotic excoriations.
   - **Primary dermatologic disorders with psychiatric comorbidities:** Patients with conditions such as acne, psoriasis, or vitiligo endure significant social stigma and decreased quality of life that can lead to the development of secondary psychiatric disorders such as depression, anxiety, or social phobia.
   - **Psychophysiologic disorders:** Psychophysiologic disorders are those dermatologic conditions such as psoriasis, atopic dermatitis, acne, and hyperhidrosis that are frequently worsened by psychological stress.
   - **Cutaneous dysesthesia:** Patients with cutaneous dysesthesia experience uncomfortable skin sensations with no primary skin pathology. They often describe their symptoms as burning, crawling, biting, stabbing, shocking, or itching. For this diagnosis, a workup for other possible organic causes must be negative, and patients must have no primary dermatologic findings.

2. How frequently do patients with dermatologic disorders have associated psychological comorbidity?
   While the exact prevalence is difficult to assess, it is estimated that up to 40% of dermatologic patients have some sort of psychiatric comorbidity. The ever-visible reminder of their disease and the social stigma associated with some conditions can have deleterious effects on patients' psyche. Even when skin lesions can be hidden with clothing, it is well known that patients can still experience significant decrement in self-esteem and self-image.

Connor CJ. Management of the psychological comorbidities of dermatological conditions: practitioners' guidelines. *Clin Cosmet Investig Dermatol.* 2017;10:117–132.

3. Define obsession, compulsion, phobia, delusion, and hallucination.
   - **Obsession:** a persistent preoccupation with an idea or impulse
   - **Compulsion:** a persistent, repetitive behavior performed in response to an obsession
   - **Phobia:** an overwhelming, irrational fear that motivates individuals to avoid particular situations
   - **Delusion:** a fixed, false, idiosyncratic belief that is impervious to rational thought
   - **Hallucination:** a sensorial experience or perception without an actual stimulus

4. What is cutaneous dysesthesia?
   Cutaneous dysesthesia is an unpleasant sensation experienced by a patient that has no identifiable biologic cause. Cutaneous dysesthesia can be broadly separated into primarily pruritic and primarily painful sensations, but patients may also complain of burning, stabbing, or shocking sensations.

5. What are some common manifestations of cutaneous dysesthesia?
   Glossodynia, burning mouth syndrome, vulvodynia, burning feet syndrome, atypical facial pain, and chronic scalp pruritus.

6. How should cutaneous dysesthesia be treated?

For patients complaining of primarily pruritic sensations, the tricyclic antidepressant (TCA) doxepin is often helpful after treatments such as topical steroids and antihistamines have failed. In order to maximize doxepin's effect, it is important to titrate the dose based on individual tolerance. Patients taking TCAs at the same dose could have up to a 20-fold variation in trough levels due to differences in metabolism. Doxepin may be used at doses of up to 300 mg per day.

If the primary symptom involves cutaneous idiopathic pain, low-dose desipramine or nortriptyline may be efficacious. The use of TCAs as analgesics has been most well documented with amitriptyline; however, amitriptyline is commonly associated with intolerable anticholinergic side effects.

Beck K, Yang E, Koo J. Dose escalation of doxepin for intractable pruritus. *J Am Acad Dermatol.* 2018;79(3):e37.

7. Name the three major categories of self-inflicted skin lesions and how they are differentiated.
   - **Obsessive-compulsive disorders (OCDs)**: Patients acknowledge being driven to self-inflict skin lesions through conscious repetitive actions.
   - **Dermatitis artefacta or factitious dermatitis**: Patients self-inflict skin lesions to satisfy a psychological need with no attempt for secondary gain.
   - **Malingering**: Patients consciously and deceitfully self-inflict skin lesions for secondary gain.

8. What are the clinical manifestations of dermatitis artefacta?

Dermatitis artefacta can mimic a variety of skin conditions, and the self-inflicted lesions vary widely in morphology and distribution. Patients often use foreign objects such as sharp instruments, caustic chemicals, or elastic bands to produce wounds. Depending on the method used, it is possible to see excoriations, blisters, burns, edema, ulcerations, purpura, and deep scars (Figs. 67.1 and 67.2). Lesions are often bizarre and irregularly rectilinear (Fig. 67.3). They are necessarily within reach.

9. How should patients with dermatitis artefacta be treated?

For the majority of patients, self-inflicting skin lesions satisfies an unconscious psychological need. The disorder often develops in response to an acute psychological stress and frequently becomes chronic. Patients should be evaluated by a qualified psychiatrist or psychologist, and antidepressants, anxiolytics, and antipsychotics are typically used to treat any underlying psychopathology. Intensive wound care may also be warranted, depending on the extent of the skin lesions.

Gattu S, Rashid RM, Khachemoune A. Self-induced skin lesions: a review of dermatitis artefacta. *Cutis.* 2009;84(5):247–251.

10. What is Munchausen syndrome?

Munchausen syndrome is a factitious disorder in which patients fabricate, self-inflict, or purposefully exacerbate a condition in order to draw attention or sympathy to themselves. Patients may undergo unnecessary and sometimes invasive tests and procedures in attempt to diagnose their often unusual complaints. If confronted, patients will

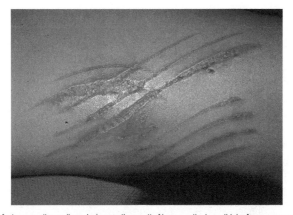

Fig. 67.1 Dermatitis artefacta presenting as linear lesions as the result of burns on the inner thigh of a young woman. (Courtesy Fitzsimons Army Medical Center teaching files.)

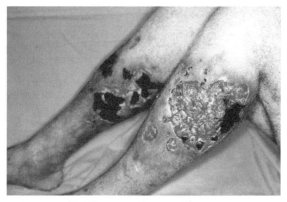

Fig. 67.2 Young man with factitial panniculitis. The patient was injecting unknown substances into his legs in an attempt to get doctors to provide him with narcotic agents. (Courtesy James E. Fitzpatrick, MD.)

frequently leave against medical advice and repeat their behavior at other institutions. In contrast, Munchausen syndrome by proxy is when a third party facilitates a condition in another individual (typically a child) in order to satisfy a psychological need.

Boyd AS, Ritchie C, Likhari S. Munchausen syndrome and Munchausen syndrome by proxy in dermatology. *J Am Acad Dermatol.* 2014;71 (2):376–381.

11. Which dermatologic conditions can result from obsessive compulsive disorder?
    Compulsive hand washing, skin picking, dysmorphophobia, and trichotillomania are all manifestations of OCD that can have dermatologic signs and symptoms.

12. How do we treat the dermatologic manifestations of OCD-spectrum disorders?
    A behavioral approach to OCD patients is the "1 minute rule." With this technique, the patient must recognize their urge and do their best to wait 1 minute before carrying out the destructive behavior. If they succeed in waiting 1 minute, they should try to extend the time resisting their urge in small increments. It is not uncommon for the patient's behavior to eventually become extinct as the exercise progresses.
    There are many effective anti-OCD medications including selective serotonin reuptake inhibitor (SSRIs). Fortunately, OCD patients are typically insightful about their condition and convincing them to see a psychiatrist for treatment of the underlying psychopathology is often easily accomplished.

Mavrogiorgou P, Bader A, Stockfleth E, Juckel G. Obsessive-compulsive disorder in dermatology. *J Dtsch Dermatol Ges.* 2015;13:991–999.

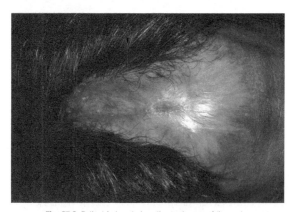

Fig. 67.3 Patient-induced ulceration and scars of the scalp.

13. What is trichotillomania?

Trichotillomania is an OCD characterized by habitual hair pulling. In this condition, patients feel rising tension just prior to or while resisting pulling hairs. They then feel a sense of pleasure or relief after completing the behavior. Scalp hairs are the most common targets, but eyebrows, eyelashes, pubic hair, and body hair can also be involved. On physical exam, hairs of varying lengths are often seen within the affected area (Fig. 67.4).

Duke DC, Keeley ML, Geffken GR, Storch EA. Trichotillomania: a current review. *Clin Psychol Rev.* 2010;30:181–193.

14. What is the differential diagnosis for trichotillomania and how are they distinguished?

The most important conditions to rule out in trichotillomania are alopecia areata, tinea capitis, and traction alopecia. In alopecia areata, exclamation point hairs are often seen on the periphery of lesions and other findings such as nail pitting may be present. Tinea capitis will typically have overlying scale with patchy alopecia and positive findings on potassium hydroxide prep or culture. Traction alopecia will correspond with the hairstyle causing the lesions.

15. What is dysmorphophobia?

Dysmorphophobia, also known as body dysmorphic disorder, is a condition in which patients have a disturbed perception of their appearance or a delusional belief about the structure or function of their skin. Frequent body sites of concern are the face, hair, breasts, and genitalia, and complaints may include excessive redness, increased sebum production, or overly large pores. The condition encompasses a spectrum of pathology, with patient's views ranging from simple preoccupations to fixed delusions. It is important to recognize these patients and to refuse any unreasonable procedures they may request. Treatment is directed at the underlying OCD or delusional disorder.

16. What are neurotic excoriations?

Patients with neurotic excoriations experience an uncontrollable desire to pick, scratch, or rub the skin. The picking behavior often begins inadvertently after the patient notices an irregularity in the shape or texture of their skin. Once initiated, the picking often proceeds in a ritualized fashion. On exam, lesions of various shapes and sizes are often noted in varying stages of healing, including ulcerations, hypertrophic nodules, and atrophic scars (Fig 67.5). Lesions are most commonly distributed on the face, scalp, upper back, buttocks, and extensor surfaces of the arms.

17. How should one approach a patient with neurotic excoriations?

The first step in treating patients with neurotic excoriations is to elucidate the underlying psychopathology that is leading to the excoriations. Frequently, the underlying pathology involves anxiety, depression, or OCD, but in some rare cases, the patient may in fact be delusional. For example, patients who excoriate and pull out their own hairs may be suffering from trichophobia, where the motivation behind the patient's actions is due to a delusion of body hairs

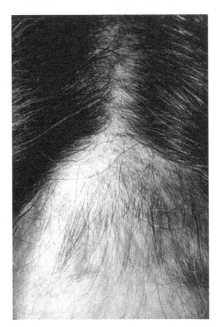

Fig. 67.4 A young girl with trichotillomania. Note hairs of varying length. (Courtesy John L. Aeling, MD.)

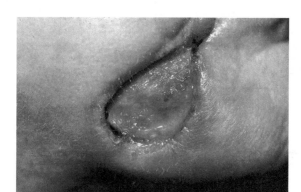

Fig. 67.5 Factitial ulcer (Courtesy John L. Aeling, MD.)

causing incomplete healing. The treatment for neurotic excoriations should be based on the nature of the underlying psychopathology.

18. What is Morgellons disease?

Morgellons disease is a widely used term but is not officially defined by any medical establishment. It includes cases of delusional parasitosis and other monosymptomatic hypochondriacal psychoses such as inanimate objects reportedly coming out of patients' skin or traveling under the skin (commonly blue fibers, black dots, etc.). Patients will often bring in specimens containing hair, lint, or organic materials for examination (Fig. 67.6). Morgellons and other similar conditions can only be diagnosed if they are a "stand-alone" entity. If a broader psychopathology such as schizophrenia or organic psychosis is responsible for the patient's skin complaints, then the diagnosis of Morgellons is not appropriate. In these cases, the treatment should be directed toward the underlying psychiatric disorder and generally requires referral to a psychiatrist.

Krooks JA, Weatherall AG, Holland PJ. Review of epidemiology, clinical presentation, diagnosis, and treatment of common primary psychiatric causes of cutaneous disease. *J Dermatolog Treat.* 2018;29(4):418–427.

19. What are synonyms for Morgellons disease?

Delusions of parasitosis, Ekbom syndrome, and monosymptomatic hypochondriacal psychosis

20. Are all patients with Morgellons delusional?

Not all patients who present with complaints of parasites or fibers are delusional. The definition of "delusional" requires that the patient be absolutely fixed in their erroneous system of beliefs. A truly delusional patient typically becomes upset when their ideations are challenged or when alternative explanations are offered. Patients with Morgellons exhibit a wide

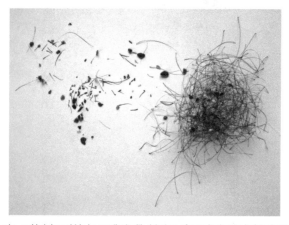

Fig. 67.6 Scale, scabs, and hair brought in by a patient with delusions of parasitosis who insists that these are parasites.

spectrum of disease. Some patients complain of crawling and biting sensations (formication) of unknown origin, while others are adamant that their symptoms are caused by some sort of infestation or contamination.

21. **What are the typical characteristics of Morgellons patients?**
    The majority of Morgellons patients are women over the age of 50. Male Morgellons patients are relatively rare. When a Morgellons syndrome-like clinical picture is seen in younger patients, they tend to have higher rates of drug use and borderline socioeconomic status. In contrast, the overwhelming majority of typical Morgellons patients are well-established women whose only disorganized behavior is related to their cutaneous delusion.

22. **What kind of workup is needed for Morgellons?**
    Formication-like symptoms can be caused by numerous etiologies; therefore, adequate physical examination and laboratory evaluation should be completed in all patients to rule out reversible causes. The differential diagnosis for Morgellons's includes actual infestation, inflammatory skin disorders, intoxication, drug abuse, diabetes, renal or hepatic failure, B_{12} or folate deficiency, lymphoma, and severe anemia. The following laboratory workup is recommended:
    - Comprehensive metabolic panel
    - Complete blood count with differential
    - Urinalysis with toxicology screen
    - Thyroid stimulating hormone
    - Vitamin B_{12} and D 25-OH levels
    - Human immunodeficiency virus, hepatitis C, and syphilis screening

23. **How can you connect with these patients?**
    It is highly likely that patients with Morgellons will already be in a defensive mindset prior to your introduction. Many of these patients have had negative experiences with other providers, and they may project that frustration. You should approach these patients with enthusiasm and empathy. Patients are often highly interested in investigating the etiology of their symptoms (insects, fibers, etc.), but pursuing this line of interaction beyond reasonable due diligence is unlikely to be of any benefit. The foremost goal for these patients is to escape the misery they experience, and it is helpful to validate the patient's symptoms while minimizing discussions about the etiology. You may explain to the patient that many conditions in medicine have no known cause and that the underlying cause is inconsequential if their suffering is able to be relieved with a safe and effective medication. Use neutral terms such as "formication" or "Morgellons disease" to avoid the negative connotation associated with "delusions of parasitosis." Offering treatment on a pragmatic trial-and-error basis is often gladly accepted by patients who simply want their symptoms to abate. If you are able to establish strong rapport with the patient, they will often agree to this therapeutic trial even if they are initially ambivalent or even skeptical. Once a patient's symptoms begin to resolve, their attitude toward treatment often shifts considerably.

24. **What medications are used to treat Morgellons?**
    Historically, the most efficacious and widely used medication for Morgellons disease has been pimozide (Orap), an atypical antipsychotic indicated by the Food and Drug Administration only for the treatment of Tourette syndrome. Because pimozide has no psychiatric indication in the United States, it may be the most acceptable medication in the view of Morgellons patients, who often have an aversion to medications with psychiatric indications. Due to more favorable side effect profiles, other atypical antipsychotics such as risperidone, aripiprazole, and olanzapine are beginning to be recommended as first-line therapies.

Campbell EH, Elston DM, Hawthorne JD, Beckert DR. Diagnosis and management of delusional parasitosis. *J Am Acad Dermatol.* 2019;80:1428–1434.

25. **What is the dosage of pimozide used in delusions of parasitosis?**
    Pimozide is started cautiously at a dose of 0.5 mg per day and is increased by 0.5 mg every 2–4 weeks as tolerated. It is important to communicate that clinical benefits are not typically seen until a dose of 3 mg per day is reached. Many patients note significant improvement at a dose lower than 3 mg per day; however, it is better to underpromise and overdeliver. Once an efficacious dose has been found and symptoms have resolved, it is important to maintain that dose for at least another 3 months. Premature discontinuation can invite recurrence of symptoms, which may be distressing to the patient. Once the patient has been on a stable dose for 3 months with no symptoms, a slow taper is begun. When this "trapezoid" strategy is utilized, patients frequently experience a "cure" of their delusion. A similar dosing strategy is recommended for risperidone, with a typical efficacious dose of 3 mg per day (Fig. 67.7).

26. **What are the common side effects of medications used to treat psychocutaneous disorders?**
    - SSRIs: headache, nausea, diarrhea, dry mouth, dizziness, nervousness/restlessness, insomnia, decreased libido, and erectile dysfunction
    - Atypical antipsychotics: anticholinergic effects (dry mouth, dry eyes, blurred vision, difficulty urinating, constipation), sedation, QT prolongation, weight gain, insulin resistance, orthostatic hypotension, extrapyramidal effects (tardive dyskinesia, akathisia, acute dystonic reactions, rigidity, stiffened gait, pill-rolling tremor, bradykinesia)

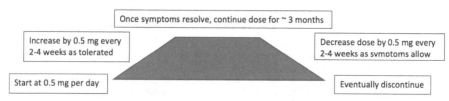

Fig. 67.7 Dosing strategy for pimozide in Morgellons disease.

For patients who experience mild rigidity or restlessness while on an atypical antipsychotic such as pimozide, as-needed diphenhydramine, or benztropine may be used for symptomatic relief. In fact, once the side effects are under control, the dosage of the antipsychotic may continue to be titrated upward until a therapeutic dose is reached. Rarely, patients may experience mild sedation or activation, which are easily accommodated by taking pimozide either at bedtime or in the morning.

Kuhn H, Mennella C, Magid M, Stamu-O'Brien C, Kroumpouzos G. Psychocutaneous disease: pharmacotherapy and psychotherapy. *J Am Acad Dermatol.* 2017;76(5):795–808.

BIBLIOGRAPHY

Beck KM, Yang EJ, Koo J. Dose escalation of doxepin for intractable pruritus. *J Am Acad Dermatol.* 2018;79(3).

Boyd AS, Ritchie C, Likhari S. Munchausen syndrome and Munchausen syndrome by proxy in dermatology. *J Am Acad Dermatol.* 2014; 71(2):376–381.

Campbell EH, Elston DM, Hawthorne JD, Beckert DR. Diagnosis and management of delusional parasitosis. *J Am Acad Derm.* 2019; 80(5):1428–1434. https://doi.org/10.1016/j.jaad.2018.12.012.

Connor CJ. Management of the psychological comorbidities of dermatological conditions: practitioners' guidelines. *Clin Cosmet Investig Dermatol.* 2017;10:117–132.

Duke DC, Keeley ML, Geffken GR, Storch EA. Trichotillomania: a current review. *Clin Psychol Rev.* 2010;30:181–193.

Gattu S, Rashid RM, Khachemoune A. Self-induced skin lesions: a review of dermatitis artefacta. *Cutis.* 2009;84(5):247–251.

Krooks JA, Weatherall AG, Holland PJ. Review of epidemiology, clinical presentation, diagnosis, and treatment of common primary psychiatric causes of cutaneous disease. *J Dermatol Treat.* 29(4):418–427.

Kuhn H, Mennella C, Magid M, Stamu-O'Brien C, Kroumpouzos G. Psychocutaneous disease. Pharmacotherapy and psychotherapy. *J Am Acad Dermatol.* 2017;76(5):795–808.

Mavrogiorgou P, Bader A, Stockfleth E, Juckel G. Obsessive-compulsive disorder in dermatology. *J Dtsch Dermatol Ges.* 2015;13:991–999.

CHAPTER 68

APPROACHING THE PRURITIC PATIENT

Emilie Fowler and Gil Yosipovitch

KEY POINTS: PRURITUS

1. Chronic pruritus can be debilitating, causing great distress to patients.
2. A patient with no obvious reason for having chronic itch and no primary skin rash needs a full workup with a thorough history, physical examination, and laboratory and/or imaging studies to rule out underlying disease.
3. The pathophysiology of chronic itch involves a phenomenon of neural sensitization, which takes place at the level of the skin, spinal cord, and brain.

1. **What is an itch?**

   Itch, or pruritus, is a sensation resulting in a desire to scratch.

2. **How is chronic itch defined?**

   Chronic itch is defined as pruritus lasting for more than 6 weeks. It can be generalized or localized to a certain area of the body and can cause great distress to patients. Suffering from chronic pruritus can lead to sleep disturbances, mood changes, symptoms of anxiety and depression, and can interfere with daily activities or work.

   Yosipovitch G, Bernhard JD. Chronic pruritus. *N Engl J Med*. 2013;368(17):1625–1634.

3. **What are the different types of chronic itch?**

   Itch can be classified into four different categories: dermatologic, systemic, neuropathic, or psychogenic (Fig. 68.1). Dermatologic causes of pruritus show primary skin lesions and include conditions such as atopic dermatitis, psoriasis, scabies, contact dermatitis, and urticaria. Systemic, neuropathic, and psychogenic causes of chronic itch do not have primary skin lesions, but lesions from scratching may be present. Systemic causes of pruritus include chronic kidney disease, cholestatic disease, human immunodeficiency virus (HIV), and Hodgkin's disease, to name a few. Neuropathic causes of pruritus include conditions such as brachioradial pruritus (BRP), notalgia paresthetica, and postherpetic pruritus. Finally, psychogenic causes include delusional infestation and substance abuse.

   Yosipovitch G, Bernhard JD. Chronic pruritus. *N Engl J Med*. 2013;368(17):1625–1634.
   Ständer S, Weisshaar E, Mettang T, et al. Clinical classification of itch: a position paper of the international forum for the study of itch. *Acta Derm Venereol*. 2007;87(4):291–294.

4. **What is neural sensitization?**

   Neural sensitization is important when discussing the pathophysiology of chronic itch. Neural sensitization refers to an increase in the sensitivity of itch-selective neurons, which decreases the threshold for itch sensation. In the skin, inflammation and abnormal innervation can lead to neural hypersensitivity. In the peripheral nervous system and skin, overactivation of nerve growth factor, substance P, and neurokinin-1 receptor also contributes to neural sensitization. Dysfunctioning inhibitory circuits and imbalance in kappa- and mu-opioid receptors, as well as overactivity of neurokinin-1 receptor, lead to neural sensitization in the spinal cord. Increased activation of certain areas of the brain, such as the anterior cingulate cortex, posterior cingulate cortex, and prefrontal area, may lead to neural sensitization in the brain. Overall, this phenomenon is part of the mechanism perpetuating chronic itch and contributes to symptoms such as alloknesis and hyperknesis.

   Yosipovitch G, Rosen JD, Hashimoto T. Itch: from mechanism to (novel) therapeutic approaches. *J Allergy Clin Immunol*. 2018;142 (5):1391.

5. **What are alloknesis and hyperknesis?**

   Alloknesis is when a nonpruritic stimulus causes itch, while hyperknesis is when a pruritic stimulus causes an enhanced, or greater than normal, sensation of pruritus.

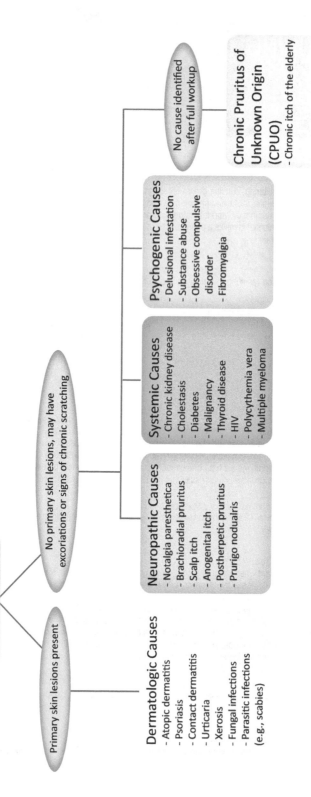

Fig. 68.1 Classification of chronic itch.

6. What are important questions to ask a patient presenting with itch without a rash?

When a patient presents with complaints of itching without a rash, a thorough history and physical examination are warranted. From there, you can decide what laboratory or imaging tests are necessary, if any. Important questions to ask include:

- When did the itch start?
- Where is the itch located? Is it localized to a certain area or is it generalized?
- In the last 24 hours, how would the patient rate the itch on a scale of 0 to 10 on average and at its worst severity?
- How many hours during the day is the patient itchy?
- Is the patient itchy in the morning, afternoon, and/or nighttime?
- Does anything alleviate the itch? What tends to aggravate the itch?
- What other medical problems does the patient have? (e.g., neuropathy, chronic kidney disease, chronic cholestatic/liver disease, diabetes, cancer, psychiatric illnesses)
- What medications is the patient taking?
- Does anyone else feel itchy around them or in their home?
- Does the patient have a history of trauma or surgeries of the back, neck, or sacral area, or any spinal cord injury or stenosis?

7. What is the recommended workup for chronic itch?

When a patient presents with itch present for more than 6 weeks, you must first take a full clinical history and physical examination. This includes a detailed medication history and review of systems, with attention to symptoms that may point to an underlying systemic illness.

On physical exam, look for primary skin lesions that may point to a dermatologic cause of pruritus, such as eczematous lesions of atopic dermatitis or silvery, scaly plaques of psoriasis. Be sure to distinguish secondary skin lesions from primary lesions, for excoriations, prurigo nodules, and nonspecific dermatitis may be simply from scratching. Undress the patient to examine the genital area to rule out scabies.

If no primary skin lesions are found, consider a nondermatologic cause for pruritus. Make sure to palpate lymph nodes in the axillary and inguinal regions. Depending on what is found on history and physical examination, you may want to order laboratory and imaging tests. Laboratory tests may include a complete blood count (CBC) with differential, liver function tests (LFTs), thyroid function tests, creatinine level, erythrocyte sedimentation rate, and HIV test. Imaging tests may include chest x-ray (CXR) or imaging of the spine if you suspect a neuropathic cause, such as notalgia paresthetica or BRP.

Yosipovitch G, Bernhard JD. Chronic pruritus. *N Engl J Med.* 2013;368(17):1625–1634.

8. Are there any other sensory symptoms associated with chronic itch?

In the setting of chronic itch, pruritus may be associated with other nociceptive symptoms, such as burning, stinging, and pain. In a recent study, patients with inflammatory itch (e.g., atopic dermatitis, psoriasis) had a significantly greater mean for the extent to which stinging, burning, sunburn-like sensation, pain, and hurting were associated with their itch compared to patients with neuropathic itch. This study suggests that not only can itch occur simultaneously with nociceptive symptoms, but that nociceptive symptoms are more often associated with inflammatory itch conditions.

Rosen JD, Fostini AC, Chan YH, Nattkemper LA, Yosipovitch G. Cross-sectional study of clinical distinctions between neuropathic and inflammatory pruritus. *J Am Acad Dermatol.* 2018;79(6):1143–1144.

9. What are the most common skin diseases causing itch?

Common causes include atopic dermatitis, psoriasis, urticaria, contact dermatitis, and xerosis (dry skin). Insect bites as well as fungal and parasitic (e.g., scabies) infections can also be common causes of pruritus.

10. What are the most common systemic diseases causing itch?

The most common systemic diseases causing itch are end-stage renal disease, cholestasis, and myeloproliferative diseases.

Common systemic diseases causing itch are listed in Table 68.1.

11. What are the most common systemic diseases causing palmar itch?

A presentation of pruritus on the palms is classic for cholestasis. Cholestasis may be present due to a number of underlying conditions, such as primary biliary cirrhosis and primary sclerosing cholangitis. Therefore, in a patient presenting with a pruritus of the palms, make sure to order LFTs, alkaline phosphatase, bilirubin levels, and antimitochondrial antibodies.

Düll MM, Kremer AE. Management of Chronic Hepatic Itch. *Dermatol Clin.* 2018;36(3):293–300.

Table 68.1 Systemic causes of pruritus and corresponding workup

SYSTEMIC CAUSE OF PRURITUS	LABORATORY AND/OR IMAGING TESTS
End stage renal disease	• Creatinine level
Cholestasis • Primary biliary cirrhosis • Sclerosing cholangitis • Pruritus gravidarum • Viral hepatitis	• Liver function tests • Alkaline phosphatase • Bilirubin level • Antimitochondrial antibodies
Thyroid disease • Hyperthyroidism	• Thyroid function tests
Malignancy • Hodgkin's lymphoma • Non-Hodgkin's lymphoma • Cutaneous T-cell lymphoma • Leukemias	• Complete blood cell count and differential • Chest x-ray
Diabetes	• Hemoglobin A1c
Polycythemia vera	• Complete blood cell count and differential • Erythrocyte sedimentation rate
Multiple myeloma	• Complete blood cell count and differential • Erythrocyte sedimentation rate • Protein electrophoresis
HIV	• HIV serologic analysis

12. What psychiatric disorders cause itch?

Common psychiatric disorders that may be the cause of pruritus include depression, generalized anxiety disorder, fibromyalgia, and obsessive-compulsive disorder. Treatment of these conditions can provide relief and improve the pruritus. Additionally, simply having increased stress in one's life can trigger development of chronic itch. Stress reduction techniques such as meditation or progressive muscle relaxation can aid in alleviating itch in these cases.

Delusional infestation, a less common psychiatric disorder, can cause severe pruritus and can be quite challenging to treat. These patients have a fixed, false belief that they are infested with some sort of "bug." Patients have associated tactile hallucinations, such as itching, and as a consequence may present with several excoriations, ulcerations, secondary infections, and lichenification. These patients have limited insight and often will not accept that they have a psychiatric disorder, so a strong therapeutic relationship is necessary in order to provide careful counseling and treatment with an antipsychotic medication.

Finally, abuse of opioids, cocaine, or amphetamines can also lead to chronic pruritus.

Vulink NC. Delusional infestation: State of the art. *Acta Derm Venereol.* 2016;96(4):58–63.

13. What is brachioradial pruritus?

A patient with BRP typically presents with pruritus localized to the dorsolateral aspects of the arms. The pruritus may be bilateral or unilateral and may spread to the shoulders, forearms, or upper trunk. Over time, pruritus may become generalized, spreading to involve other areas of the body.

The pathophysiology of BRP involves damage or impingement of the cervical nerves C4–C8. This may be a result of cervical spinal stenosis or previous trauma, so be sure to inquire about these and consider ordering imaging. Additionally, patients typically endorse relief of pruritus upon application of ice to the area. This has been dubbed the "ice-pack sign."

Kwatra SG, Stander S, Bernhard JD, Weisshaar E, Yosipovitch G. Brachioradial pruritus: a trigger for generalization of itch. *J Am Acad Dermatol.* 2013;68(5):870–873.
Rosen JD, Fostini AC, Yosipovitch G. Diagnosis and management of neuropathic itch. *Dermatol Clin.* 2018;36(3):213–224.

14. What is the most common pathophysiology of itch in cutaneous T-cell lymphoma (CTCL)?

CTCL patients are often plagued with pruritus. Interleukin-31 (IL-31) has been implicated as the main culprit of itch in CTCL. Its presence in the skin has been shown to directly correlate with itch severity.

Nattkemper LA, Martinez-Escala ME, Gelman AB, et al. Cutaneous T-cell lymphoma and pruritus: the expression of IL-31 and its receptors in the skin. *Acta Derm Venereol.* 2016;96(7):894–898.

15. What is aquagenic pruritus?

Aquagenic pruritus occurs when a patient develops itch shortly after their skin makes direct contact with water. The water can vary in temperature and the patients have no visible rash or urticaria. Presentation of aquagenic pruritus may be associated with lymphoproliferative diseases, such as polycythemia vera and myelodysplasia, as well as malignant diseases such as lymphomas. To rule out any serious underlying conditions, perform a thorough history and physical exam and check for palpable lymph nodes. Additionally, order a complete blood cell count (CBC) with differential and a CXR. If negative, monitoring with yearly CBCs and CXRs is recommended.

Yosipovitch G. Chronic pruritus: a paraneoplastic sign. *Dermatol Ther.* 2010;23(6):590–596.

16. What are some common areas of itch seen in neuropathy?

Nerve damage can cause pruritus. When nerves are damaged by a direct force, as seen in compression or trauma, a dermatomal distribution of pruritus may be seen. This, however, is not the case with lesions in the central nervous system or when there is extensive damage of peripheral nerves.

Common causes of neuropathic itch have distinctive locations. BRP, as mentioned above, is typically distributed along the dorsolateral arms. In notalgia paresthetica, pruritus is localized to a discrete location on the back, usually in the midthoracic dermatomes. Postherpetic pruritus occurs unilaterally and in a dermatomal distribution.

Scalp itch may also result from neuropathy, for example, in cases of cervical neck trauma or chronic diabetes.

Rosen JD, Fostini AC, Yosipovitch G. Diagnosis and management of neuropathic itch. *Dermatol Clin.* 2018;36(3):213–224.

17. What are common causes of scalp itch?

Often, there is no obvious etiology of scalp itch. If the scalp is itchy and appears erythematous with flaking, consider a diagnosis of seborrheic dermatitis. Seborrheic dermatitis is one of the most common causes of scalp itch. Additionally, psoriasis, distinguished by raised, red, scaly plaques, is a common cause of scalp itch.

If there is no apparent rash present on the scalp, consider old age, a manifestation of chronic diabetes, or neuropathic or psychogenic etiologies. Inquire about cervical neck trauma, which could lead to symptoms of scalp pruritus.

Vázquez-Herrera NE, Sharma D, Aleid NM, Tosti A. Scalp itch: a systematic review. *Skin Appendage Disord.* 2018;4(3):187–199.

18. What is "old age itch"?

Chronic itch is quite prevalent (up to 30%) in the elderly population. It may be the result of a number of conditions or may be idiopathic. In general, the geriatric population is predisposed to the development of itch due to changes relating to their skin causing skin barrier damage, changes in their immune system, and dysfunctions of their nervous system. In addition, the older population is more likely to suffer from skin conditions such as seborrheic dermatitis, systemic conditions such as diabetes and chronic kidney disease, and psychiatric ailments such as dementia. These patients are also susceptible to taking many medications, so a thorough evaluation of their current prescriptions and potential side effects of pruritus is warranted.

Shevchenko A, Valdes-Rodriguez R, Yosipovitch G. Causes, pathophysiology, and treatment of pruritus in the mature patient. *Clin Dermatol.* 2018;36(2):140–151.

19. What are common causes of localized pruritus?

Localized chronic pruritus is often attributed to a neuropathic etiology; however, dermatologic (if there is a corresponding rash) or psychogenic causes may also be sources of localized itch. The specific location of the pruritus is critical in making the diagnosis. If a patient presents with pruritus affecting the bilateral upper arms, consider BRP. If a patient endorses itch in a unilateral spot on their back, which may be visualized as a hyperpigmented patch, consider notalgia paresthetica. Itch localized to the genital area may be associated with pathology in the lumbosacral spine, such as lumbosacral radiculopathy.

Cohen AD, Vander T, Medvendovsky E, et al. Neuropathic scrotal pruritus: anogenital pruritus is a symptom of lumbosacral radiculopathy. *J Am Acad Dermatol.* 2005;52(1):61-66.

20. What is chronic pruritus of unknown origin (CPUO)?

CPUO is pruritus that has undergone a full workup and no underlying cause has been identified.

21. **How do you treat a patient with CPUO?**

Initially, treat with topical therapies such as emollients, topical anesthetics, and cooling agents (e.g., menthol). A combination of topical ketamine-amitriptyline-lidocaine has proven effective for patients with pruritus of varying origins. If ineffective, oral agents such as gabapentin may be added. Next, oral medications such as antidepressants, kappa opioid agonists, mu opioid antagonists, and neurokinin-1 inhibitors may be helpful. Fig. 68.2 outlines a stepwise approach for treating CPUO.

Fowler E, Yosipovitch G. Chronic itch management: therapies beyond those targeting the immune system. *Ann Allergy Asthma Immunol.* 2019;123:158–165.

22. **What are the most effective treatments for pruritus in patients with end-stage renal failure on hemodialysis?**

Pruritus in patients with end-stage renal disease is a significant problem. It has been reported that up to 66% of patients on hemodialysis are affected by itch. Unfortunately, there is no standardized therapeutic ladder for the treatment of uremic pruritus, but there are small studies and case reports that have identified potential therapies for relief.

Gabapentin in low doses, postdialysis, has been successful in providing relief to patients suffering from uremic pruritus. Topical pramoxine 1% cream, an anesthetic, has been shown to significantly reduce pruritus in patients with chronic kidney disease. Topical capsaicin has also shown a beneficial effect. In Japan, the kappa opioid agonist nalfurafine is approved for the treatment of uremic pruritus. In the United States, intranasal butorphanol can be used. Finally, it is important to remember to heavily moisturize these patients' skin, as xerosis is a common problem in end-stage renal disease and can contribute to pruritus but is not the main cause.

Zucker I, Yosipovitch G, David M, Gafter U, Boner G. Prevalence and characterization of uremic pruritus in patients undergoing hemodialysis: uremic pruritus is still a major problem for patients with end-stage renal disease. *J Am Acad Dermatol.* 2003; 49(5):842–846.
Simonsen E, Komenda P, Lerner B, et al. Treatment of uremic pruritus: a systematic review. *Am J Kidney Dis.* 2017;70(5):638–655.

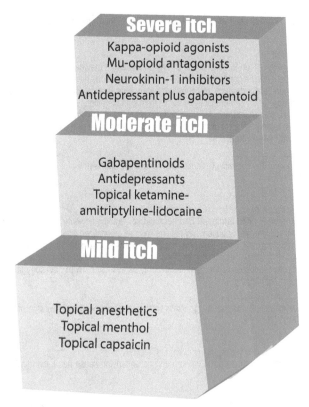

Fig. 68.2 Therapeutic ladder for treatment of chronic pruritus of unknown origin.

23. What is the most effective treatment for itch of atopic dermatitis?

Itch is a tremendous problem in atopic dermatitis. Dubbed "the itch that rashes," atopic dermatitis treatment centers on breaking the itch-scratch cycle. A variety of medications have been developed over the years, with some more effective than others. Currently, the most effective therapy for severe atopic dermatitis is dupilumab, a biologic drug targeting the IL-4 alpha receptor. Other treatments for atopic dermatitis are listed in Table 68.2.

24. What are the most effective treatments for itch secondary to psoriasis?

Biologic therapies targeting IL-17 have emerged as effective treatments for itch secondary to psoriasis. These drugs include secukinumab, ixekizumab, and brodalumab. Other biologics and small molecules such as janus kinase (JAK) inhibitors are also very effective. Apremilast, an oral phosphodiesterase inhibitor, has shown to be effective in relieving itch associated with psoriasis.

Sobell JM, Foley P, Toth D, et al. Effects of apremilast on pruritus and skin discomfort/pain correlate with improvements in quality of life in patients with moderate to severe plaque psoriasis. *Acta Derm Venereol.* 2016;96(4):514–520.

Table 68.2 Treatments for AD and corresponding levels of severity

AD SEVERITY	MEDICATION
Mild	Emollients
	Low-potency topical corticosteroids
	Topical calcineurin inhibitors
Mild to moderate	Crisaborole
	Medium- to high-potency topical corticosteroids
	Phototherapy
Moderate to severe	Dupilumab
	Nonspecific systemic immunosuppressants (e.g., cyclosporine, methotrexate, azathioprine) *short-term only!*

AD, Atopic dermatitis.

CHAPTER 69

NAIL DISORDERS

Whitney A. High

1. List the functions of the nails.
   - Nails protect the terminal phalanx and fingertip from traumatic impact
   - Nails help to perform tasks that require manual dexterity
   - Nails, while unparalleled in their ability to relieve itching, cause trauma to the skin
   - Nails may serve an esthetic (beauty) function

2. Why are nails important in dermatology?
   Nails are observable and serve as a window into body function and homeostasis. Nail health and appearance may be affected by numerous internal (heart, liver, kidney) and external (infection, trauma, and drugs) factors. Nail changes may also serve to diagnose other skin disorders.

3. What systemic diseases have specific nail findings?
   Many systemic diseases have characteristic nail findings. Most nail changes are part of a symptom complex or a reaction pattern that may be of use in rendering a diagnosis (Table 69.1).

4. What are Beau lines? How are they formed?
   Beau lines are forward-pointing, wedge-shaped depression in the nail plate of variable depth and obliquity that while not entirely specific, point to certain disease associations. These lines are caused by temporarily diminished nail growth. Beau lines may also be caused by mechanical trauma or diseases of the proximal nail fold. When all the nails are affected, a systemic cause is suggested (Fig. 69.1), while localized events (trauma) yield isolated lines. An exaggerated form of Beau lines is onychomadesis, which is an insult so severe that nail growth is halted. When nail growth begins again, there is a visible separation between the old nail and the new growing nail. Onychomadesis is most often seen in children after an episode of hand, foot, and mouth disease.

5. What is a splinter hemorrhage?
   A splinter hemorrhage is a nonspecific finding that results from extravasation of blood from the vessels of the nail bed. The blood becomes entrapped by the overlying nail plate and moves distally with it. This is often caused simply by trauma or medications. The occurrence of hemorrhage close to the lunula, and in multiple nails, simultaneously, can be indicative of systemic disease, such as endocarditis or vasculitis, but certainly, these represent uncommon causes of splinter hemorrhage (even if oft taught in medical school as major concerns).

Haber R, Khoury R, Kechichian E, Tomb. Splinter hemorrhages of the nails: a systematic review of clinical features and associated conditions. *Int J Dermatol.* 2016;55:1304–1310.

6. What is the difference between Mees lines and Muehrcke lines?
   Mees lines represent single or multiple transverse white lines that occur in the nail plate and move distally with nail growth. Arsenic intoxication is the "classic" cause, but many systemic insults, including chemotherapy, may cause Mees lines. **Muehrcke lines** represent transverse, double white lines that are caused by an abnormality of the vascular bed, probably localized edema due to the hypoalbuminemia. Muehrcke lines have been reported in over 70 different illnesses, including rheumatoid arthritis, nephrotic syndrome, liver disease, malnutrition.

Chávez-López MA, Arce-Martínez FJ, Tello-Esparza A. Muehrcke lines associated to active rheumatoid arthritis. *J Clin Rheumatol.* 2013;19:30–31.

7. What are "half-and-half" (Lindsay) nails, and with what diseases are they associated?
   Half-and-half nails (Lindsay nails) are characterized by leukonychia (white color that disappears with pressure) that affects the proximal half of the nail (Fig. 69.2). The condition may occur idiopathically in normal individuals, but it may also be associated with chronic renal disease in about 10% of patients.

8. What are Terry nails and how does this differ from "half-and-half" (Lindsay) nails?
   Distinction between half-and-half nails (Lindsay nails) and Terry nails is difficult. In Lindsay nail, the proximal part of the nail is white, while the distal portion is normal in appearance. A Terry nail is defined as a white nail bed that affects at least 80% of the nail bed. Terry nails are frequently associated with cirrhosis, chronic congestive heart failure, and adult-onset diabetes.

Table 69.1 Nail disorders in systemic disease

NAIL ABNORMALITY	AREA INVOLVED	ASSOCIATED DISEASE
Splinter hemorrhages	Bed	Bacterial endocarditis
Mees' lines	Plate	Arsenic exposure
Muehrcke's lines	Bed	Nephrotic syndrome
Terry's nails	Bed	Cirrhosis
Half-and-half nails	Bed	Chronic renal failure
Blue lunulae	Matrix	Wilson's disease
Red lunulae	Matrix	Rheumatoid arthritis
Clubbing	Plate/matrix	Pulmonary disorders
Spoon nails	Plate/matrix	Iron deficiency
Nail fold telangiectasias	Nail fold	Scleroderma, systemic lupus
Yellow nails	Plate	Pulmonary disorders, sinusitis

Pitukweerakul S, Pilla S. Terry's nails and Lindsay's nails: two nail abnormalities in chronic systemic diseases. *J Gen Intern Med.* 2016;31:970.

9. What is nail fold dermoscopy (capillaroscopy) and how is it useful in dermatology?

Nail fold dermoscopy, with the *in vivo* examination of nail fold and finger cuticle capillaries by magnification (capilloroscopy), to detect anomalies in pattern, is of diagnostic utility in dermatology. For example, connective tissue disorders can have distinct changes in the capillaries of the proximal nail fold. The technique can be useful in predicting the development of progressive systemic sclerosis (PSS) in those with Raynaud phenomenon. In those already with PSS, the severity of capillary anomalies may correlate with the degree of visceral disease. Patients with dermatomyositis have capillary changes within "ragged" cuticles. In systemic lupus, paronychial inflammation may be prominent with distinctive dilated and tortuous capillaries.

Fueyo-Casado A, Campos-Muñoz L, Pedraz-Muñoz J, Conde-Taboada A, López-Bran E. Nail fold dermoscopy as screening in suspected connective tissue diseases. *Lupus.* 2016;25:110–111.

10. What is nail clubbing?

Nail clubbing or digital clubbing is a deformity of the fingernails or toenails associated with many diseases. It is caused by increased bilateral curvature of the nails with proliferation of the soft tissues beneath the distal phalanges (Fig. 69.3). The result is an emergence angle of the nail (Lovibond angle) that is equal or greater than 180 degrees.

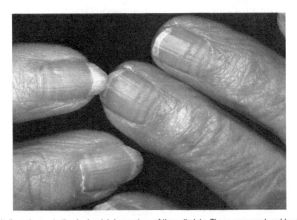

Fig. 69.1 Multiple Beau's lines demonstrating horizontal depressions of the nail plate. These were produced by chemotherapy with CHOP (**c**yclophosphamide, **h**ydroxydaunorubicin, **o**novin, **p**rednisone/prednisolone). (Courtesy Fitzsimons Army Medical Center teaching files.)

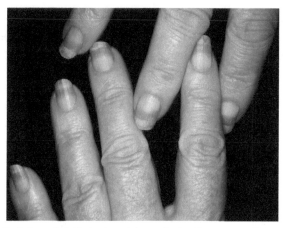

Fig. 69.2 Half-and-half nails in a patient with chronic renal disease. (Courtesy Fitzsimons Army Medical Center teaching files.)

There are diverse causes of clubbing, including idiopathic and inherited forms, but up to 80% of clubbing is associated with hypoxia from cardiothoracic ailments.

11. What is hypertrophic osteoarthropathy?

Hypertrophic osteoarthropathy is an uncommon but important condition that consists of digital clubbing (including toes) and periostitis of the distal interphalangeal. There may also be hypertrophy of the upper and lower extremities, peripheral neurovascular disease, acute bone pain, other joint problems, and muscle weakness. The syndrome can be associated with malignant tumors of the chest, particularly non–small cell lung carcinoma. Sometimes, the only presenting signs/symptoms are clubbing and painful ankles.

Carlson S, Rauchenstein J. Hypertrophic osteoarthropathy. *J Am Osteopath Assoc.* 2015;115:745.

12. What is yellow nail syndrome?

Yellow nail syndrome (YNS) is another rare condition that presents with a triad of chronic respiratory symptoms, lymphedema, and dystrophic yellowed nails. The diagnosis is made when two of three characteristic features are present, and only one-third of patients simultaneously possess all three features. The nails may also be curved from side to side, with absent lunulae and diminished cuticles (Fig. 69.4). The disease is thought to be due to problems with lymphatic drainage. YNS is associated with many pulmonary diseases including tuberculosis, asthma, and respiratory tract cancers. The condition is treated with vitamin E and oral antifungals, although the disease is not thought to be caused by fungal organisms.

Preston A, Altman K, Walker G. Yellow nail syndrome. *Proc (Bayl Univ Med Cent).* 2018;31:526–527.

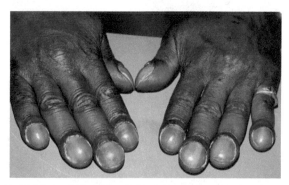

Fig. 69.3 Benign clubbing of the nails inherited in an autosomal dominant fashion.

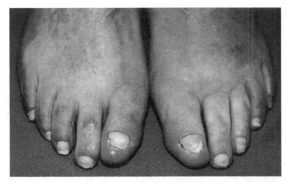

Fig. 69.4 Yellow nail syndrome, demonstrating typical thick, yellow, and curved nails. (Courtesy James E. Fitzpatrick, MD.)

13. **What characteristic nail changes are associated with primary dermatologic diseases?**
    There are a limited number of ways that the nail unit may respond to pathologic insults, and hence, pathognomonic changes are seldom encountered, but examination of the nails is imperative in dermatology because there are certain changes, when viewed in context with the entire clinical picture, that help to establish a diagnosis (Table 69.2).

Rich P. Nail disorders: diagnosis and treatment of infectious, inflammatory, and neoplastic nail conditions. *Med Clin North Am.* 1998;82:1171–1182.

14. **What are nail pits?**
    Nail pits are shallow depressions in the nail plate that are the result of abnormally retained nuclei of the keratin-forming cells (parakeratosis), which are then shed with growth. Nail pits are associated with psoriasis (large, deep, and random pitting) and alopecia areata (small, uniform pitting arranged in a "cross-hatched" or geometric pattern).

15. **What other nail findings are seen in psoriasis? What is the significance of nail changes?**
    Psoriasis can affect all parts of the nail unit, and this results in a variety of nail changes. Nail abnormalities may even be the only manifestation of psoriasis. In descending order of frequency, the nail findings of psoriasis are:
    - Nail pits
    - Oil spots (brownish-yellowish discolorations) (Fig. 69.5)
    - Onycholysis (separation of the distal nail plate from the nail bed)
    - Subungual hyperkeratosis
    - Splinter hemorrhages.

16. **How does a pterygium differ from pterygium inversum unguis?**
    A **pterygium** (Greek for "wing") is classically associated with lichen planus. Lichen planus attacks the nail matrix, and this leads to permanent scarring. Because the nail plate is no longer made areas of scar, the proximal nail fold grows out on to the nail bed; this produces a triangular protuberance with a "wing-like" appearance. **Pterygium inversum unguius** occurs when the distal nail plate does not separate from the underlying digital bed skin, resulting in a subungual extension of the hyponychium. The condition is related to systemic connective tissue diseases, including PSS and systemic lupus erythematosus. Fingertip ulcerations and scarring seen in PSS contribute to the inability of the nail to separate (Fig. 69.6).

Table 69.2 Dermatologic disorders with nail changes

DISEASE	INCIDENCE	FINDINGS
Psoriasis	10%–50%	Pits, "oil spots"
Alopecia areata	20%–50%	Pits
Lichen planus	10%	Pterygium
Scleroderma	Frequent	Pterygium inversus unguium
Darier's disease	High	Wedge shaped, hyperkeratosis
Pityriasis rubra pilaris	Majority	Yellow-brown, hyperkeratosis

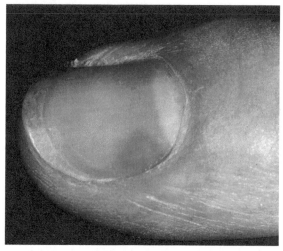

Fig. 69.5 Typical "oil spot" on the nails of a patient with psoriasis. (Courtesy James E. Fitzpatrick, MD.)

17. **What is the most common cause of a subungual hematoma? How is the condition treated and what are the sequelae?**

The most common cause is trauma. Most acute subungual hematomas are accompanied by a throbbing pain caused by pressure on the underlying nail bed due to the accumulation of blood (Fig. 69.7). A simple and effective treatment is trephination with the heated filament of a cautery pen (or a heated paper clip) that is pressed through the nail plate into the hematoma. Immediate pain relief results, making you a hero!

18. **Does melanoma occur in the nail unit?**

Nail unit melanoma does occur, but it accounts for only about 1% of all melanomas occurring in light-skinned persons. However, nail unit melanomas are more common in darker skinned persons. Moreover, nail unit melanoma tends to be discovered late, and it has a worse overall prognosis than melanoma occurring glabrous skin.

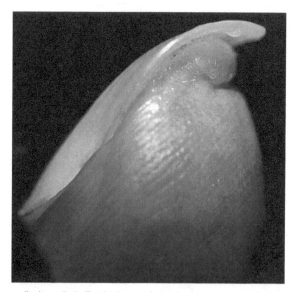

Fig. 69.6 Lack of distal separation in a patient with scleroderma and pterygium inversus unguium. (Courtesy James E. Fitzpatrick, MD.)

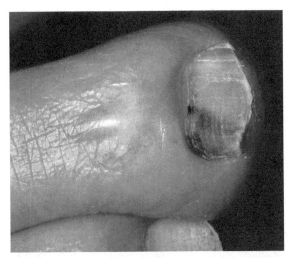

Fig. 69.7 Subungual hematoma. (Courtesy Walter Reed Army Medical Center teaching files.)

19. How do you tell the difference between a subungual hematoma and a malignant melanoma?

Distinction of melanoma from subungual hematomas is important, as the former can have a higher mortality if the diagnosis is delayed. One should be suspicious for melanoma when a pigment lesion develops in a single nail in a person greater than 50 years of age. Longitudinal melanonychia (pigmented nail bands) that are wider toward the base, or darken toward the base, are worrisome, as this is where the most recent nail growth lies. Longitudinal melanonychia is common in individuals with darker skin and is less concerning if multiple nails are involved, if width is less than 3 mm, and if coloration is uniform. Hutchinson sign is the leaching of pigment into the surrounding nail fold, and it is a concerning finding. Pigment due to subungual hematoma remains confined to the nail bed and gradually grows out with the nail. The following is an ABCDEF mnemonic for features of longitudinal melanonychia:

A—**A**ge at presentation, with melanoma more common in older age
B—**B**and width >3 mm and with **b**lurred borders
C—**C**hange (change in width/size of pigmented band)
D—single **D**igit involved with the thumb, then great toe or index finger being higher risk
E—**E**xtension of pigment into the perionychium (Hutchinson's sign)
F—**F**amily or personal history of melanoma and/or dysplastic nevus syndrome.

20. What nail changes are associated with human immunodeficiency virus (HIV) infection?

Patients with HIV may develop acromelanosis, in which hyperpigmented macules occur on the fingers, palms, and soles. In the nails, there may be longitudinal melanonychia. An older drug, zidovudine, may yield pigmented nails. Proximal subungual onychomycosis and candidal onychomycosis are also associated with HIV infection. Long-standing, treatment-resistant, periungual warts are common in HIV/AIDS, and progression to squamous cell carcinoma can occur.

High WA, Tyring SK, Taylor RS. Rapidly enlarging growth of the proximal nail fold. *Dermatol Surg*. 2003;29:984–986.

21. What is onychocryptosis? Why does it occur?

Onychocryptosis is the medical term for an ingrown toenail. It occurs when the free edge of the nail plate penetrates the soft tissue of the nail bed/fold. The condition may be caused by congenital malalignment, excessive rotation of the toe, onycholysis at the nail margin, ill-fitting shoes, hyperhidrosis, and poor hygiene practices (rounding the edges during nail trimming). Infection is a secondary complication.

22. What is a paronychia?

Paronychia is inflammation of the nail fold and it may present as an acute or chronic problem. Acute forms are precipitated by trauma or chemical damage and present with pain and inflammation (Fig. 69.8). Chronic paronychia tends to occur in several fingers simultaneously and it results from activities that leave the hands wet. An exception to this rule is the chronic paronychia caused by the habitual sucking of a finger, which often affects one digit. Coexisting skin disease, such as eczema or onychomycosis, can contribute to chronic paronychia.

Relhan V, Goel K, Bansal S, Garg VK. Management of chronic paronychia. *Indian J Dermatol*. 2014;59:15–20.

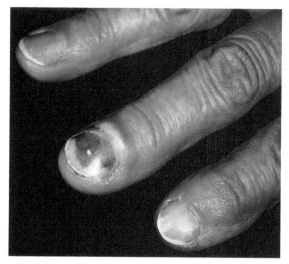

Fig. 69.8 Acute paronychia demonstrating swelling, pus, and hemorrhage.

23. Which infectious organisms cause paronychia?

Acute lesions are often caused by bacteria, such as *Staphylococcus*, *Streptococcus*, and *Escherichia coli*. Chronic infectious paronychia is more often due to *Candida* species, other molds (*Scytalidium*), or, rarely, syphilis, tuberculosis, and leprosy.

24. How do you treat acute paronychia?

A method to relieve pain and hasten healing is to drain the purulent area with a #11 scalpel blade to discharge the pus. A topical refrigerant spray can be used to temporarily numb the area prior to incision. Antibiotics and soaks should be instituted, with appropriate coverage for *Staphylococcus aureus* until the culture is back.

25. What is the most common cause of green nails?

Pseudomonas aeruginosa can colonize nail plates with onyholysis, and the pyocyanin pigment produced by this organism imparts a greenish discoloration (Fig. 69.9). All that is typically needed for therapy is a topical antiseptic/antibiotic.

26. What is the difference between onychomycosis and tinea unguium?

Onychomycosis is an umbrella term that refers to all fungal infections of the nail, whereas tinea unguium refers specifically to a dermatophyte infection of the nail. The most common dermatophyte infections are caused by *Trichophyton rubrum*, *T. mentagrophytes*, and *Epidermophyton floccosum*. Most fungal nail infections start at the distal end of the nail (distal subungual infection). Proximal subungual infections are rare in persons with normal immune systems but can be seen in the setting of HIV/AIDS.

KEY POINTS: NAIL DISORDERS

1. Nails can serve as window into the overall health of a person.
2. Trauma is the most common cause of splinter hemorrhages.
3. Squamous cell carcinoma is the most common malignancy of the nail unit.
4. The diagnosis of connective tissue diseases may be enhanced by nail fold dermoscopy/capillaroscopy.
5. Any perceived mass that distorts the nail plate should lead to imaging studies.

27. List the antifungal medications most often used in the treatment of toenail onychomycosis.

See Table 69.3.

28. What should patients expect when undergoing treatment of onychomycosis?

The cure rate, particularly the 5-year cure rate, may be just slightly better than 50% (certainly *not* 100%), and a cure may never be achieved in 20%–25% of patients. Oral terbinafine deposits in the nail near the matrix, and then grows forward, displacing the fungal-infected nail. Fingernails grow ~3 mm per month, with complete replacement in about 6 months. Toenails grow ~1 mm per month with replacement in 12 to 18 months. At the end of a typical 12-week treatment course, the nails will not appear normal, but there typically some healthy-appearing nail proximally. The high

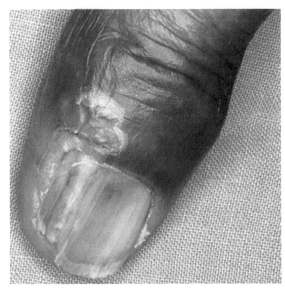

Fig. 69.9 Green nail with onycholysis secondary to *Pseudomonas aeruginosa* infection. (Courtesy Fitzsimons Army Medical Center teaching files.)

risk of recurrence for fungal infections of the toenail may be lessened by use of daily topical antifungal powders, or other preventative use of antifungal creams, lacquers, and sprays.

Christenson JK, Peterson GM, Naunton M, et al. Challenges and opportunities in the management of onychomycosis. *J Fungi (Basel)*. 2018;4:87.

29. What is "habit tic" deformity? How is it different from median nail dystrophy?

   "Habit tick deformity" is a common self-induced condition of the thumbnail characterized by horizontal parallel ridges of the nail plate caused by near-constant manipulation of the cuticle and proximal nail fold (Fig. 69.10). Median nail dystrophy is a similar-appearing idiopathic disorder that is unassociated with self-inflicted trauma, maintains a normal cuticle, and yields an inverted fir tree appearance to center of the nail plate.

30. List the common benign "tumors" that occur in and around the nail unit.
   - Acquired digital fibrokeratoma
   - Exostosis
   - Glomus tumor
   - Periungual fibroma
   - Pyogenic granuloma

Table 69.3 Antifungal medications for treatment of toenail onychomycosis

DRUG	BRAND NAME	DOSE
Itraconazole	Sporanox	Continuous: 200 mg qd for 12 weeks Pulse: 200 mg bid 1 week per month for 12 weeks
Terbinafine	Lamisil	Continuous: 250 mg qd for 12 weeks Pulse: 250 mg qd 1 week per q 3 months for 6–12 months
Fluconazole	Diflucan	150–200 mg every week for 12 months or until nails clear
Efinaconazole	Jublia	Topical daily for 48 weeks
Ciclopirox	Penlac	Topical lacquer daily for 48 weeks
Tavaborole	Kerydin	Topical daily for 48 weeks

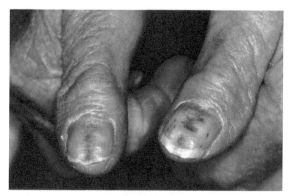

Fig. 69.10 Habit tic deformity. Both thumb nails demonstrate multiple centrally place ridges of varying size. Also note that the nail on the right also demonstrates multiple splinter hemorrhages. (Courtesy Fitzsimons Army Medical Center teaching files.)

- Myxoid (mucous) cyst
- Lentigo (melanonychia striata)
- Subungual nevus

Baran R, Richert B. Common nail tumors. *Dermatol Clin.* 2006;24:297–311.

31. What is an exostosis?

An exostosis is a common and benign bony growth of the distal phalanx, usually on the great toe. It involves the bone first and secondarily the nail. Trauma is thought to play a role in its development. It most often affects adolescent females. It presents as a slow-growing painful mass under the nail that can develop a secondary infection (Fig. 69.11). Plain radiographs easily delineate the pathology.

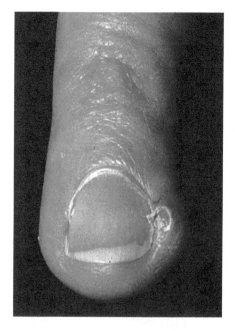

Fig. 69.11 Subungual exostosis. (Courtesy James E. Fitzpatrick, MD.)

32. Name the four most common malignant tumors of the nail unit.

    Squamous cell carcinoma in situ and squamous cell carcinoma are the most common malignant tumors of the nail unit and digit. The next most common is malignant melanoma, followed by basal cell carcinoma, and this pattern differs from that of the glabrous skin.

33. How common are nail side effects in the setting of epidermal growth factor receptor inhibitors, and what types of problems are seen?

    The nails are adversely affected approximately 17% of the time. Onycholysis, paronychia, granulation tissue response, nail fragility, and abnormal pigmentation are some of the more common problems seen. Given the critical importance of these medications, only a minority of patients with nail-related side effects need to discontinue the medication.

Miller KK, Gorcey L, McLellan BN. Chemotherapy-induced hand-foot syndrome and nail changes: a review of clinical presentation, etiology, pathogenesis, and management. *J Am Acad Dermatol.* 2014;71:787–794.

34. What is "disappearing digit"?

    Prolonged use of potent topical corticosteroids on the nail unit for inflammatory conditions can result in permanent absorption of the bone of the distal phalanx.

Wolf R, Tur E, Brenner S. Corticosteroid-induced "disappearing digit." *J Am Acad Dermatol.* 1990;23:755–756.

35. What is the role of lasers in treating onychomycosis?

    Lasers are currently approved by the Food and Drug Administration (FDA) to temporarily increase the clear-appearing nail in onychomycosis patients. Lasers can theoretically elicit fungicidal effects, through selective photolysis, but in practice yield mixed results. This review compared laser-induced improvement rates to FDA-approved indications and traditional onychomycosis treatments. A recent systemic review indicated that lasers provide a clinical improvement in the form of clear nail growth in toenail onychomycosis, which is consistent with the FDA clearance for aesthetic, but it found that mycologic cures were less that those achieved with traditional oral therapy.

Gupta AK, Versteeg SG. A critical review of improvement rates for laser therapy used to treat toenail onychomycosis. *J Eur Acad Dermatol Venereol.* 2017;31:1111–1118.

CHAPTER 70

DERMATOLOGIC TRIVIA

Scott A. Norton, Ali Damavandy, and Karl M. Saardi

"I'm terrible at Trivial Pursuit. Everything I know is significant."

"There are three levels of knowledge: trivia, significa, and necessaria. Information that you may regard as trivial is likely to be regarded by your attending as necessary."

1. The suffix -itis has come to mean inflammation. What is inflamed in "pruritis?"
Nothing. The word is *pruritus*, not *pruritis*. It is derived from the Latin *prurire*, "to itch." Pruritus is commonly misspelled; please learn how to spell it correctly.

Bernhard JD. *Itch: Mechanisms and Management of Pruritus.* New York: McGraw-Hill; 1994.

2. What is the difference between pruritus and itch?
There is none; the words are clinically interchangeable. Their International Classification of Diseases, Tenth Revision (ICD-10), codes are the same (L29.9), as were their ICD-9 codes (698.9) and all of the previous codes back to the Dawn of ICDs.

3. What is a Dąbska tumor and who was Dąbska?
Also known as an endovascular papillary hemangioendothelioma, Dąbska tumors are thought to be a subtype of hobnail hemangioendotheliomas that exhibit indolent behavior. Maria Dąbska was a Polish pathologist—and a member of the Polish Home Army who fought the Nazis during the failed Warsaw Uprising of 1944. Dąbska tumors and Spitz nevi are the only two neoplasms named after female physicians. Hobnails are tack-like metal inserts placed into the soles of shoes to add traction. They have small metal projections that dig into terrain, similar to how to nuclei in hemangiomas project into the vessel lumens.

Schwartz RA, Janniger EJ. On being a pathologist: Maria Dąbska—the woman behind the eponym, a pioneer in pathology. *Hum Pathol.* 2011;42(7):913–917.

4. There are only two prescription medications on the market with single-syllable brand names and both are relevant to dermatology. What are they?
Yaz (ethinyl estradiol and drospirenone, acne) and *Taltz* (psoriasis)

5. Where was sirolimus discovered and what is it used to treat?
Sirolimus (rapamycin) was discovered on Easter Island (also known as Rapa Nui to the native Polynesiasns, hence the name RAPAmycin) when *Streptomyces hygroscopicus* bacteria grown from a sample was found to have antifungal properties in culture media. It was isolated from bacterial cultures of *S. hygrascopicus*. It has been used in dermatology to treat angiofibromas in tuberous sclerosis and certain types of vascular malformations.

Sehgal SN. Sirolimus: its discovery, biological properties, and mechanism of action. *Transplant Proc.* 2003;35(3 suppl):7S–14S.

6. What is St. Anthony's fire?
St. Anthony's Fire is an eponym primary used for erysipelas. St. Anthony was an 11th-century Egyptian monk who was thought able to both inflict and cure this condition. Considerable confusion exists with regard to the true disease thought to embody his powers, as both ergot poisoning and bubonic plaque have been called St. Anthony's fire.

Asensi V, Asensi JM. Saint Anthony's fire. *JAMA Dermatol.* 2016;152(7):850.
Long V. The myth of erysipelas: fire, water, and blood. *JAMA Dermatol.* 2017;153(1):48.

7. What is "the clap" and where did the name come from?
Gonorrhea. The origins of the word "clap" and its introduction into English slang are unclear, but it is thought to be a shortened form of "*les clapiers*" and was first recorded in the 1300s. Some claim that "Les Clapiers" was a neighborhood in Paris known for prostitution, while others suggest the term means "rabbit hutch," or another word for

the small buildings where prostitutes often serviced clients. The term "gonorrhea" itself comes from *gonos-* (Greek: semen) and *-rrhea* (Greek: flow).

Lee KC, Ladizinski B. The clap heard round the world. *Arch Dermatol.* 2012;148(2):223.
Unemo M, Shafer WM. Antimicrobial resistance in *Neisseria gonorrhoeae* in the 21st century: past, evolution, and future. *Clin Microbiol Rev.* 2014;27(3):587–613.

8. What other disease in dermatology is named after rabbits?

Carcinoma cuniculatum is a rare presentation of squamous cell carcinoma of the foot, usually occurring in chronic ulcers. The "cuniculatum" portion of the term comes from the numerous sinuses and tracts that often occur within these lesions. *Cuniculum* means "rabbit warren" in Latin. Going even further down the proverbial rabbit hole, a warren is a network of interconnected passageways and can be used figuratively to describe buildings and cities.

Coldiron BM, Brown FC, Freeman RG. Epithelioma cuniculatum (carcinoma cuniculatum) of the thumb: a case report and literature review. *J Dermatol Surg Oncol.* 1986;12(11):1150–1155.

9. What are "cooties?"

The term "cooties" refers to lice and originally appeared in English during World War I, where pediculosis (human head lice due to *Pediculus capitis*) or body louse (*Pediculus corporis*) proliferated widely. The term "cootie" has unclear etymology but may be related to the term **utu* (meaning "louse") in one of a variety of southeast Asian languages such as Malay or Māori.

Taylor SJ. Got Cooties? Try P.D.Q. *Hoosier State Chronicles;* 2015. https://blog.newspapers.library.in.gov/got-cooties-try-p-d-q/. Accessed 25 February, 2019.

10. What is the definition of a "biologic" medication?

The Food and Drug Administration (FDA) defines a "biologic" as any agent that is derived from or created entirely by a living organism. Colloquially, it refers to antibody-based medications but could refer to anything from insulin to packed red blood cells to vaccines to gene therapy!

U.S. Food & Drug. *What Are "Biologics"—Questions and Answers.* 2018. https://www.fda.gov/aboutfda/centersoffices/officeofmedicalproductsandtobacco/cber/ucm133077.htm.

11. What does the word *pityriasis* mean in conditions such as pityriasis alba, pityriasis rosea, pityriasis versicolor, and pityriasis rubra pilaris?

It originates from the Greek word *pituron*, meaning bran, which refers to conditions that cause branlike scaling of the skin (but not the kind you would want in your morning cereal!).

12. What does the X in "histiocytosis X" mean?

It expresses the common etiologic link among the three clinical forms of the disease: eosinophilic granuloma, Hand-Schüller-Christian disease, and Letterer-Siwe disease. When Louis Lichtenstein coined the name *histiocytosis X* in 1953, he chose the X to represent the then-undetermined cause of the disorders. He wrote that the suffix X "has the advantage of brevity and, by implication, emphasizes the necessity for an intensive search for the etiologic agent." We now know that the common link is a proliferation of Langerhans cells, as reflected in the current name for histiocytosis X: Langerhans cell histiocytosis. Much about the disorder is still unknown, so perhaps Langerhans cell histiocytosis deserves to keep an X-designation. Maybe we should we call it LCH-X?

Lichtenstein L. Histiocytosis X. *Arch Pathol.* 1953;56:84–102.

13. Several names are used for the disease caused by *Bartonella bacilliformis*: bartonellosis, verruga peruana, Peruvian warts, Oroya fever, and Carrión disease. Who was Carrión?

Daniel Carrión studied the relationship between the disfiguring, but seemingly benign, cutaneous disease verruga peruana and the often-deadly disease Oroya fever. As part of a student research competition in 1885, the 26-year-old medical student inoculated himself with the blood of a patient with verruga peruana. Carrión soon developed the malignant form of *Bartonella* infection, Oroya fever, characterized by high fevers, severe myalgias, and profound hemolytic anemia. He postulated that the two conditions were related, but his experiment sadly ended fatally. A few decades later, his theory was proven correct, and now Carrión is the hero of the Peruvian medical profession.

Pamo OG. Daniel Carrion's experiment: the use of self-infection in the advance of medicine. *J R Coll Physicians Edinb.* 2012;42:81–86.

14. **What other illnesses are caused by *Bartonella* species?**
Cat-scratch disease is caused by *B. henselae*, and trench fever is caused by *B. quintana*. Some conditions caused by various *Bartonella* species (including *B. henselae* and *B. quintana*) are most common in immunocompromised individuals, particularly those with advanced human immunodeficiency virus infection. These conditions include bacillary angiomatosis, peliosis hepatis, and a form of culture-negative endocarditis.

15. **We all know about Lyme disease and its association with *Borrelia* infection, but what are some other Borrelial infections that occur in humans?**
B. burgdorferi, B. afzelii, B. garinii—Lyme disease, cutaneous "borrelioma," acrodermatitis chronic a atrophicans (spp. *afzelii*)
    B. recurrentis, B. hermsii, B. parkari, and the more recently discovered *B. miyamotoi*—Tick-borne relapsing fever

16. **Name some other diseases whose etiology (infectious or noninfectious) was determined through intrepid self-experimentation**
    - *Helicobacter pylori*—Barry Marshall, an Australian infectious disease specialist, resorted to drinking broth containing *H. pylori* to prove that it caused gastritis, after the scientific world did not believe that bacteria could cause a chronic disease. Marshall was awarded the 2005 Nobel Prize in Physiology or Medicine for his iconoclastic ideas and discoveries.
    - Pellagra—In the early 1910s, Joseph Goldberger invited his wife and several of their friends to consume (imbibe, ingest, and inject) various bodily fluids and excretions from pellagra sufferers to prove that the disease was not communicable, despite its frequent appearance in epidemic-like clusters among populations who subsisted on a corn-based, protein-deficient diet.
    - Yellow fever—Stubbins Ffirth conducted a similar experiment on himself with bodily fluids from patients suffering from yellow fever. When Ffirth remained healthy, he wrongly concluded that yellow fever was not a communicable disease.
    - Gonorrhea/syphilis—Jonathan Hunter, a British surgeon made famous by his study of anatomy on exhumed corpses, tried to prove that gonorrhea's urethral discharge and the myriad manifestations of syphilis were signs of the same disease. Hunter inoculated his own genitals with a patient's urethral discharge and soon developed signs of both gonorrhea and syphilis, "proving" his theory. It is now believed that the source patient was coinfected, which is a good reminder that sexually transmitted infections rarely travel alone. There have been rare case reports of gonorrhea being transmitted through fomites, including a fishing captain who contracted the disease from an engineer while at sea through a shared inflatable doll.

Gamble M, Kaufman B, Norton SA. The pus pioneers. *JAMA Dermatol.* 2016;152(3):298.
Marshall BJ, Armstrong JA, Mcgechie DB, Glancy RJ. Attempt to fulfil Koch's postulates for pyloric *Campylobacter. Med J Aust.* 1985; 142(8):436–439.
Kleist E, Moi H. Transmission of gonorrhea through an inflatable doll. *Genitourin Med.* 1993;69(4):322.

17. **What is ciguatera poisoning?**
Ciguatera poisoning is caused by ingestion of ciguatoxin, a tasteless toxin produced by dinoflagellates (*Gambierdiscus toxicus*). Humans are affected by eating carnivorous fish (such as barracuda or red snapper) that have accumulated the toxin as it is passed along the oceanic food chain. Ciguatera occurs in areas where people consume fish caught along coral reefs in tropical or warm subtropical waters. Ciguatoxin interferes with sodium channels in mammalian cell membranes. There are a number of gastrointestinal symptoms, but the occasional fatality is usually due to cardiorespiratory involvement.

Friedman MA, Fleming LE, Fernandez M, et al. Ciguatera fish poisoning: treatment, prevention and management. *Mar Drugs.* 2008;6:456–479.

18. **What are the neurocutaneous manifestations of ciguatera poisoning?**
Pruritus is noted in about half of the cases, often confined to palms and soles, and is exacerbated by exercise or alcohol consumption. There are often perioral and acral dysesthesias that most distinctively demonstrate a heat-cold reversal phenomenon. Dry mouth may also occur.

19. **From what is cantharidin made?**
Cantharidin ($C_{10}H_{12}O_4$), a vesicant therapy for molluscum contagiosum and warts, is a semipurified extract from blister beetles. The compound induces a blister at the epidermal-dermal junction. Blister beetles, mostly in the family Meloidae, have been used in Asian folk medicine for millennia. In the southern United States, horses are often afflicted with cantharidin toxicity after inadvertently eating the blister beetles that live in mowed alfalfa.

20. **What is Spanish fly?**
It is the legendary aphrodisiac powder made from crushed blister beetles (*Lytta* [syn. *Cantharis*] *vesicatoria*). Supposedly, it serves as an excitatory rubefacient when applied to an uncooperative male appendage.

21. Seriously now, cantharidin has been confirmed as an aphrodisiac. Who uses it and how does it work?

Male beetles of the species *Neopyrochroa flabellata* secrete cantharidin from a gland on their heads as a courtship or prenuptial offering. Females prefer to mate with males who offer cantharidin, which the female consumes and then uses to protect her eggs from predacious grubs.

Eisner T, Smedley SR, Young DK, et al. Chemical basis of courtship in a beetle *(Neopyrochroa flabellata):* cantharidin as "nuptial gift." *Proc Natl Acad Sci U S A.* 1996;93:6499–6503.

22. Who is generally considered the father of modern dermatology?

Robert Willan (1757–1812), a Yorkshireman, was awarded the Fothergillian Gold Medal in 1790 for establishing a classification of skin disease that is still used today.

Clendening L. Robert Willan. In: Clendening L, ed. *Source Book of Medical History.* New York: Dover; 1960:560–563.

23. Name the eight orders in which Willan classified cutaneous disease.

Papules, scaling disorders, rashes (exanthems), bullae, vesicles, pustules, tubercles, and maculae. The terms are retained today in the daily parlance of the dermatologist. Interestingly, he also specified four subtypes of pustules called phlyzacium, psydracium, achor, and cerion. Willan distinguished pustules by differences in size, characteristics of the pus, and quality of the scab. These terms have been abandoned. (Now *this* is trivia.)

24. Mucicarmine is a histologic stain used to detect mucin. From what natural source is mucicarmine obtained?

Cochineal, which is produced by a mealybug-like insect (*Dactylopius coccus*) that lives on several species of cacti (Fig. 70.1). The pigment's chemical properties serve as deterrents against predation by other insects. Cochineal dye is crimson and has long been used as a traditional textile dye in Mexico. Emily Dickinson described the colors of a ruby-throated hummingbird as "A resonance of Emerald/A rush of Cochineal." Check the ingredients on bottles of pink grapefruit juice and you're likely to discover that the pinkish-red color is conferred by cochineal-laden bug poop.

25. How does the FDA differentiate between an underarm deodorant and an underarm antiperspirant?

Deodorants are cosmetics that control, obscure, or mask body odor. As a cosmetic, it has no claim to alter the body's physiologic process of perspiring. Antiperspirants alter the natural process of sweating and are therefore considered an over-the-counter drug. Antiperspirants are often deodorants, too.

Schoen LA, Lazar P. *The Look You Like.* New York: Marcel Dekker; 1990.

26. What is Compound 606?

Also called *salvarsan*, Compound 606 was introduced to clinical medicine by future Nobel laureate Paul Ehrlich in 1909. It was long considered the drug of choice for treponemal infections such as syphilis and yaws. The name reflects

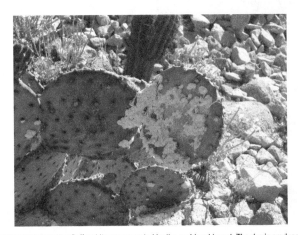

Fig. 70.1 Prickly pear cactus demonstrating fluffy white wax secreted by the cochineal insect. The dye is produced from the dried crushed bodies of the actual insect.

its place as the 606th compound tested by Ehrlich and his partner Sahachiro Hata. Ironically, salvarsan was developed not as a treatment for human syphilis but as part of an experiment on murine trypanosomiasis.

27. **Who was James Lind?**
    James Lind (1716–1794), a British naval surgeon, has received an inordinate share of credit in establishing the preventive and curative role of citrus products in the management of scurvy. Although Lind believed scurvy was caused by clogged skin pores, he conducted several shipboard trials of alleged antiscorbutic substances, leading to the use of citrus products (limes) by the Royal Navy during long voyages, hence the moniker "limeys" for British sailors.

Milne I. Who was James Lind, and what exactly did he achieve? *J R Soc Med.* 2012;105:503–508.

28. **If citrus products prevent scurvy, why did the Royal Navy suffer from so many scurvy outbreaks a century after Lind?**
    Not all citrus fruits have high amounts of vitamin C. In the mid-1800s, long before Casimir Funk's theory of vital amines (vitamins), the Royal Navy changed its fruit supplier and started receiving a strain of Caribbean lime that has very little vitamin C. Several polar exploring expeditions used the nonprotective limes and consequently suffered severe losses from scurvy. This led many to doubt the efficacy of citrus fruit in the management of scurvy. After the discoveries of Pasteur and Koch, a paradigm swept through medicine that most diseases were caused by bacteria, either by direct infection or by ptomaine, a bacteria-induced food poisoning. Indeed, several nutritional diseases had their "offending bacteria" identified, including scurvy, pellagra, and beriberi.

29. **Hansen's disease (leprosy) is generally considered a tropical condition. Where was G.H. Armauer Hansen working when he discovered the causative bacillus of leprosy?**
    Norway. Leprosy was abundant in coastal Norway in the mid-1800s, so Hansen did not leave his country to study this "tropical" disease. Bergen, Norway, was the world's center for leprosy research (Fig. 70.2). Leprosy may have been carried to Norway by Viking voyagers a millennium earlier. The biblical condition *tsara'ath*, which is often construed to be leprosy, may in fact be a disorder of hypopigmentation, such as vitiligo, or a generalized papulosquamous eruption, such as psoriasis.

Irgens LM. The discovery of *Mycobacterium leprae*. Am J Dermatopathol. 1984;6:337–343.
Shenefelt PD, Shenefelt DA. Spiritual and religious aspects of skin and skin disorders. *Psychol Res Behav Manag.* 2014;7:201–212.

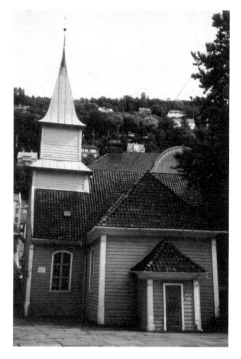

Fig. 70.2 Photograph of St. George's hospital in Bergen, Norway, where Dr. Hansen treated and did research on leprosy. The hospital is now the site of a leprosy museum. (Courtesy Fitzsimons Army Medical Center teaching files.)

30. In the United States, most persons with newly diagnosed Hansen's disease are immigrants from Southeast Asia, but in one region of the country, Hansen's disease is endemic. Where is this region of endemic Hansen's disease?

The southeastern quadrant of the United States from Georgia to Texas—and most particularly Louisiana. Individuals in this region can acquire the disease autochthonously, apparently with no contact with any other infected persons.

31. What seems to be the natural reservoir of Hansen's disease in these states?

In the past several decades, the nine-banded armadillo (*Dasypus novemcinctus*) has been found naturally infected with *Mycobacterium leprae*. The disease manifests itself similarly to lepromatous leprosy. Persons who handle armadillos for work or sport are at increased risk for acquiring Hansen's disease. Curiously, the first reports of naturally occurring armadillo leprosy emerged from southern Louisiana several years after the animals started being used for experimental infections at two nearby sites.

32. Has there ever been a "leper colony" in the United States?

Yes. There have been two leprosaria in the United States, one in Carville, LA, and the other on Kalaupapa, HI. Both leprosaria are closed; however, the National Hansen's Disease Museum is open to the public and still located in Carville.

33. Who was Father Damien?

Father Damien de Veuster was a Catholic missionary priest from Belgium who went to the leprosarium on Kalaupapa, HI, in 1873. At the time of his arrival, the leprosy colony did not have any buildings or potable water, and patients lived in caves and rudimentary shacks made of sticks and leaves. It was supplied by ships that would throw supplies into the water and rely on either currents or leprosy patients to swim out to retrieve the materials. Father Damien was responsible for building permanent structures, including churches, and organizing the leprosarium. Ironically, Father Damien developed leprosy and later died from it in 1889.

Tayman J. *The Colony: The Harrowing True Story of the Exiles of Molokai.* New York: Scribner; 2007.

34. Urology textbooks list about 50 causes of discolored urine. If an infant's diapers have a black discoloration, what genodermatosis should you include in your differential diagnosis?

Alkaptonuria, or hereditary ochronosis. This is a rare, autosomal recessive disorder due to the absence of an enzyme, homogentisic acid oxidase, which normally helps metabolize tyrosine and phenylalanine. Much of the excess metabolite, homogentisic acid, is excreted in the urine. The urine turns dark on oxidation; hence, a freshly removed, urine-soaked diaper may have a normal color but will quickly turn black upon exposure to air. Homogentisic acid is also accumulated in cartilage, leading to arthritis and characteristic darkening of the sclera and pinnae.

35. What disease should you consider in an elderly patient with new onset of photo-induced extensive dermatoheliosis and the same sign?

Metastatic melanoma. In some cases, the melanin-type pigments are excreted by the kidneys—and these turn black upon exposure to sunlight. The term "melanogenuria" is used when the urine turns black after oxidation. Melanuria is used when the urine appears black on excretion. Pigment-laden macrophages and melanin casts can be detected in this situation.

Aivaz O, Gaertner EM, Norton SA. Metastatic melanoma and melanogenuria. *Cutis.* 2012;89(3):125–128.
Valente PT, Atkinson BF, Guerry D. Melanuria. *Acta Cytol.* 1985;29(6):1026–1028.

36. Several inherited metabolic disorders with cutaneous manifestations can cause discolored urine. If an infant's diapers have a reddish discoloration, what genodermatosis should you include in your differential diagnosis?

Erythropoietic porphyria. This is another very rare autosomal recessive disorder due to an absence in uroporphyrinogen III cosynthase, an enzyme required early in the heme synthesis pathway. Much of the excess substrate is excreted in the urine and may give diapers a distinctive reddish color. Patients develop a destructive, scarring photodermatitis and a variety of hematologic abnormalities. In acute intermittent porphyria, the urine of adolescents and adults may also turn red when exposed to air. Do not confuse this condition with erythropoietic protoporphyria (EPP), in which a deficiency in the ferrochelatase enzyme leads to increased protoporphyrins in the blood and feces but no significant biochemical findings in the urine, hence the mnemonic EPP = empty pee pee.

37. What is the eponymic name for erythropoietic porphyria?

Günther's disease. Some authorities believe that people with this disease are the basis for reports of "werewolves" in Europe. Individuals afflicted with this disorder avoid light, because it produces burning, and they demonstrate marked diffuse hypertrichosis, scarring, and erythrodontia (red-stained teeth). Many other diseases have been associated with lycanthropy and vampirism—but this is pure speculation.

38. What is the carrier protein of a hapten called?

Schlepper, from the German word for "drag" or "haul." The molecular weight of a hapten is too low to induce an allergenic response. The schlepper protein provides the molecular muscle to allow the hapten to serve as an antigen.

39. Fifth disease is the common childhood exanthem also known as erythema infectiosum and is caused by parvovirus B19. But what is fourth disease? And what about sixth disease?

A century ago, common childhood exanthems were assigned numbers one through six for ease of classification. Only *fifth disease* retains its numeric name. **Fourth disease**, also called *Dukes' disease* or *Filatov-Dukes disease*, purportedly consisted of a nonspecific febrile illness accompanied by a cutaneous eruption. It may have been a streptococcal toxin–mediated disease, but it is not considered a precise or specific disease description. The term has been abandoned as a nosologic entity. **Sixth disease** is another name for roseola infantum (also known as exanthem subitum)—but no one uses the numeric moniker any more.

Bialecki C, Feder HM, Grant-Kels JM. The six classic childhood exanthems: a review and update. *J Am Acad Dermatol.* 1989;21:891–903.

40. Your esteemed attending overhears you using modern slang to refer to a particularly difficult patient as "cray cray." Intrigued (or perhaps simply confused), he challenges you by suggesting the patient probably just suffers from craw-craw. What is craw-craw?

Craw-craw is a term used in Africa to describe the intensely pruritic papular eruption that forms as a reaction to microfilariae during cutaneous onchocerciasis infection.

41. Onchocerciasis is found in both Africa and South America. Where did the disease originate, and how did it cross the Atlantic?

The disease caused by *Onchocerca volvulus* is endemic to tropical regions of west and central Africa. The human cargo of the slave trade carried the disease to the Americas, where there were natural populations of native black flies and an awaiting ecological niche.

Hoeppli R. *Parasitic Disease in Africa and the Western Hemisphere: Early Documentation and Transmission by the Slave Trade.* Basel: Verlag Recht Gesellschaft; 1969.

42. What skin disease does the sailor's curse, "I'll be jiggered" refer to?

It refers to parasitization by the jigger (*Tunga penetrans*). The gravid female flea burrows into mammalian skin. After a few weeks, the maternal flea extrudes the eggs via her uterine pore and out into the world. Larvae emerge from the eggs and mature in damp sandy soil. In most cases, only one or two embedded fleas are present, but dozens to hundreds of lesions are not uncommon.

43. Tungiasis (jiggers) was originally confined to the subtropical and tropical regions of the New World. How did it get to Africa, where it is now extensively entrenched in the sub-Sahara region?

European ships returning from the New World sometimes took on sand for ballast. In 1872, the *Thomas Mitchell* dropped infested sand ballast on the coast of West Africa, thereby introducing the noxious pest to this region. It is likely that it was introduced more than once and it is hyperendemic in many parts of coastal east Africa, especially Mozambique.

44. The first written account of poison ivy appeared in 1609 in the journal of this famous settler of the New World. Who wrote this account?

Poison ivy, referring to the plant and its dermatitis, was first described in Western literature by Captain John Smith (of Pocahontas fame). Captain Smith was the leader of the mercantile colony at Jamestown, VA. His journal described this as "The poisonous weed, being in shape but little different from our English yvie; but being touched causeth redness, itchinge, and lastly blysters, the which howsoever, after a while they passe awaye of themselves without further harme…" Modern dermatology textbooks can add little to his very accurate description!

Crissey JT, Parish LC, Holubar K. *Historical Atlas of Dermatology and Dermatologists.* Boca Raton, FL: Parthenon Publishing Group; 2002.

45. What is the name of the dermatologist who invented adhesive tape?

We often take adhesive tape for granted, but it did not exist until it was invented by a German dermatologist, Paul Gerson Unna, a renowned dermatologist of the late 19th and early 20th centuries. He was a brilliant clinician and therapeutic innovator, devising many treatments including the Unna boot, which is still used today, and Unna's paste (made of zinc oxide, gelatin, and glycerin) and ichthammol (used for psoriasis and many forms of dermatitis). He was also a great dermatopathologist and teacher. Some sources credit Beiersdorf for Unna's paste, a compound similar to modern day Eucerin. In all probability, they worked together.

Crissey JT, Parish LC, Holubar K. *Historical Atlas of Dermatology and Dermatologists.* Boca Raton, FL: Parthenon Publishing Group; 2002.

46. How many keratinocytes (skin cells) do you shed per minute?

It has been calculated that we shed about 35,000 skin cells per minute, which calculates to more than 50 million per day! In 1 year, the total number of shed keratinocytes would weigh almost 9 pounds. While this is truly trivia, it does highlight the fact that the skin is an amazingly active structure. Many of those shed keratinocytes wind up as a component of house dust.

47. Has there ever been a Nobel prize winner in the field of dermatology?

Yes. Niels Ryberg Finsen (1860–1904), a Faroese-Danish physician of Icelandic descent, won the Nobel Prize in Medicine and Physiology in 1903. Dr. Finsen suffered from Niemann-Pick disease and became interested in the role of light to treat this and other diseases including cutaneous tuberculosis (lupus vulgaris). He developed the Finsen lamp and won the prize for "his contribution to the treatment of diseases, especially lupus vulgaris, with concentrated light radiation." Phototherapy is no longer used in the treatment of any form of tuberculosis; however, Finsen is considered a founder of phototherapy in dermatology.

Grzybowski A, Pietrzak K. From patient to discoverer: Niels Ryberg Finsen (1860–1904), the founder of phototherapy in dermatology. *Clin Dermatol.* 2012;30:451–455.

INDEX

Note: Page numbers followed by *f* indicate figures, *t* indicate tables, and *b* indicate boxes.